PULMONARY/ RESPIRATORY THERAPY SECRETS

PULMONARY/ RESPIRATORY THERAPY SECRETS

POLLY E. PARSONS, MD
Associate Professor
Department of Medicine
University of Colorado Health Sciences Center
Medical Director, Intensive Care Unit
Denver Health Medical Center
Denver, Colorado

JOHN E. HEFFNER, MD
Professor of Clinical Medicine
University of Arizona Health Sciences Center
Tucson, Arizona
Chairman, Academic Internal Medicine
St. Joseph's Hospital and Medical Center
Phoenix, Arizona

HANLEY & BELFUS, INC./ Philadelphia
MOSBY/ St. Louis • Baltimore • Boston • Carlsbad • Chicago • London
Madrid • Naples • New York • Philadelphia • Sydney • Tokyo • Toronto

Publisher: HANLEY & BELFUS, INC.
                    Medical Publishers
                    210 South 13th Street
                    Philadelphia, PA 19107
                    (215) 546-7293; 800-962-1892
                    FAX (215) 790-9330

North American and worldwide sales and distribution:

                    MOSBY
                    11830 Westline Industrial Drive
                    St. Louis, MO 63146

In Canada: Times Mirror Professional Publishing, Ltd.
                    130 Flaska Drive
                    Markham, Ontario L6G 1B8
                    Canada

Library of Congress Cataloging-in-Publication Data

Pulmonary/Respiratory Therapy Secrets / [edited by] Polly E. Parsons, John E. Heffner.
        p.   cm. – (The Secrets Series®)
     Includes bibliographical references and index.
     ISBN 1-56053-163-0 (alk. paper)
     1. Lungs–Diseases–Miscellanea.   2. Respiratory Therapy–Miscellanea.
  I. Parsons, Polly E., 1954-.   II. Heffner, John E.,   III. Series.
     [DNLM: 1. Respiratory Tract Diseases–examination questions.
WF 18.2 P982 1996]
RC756.P84 1996
  616.2' 0076–dc21
  DNLM/DLC
  for Library of Congress   96-47624
                                                                   CIP

PULMONARY/RESPIRATORY
THERAPY SECRETS   ISBN 1-56053-163-0

Last digit is the print number: 9 8 7 6 5 4 3 2 1

DEDICATION

To our spouses, Jim Jacobson and Ann Heffner, for their support and understanding, and to our children, Alec and Chandler Jacobson and John and Jim Heffner, for their inspiration and patience.

CONTENTS

VII. PULMONARY COMPLICATIONS OF AIDS

VIII. PULMONARY VASCULAR DISEASES

IX. INTERSTITIAL LUNG DISEASES

X. VASCULITIS AND IMMUNOLOGIC DISORDERS

XI. VENTILATORY DISORDERS

XII. OCCUPATIONAL AND ENVIRONMENTAL LUNG DISEASES

CONTRIBUTORS

Antonio Anzueto, M.D.
Assistant Professor of Medicine, Pulmonary Disease Section, University of Texas Health Sciences Center at San Antonio, San Antonio, Texas

Selim M. Arcasoy, M.D.
Fellow, Pulmonary and Critical Care Medicine, University of Pittsburgh School of Medicine, Pittsburgh, Pennsylvania

Elizabeth L. Aronsen, M.D.
Clinical Assistant Professor, Department of Medicine, University of Colorado Health Sciences Center, Denver, Colorado

Alejandro C. Arroliga, M.D.
Director, Fellowship Program, Department of Pulmonary and Critical Care Medicine, Cleveland Clinic Foundation, Cleveland, Ohio

Ronald C. Balkissoon, M.D., FRCP(C), MSc, DIH
Assistant Professor, Departments of Medicine and Preventive Medicine, and Biometrics, University of Colorado School of Medicine, Denver, Colorado

Robert D. Ballard, M.D.
Associate Professor, Department of Medicine, Division of Pulmonary Sciences and Critical Care, University of Colorado Health Sciences Center, Denver, Colorado

Rafael Barrera, M.D.
Fellow, Pulmonary and Critical Care Medicine, Memorial Sloan Kettering Cancer Center, New York, New York

Gideon Besson, M.D.
Fellow, Department of Pulmonary and Critical Care Medicine, Hospital of the University of Pennsylvania, Philadelphia, Pennsylvania

Jamie M. Bigelow, M.D.
Assistant Clinical Professor, Department of Medicine, Highland Hospital of Rochester, Rochester, New York

Douglas W. Booth, B.A., R.R.T.
Director of Respiratory Care, Highland Hospital of Rochester, Rochester, New York

V. Courtney Broaddus, M.D.
Associate Professor, Department of Medicine, University of California at San Francisco School of Medicine, San Francisco, California

Roy G. Brower, M.D.
Associate Professor, Department of Medicine, Division of Pulmonary and Critical Care, Johns Hopkins University School of Medicine, Baltimore, Maryland

Lee K. Brown, M.D.
Associate Professor of Clinical Medicine, Department of Internal Medicine, University of Arizona College of Medicine, Tucson; Director, Pulmonary and Exercise Physiology Laboratory; Director, Sleep Disorders Center; Associate Program Director, Department of Internal Medicine, St. Joseph's Hospital and Medical Center, Phoenix, Arizona

G. Douglas Campbell, Jr., M.D.
Professor of Medicine, and Chief, Division of Pulmonary and Critical Care Medicine, Louisiana State University Medical Center, Shreveport, Louisiana

Hugh A. Cassiere, M.D.
Assistant Clinical Instructor of Medicine, Department of Pulmonary and Critical Care Medicine, Winthrop-University Hospital, Mineola, New York

Bartolome R. Celli, M.D.
Professor, Tufts University School of Medicine, Boston, Massachusetts; Chief of Pulmonary and Critical Care Medicine, St. Elizabeth's Medical Center, Boston, Massachusetts

Kevin G. Connelly, M.D.
Fellow, Division of Pulmonary Sciences and Critical Care, University of Colorado Health Sciences Center, Denver, Colorado

Thomas Corbridge, M.D.
Director, Medical Intensive Care Unit, and Assistant Professor of Medicine, Pulmonary Division, Northwestern University Medical Center, Chicago, Illinois

Anthony M. Cosentino, M.D., FACP, FCCP
Clinical Professor, Department of Medicine, University of California at San Francisco School of Medicine, San Francisco, California

Feroza M. Daroowalla, M.D.
Fellow, Pulmonary/Critical Care and Occupational Medicine, University of Washington School of Medicine, Seattle, Washington

Gregory B. Diette, M.D.
Postdoctoral Fellow, Pulmonary and Critical Care Medicine, Johns Hopkins University School of Medicine, Baltimore, Maryland

Thomas James Donnelly, M.D.
Fellow, Division of Pulmonary Sciences and Critical Care, University of Colorado Health Sciences Center, Denver, Colorado

Robert B. Dreisin, M.D.
Clinical Professor of Medicine (Pulmonary and Critical Care), Oregon Health Sciences University School of Medicine, Portland, Oregon

James Duke, M.D.
Assistant Professor of Anesthesiology, University of Colorado Health Sciences Center, Denver; Associate Director, Department of Anesthesiology, Denver Health Medical Center, Denver, Colorado

Karen A. Fagan, M.D.
Fellow, Pulmonary Sciences and Critical Care, University of Colorado Health Sciences Center, Denver, Colorado

Bonnie F. Fahy, R.N., M.N.
Coordinator, Pulmonary Rehabilitation, and Pulmonary Clinical Nurse Specialist, St. Joseph's Hospital and Medical Center, Phoenix, Arizona

Kevin P. Fennelly, M.D., M.P.H.
Assistant Professor, Pulmonary/Occupational-Environmental Medicine, University of Colorado Health Sciences Center, Denver, Colorado

Carla J. Fenton, M.D.
Resident, Department of Family Medicine, University of Colorado, Lafayette, Colorado

Enrique Fernandez, M.D.
Professor of Medicine, University of Colorado Health Sciences Center, Denver, Colorado

Philip J. Fracica, M.D.
Associate Professor of Clinical Medicine, University of Arizona; Director of Medical Critical Care, St. Joseph's Hospital and Medical Center, Phoenix, Arizona

Mark W. Geraci, M.D.
Assistant Professor of Medicine, University of Colorado Health Sciences Center, Denver, Colorado

Mary E. Gilmartin, B.S.N., R.R.T.
Clinical Nurse Specialist, and Instructor, Department of Medicine, University of Colorado Health Sciences Center, Denver, Colorado

Carlos E. Girod, M.D.
Assistant Professor, Department of Internal Medicine, Division of Pulmonary Sciences and Critical Care, University of Colorado Health Sciences Center, Denver, Colorado

Jeffrey Glassroth, M.D.
Thomas J. Vischer Professor and Chair, Department of Medicine, Allegheny University of the Health Sciences, MCP-Hahnemann School of Medicine, Philadelphia, Pennsylvania

Philip L. Goodman, R.R.T.
Director of Respiratory Therapy, Department of Medicine, Denver Health Medical Center, Denver, Colorado

Marc Vincent Gosselin, M.D.
Resident, Department of Radiology, Medical Center Hospital of Vermont and University of Vermont College of Medicine, Burlington, Vermont

E. Brigitte Gottschall, M.D.
Fellow, Pulmonary/Occupational-Environmental Medicine, University of Colorado Health Sciences Center, Denver, Colorado

Christopher Gregory, M.D.
Assistant Professor, Department of Medical Imaging, University of Colorado Health Sciences Center, Denver, Colorado

Susan W. Grey, M.D.
Senior Fellow, Division of Pulmonary and Critical Care Medicine, University of Tennessee, Memphis, Tennessee

Michael E. Hanley, M.D.
Associate Professor of Medicine, University of Colorado Health Sciences Center, Denver, Colorado

John E. Heffner, M.D.
Professor of Clinical Medicine, Department of Medicine, University of Arizona Health Sciences Center, Tucson, Arizona; Chairman, Academic Internal Medicine, St. Joseph's Hospital and Medical Center, Phoenix, Arizona

Richard A. Helmers, M.D.
Section Chair and Consultant, Thoracic Diseases and Critical Care Medicine, Mayo Clinic Scottsdale, Scottsdale, Arizona

Dean Hess, Ph.D., R.R.T.
Assistant Professor of Anesthesia, Harvard Medical School, Boston; Assistant Director of Respiratory Care, Massachusetts General Hospital, Boston, Massachusetts

Nicholas S. Hill, M.D.
Professor of Medicine, Division of Pulmonary and Critical Care Medicine, Brown University School of Medicine, Providence; Director, Medical Intensive Care Unit, Rhode Island Hospital, Providence, Rhode Island

Tony N. Hodges, M.D.
Fellow, Pulmonary Sciences and Critical Care, University of Colorado Health Sciences Center, Denver, Colorado

R. Hal Hughes, M.D.
Senior Fellow, Department of Medicine, Division of Pulmonary Diseases and Critical Care Medicine, The University of Texas Health Sciences Center at San Antonio, San Antonio, Texas

Michael C. Iannuzzi, M.D.
Associate Professor of Internal Medicine, Department of Pulmonary and Critical Care Medicine, Case Western Reserve University, and Senior Staff Physician, Henry Ford Hospital, Detroit, Michigan

David H. Ingbar, M.D.
Associate Professor of Medicine, Division of Pulmonary and Critical Care Medicine, University of Minnesota Medical School, Minneapolis, Minnesota

James R. Jett, M.D.
Professor of Medicine, University of Pittsburgh School of Medicine, Pittsburgh, Pennsylvania

David A. Kaminsky, M.D.
Assistant Professor of Medicine, University of Vermont College of Medicine, Burlington, Vermont

Robert J. Karman, M.D.
Pulmonary Fellow, Indiana University School of Medicine, Indianapolis, Indiana

Carol A. Kauffman, M.D.
Professor of Internal Medicine, Division of Infectious Diseases, University of Michigan Medical School, Ann Arbor, Michigan

Hyun Joo Kim, M.D.
Instructor, Department of Medicine, Division of Pulmonary and Critical Care Medicine, University of Minnesota Medical School, Minneapolis, Minnesota

Talmadge E. King, Jr., M.D.
Professor of Medicine, National Jewish Center for Immunology and Respiratory Medicine, Denver, Colorado

Jeffrey S. Klein, M.D.
Associate Professor of Radiology, University of Vermont College of Medicine, Burlington, Vermont

Monica Kraft, M.D.
Assistant Professor of Medicine, University of Colorado Health Sciences Center, Denver, Colorado

Jeon W. Lee, M.D.
Department of Pulmonary/Critical Care Medicine, St. Elizabeth's Medical Center, Boston, Massachusetts

Teofilo L. Lee-Chiong, Jr., M.D.
Medical Director, Intensive Care Unit and Cardiopulmonary Services, Androscoggin Valley Hospital, Berlin, New Hampshire

David L. Levin, M.D.
Chief of Chest Radiology, Department of Radiology, Beth Israel Hospital, Boston, Massachusetts

Stephanie M. Levine, M.D.
Associate Professor of Medicine, Division of Pulmonary Diseases and Critical Care Medicine, The University of Texas Health Sciences Center at San Antonio, San Antonio, Texas

Andrew H. Limper, M.D.
Associate Professor of Pulmonary and Critical Care and Internal Medicine, Mayo Clinic, Rochester, Minnesota

David A. Lynch, M.B.
Associate Professor of Radiology and Medicine, University of Colorado Health Sciences Center, Denver; Codirector, Thoracic Imaging, National Jewish Center for Immunology and Respiratory Medicine, Denver, Colorado

Joseph P. Lynch III, M.D.
Professor of Internal Medicine (Pulmonary), University of Michigan Medical School, Ann Arbor, Michigan

Thomas D. MacKenzie, M.D.
Assistant Professor of Medicine, Division of General Internal Medicine, University of Colorado Health Sciences Center, Denver, Colorado

Lisa A. Maier, M.D.
Fellow, Division of Pulmonary Sciences and Critical Care, and Fellow, Occupational and Environmental Medicine, Departments of Medicine and Preventive Medicine and Biometrics, University of Colorado Health Sciences Center, Denver, Colorado

Richard J. Martin, M.D.
Professor of Medicine, University of Colorado Health Sciences Center, Denver, Colorado

Praveen N. Mathur, M.B.B.S.
Associate Professor of Medicine, Department of Pulmonary and Critical Care Medicine, Indiana University School of Medicine, Indianapolis, Indiana

Richard A. Matthay, M.D.
Boehringer Ingelheim Professor and Associate Director, Pulmonary and Critical Care Section, Department of Medicine, Yale University School of Medicine, New Haven, Connecticut

Janet R. Maurer, M.D.
Head, Section of Lung Transplantation, Department of Pulmonary and Critical Care Medicine, The Cleveland Clinic Foundation, Cleveland, Ohio

Culpepper Hewitt McCuller, Jr., M.D.
Assistant Professor of Medicine, Department of Pulmonary and Critical Care Medicine, Louisiana State University Medical Center, Shreveport, Louisiana

G. Umberto Meduri, M.D.
Associate Professor of Medicine, Division of Pulmonary and Critical Care Medicine, University of Tennessee, Memphis, Tennessee

Sangeeta Mehta, M.D.
Research Fellow, Division of Pulmonary and Critical Care Medicine, Brown University School of Medicine, Providence, Rhode Island

Rebecca L. Meredith, R.R.T.
Supervisor, Respiratory Therapy, Department of Emergency Services, The Cleveland Clinic Foundation, Cleveland, Ohio

Albert Miller, M.D.
Professor of Clinical Medicine, Albert Einstein College of Medicine of Yeshiva University, New York; Clinical Professor of Occupational Medicine, Mount Sinai School of Medicine, New York, New York

York E. Miller, M.D.
Professor of Medicine, Division of Pulmonary Sciences and Critical Care, University of Colorado Health Sciences Center, Denver, Colorado

Melvin L. Morganroth, M.D.
Clinical Associate Professor, Department of Internal Medicine, Division of Pulmonary and Critical Care Medicine, Oregon Health Sciences University, Portland, Oregon

Marc Moss, M.D.
Assistant Professor of Medicine, Division of Pulmonary and Critical Care Medicine, Emory University School of Medicine, Atlanta, Georgia

Steve Nelson, M.D.
John H. Seabury Professor of Medicine, Department of Pulmonary/Critical Care Medicine, Louisiana State University Medical Center, New Orleans, Louisiana

Lee Scott Newman, M.D., M.A.
Associate Professor, Departments of Medicine and Preventive Medicine and Biometrics, University of Colorado Health Sciences Center, Denver, Colorado

Michael S. Niederman, M.D.
Associate Professor of Medicine, Department of Pulmonary and Critical Care Medicine, State University of New York at Stony Brook, Stony Brook, New York

C. Martin O'Driscoll, M.B.
Fellow in Thoracic Radiology and Mammography, University of Colorado Health Sciences Center and National Jewish Center for Immunology and Respiratory Medicine, Denver, Colorado

Gerald Norman Olsen, M.D.
Professor of Medicine, Assistant Dean for Clinical Curriculum, Curricular Affairs and Faculty Support, University of South Carolina School of Medicine, Columbia, South Carolina

David Ost, M.D.
Instructor of Medicine, New York University School of Medicine, New York, New York

Harold I. Palevsky, M.D.
Associate Professor of Medicine, Division of Pulmonary and Critical Care Medicine, University of Pennsylvania School of Medicine, Philadelphia, Pennsylvania

Polly E. Parsons, M.D.
Associate Professor, Department of Medicine, University of Colorado Health Sciences Center, Denver; Medical Director, Intensive Care Unit, Denver Health Medical Center, Denver, Colorado

Robert H. Poe, M.D.
Professor of Medicine, University of Rochester School of Medicine and Dentistry, Rochester, New York

Udaya B. S. Prakash, M.D.
Edward W. and Betty Knight Scripps Professor of Medicine, Mayo Medical School and Mayo Graduate School of Medicine; Consultant in Pulmonary and Critical Care Medicine, and Director of Bronchoscopy, Mayo Clinic and Mayo Medical Center, Rochester, Minnesota

Ganesh Raghu, M.D.
Chief, Chest Clinic, and Associate Professor of Medicine, University of Washington School of Medicine, Seattle, Washington

Carrie A. Redlich, M.D., M.P.H.
Associate Professor of Internal Medicine, Yale University School of Medicine, New Haven, Connecticut

Cecile Rose, M.D., M.P.H.
Associate Professor of Medicine, National Jewish Center for Immunology and Respiratory Medicine, and University of Colorado Health Sciences Center, Denver, Colorado

Stuart G. Rosenberg, M.D.
Assistant Professor and Director, Department of Anesthesiology, Denver Health Medical Center, University of Colorado Health Sciences Center, Denver, Colorado

Edward C. Rosenow, III, M.D.
Arthur M. and Gladys D. Gray Professor of Medicine, Department of Pulmonary and Critical Care and Internal Medicine, Mayo Clinic, Rochester, Minnesota

Lewis J. Rubin, M.D.
Professor and Head, Division of Pulmonary and Critical Care Medicine, Department of Medicine, University of Maryland School of Medicine, Baltimore, Maryland

Steven A. Sahn, M.D.
Professor of Medicine, and Director, Division of Pulmonary and Critical Care Medicine, Medical University of South Carolina, Charleston, South Carolina

Catherine S. H. Sassoon, M.D.
Associate Professor of Medicine, Pulmonary and Critical Care Section, University of California at Irvine School of Medicine, Irvine, California

Neil W. Schluger, M.D.
Assistant Professor of Medicine, New York University School of Medicine, New York, New York

Marvin I. Schwarz, M.D.
Professor of Medicine, and Head, Division of Pulmonary Sciences and Critical Care, University of Colorado Health Sciences Center, Denver, Colorado

Om P. Sharma, M.D.
Professor, Department of Pulmonary and Critical Care Medicine, University of Southern California School of Medicine, Los Angeles, California

Thomas E. Shaughnessy, M.D.
Assistant Clinical Professor of Anesthesia, University of California at San Francisco School of Medicine, San Francisco, California

Amy A. Silverthorn, M.D.
Medical Director, Pulmonary Rehabilitation, and Section Chief, Pulmonary Medicine, St. Joseph's Hospital and Medical Center, Phoenix, Arizona

Akshay Sood, M.B.B.S.
Postdoctoral Fellow, Pulmonary, Critical Care, Occupational and Environmental Medicine, Department of Internal Medicine, Yale University School of Medicine, New Haven, Connecticut

John L. Stauffer, M.D.
Professor, Division of Pulmonary and Critical Care Medicine, Department of Medicine, The Pennsylvania State University, The Milton S. Hershey Medical Center, Hershey, Pennsylvania

James K. Stoller, M.D.
Head, Section of Respiratory Therapy, Department of Pulmonary and Critical Care Medicine, The Cleveland Clinic Foundation, Cleveland, Ohio

Eugene J. Sullivan, M.D.
Staff Physician, Department of Pulmonary and Critical Care Medicine, The Cleveland Clinic Foundation, Cleveland, Ohio

Kathleen Sutherland, M.D.
Senior Fellow, Pulmonary and Critical Care Medicine, Oregon Health Sciences University, Portland, Oregon

David J. Tardio, M.D.
Private Practice, Prince Frederick, Maryland

Omar Tirmizi, M.D.
Fellow, Division of Pulmonary and Critical Care Medicine, University of Southern California School of Medicine, Los Angeles, California

Yuan-Po Tu, M.D.
Staff Physician, The Everett Clinic, Everett, Washington

Allan R. Tunkel, M.D., Ph.D.
Associate Professor of Medicine, Allegheny University of the Health Sciences, MCP-Hahnemann School of Medicine, Philadelphia, Pennsylvania

Thomas R. Vendegna, M.D.
Pulmonary Fellow, Division of Pulmonary Sciences and Critical Care, Department of Medicine, University of Colorado Health Sciences Center, Denver, Colorado

Elcio Oliveira Vianna, Ph.D., M.D.
Visiting Scientist, Department of Medicine, National Jewish Center for Immunology and Respiratory Medicine, Denver, Colorado

Ann Weinacker, M.D.
Assistant Professor of Medicine, Department of Pulmonary/Critical Care Medicine, Louisiana State University Medical Center, New Orleans, Louisiana

Idelle M. Weisman, M.D.
Chief, Department of Clinical Investigation, and Director, Human Performance Laboratory and Pulmonary/Critical Care Services, William Beaumont Army Medical Center; Associate Professor of Medicine and Anesthesiology, Texas Tech University Health Sciences Center, El Paso, Texas

Dorothy A. White, M.D.
Associate Attending, Department of Medicine, Cornell University College of Medicine and Memorial Sloan Kettering Cancer Center, New York, New York

Jeanine P. Wiener-Kronish, M.D.
Professor, Departments of Anesthesia and Medicine, University of California at San Francisco School of Medicine, San Francisco, California

Ann M. Wierman, M.D.
Clinical Instructor, Department of Medicine, University of Colorado Health Sciences Center, Denver, Colorado

John P. Wilkins, M.D.
Senior Fellow in Pulmonary and Critical Care Medicine, Oregon Health Sciences University, Portland, Oregon

Roxana Zulauf Witter, M.D.
Resident, Department of Medicine, St. Joseph Hospital, Denver, Colorado

Robert F. Wolken, B.S., R.R.T.
Critical Care Respiratory Specialist, Department of Medicine, Denver Health Medical Center, Denver, Colorado

Marie E. Wood, M.D.
Assistant Professor of Medicine, University of Colorado Health Sciences Center, Denver, Colorado

Shawn Wright, M.D.
Clinical Instructor, Pulmonary Medicine, St. Joseph's Hospital and Medical Center, Phoenix, Arizona

Inchel Yeam, M.D.
Fellow, Department of Pulmonary and Critical Care Medicine, University of California at Irvine Medical Center, Orange, California

Nelson C. Yu, M.D.
Fellow, Department of Pulmonary and Critical Care Medicine, The Cleveland Clinic Foundation, Cleveland, Ohio

R. Jorge Zeballos, M.D., D.M.Sc.
Associate Professor, Departments of Anesthesiology and Internal Medicine, Texas Tech University Health Sciences Center; Co-Director, Human Performance Laboratory, Department of Clinical Investigation, William Beaumont Army Medical Center, El Paso, Texas

PREFACE

The basic theme of this book is that pulmonary clinicians and respiratory therapists must first pose proper questions before they can formulate effective answers to their patients' respiratory problems. Perhaps in no field of medicine is this twin challenge of identifying essential questions and deriving appropriate answers more fundamentally important than in the management of pulmonary disorders. The broad-based nature of pulmonary medicine requires a masterly understanding of diverse immunologic, infectious, traumatic, neoplastic, and inflammatory conditions. Some respiratory conditions arise primarily in the lungs, whereas others pose as "lung diseases" but actually represent pulmonary manifestations of underlying "occult" systemic disorders. Moreover, effective application of respiratory therapeutics requires proficiency in diverse pharmacologic and surgical interventions in addition to a mechanic's (or sometimes an engineer's) grasp of ventilator tubes, principles of gas and fluid flow, and electronic circuitry of ventilatory and monitoring devices. It is no wonder that this complex field presents clinicians with major challenges in identifying the appropriate questions let alone providing correct answers to patients' clinical problems.

In this book we have brought many of the present day leaders in pulmonary medicine and respiratory therapy to present their fields of expertise in question-and-answer format. We believe that they have succeeded in preserving the "cutting edge" nature of their content while presenting information in a readable and retainable manner that will benefit a broad readership. Like other texts in The Secrets Series®, we hope that this book will represent a valuable resource to medical students, residents, fellows, and experienced clinicians alike in their efforts to ask the right questions and discover the best answers.

Polly E. Parsons, M.D.
John E. Heffner, M.D.

I. Bedside Evaluation

1. TAKING THE PULMONARY HISTORY

Karen A. Fagan, M.D.

1. What is dyspnea and what causes it?

Dyspnea is the subjective sensation of uncomfortable or difficult breathing. Although it is not painful, it is unpleasant. Most patients report dyspnea as "shortness of breath" or "breathlessness." Patients experience dyspnea when their breathing is excessive for the activity that they are doing. The sensation of dyspnea is produced by stimulation of both central and peripheral receptors that monitor respiratory muscle activity, hypoxia, hypercapnia, acid-base status, airway irritation, and changes in the pressure volume characteristics of the lung (i.e., lung fibrosis or emphysema).

Several systems are involved in causing shortness of breath, including cardiopulmonary, hematologic, psychosocial, environmental (i.e., high altitude), body habitus (obesity), fever, and level of exercise. Any situation that increases the work of breathing (i.e., airway obstruction, decreased lung compliance) also contributes to the sensation of dyspnea.

2. What features of dyspnea are important to distinguish in the pulmonary/respiratory history?

Shortness of breath is a common complaint. Distinguishing features of this complaint will help the physician develop a differential diagnosis during the patient interview.

The **onset of dyspnea** is crucial to determine, because it can present as acute, subacute, or progressive over time. Acute dyspnea is readily recognized by both patient and physician. Chronic and progressive dyspnea, however, may be more difficult to characterize. Exercise tolerance or limitation over time may be the most useful way to establish the duration of symptoms in this situation. The patient's report of changes in exercise capacity over time (i.e., months to years) may identify the onset of symptoms. Dyspnea at rest is a late complaint in many diseases of the respiratory system.

Positional complaints of dyspnea, if present, may identify causes of dyspnea. Platypnea, shortness of breath experienced upon assuming the upright position, is most commonly seen in patients with hepatic disease and intrapulmonary shunts. Orthopnea, dyspnea occurring in the supine position, is most commonly a symptom of cardiac dysfunction. Paroxysmal nocturnal dyspnea is also a feature of many cardiac diseases. Occasionally, patients with upper airway lesions may present with complaints of dyspnea or cough while recumbent.

Reliable precipitants of dyspnea should be elicited such as environmental or occupational activities, exposure to animals, and exposure to inhalational agents (industrial or recreational). Associated symptoms of cough, wheeze, chest pain, and so forth also need careful attention.

3. What should patients be asked about their smoking history?

Smoking-related lung disease is common; thus, a complete, reliable smoking history, including the following information, is important in the initial assessment of any patient, especially the patient with pulmonary disease:

Age at which smoking began	Type of tobacco used
Breaks in smoking history	Amount of smoking

A physician caring for a smoking patient should assess previous attempts at smoking cessation and determine ways to improve the patient's success. Information should be sought about presence of other smokers in the patient's environment, the use of support groups, and prior input from medical personnel.

4. What are *pack years*?

Pack years refers to the amount of cigarette tobacco consumed as packs per day times the number of years smoked.

5. How is the severity of hemoptysis assessed?

Hemoptysis is the expectoration of blood with coughing; it is a manifestation of an underlying problem of a number of causes. It is a frightening, occasionally life-threatening complaint that brings patients to medical attention promptly. Most important in the patient interview is assessment of the quantity and quality of blood and the presence of any associated symptoms. Massive hemoptysis is usually easily assessed. It is generally greater than 600 cc in a 24-hour period and can be quite dramatic. More commonly, patients will complain of lesser quantities such as streaks, specks, or clots. It may be difficult to estimate the amount of blood based on such reports. Use of collection containers may be the best way to establish the amount of blood produced.

6. How is the differential diagnosis of hemoptysis developed?

There are numerous causes of hemoptysis. The presence of associated symptoms may greatly enhance the physician's ability to form a differential diagnosis of the cause. Sputum production, especially purulent, may point to an infectious cause of the hemoptysis. Weight loss and chronic cough in a patient with hemoptysis who smokes may be an indication of malignancy. Tuberculosis may present with similar symptoms in a patient exposed to the mycobacterium. Hemoptysis in a patient with heart disease and dyspnea while recumbent is probably caused by pulmonary edema. Hemoptysis also may be a symptom of a pulmonary complication of a coexistent systemic disease such as systemic lupus erythematosus. The presence of chest pain and acute dyspnea may suggest pulmonary embolism.

7. Can the causes of chest pain be reliably differentiated from one another?

No. Chest pain arises from several sites in the thorax and surrounding organs. Although there are features that suggest a particular cause of chest pain, it can be frustrating to accurately establish and treat the cause of the chest pain. History alone can rarely identify the cause of chest pain, but attention to the quality, onset, duration, related symptoms, and precipitating and alleviating factors may help the observant historian more carefully evaluate this serious complaint.

8. What is pleuritic chest pain?

Pleuritic chest pain, or pain arising from the parietal surface of the pleura, usually can be distinguished easily from other chest pain syndromes by history. It is usually sharp and relates to respiratory muscle movement such as that with inspiration or cough. It is frequently sudden in onset and may be episodic. Causes of pleuritic chest pain include pneumonia, pleural effusion, pulmonary infarction, chest wall muscle inflammation, rib fractures, pneumothorax, and inflammation of the pleura in systemic diseases such as systemic lupus erythematosus and rheumatoid arthritis.

9. What are the causes of nonpleuritic chest pain?

Nonpleuritic chest pain can be more difficult to characterize than pleuritic chest pain because both pulmonary and cardiac disease may present in similar ways. Classic anginal chest pain with pressure-like pain, radiation to the arm and jaw with associated shortness of breath, nausea, and diaphoresis may be difficult to distinguish from similar symptoms seen in pulmonary hypertension. Careful attention to medical history of other conditions and risk factors for coronary artery disease may distinguish the cause of this type of pain. Other important causes of non-pleuritic chest pain include musculoskeletal, gastroesophageal, pericardial, and aortic disorders. Subdiaphragmatic processes can also present with referred pain to the chest through irritation of the diaphragm and its surfaces.

10. What information should be obtained in the history of exposure and the occupational history?

Occupational and exposure histories are important in the evaluation of the patient with pulmonary disease. Two distinct environments must be considered when considering a possible exposure that may be causing or exacerbating a particular medical problem: the home environment and the work environment. Before a detailed history of either of these locations is undertaken, it is important to have a clear understanding from the patient of the primary symptoms and whether they relate to a particular location or activity.

A detailed history of potential exposures in the home encompasses the construction, site, furnishings, heating and cooling systems, damage to the home (i.e., water damage), presence of carpeting, type of linens, and pets. This information is of particular interest in patients with hypersensitivity syndromes and asthma or other allergic syndromes. Molds can grow in damp spots that include wet carpeting or padding, water-damaged walls, and swamp cooling systems. Down pillows and comforters may cause worsening of allergic symptoms. The presence of pets and other animals, currently or previously, may help the clinician identify potential causes and develop management plans for some illnesses. Pet birds are frequently overlooked in reports of animals in the home, so it is important to ask about these specifically.

The work environment is fraught with potential exposures that may cause illness and disease. A detailed history includes attention to all past and current jobs, specific responsibilities at each location, and information regarding chemicals and other hazardous materials at the workplace. It is especially important to ascertain whether respiratory protection was worn and if so, what type. Documented exposures should be thoroughly reviewed. If necessary, the patient or physician may request material safety data sheets from the work site.

11. What is the most important information to obtain when a patient is being evaluated for an abnormal chest radiograph?

The most important questions to be addressed when a patient has been referred for evaluation of an abnormal chest radiograph are:
- Does the patient have any previous chest radiographs?
- Are they available for comparison with the current films?
- Can they be obtained?

Other aspects of the history and physical examination are equally important, but direct comparison of prior radiographs may establish a lesion as benign or suggest that a further evaluation is necessary.

12. What information should be obtained from a patient who complains of coughing?

Coughing is the most common complaint of patients who seek care from a pulmonologist. The onset of the cough and the associated features are necessary components of any patient history. Although cough can be a nonspecific symptom of many diseases, a good history should begin to limit the differential diagnosis. The history includes descriptions of the onset, quality, duration, associated expectoration, presence of other respiratory symptoms, and changes in voice. Cough may be caused by inflammatory, chemical, mechanical, or psychosocial mechanisms.

Sputum production is a key feature of cough. Healthy adults generally do not expectorate any sputum during the course of the day; thus, sputum production may be considered abnormal. The consistency and color of the sputum may help identify the source, as purulent sputum usually correlates with infectious causes. The presence and quantity of blood are also important. Fetid-smelling, purulent sputum may indicate the presence of an anaerobic infection or lung abscess. Large quantities of sputum (i.e., bronchorrhea) can be seen in some malignancies, bronchiectasis, and inflammatory airway disease. Thick, tenacious sputum associated with mucous plugs can be seen in patients with cystic fibrosis and asthma (especially allergic bronchopulmonary aspergillosis). Rarely, patients report expectoration of a chalky or stone-like object, a broncholith, that can be associated with tuberculosis and some fungal infections.

The time of day during which the cough is worse may help identify a cause. Chronic sinusitis may cause a nocturnal or morning cough but can be a cause of cough throughout the day. Similarly, gastroesophageal reflux may cause symptoms that are worse at night or when the patient is supine. Upper airway obstruction has the same pattern. Cough after exercise may indicate reactive airway disease. Cough, shortness of breath, and other systemic symptoms at the end of a workday may indicate hypersensitivity pneumonitis. Nocturnal coughing may indicate the presence of cardiac disease, especially when associated with paroxysmal nocturnal dyspnea. Cough that occurs during eating may indicate the presence of a tracheoesophageal fistula.

A careful list of past and present medication use is important in evaluating a cough. Chronic dry coughing is seen with the use of angiotensin-converting enzyme inhibitors is as many as 20% of patients treated with these antihypertensive agents. Fortunately it resolves with cessation of the drug. Chronic dry coughing with dyspnea may also be a feature of the pulmonary fibrosing diseases.

Aspiration of foreign bodies may also produce both acute and chronic coughing; this possibility should be considered in children with cough and in adults with a history of impaired consciousness. Hoarseness may be associated with laryngeal sources of cough. An often overlooked cause of chronic cough is hair or wax in the external auditory canal causing stimulation of the vagus nerve.

13. A patient's wife complains that he snores and "sputters" at night and that he falls asleep at embarrassing times during the day; what else do you want to know about the patient?

- Does he stop snoring for brief intervals in the night? If so, how does he resume snoring?
- Does he ever have quick, jerky limb movements while asleep?
- Does he complain of not sleeping well or feeling very sleepy during the day?
- Does he frequently take naps?
- Does he have headaches in the morning?
- Has he experienced sexual dysfunction?

These questions may help characterize several sleep disorders, especially obstructive sleep apnea. Although the patient can frequently provide adequate information to the interviewer, it is always important to obtain additional data from family and sleep partners because the patient may have frequent wakenings that do not fully arouse him but that significantly disturb his sleep.

BIBLIOGRAPHY

1. Glauser FL: Signs and Symptoms in Pulmonary Medicine. Philadelphia, J.B. Lippincott, 1983.
2. Karlinsky JB, Lau J, Goldstein RH: Decision Making in Pulmonary Medicine. Philadelphia, B.C. Decker, 1991.
3. Kiss GT: Diagnosis and Management of Pulmonary Disease in Primary Practice. Menlo Park, CA, Addison-Wesley, 1982.
4. Sackner MA: Diagnostic Techniques in Pulmonary Disease: Part 1. New York, Marcel Dekker, 1980.

2. PHYSICAL EXAMINATION

Om P. Sharma, M.D., and Omar Tirmizi, M.D.

Although the physical examination of the chest should be pursued in an orderly manner through inspection, palpation, percussion, and auscultation, the physician must continue to sift the gathered information and look for the cardinal features. The physical examination is not just a routine exercise, but rather a systematic intellectual activity that should be pursued logically and diligently.

1. Which clinical signs best indicate respiratory distress?

Rapid respiratory rate and the use of accessory muscles of respiration denote the presence of respiratory discomfort. The rate of normal quiet respiration varies from 12 to 18 breaths per minute. The diaphragm and the intercostal muscles perform respiration. Accessory muscles of respiration include the scalene and pectorals. During their use the nostrils flare, the alae nasi contract, and the sternomastoids elevate the clavicles and sternum. Large changes in intrathoracic pressure during inspiration and expiration produce retraction of the intercostal muscles during inspiration, particularly if tracheal obstruction exists. Patients with advanced emphysema often breathe through pursed lips, a maneuver that helps to increase expiratory flow time.

2. What is the significance of paradoxical respiration?

Normal respiration is of two types, thoracic and abdominal. Thoracic respiration, performed by the upper part of the chest, is seen in normal women, anxious subjects, patients with ascites, and patients with diaphragmatic paralysis. In men and young children, respiration is abdominal. During normal respiration the diaphragm moves down in inspiration (seen as an outward movement of the abdominal viscera) and upward in expiration. In paradoxical respiration, the diaphragm moves down in expiration and is sucked in during inspiration. This finding represents diaphragmatic fatigue or paralysis and indicates impending respiratory arrest. In ventilated patients, it reflects ventilator-patient dysynchrony and requires either adjustment of the ventilator or sedation of the patient.

3. Is the inspection of the chest a useful technique?

Yes, but looking is not enough; the patient must be observed. The patient with a barrel-shaped chest whose supraclavicular spaces are retracted on inspiration clearly has emphysema. A pale, elderly man who is a smoker with recent weight loss and chest pain is a prime candidate for bronchogenic carcinoma. The presence of dilated veins on the chest wall is pathognomonic of superior vena cava syndrome. Impaired movement of part or all of the hemithorax may result from pleural effusion, pneumothorax, pleural tumor, or fibrosis. Gynecomastia in a man with cigarette stains on the fingers is a telltale sign of lung cancer.

4. What does tracheal shift denote?

The trachea is normally palpated in the suprasternal notch. Its displacement to either the left or the right of the midline indicates a shift in the mediastinum. Conditions that push the mediastinum away from the affected side include pleural effusion, pneumothorax, and massive tumors. Fibrosis of the lung or collapse of one or more lobes pulls the mediastinum and trachea toward the affected side.

5. Define subcutaneous emphysema.

Subcutaneous emphysema is the presence of air in the subcutaenous tissues. It may be caused by the following: air leaking from within the pleura, for example, from a pneumothorax;

mediastinal air, for example, from a ruptured esophagus; or gas-forming organisms. Sub-cutaneous emphysema also may be caused iatrogenically by insertion of chest tubes and central lines.

6. What is Tietze's syndrome?

Careful palpation of the chest sometimes reveals costochondral tenderness that may be the source of unexplained pain in the chest. The condition, also called *relapsing polychondritis*, may be caused by stress or trauma to rib structures at one or more costochondral junctions.

7. How is consolidation distinguished from pleural effusion on pulmonary examination?

A combination of percussion and auscultatory findings distinguishes consolidation from effusion.

Physical Findings in Pulmonary Consolidation and Pleural Effusion

CONDITION	INSPECTION	PALPATION	PERCUSSION NOTE	AUSCULTATION
Consolidation	Respiratory rate increased; movements decreased on affected side	No mediastinal shift; tactile (vocal) fremitus increased	Dull	Bronchial breathing; bronchophony; whispering pectoriloquy; fine crepitations
Pleural effusion	Movements diminished	If large, mediastinum shifted to opposite side; tactile (vocal) fremitus absent	Flat or stony, dull	Breath sounds absent; sometimes bronchial and egobronchophony above upper level of fluid

8. Describe egobronchophony.

Egobronchophony is a nasal character imparted to the spoken word because of the presence of overtones. It is easily recognized. When a patients says "E," it sounds like "A." Egobronchophony is heard best over the effusion.

9. What are rales, or crackles?

Crepitations sound like bursting of air bubbles and indicate that secretions are present.

Differences Between Fine and Coarse Crackles

FEATURES	FINE CRACKLES	COARSE CRACKLES
Sound	Explosive interrupted sounds (< 250 msec); higher in pitch, simulated by rubbing a lock of hair between the fingers	Explosive interrupted sounds (< 250 msec); lower in pitch, simulated by bubbling liquid
Cause	Sudden opening up of previously collapsed alveoli and small airways	Sudden opening up of previously collapsed bronchi and large airways; air bubbling through secretions
Phase of respiratory cycle	End inspiration	Early inspiration; often expiration
Effect of cough	Does not clear	May clear
Settings	Pulmonary fibrosis Pneumonia Heart failure	Acute bronchitis Severe pulmonary edema Chronic bronchitis

Adapted from Boyars MC: J Respir Dis 12:627–636, 1993.[3]

10. How is airway obstruction identified?

The presence of wheezes or rhonchi is suggestive of airway obstruction. Both are produced by the rapid flow of air through narrowed bronchi. The walls and secretions of the bronchus vibrate between the closed and barely open positions similar to the way a reed vibrates in a musical instrument. Wheezes tend to be of a higher pitch and greater intensity than rhonchi, which have a snoring or moaning quality.

Differences Between Wheezes and Rhonchi

FEATURES	WHEEZES	RHONCHI
Sound	Continuous (> 250 msec), high-pitched musical sound; usually polyphonic	Continuous (> 250 msec), low-pitched moaning sound; frequently monophonic
Cause	Vibration of small airways at point of closure	Vibration of larger airways at point of closure
Phase of respiratory cycle	Almost always inspiratory; occasionally expiratory	Almost always inspiratory; occasionally expiratory
Effect of cough	May change with cough	Clears, at least temporarily
Diseases	Asthma Extrinsic compression of airway Obstruction of airway by foreign body, tumor, or secretions	Acute bronchitis Chronic obstructive pulmonary disease Extrinsic compression of airway Obstruction of airway by foreign body, tumor, or secretions

Adapted from Boyars MC: J Respir Dis 12:627–636, 1991.[3]

11. Which findings in bronchospasm are most ominous?

A silent chest in a tired and lethargic patient with airway obstruction signifies exhaustion and impending respiratory arrest. Previously heard wheezes disappear because airflow velocity is decreased in obstructed airways and no sounds are produced. Such a situation requires prompt intervention with intubation and mechanical ventilation.

12. How is the severity of bronchospasm assessed?

Although respiratory rate and pulsus paradoxus are useful indicators, they are neither sensitive nor specific for assessing the severity of airway obstruction. The only way to reliably measure airway obstruction is by measuring flow rates either by spirometry or peak flow meters.

13. Name the five most common pulmonary causes of clubbing.

Clubbing is a bilateral, symmetric fingernail deformity, originally described by Hippocrates. When associated with periostitis and arthritis, this syndrome is called *hypertrophic pulmonary osteoarthropathy*. Pulmonary causes of clubbing include bronchiectasis, lung abscesses, pulmonary malignancy, pulmonary fibrosis, and sarcoidosis. Clubbing is not a feature of chronic bronchitis, emphysema, or bronchial asthma.

14. What are the usual clinical signs in emphysema?

Patients with emphysema present with a relatively quiet chest that is often barrel shaped. Chest percussion is diffusely hyperresonant. Breath sounds are vesicular but significantly reduced in intensity. Adventitious sounds are unusual unless there is concomitant bronchitis or asthma. The expiratory phase of respiration is usually prolonged.

15. Describe the skin findings associated with pulmonary disease.

Although not specific for pulmonary disease, cyanosis is a reliable marker of hypoxemia. It presents as bluish discoloration of extremities, usually the tips of fingers or the lips. It may be seen in various forms of heart disease or conditions giving rise to peripheral vascular disease.

Lupus pernio is the most characteristic of all cutaneous lesions of sarcoid. It is a chronic, bluish, granulomatous infiltration of the nose, cheeks, ears and sometimes the lips and chin.

Erythema nodosum consists of painful red nodules occurring mainly on the shins. It is an important, albeit nonspecific, manifestation of many pulmonary diseases.

Lupus vulgaris is the cutaneous lesion of tuberculosis. It consists of reddish-brown, flat plaques with yellowish brown nodules on the head, face, neck, arms, and legs, in descending order of frequency. Ulceration and scarring are characteristic findings.

Some pneumonias have characteristic skin findings. Patients with psittacosis pneumonia may have splinter hemorrhages or faint pink spots on their trunk (Horder's spots). Varicella pneumonia may present with eruption of clear vesicles ranging from 2 to 5 mm. Cutaneous ulcers are seen in 60% of patients with tularemia pneumonia.

16. Which eye disorders are seen in patients with pulmonary diseases?

Episcleritis and uveitis may be seen in patients with systemic lupus erythematosus and other autoimmune disorders. Patients with ankylosing spondylitis and up to 25% of patients with sarcoidosis have uveitis. Optic nerve involvement with gradual progressive visual loss is also seen in sarcoidosis.

Keratoconjunctivitis sicca is seen in patients with Sjögren's syndrome, who may also have chronic interstitial lung disease. Choroid tubercles may be seen in patients with tuberculosis. Wegener's granulomatoses may produce lid edema, nasolacrimal duct obstruction, proptosis, and conjunctival chemosis.

BIBLIOGRAPHY

1. Badgett RG, Tanaka DJ, Hung DK, et al: Can moderate chronic obstructive pulmonary disease be diagnosed by historical and physical findings alone? Am J Med 94:188–196, 1993.
2. Bohadana AB, Peslin R, Uffholtz R: Breathsounds in the clinical assessment of airway obstruction. Thorax 33:345–351, 1978.
3. Boyars MC: Getting the most out of chest auscultation. J Respir Dis 12:627–636, 1993.
4. Isselbacher KJ, Braunwald E, et al (eds): Harrison's Principles of Internal Medicine, 13th ed. New York, McGraw-Hill, 1994.
5. Jamison JP, McKinley RK: Validity of peak expiratory flow rate variability for the diagnosis of asthma. Clin Sci 85:367–371, 1993.
6. Mangione S, Fiel SB: Lung auscultation among physicians in training: A lost art. Chest 106(Suppl):855, 1994.
7. Murray JF, Nadel JA: Textbook of Respiratory Medicine. Philadelphia, W.B. Saunders, 1988.
8. Nairn JR, Tuner-Warwick M: Breath sounds in emphysema. Br J Dis Chest 63:29–37, 1969.
9. O'Donnell DE: Breathlessness in patients with chronic airflow obstruction. Mechanisms and management. Chest 106:904–912, 1994.
10. Rish RJ, Shore A: Hypertrophic pulmonary osteoarthropathy system complex. In Cannon GW, Zimmerman GA (eds): The Lung in Rheumatic Diseases. New York, Marcel Dekker, 1990, pp 415–432.
11. Schneider IC, Anderson AE Jr: Correlation of clinical signs with ventilatory function in obstructive lung disease. Ann Intern Med 62:477–485, 1965.
12. Sharma OM: Symptoms and signs in pulmonary medicine. Dis Mon 41:577–640, 1995.
13. Shin C, Williams MH Jr: Evaluation of the severity of asthma. Am J Med 68:11–13, 1990.
14. Shneerson JM, Jones BM: Ferritin, finger clubbing and lung disease. Thorax 36:688–692, 1981.

II. Diagnostic Imaging

3. CHEST RADIOGRAPHS

David Levin, M.D., and Jeffrey S. Klein, M.D.

ORDERING

1. When should a portable chest radiograph be ordered?

Portable chest radiographs are inferior to films obtained in the radiology department because of technical limitations. Portable radiographic equipment uses lower energy (kVp), which requires a longer exposure time to adequately penetrate the patient and results in greater motion artifact. The focal length (distance between x-ray source and film) is reduced in portable radiography, which leads to magnification of the heart and thoracic structures, making assessment of cardiac size difficult. Poor contact between the patient and the film cassette produces further magnification and causes indistinctness of margins. Portable chest radiography is often performed with the patient in the supine or semierect position, which limits the degree of inspiration.

Given these limitations, portable radiographs should be obtained only when it is impossible for the patient to be brought to the radiology department. This occurs most commonly in the intensive care and postoperative settings.

2. What are the indications for an expiratory chest radiograph?

They are usually obtained to evaluate for possible pneumothorax. In full expiration, the density of lung is increased while the amount of pleural air is unchanged. Therefore, the greater contrast between the lung and the air in the pleural space should enhance detection of pneumothorax. Additionally, the greater volume of pleural air relative to lung at end expiration displaces the visceral pleural reflection away from the inner ribs and should enhance its visibility. Despite these theoretical advantages, clinical studies have shown no improvement in the rate of pneumothorax detection using expiratory radiographs.

Expiratory radiographs can assess for unilateral air trapping, as might be seen with an aspirated foreign body. In this situation, a normal lung increases in density and decreases in volume on the expiratory film, whereas an obstructing foreign body produces a lucent lung that remains unchanged in volume.

3. When should a lateral decubitus film be ordered?

For a lateral decubitus film, the patient lies on his or her side and the x-ray beam is directed horizontally toward the body. This study is usually obtained to determine the presence and size of a pleural effusion. A free-flowing effusion will layer between the inner cortex of the ribs and the lung, producing a sharply defined homogeneous opacity traversing the length of the chest. A loculated pleural effusion is immobile and will not layer dependently.

An additional indication for a decubitus chest radiograph is the evaluation of possible pneumothorax. Although an upright expiratory chest film is usually obtained for this purpose, a decubitus radiograph made with the affected side up may detect a pneumothorax in a patient who cannot sit or stand. On decubitus radiographs, the pleural air is seen as a lucency in the nondependent thorax that outlines the visceral pleura medially and the inner surface of the ribs laterally.

4. Should the radiology requisition include a clinical history?

The request for a radiologic study is a request for consultation with a radiologist. Although some physicians believe that providing clinical information on the radiograph requisition will bias the radiologist, studies show that awareness of the clinical data aids the radiologist in accurate interpretation of the study. The clinical history also may suggest alternative imaging modalities that may prove more useful.

INTERPRETATION

5. What should be examined first on a chest radiograph?

The most important initial observation to make on any radiographic study is the demographic data provided on the corner of the film: the patient's name, gender, date of birth, and date of the study. The metallic marker indicating the right or left side of the patient should be identified to guide proper film display (the patient's right should correspond to the viewer's left) and to detect congenital abnormalities of organ migration that may be associated with disease. Use of this routine before the radiograph is interpreted prevents mistakes and provides useful information that may aid in image interpretation.

6. How should a chest radiograph be evaluated?

After the patient data are verified, the films should be examined in a systematic manner. Any pattern that examines all regions of the film is acceptable. A reasonable method would begin with evaluation of the soft tissues of the neck, shoulders, breasts, axillae, diaphragms, and upper abdomen. The skeletal structures are examined next. The pleural surfaces are evaluated for presence of effusion, pneumothorax, focal or diffuse thickening and calcification. The mediastinal, hilar, and cardiac interfaces are assessed for contour abnormalities. The trachea and main bronchi are studied for displacement, narrowing, or intraluminal masses. Finally, the lung parenchyma is examined for abnormally increased or decreased density, either localized or diffuse. A comparison with the opposite lung is helpful to detect subtle localized parenchymal disease. Both frontal and lateral radiographs should be evaluated in this fashion.

7. How are the anterior, middle, and posterior mediastinal compartments defined?

The mediastinum is often divided into anterior, middle, and posterior compartments to aid in the differential diagnosis of masses. The division used by radiologists is based on the lateral radiograph. The anterior mediastinum includes the region posterior to the sternum and anterior to the heart and great vessels. The posterior mediastinum extends posteriorly from the posterior margins of the trachea and heart. This compartment includes the descending aorta, esophagus, sympathetic chain, thoracic duct, azygos and hemiazygos veins, and paravertebral spaces. The middle mediastinum includes the heart, great vessels, pericardium, pericardial spaces, trachea, and main bronchi.

8. What are the most common causes of mediastinal masses?

Common Mediastinal Masses

ANTERIOR MEDIASTINUM	MIDDLE MEDIASTINUM	POSTERIOR MEDIASTINUM
Lymphoma	Lymphadenopathy	Neurofibroma (schwannoma)
Thymoma	Tracheobronchial duplication cyst	Vertebral tumors (metastases, myeloma)
Thyroid goiter	Vascular lesions (aneurysm, etc.)	
Germ cell tumor (teratoma)	Tracheobronchial tumors	Paraspinal abscess or hematoma
		Descending aortic aneurysm
		Esophageal neoplasms

9. What lung diseases are associated with increased radiographic density?

Lung disease can produce increased radiographic density (the lungs are too white or opaque) or decreased radiographic density (the lungs become too black or lucent). Increased radiographic density due to air space filling reflects replacement of alveolar air with water (edema), pus (pneumonia), or blood (hemorrhage). Uncommon causes of air space disease include alveolar filling with malignant cells (that is, bronchoalveolar cell carcinoma, lymphoma) or proteinaceous material (pulmonary alveolar proteinosis, acute silicosis). Air space disease is confluent and ill-defined at its margins. It obscures pulmonary vessels and tends toward lobar or segmental distribution as the process extends from involved to uninvolved lung via interalveolar channels (pores of Kohn). Branching tubular lucencies coursing through regions of confluent opacity represent patent, air-filled bronchi surrounded by consolidated lung and are termed air bronchograms.

Increased radiographic density also may be caused by interstitial disease. In contrast to air space disease, which usually reflects an acute process, interstitial disease may reflect either acute or chronic infiltration of the supporting structures of the lung. The most common cause of acute interstitial disease is pulmonary edema, although viral or atypical pneumonias can produce similar findings. Chronic interstitial disease most often results from noninfectious interstitial inflammation and fibrosis or metastatic tumor infiltration. The conditions most often associated with chronic interstitial inflammation are collagen vascular diseases (such as scleroderma or rheumatoid arthritis), asbestos exposure, sarcoidosis, and drug reactions. Interstitial edema or inflammation appears radiographically as curvilinear (reticular) or linear opacities, whereas granulomatous processes and metastatic neoplasms can cause diffuse small (miliary) nodules.

10. What lung diseases are associated with decreased radiographic density?

Decreased radiographic lung density is difficult to detect. When generalized, it is most often associated with chronic obstructive pulmonary disease (i.e., emphysema). Generalized decreased density (hyperlucency) is usually associated with findings of hyperinflation such as flattening or inversion of the diaphragms and an increased anteroposterior diameter of the chest.

11. What should be examined on the lateral chest radiograph?

The lateral film is useful in evaluating regions of the chest not well displayed on the frontal projection. Such regions include the retrosternal clear space (the lucent region behind the sternum and anterior to the heart and great vessels) and the posterior lung bases. On the lateral film, these regions are roughly triangular in shape and are radiolucent (black). An opacity in either region is abnormal and should prompt further evaluation. The lateral film helps confirm the intrathoracic location of focal lesions and aids in accurate compartmentalization of mediastinal masses detected on the frontal radiograph.

12. How is the size of a pneumothorax determined?

A pneumothorax is usually estimated from the frontal radiograph as small, moderate, or large. If a more precise determination is needed, three measurements are obtained from an upright film: the vertical height of the pneumothorax at the lung apex and the lateral width of the pneumothorax at 25% and 75% of the height of the thorax. The average of the three measurements expressed in millimeters corresponds to the percentage pneumothorax present. An average of 10 mm indicates a 15% pneumothorax, 15 mm indicates a 20% pneumothorax, and 40 mm corresponds to a 40% pneumothorax.

13. How is the size of a pleural effusion estimated?

A 50-ml pleural fluid collection will produce blunting of the posterior costophrenic sulcus on the lateral film. A pleural effusion of 200 ml will blunt the lateral costophrenic angle on the frontal radiograph. A pleural collection of 500 ml is necessary to obscure the diaphragmatic contour. On a lateral decubitus view, pleural collection 1 cm thick represents approximately 200 ml of fluid.

CLINICAL USES

14. Describe the radiologic evaluation of a solitary pulmonary nodule.

A solitary pulmonary nodule is detected on approximately 0.2% of chest radiographs. The majority of solitary pulmonary nodules are caused by four entities: granuloma, bronchogenic carcinoma, hamartoma (a benign pulmonary neoplasm), and solitary metastasis. The radiographic evaluation should result in classifying the nodule as benign (not requiring further evaluation) or possibly malignant (requiring a pathologic diagnosis).

The initial step in the evaluation of a nodule is a comparison with the patient's prior chest films. A complete lack of growth for at least 2 years is an accurate indication of benignancy. If old films are unavailable, the nodule should be studied for its size, margins, and the presence of calcification or fat. Nodules exceeding 3 cm in diameter have a high likelihood of malignancy regardless of their density and usually require biopsy. Similarly, a lobulated or spiculated margin is highly suggestive of malignancy. Benign patterns of calcification in a smoothly marginated nodule include complete, central, laminated, and popcorn calcification. Although a benign pattern of calcification is occasionally recognized on plain radiographs, thin-section CT is usually necessary for definitive evaluation. The detection of fat in a smooth nodule is indicative of a hamartoma.

15. What is the best method for detection of a fractured rib?

In patients sustaining blunt chest trauma, rib fractures are common and simply indicate significant trauma. A rib series can be performed to detect rib fractures, but the results rarely alter the patient's management. It is more appropriate to obtain frontal and lateral chest radiographs to detect complications of blunt trauma that require emergency intervention such as pneumothorax, hemothorax, and hemomediastinum.

16. What is the proper radiographic position for indwelling tubes, lines, and catheters?

The tip of an **endotracheal tube** should lie between 3 and 6 cm above the tracheal carina when the patient's head is in a neutral position (that is, with the mandible overlying C6 or C7). This position allows the tube to move 2 cm superiorly (with full neck extension) or inferiorly (with full neck flexion) while remaining safely within the trachea.

A **central venous catheter** is optimally placed with its tip in the superior vena cava, although a position within a brachiocephalic, central internal jugular, or subclavian vein is acceptable. Positioning of the catheter tip within the right atrium increases the incidence of cardiac perforation and arrhythmia. The tip of a Swan-Ganz catheter should be located within the right or left main pulmonary artery. A tip positioned more than 1.5 cm from the lateral margin of the hilum may lead to vessel injury or occlusion.

An **intraaortic balloon pump** is ideally placed with its radiopaque tip just inferior to the aortic knob, which ensures that the catheter tip will not occlude the origin of the left subclavian artery. Placement of the pump too far distally in the aorta may lead to obstruction of the origins of the celiac, mesenteric, or renal arteries during balloon insufflation.

BIBLIOGRAPHY

1. Blackmore CC, Black WC, Dallas RV, et al: Pleural fluid volume estimation: A chest radiograph prediction rule. Acad Radiol 3:103–109, 1996.
2. Brant WE, Helms CA (eds): Fundamentals of Diagnostic Radiology. Baltimore, Williams & Wilkins, 1994, p 1308.
3. Forrest JV, Feigin DS: Essentials of Chest Radiology. Philadelphia, W.B. Saunders, 1982, p 152.
4. Groskin S (ed): Heitzman's The Lung. Radiologic-Pathologic Correlations, 3rd ed. St. Louis, Mosby-Year Book, 1993, pp 70–104.
5. Klein JS: Intensive and coronary care radiology. In Higgins CB (ed): Essentials of Cardiac Radiology and Imaging. Philadelphia, J.B. Lippincott, 1992, pp 92–103.
6. Proto AV, Speckman JM: The left lateral radiograph of the chest. Part I. Med Radiog Photogr 55:30–74, 1979.
7. Proto AV, Speckman JM: The left lateral radiograph of the chest. Part II. Med Radiog Photogr 56:38–64, 1980.
8. Webb WR: Radiologic evaluation of the solitary pulmonary nodule. Am J Roentgenol 154:701–708, 1990.

4. CT SCANS AND ULTRASOUND

David A. Lynch, M.B., and C. Martin O'Driscoll, M.B.

1. When can biopsies be performed under ultrasound guidance?

Ultrasound cannot "see" through bone or aerated lung parenchyma, and therefore lesions accessible to ultrasound are usually apical, juxta-diaphragmatic, involving the chest wall, in the anterior mediastinum, or having a broad area of contact with the pleura. As a general rule with ultrasound, "If it can be seen, it can be biopsied."

2. Which modality is better for assessing diaphragmatic disease, CT or ultrasound?

This is one area where ultrasound has several advantages over CT. These include multiplanar imaging, portability, lack of ionizing radiation, and real-time imaging that can be used to detect paralysis or loss of integrity of either hemidiaphragm. Evaluation of the diaphragm is facilitated in patients who have pleural effusions and is made more difficult in patients with a pneumothorax or distended bowel adjacent to the area of interest.

3. When is ultrasound needed in thoracentesis?

Image-guided pleural drainage is the recommended primary management of empyema, but most pleural collections may be aspirated without image guidance by experienced clinicians. Failure of "blind" thoracentesis is an indication for image-guidance, most conveniently under ultrasound, which allows additional diagnostic information regarding the nature, extent, mobility, and precise position of pleural fluid to be obtained. In addition, ultrasound may identify local pleural abnormalities (e.g., metastases) when present.

In some clinical settings the risk of nonguided aspiration of small pleural collections is increased because a pneumothorax on that side would seriously compromise the patient's respiratory function—e.g., following pneumonectomy, unilateral lung transplantation, and bilateral lung transplantation, where there is effectively one common pleural space within the thorax ("buffalo chest"). In these and other settings, when thoracentesis is indicated on the side providing maximal gas exchange, the procedure should be conducted under image-guidance to maximize yield and minimize complications.

4. How safe is CT-guided transthoracic needle biopsy (TNB)?

Mortality from CT-guided TNB is reported to be 0.02%. Pneumothorax is the most common morbidity (typically 5–30%), but less than half of all patients who develop a pneumothorax require treatment with chest tube drainage. Postprocedure surveillance is critical in the first hour because > 90% of pneumothoraces requiring intervention will be evident within that time. This is one of the reasons TNB can be safely performed on an outpatient basis.

Hemorrhage, with or without hemoptysis, occurs in 1–10% of cases and in the absence of a bleeding diathesis is usually self-limiting. Other complications are uncommon and include vasovagal reactions, subcutaneous emphysema, malignant seeding of the biopsy track, and air embolism (which may be fatal).

5. Can one predict who will get a pneumothorax after TNB?

Several prospective and retrospective studies have identified factors associated with *increased* risk of pneumothorax. These can be divided into three general categories, but many of these are inter-related:

Patient	Increasing age, increased total lung capacity, $PaO_2 < 59$ mmHg, FEV_1/FVC ratio < 70% predicted, intractable cough, mechanical ventilation
Target (lesion)	Deeper lesions, smaller lesions, cavitary lesions, lymphangitic carcinoma

Technique   Number of pleural passes, increasing external diameter of biopsy nee-
                     dles, use of core-cutting needles rather than aspiration needles, increased
                     duration of the procedure, inexperience of operator

6. Are there any contraindications to CT-guided TNB?

Absence of informed consent from the patient or his or her representative

Biopsy by an inexperienced person without direct supervision

Lack of adequate personnel and equipment to effectively manage all potential complications, including cardiopulmonary arrest

Situations in which biopsy results, whether positive or negative, would have no effect on the patient's management or prognosis

Severe obstructive lung disease ($FEV_1 < 1.0$ liter)

A patient who is uncooperative or unable to maintain a constant position

Intractable cough

Bullae in the needle path

Patients on positive end-expiration pressure (PEEP) ventilation

Possible echinococcal cyst

Possible pulmonary arteriovenous malformation or other vascular lesion

Severe pulmonary hypertension

Uncorrectable bleeding diathesis or thrombocytopenia

Recent myocardial infarction, unstable angina, cardiac decompensation, or uncontrolled cardiac arrhythmia

Uremia

Superior vena cava obstruction

The risk-benefit ratio should be assessed in each individual in whom there are relative contraindications to TNB.

7. What general problems may be encountered in CT scanning of the chest?

1. Patients who are claustrophobic may be unable to lie still in the scanner or may refuse to enter the scanner (uncommon with today's machines having wider apertures).

2. Patients who are morbidly obese may exceed the maximal weight allowed on the table portion of the scanner (usually 300–350 pounds) or may be too large to fit in the scan aperture, particularly with their arms elevated.

3. Patients with restricted shoulder-girdle movements, e.g., frozen shoulder, may not be able to place or maintain their arms in optimal position.

4. Trauma patients may have orthopedic external fixation devices or multiple thoracostomy tubes which may need to be repositioned to allow the patient to enter the scanner or may dictate a customized scan protocol, e.g., scanning from the feet up with arms by the sides.

5. Spinal fixation devices, e.g., Harrington rods or metallic shoulder replacements, may cause significant artifact on images acquired in standard fashion (the presence of metallic material in the region to be scanned should always be mentioned on the request form).

6. Supplemental analgesia or sedation may be required in young children or patients who are uncooperative by virtue of uncontrolled pain, decreased cerebral function, or fear.

8. What respiratory complications may arise when performing a CT scan of the chest in a critical care patient? When might a patient need to be intubated?

A patient's respiratory status may deteriorate due to positioning; due to administration of contrast media, sedative, or analgesic drug; or as a direct complication of a related procedure (e.g., pneumothorax following CT-guided TNB). Patients in left-heart failure or congestive heart failure do not always tolerate the supine position well, and their increased dyspnea may preclude breath-holding, resulting in a poor-quality image. Benzodiazepines depress consciousness and decrease muscle tone, which predispose to aspiration in the supine position with an unprotected airway.

Narcotic analgesics depress central respiratory drive, which may lead to arterial desaturation and hypercapnia, particularly when combined with intravenous benzodiazepine. In these situations, intubation and mechanical ventilation should be anticipated and considered in the assessment of the patient before transfer to the scanning suite. Finally, if TNB is to be performed on a patient on mechanical ventilation, close cooperation is required between the radiologist and respiratory therapist to ensure the lungs are not in motion when a transpleural needle pass is performed.

9. Are all CT scans of the thorax performed in the supine position?

Although the supine position with the arms elevated above the head is the standard position for a CT examination of the thorax, **prone** imaging is often included in high-resolution scan protocols to negate gravitational effects on the dependent portions of the lungs, particularly in interstitial lung diseases that have a predilection for the posterior lungs (e.g., asbestosis). The **lateral decubitus** position is particularly useful in the evaluation of pleural fluid collections, notably when there is associated consolidation.

10. Should all CT scans of the respiratory system be performed in the same phase of arrested respiration?

Routine scanning of the thorax is performed at the end of quiet inspiration. If the patient cannot hold his or her breath for the required length of time for the particular scanner, the scan may be performed during gentle mouth-breathing to minimize motion artifact. Breath-holding is facilitated in a proportion of patients by prior gentle hyperventilation. Scans done prior to TNB are most often done at the end of normal expiration (functional residual capacity), as this is the preferred phase of arrested respiration for traversing the pleural space. A specific case is the examination of the larynx; this is usually a two-phase study done initially during continuous quiet mouth-breathing (larynx relaxed and true cords abducted) followed by an identical examination during phonation of a low-pitched *e* (true cords adducted and piriform sinuses distended).

11. Is CT of value in patients with blunt laryngeal trauma?

The primary goal in this clinical situation is to secure an adequate airway. This should then be followed by endoscopic evaluation of the injuries, following which CT is indicated only if exploratory surgery and repair are planned. CT not only documents the injuries to both the cartilaginous and soft-tissue components of the larynx, but also helps to exclude associated injuries to the cervical spine and cervical esophagus.

12. What is meant by "spiral CT"?

Newer CT systems have a design modification called **slip-ring technology** which allows faster dynamic scanning compared to older designs. In conventional CT, data are acquired separately at each slice location, with movement of the patient only between images. In spiral scanning, the image data are acquired continuously, as the tube and detector rotate within the gantry and the patient moves continuously through the gantry. The combined movements generate spiral relative motion between patient and image receptor; hence, this technique is called spiral scanning. This type of scanning is also called **helical scanning**.

13. What are the advantages of spiral scanning?

The **faster scan times** available with spiral scanning are of particular importance in critically ill patients, children, and patients in whom reduced image acquisition times result in reduced cardiac and respiratory motion artifact. A further advantage is the need for **reduced volumes of intravenous contrast** for a given study, especially in children and patients with renal impairment. Finally, scanning in spiral mode permits **greater processing of the raw data** with slice reconstruction at variable increments and the ability to reconstruct studies in sagittal, coronal, and oblique planes.

14. How long does it take to acquire a single CT image?

This depends on the type of scanner used and the mode in which it is operated. Typically, newer slip-ring designs acquire a routine image in 1 sec or less. Many scanners also have a partial or

half-scan mode, which may reduce scan time by up to 50%. However, the trade-off is reduced resolution of the image. When scanning in spiral dynamic mode, the entire thorax may be imaged in a
single breath-hold of 30 sec or less. Cine-CT scanners can obtain images in as little as 0.05 sec, but
these are relatively expensive and not widely available.

15. What is meant by high resolution CT (HRCT)?
The HRCT technique is designed for detailed evaluation of the interstitial structures of the
lung. It requires the use of narrow slice thickness (1–2 mm compared with 5–10 mm for routine
scans) with high-resolution, edge-enhancing reconstruction algorithms and separate reconstruc-
tions of each lung.

16. What are the principal indications for HRCT?
- Evaluation for suspected interstitial lung disease in patients with normal or nonspecific
  chest radiographs
- Characterization of interstitial lung disease
- Characterization of solitary pulmonary nodules
- Diagnosis of bronchiectasis

CONTROVERSIES

17. What is the role of ultrasound in the diagnosis of pulmonary thromboembolic disease?
Ultrasound is very accurate in the diagnosis of above-calf deep vein thrombosis (DVT). The
sensitivity of compression scanning is > 90% with a specificity of > 98%, and sensitivity can be
increased by the addition of Doppler and color-flow imaging. These additional techniques are essential in evaluating pelvic veins.

The calf veins are more difficult to image but are well-visualized in 50–90% of cases, with a
sensitivity for DVT diagnosis of approximately 80%, at the expense of an additional 15–30 minutes of scanning time.

The finding of DVT in a patient with an equivocal/indeterminate ventilation-perfusion (V/Q)
scan raises the pre-test probability of a positive pulmonary angiogram to > 90%. However, approximately 30% of patients with angiographically proven pulmonary embolism will have normal bilateral lower-limb venograms. It is therefore useful to evaluate the lower-limb and pelvic veins in
patients with indeterminate V/Q scan findings, as the documentation of lower-extremity DVT may
reduce the need for angiography, though negative studies do not alter the need for further investigations. Ultrasound is preferable to contrast venography because it is noninvasive, portable, and does
not require intravenous contrast administration. It is, however, relatively time-consuming.

18. Is CT superior to fiberoptic bronchoscopy in the investigation of patients with hemoptysis?
The most commonly identified causes of hemoptysis are bronchogenic carcinoma and
bronchiectasis. Most patients with carcinoma can be diagnosed with either CT or bronchoscopy,
but **bronchoscopy** has the advantage of detecting early mucosal abnormalities, inflammation,
and squamous metaplasia and may identify blood in an airway when an actual bleeding point is
not identified. **CT** has the advantage of being noninvasive, less operator-dependent, and better at
diagnosing peripheral tumors and bronchiectasis, which are usually beyond the reach of the
endoscopist. Spiral scanning with reformatting targeted to the central airways will increase sensitivity for endobronchial lesions but is not recommended as routine practice.

Therefore, while plain radiographs and bronchoscopy are the primary investigations for hemoptysis, CT is a complementary investigation. Specific instances in which CT is of value include:
1. Planning of biopsy sites to maximize bronchoscopic yield
2. To identify and characterize abnormalities outside the endoscopic range
3. When radiographs and bronchoscopy are negative
4. To stage known tumors
5. When there are contraindications to bronchoscopy and transbronchial biopsy

19. Is spiral CT as accurate as pulmonary angiography in detecting pulmonary emboli (PE)?

Contrast-enhanced spiral CT scanning, with meticulous attention to scan technique, when read by experienced observers can reliably detect PE in second to fourth division pulmonary arteries. Reported sensitivities and specificities for CT diagnosis of central PE are both > 90%. Sensitivity falls to approximately 60% for CT diagnosis of subsegmental PE. However, interobserver agreement on arteriographic diagnosis of subsegmental PE is approximately 70%. Therefore, neither test is perfect.

CT does not replace standard noninvasive tests, such as ventilation-perfusion (V/Q) imaging and lower-limb venous sonography, nor does it replace pulmonary arteriography as the definitive diagnostic test. CT appears to have a role in the evaluation of patients with an acute presentation and an equivocal or indeterminate V/Q scan, as the technique is noninvasive and has lower morbidity and mortality than arteriography. Approximately one-third of patients with PE have involvement of subsegmental vessels alone. Therefore, two-thirds of patients have more central PE, in which CT should provide a diagnosis without the need for angiography.

CT also provides a noninvasive means of evaluating thrombolytic therapy of central PE, has a role in the preoperative evaluation of patients with chronic PE disease, and provides an alternative diagnostic test in patients who refuse pulmonary arteriography.

20. How accurate is CT staging of primary lung cancer?

The purpose of staging non-small-cell primary lung cancer is to determine resectability, largely by detecting enlarged lymph nodes or invasion of critical structures or the chest wall. Definitive staging may involve the radiologist, bronchoscopist, surgeon, and pathologist. CT is the best noninvasive staging procedure, although it is not 100% accurate. CT lacks sensitivity in assessing mediastinal and chest wall invasion. In superior sulcus tumors, MRI may be preferred. Sensitivity and specificity of CT nodal staging are primarily related to nodal size, but other factors also must be considered, including short versus long axis measurements, nodal location, nodal calcification, location of the primary tumor, tumor cell type, associated atelectasis, prevalence of nonneoplastic nodal enlargement in the patient population, and scan technique. Reported accuracies for CT nodal staging compared to mediastinoscopy using a 15-mm size threshold vary from approx 75–92%. As the size threshold is lowered, sensitivity increases but specificity decreases. Furthermore, in 10% of patients with primary lung carcinoma adrenal abnormalities are noted on CT, the majority of which prove to be benign, further reducing specificity. Nonetheless, a staging CT that does not identify enlarged nodes has sufficient negative predictive value to obviate the need for mediastinoscopy before resection at thoracotomy. When enlarged nodes are identified on CT, the radiologist can guide the mediastinoscopist to the areas to be sampled.

BIBLIOGRAPHY

1. American College of Radiology Task Force on Appropriateness Criteria: Appropriateness Criteria for Imaging and Treatment Decisions. Reston, VA, American College of Radiology, 1995.
2. American College of Radiology Standards. Reston, VA, American College of Radiology, 1995.
3. Goodman LR, et al: Detection of pulmonary embolism in patients with unresolved clinical and scintigraphic diagnosis: Helical CT versus angiography. AJR 164:1369–1374, 1995.
4. Moss AA, Gamsu G, Genant HK: Computed Tomography of the Body with Magnetic Resonance Imaging, 2nd ed. Philadelphia, W.B. Saunders, 1992.
5. Muller NL, Miller RR: Computed tomography of chronic diffuse infiltrative lung disease. Ann Rev Respir Dis 142:1206–1215, 1990.
6. Muller NL: Imaging of the pleura. Radiology 186:297–309, 1993.
7. Newell JD, Tarver RD: Thoracic Radiology. New York, Raven Press, 1993.
8. Remy-Jardin M, et al: Central pulmonary thromboembolism: Diagnosis with spiral volumetric CT with the single-breath-hold technique—Comparison with pulmonary angiography. Radiology 185:381–387, 1992.
9. Set PAK, et al: Hemoptysis: Comparative study of the role of CT and fiberoptic bronchoscopy. Radiology 189:677–680, 1993.
10. Staples CA, et al: Mediastinal nodes in bronchogenic carcinoma: Comparison between CT and mediastinoscopy. Radiology 167:367–372, 1988.
11. Swensen SJ, et al: High-resolution CT of the lungs: Findings in various pulmonary diseases. AJR 158:974–979, 1992.
12. Westcott JL: Percutaneous transthoracic needle biopsy. Radiology 169:593–601, 1988.

5. PULMONARY ANGIOGRAPHY AND MRI OF THE CHEST

Marc Gosselin, M.D., and Jeffrey S. Klein, M.D.

PULMONARY ANGIOGRAPHY

1. What are the indications for pulmonary angiography?

The most common indication is the detection of pulmonary embolism when lung ventilation/perfusion scanning is nondiagnostic. Additional indications include the diagnosis and treatment (by embolization) of pulmonary arteriovenous malformations, aneurysms, and congenital vascular anomalies.

2. List the contraindications to pulmonary angiography.

Contraindications to pulmonary angiography relate to one of the following three factors:

1. **Iodinated contrast.** A previous severe contrast reaction warrants pretreatment with oral corticosteroids (32 mg of methylprednisolone 12 and 2 hours before the procedure) and the use of nonionic contrast. This regimen limits the overall incidence of contrast reactions to less than 2%. Pulmonary angiography is also contraindicated in patients with renal insufficiency (i.e., those with serum creatinine levels over 2.5 mg/dl), who have an increased risk of contrast-induced nephrotoxicity and progressive renal failure.

2. **Cardiac disease.** Patients with left bundle branch block are at risk for complete heart block if the angiographic catheter induces a right bundle branch block as it courses through the heart. In such patients, prophylactic placement of a transvenous pacemaker is necessary before the procedure. Patients susceptible to frequent ventricular tachyarrhythmias may require intravenous lidocaine treatment to suppress ventricular ectopy induced by the tip of the catheter as it traverses the right ventricle.

3. **Pulmonary arterial hypertension and cor pulmonale.** Pulmonary artery systolic pressure exceeding 80 mmHg or right ventricle end-diastolic pressure exceeding 20 mmHg is associated with an increased risk of death from pulmonary angiography. The vasoconstrictive effects of the hypertonic contrast on the pulmonary arteries produces a sudden elevation in pulmonary pressures and can result in right heart failure. The use of nonionic contrast with selective right or left pulmonary artery injection and the injection of a lower osmolarity contrast agent at a reduced rate can minimize this risk.

3. How is a pulmonary angiogram performed?

This procedure is usually performed under fluoroscopic guidance in the angiography suite of the radiology department. It entails puncturing the femoral vein and placing a pigtail or balloon-tipped catheter into the inferior vena cava (IVC). Contrast is then injected to assess for the presence of IVC thrombus. Under fluoroscopic guidance, the catheter is advanced into the right atrium, through the tricuspid valve, and into the right ventricle as the ECG is monitored closely for ventricular arrhythmias. The catheter is then advanced into the pulmonary artery and the pressure is measured. The side with the largest perfusion defects on perfusion scintigraphy is studied first. Routinely, direct anteroposterior and ipsilateral posterior oblique projections are obtained, each using an injection of 40–50 cc at a rate of 20–25 cc/second. The study is performed with conventional radiographs, which have superior spatial resolution and are less susceptible to motion artifact compared with digital subtraction angiography. The procedure is complete when an embolus is detected or all pulmonary arteries in question have been visualized. Since the angiogram may be complete after a single injection or may require six to eight injections to evaluate the entire arterial system, the procedure may require 30 minutes to 2 hours. No sutures are needed at the incision site after the catheter is removed. The patient must remain supine with the leg extended for 3–5 hours after the procedure to ensure healing of the vein at the puncture site.

If pulmonary embolism is diagnosed in a patient with a contraindication to anticoagulant therapy, an IVC filter can be placed immediately following the angiogram. This requires an additional 30 minutes and is performed via the same venotomy site. A properly positioned IVC filter limits the rate of recurrent pulmonary embolism to 2–5%.

4. What monitoring is recommended during a pulmonary angiogram?

Cardiac monitoring is necessary during pulmonary angiography, particularly since catheter manipulation through the right ventricle often induces ventricular ectopy. Blood pressure and oxygen saturation are monitored continuously during the procedure.

Once the catheter has been placed into the pulmonary artery, a transducer is used to measure pulmonary artery pressure. If pulmonary hypertension (defined as systolic pressure exceeding 40 mmHg) is present, the rate and volume of contrast injected are reduced to prevent sudden right ventricular overload.

5. Describe the angiographic findings of acute and chronic thromboembolism.

There are two direct angiographic findings that are considered specific for acute pulmonary embolus: a central intraluminal filling defect, which is the most common appearance (94%), and an abrupt contrast cut-off outlining the proximal convex margin of the embolus. In 65% of patients multiple emboli are found; bilateral emboli are seen in 42%, most commonly in the lower lobes. Secondary findings include diminished peripheral perfusion, delayed or absent venous filling, and the presence of tortuous arterial collaterals. Unfortunately, these findings are nonspecific; they are seen in several other disease processes, including vasculitis and COPD.

Chronic pulmonary thromboembolism exists when intraluminal organization of thrombus is incomplete. This can produce several angiographic findings, including proximal arterial dilatation and distal occlusion with a tapered or rounded edge, stenosis, webs, or eccentric plaques.

6. How accurate is pulmonary angiography?

Although pulmonary angiography is considered the gold standard for the diagnosis of pulmonary embolism, there are no studies that compare the accuracy of pulmonary angiography with autopsy findings. Studies comparing interobserver variability in pulmonary angiographic interpretation show a 98% agreement rate for lobar emboli, 90% for segmental emboli, and 66% agreement for subsegmental emboli. These data suggest that the sensitivity of pulmonary angiography is limited when only subsegmental emboli are present. The significance of small subsegmental emboli is controversial. It is likely that they are occasionally missed, yet follow-up of untreated patients with subsegmental emboli shows a recurrence rate of symptomatic embolism of only 0.6%. For this reason, a negative pulmonary angiogram is associated with an excellent prognosis.

7. List some complications of pulmonary angiography.
• Mild, moderate, or severe contrast reaction.
• Serious cardiac arrhythmias or cardiac arrest (1%).
• Death (0.2-0.5%); occurs almost exclusively in patients with severe pulmonary arterial hypertension and right ventricular failure.
• Cardiac perforation or endocardial injury from end-hole catheters has been virtually eliminated by the use of pigtail-tipped catheters.
• Papillary muscle/tricuspid valve injury may occur when the pigtail catheter is not carefully withdrawn upon completion of the angiogram.

8. What are the risk factors for a contrast reaction and how is it treated?

There are two forms of contrast reaction: nonidiosyncratic and idiosyncratic (anaphylactoid). Nonidiosyncratic reactions are related to the chemical properties of contrast agents and include nausea, vomiting, arrhythmias, congestive heart failure, angina, renal failure, and seizures. Patients at greatest risk for contrast-induced nephrotoxicity and renal failure include those with diabetes, cardiac disease, and multiple myeloma. The use of a smaller volume of nonionic contrast and adequate preprocedural hydration can reduce the incidence of nephrotoxicity.

Symptoms of a mild idiosyncratic reaction occur in 5–10% of patients and include pruritus, urticaria, and flushing. Antihistamines may be administered to symptomatic patients. Moderate reactions, including bronchospasm or angioedema, are treated with supplemental oxygen and parenteral bronchodilators and antihistamines.

Major reactions include arrhythmias, myocardial infarction, hypotension, anaphylactoid shock, and death. The fatality rate from intravascular contrast injection is less than 1 in 10,000 patients. Patients at risk for severe idiosyncratic contrast reaction include those with a history of prior contrast reaction (elevenfold more likely than the general population), asthma (fivefold increase), and multiple food or medication allergies (fourfold increase). If a patient is considered to be at high risk for a contrast reaction, pretreatment with corticosteroids 12 and 2 hours before the procedure and the use of nonionic contrast decrease the incidence and severity of reactions.

Hypotension due to a vasovagal reaction is not uncommon; the presence of bradycardia helps distinguish this form of hypotensive reaction from anaphylactoid shock. Severe hypotension from anaphylaxis is treated with vasopressors (epinephrine, 1–3 mg of 1:10,000 IV, or 0.1–0.3 mg of 1:1,000 subcutaneously); vasovagal hypertension is effectively managed with atropine (0.5–1.0 mg IV to a total of 2 mg).

Severe respiratory complications are managed by airway maintenance and may require intubation and mechanical ventilation in severe cases.

9. How long after the onset of pulmonary embolism symptoms will an angiogram remain positive?

Animal experiments show partial resolution of a nonmassive pulmonary embolus within 24 hours of embolization. Often, a large embolus fragments and embolizes to more distal arterial branches. Depending on embolus size and assuming no additional embolic events, however, the pulmonary angiogram will remain abnormal for 3–4 weeks after the initial embolism. Although angiography is best performed within 24 hours of the onset of symptoms, an accurate angiographic diagnosis of acute pulmonary embolism is possible after 48 to 72 hours. Therefore, emergency pulmonary angiography is rarely necessary.

MRI

10. How does MRI work?

MRI uses the effects of magnetism on the hydrogen protons in the body. The patient is placed within a large magnetic field that aligns the spinning hydrogen protons with respect to the magnetic field, producing a net electromagnetic vector from the protons. The magnet then disrupts this proton alignment with different sequences of superimposed electromagnetic excitations over a period of milliseconds. As the protons return to the original configuration within the large magnetic field, they release an electromagnetic signal that is sensed by receiving coils within the unit and sent to a computer. After several repetitions over a preset region, the total information is processed mathematically (using a process called *Fourier transformation*) and converted to a cross-sectional image. Tissue differentiation is based not on density but on several other factors: the number of protons, local heterogeneities within the magnetic field, the relaxation of excited photons inherent within various tissues (known as the T1 and T2 relaxation times), and the type of electromagnetic pulse sequence used. Because there are many different pulse sequences available to depict different information, the radiologist requires an adequate clinical history to tailor the MRI examination to the patient.

11. What are the advantages of thoracic MRI versus CT?

Although CT is the most widely used cross-sectional imaging modality for depicting chest disease, there are situations in which MRI is preferred. MRI provides superior tissue contrast that helps detect mediastinal or chest wall invasion by lung cancer. In addition, residual or recurrent mediastinal lymphoma is readily differentiated from posttreatment fibrosis. Another advantage of

MRI is its ability to demonstrate blood flow without the use of intravenous contrast, which is particularly useful in patients with renal insufficiency or severe contrast allergy. Because of its superior depiction of vascular anatomy and direct multiplanar imaging capabilities, MRI is the primary modality in the evaluation of congenital cardiovascular disease, aortic dissections and aneurysms in stable patients, and the relationship of a mediastinal or hilar mass to central vascular structures. The ability of MRI to perform direct coronal and sagittal imaging is particularly useful in the evaluation of brachial plexus involvement by a superior sulcus (Pancoast's) tumor, posterior mediastinal masses, and diaphragmatic and juxtacardiac lesions.

12. What are the disadvantages of thoracic MRI?

The thorax is the most difficult region of the body to image with MRI. Since only 10–20% of the lung parenchyma is composed of tissue and blood vessels, there are few protons available to generate a signal. Also, the innumerable tissue-air interfaces give the local magnetic field tremendous heterogeneity, which limits the utility of the T2-weighted spin-echo pulse sequence. The final major limitation is motion artifact from the heart, great vessels, and respiration, which results in poor spatial resolution.

13. List the clinical situations in which MRI of the chest has been shown to be useful in the patient's evaluation.

- Assessment of neurovascular involvement by superior sulcus tumor
- Differentiation between recurrent lymphoma and posttherapeutic fibrosis
- Chest wall, hilar, and mediastinal invasion by tumor
- Congenital cardiovascular disease
- Diagnosis of constrictive pericarditis
- Aortic dissection or aneurysm (in stable patients)

14. What are the absolute and relative contraindications to MRI?

Absolute. Pacemakers and even inactive pacing leads act like an antenna to induce arrhythmias from the strong electromagnetic field. Any ferromagnetic metal within or adjacent to vital structures can shift in the strong magnetic field and cause tissue damage. Before the MRI examination, the patient should be questioned about the presence of such devices, which include older aneurysm clips, metallic foreign bodies in the orbit, cochlear implants, and older Starr-Edwards cardiac valve prostheses.

Relative. Since the MRI tunnel is confining, a claustrophobic patient must be sedated before entering the MRI area, or an alternative imaging modality should be selected. Similarly, uncooperative patients and children need to be sedated to reduce motion artifacts. As a result of the rapidly changing magnetic fields, the MRI machine generates a repetitive loud banging noise that can agitate a disoriented patient or child. Although there is no evidence of any harmful effects on the fetus, elective MRI examinations on pregnant patients should be postponed until the postpartum period.

15. What techniques are used to reduce motion artifacts?

Cardiac motion is reduced with the use of ECG cardiac gating. The electromagnetic pulses are synchronized to set points in the cardiac cycle, usually the R-wave of the QRS complex. This allows imaging to occur at the same phase of the cardiac cycle, which substantially diminishes motion artifact and adds only 10–15% to the length of the examination. Cardiac gating can be implemented only in patients with a regular cardiac rate and rhythm; it cannot be used in patients with frequent ectopy or atrial arrhythmias such as atrial fibrillation.

Respiratory compensation is usually accomplished with a sensor device on the chest wall that matches chest wall motion with the acquisition of images, thereby allowing the computer to compensate for significant respiratory motion. Finally, although flowing blood within vessels normally produces no identifiable signal, nonuniform flow may produce intravascular signal on the spin-echo sequences. This artifact can be reduced by "presaturating" the blood flowing into the imaging volume, thereby eliminating intravascular signal within the image.

16. How is the ventilated patient managed in the MRI room?

The most important consideration in scanning a ventilated patient is to ensure the use of the proper equipment in the MRI suite. Most MRI areas have a dedicated ventilator composed of nonferromagnetic material. When general anesthesia is required to scan a patient, the anesthesia department usually provides a similar MRI-compatible machine. A resident, attending physician, or nurse should monitor the ventilated patient during the study.

17. Define the role of MRI in the diagnosis of pulmonary embolism.

New MRI-software and pulse sequences are currently being developed to perform two- and three-dimensional MR pulmonary angiography. Under ideal circumstances, fourth or fifth order branches of the pulmonary arteries can be visualized. Although MR pulmonary angiography is noninvasive and requires no intravascular contrast, limitations in spatial resolution, accessibility, and expense must be overcome if it is to become a practical alternative to conventional angiography in the diagnosis of pulmonary embolism.

BIBLIOGRAPHY

1. Armstrong P, Wilson A, Dee P, et al: Imaging of Diseases of the Chest, 2nd ed. St. Louis, Mosby, 1995, pp 9–13, 369–393.
2. Kadir S: Diagnostic Angiography. Philadelphia, W.B. Saunders, 1986, pp 584–603.
3. Lasser EC, Berry CC, Mishkin MM, et al: Pretreatment with corticosteroids to prevent adverse reactions to nonionic contrast media. Am J Roentgenol 162:523–526, 1994.
4. Link KM, Samuels LJ, Reed JC, et al: MR imaging of the mediastinum. J Thorac Imaging 8:34–53, 1993.
5. Nadich DF, Zerhouni EA, Siegelman SS: Computed Tomography and MRI of the Thorax, 2nd ed. New York, Raven Press, 1991, pp 19–32.
6. Newman GE: Pulmonary angiography in pulmonary embolic disease. J Thorac Imaging 4:28–39, 1989.
7. Stein PD, Athanasoulis C, Alavi A, et al: Complications and validity of pulmonary angiography in acute pulmonary embolism. Circulation 85:462–468, 1992.

6. LUNG SCANS

Christopher Gregory, M.D.

1. How is a nuclear medicine lung perfusion scan performed and what is the pathophysiologic basis of the study?

Technetium (Tc) 99m radionuclide is "tagged" to either macroaggregated albumin (MAA) or human albumin microspheres (HAM) to make small radioactive particles. When Tc decays, it emits a gamma ray that is detected by the nuclear medicine gamma camera; a nuclear medicine image is formed by detection of many gamma rays.

MAA is between 10 and 100 μ and HAM is between 15 and 45 μ in size. Because Tc-MAA and Tc-HAM are larger than a red blood cell (which is approximately 6 μ), these particles are trapped by "capillary blockage" at the first capillary bed they encounter. When these radioactive particles are injected via a peripheral venous site, the first capillaries encountered (assuming no right to left intracardiac shunt) are the pulmonary capillaries. Therefore, if perfusion is present at the capillary level of the lungs, the nuclear medicine perfusion image demonstrates activity in the periphery of the lungs. If there is a proximal (upstream) obstructing vascular lesion in the pulmonary arterial circulation resulting in blocked perfusion to the distal (downstream) capillary level, the nuclear medicine perfusion image demonstrates no activity in the periphery of the lungs; thus a perfusion defect is seen.

2. Does a lung perfusion scan introduce emboli in the pulmonary circulation?

Yes. A lung perfusion scan introduces tiny (10–100 μ) particles that are trapped at the capillary level and cause, in a sense, pulmonary emboli. These tiny distal (downstream) capillary emboli, however, cause blockage of less than 0.1% of all lung capillaries and do not produce any clinical signs or symptoms. The presence of these downstream emboli results in gamma activity in the periphery of the lung that is detectable by a lung scan and indicates that no proximal arterial blockage exists. Clinically significant pulmonary emboli are much larger than the Tc-tagged particles and cause blockage of segmental and subsegmental proximal pulmonary arteries. The presence of these obstructing emboli prevents the distribution of Tc-tagged particles into distal pulmonary capillaries and thereby produces a region in which perfusion activity is absent on the lung scan.

3. How is a nuclear medicine lung ventilation scan performed and what is the pathophysiologic basis of the study?

Tc radionuclide is tagged to aerosolized diethylenetriamine pentaacetic acid (DTPA) macromolecules. The aerosolized particles are then inhaled by the patient. Alternatively, a ventilation scan can be performed using xenon (Xe) 133 radionuclide gas molecules that are inhaled by the patient. When Xe decays, it emits a gamma ray that is detected by the nuclear medicine gamma camera. A nuclear medicine image is formed by the detection of many gamma rays.

The Tc-DTPA macromolecule or the Xe gas migrates by "bulk flow" within the lung. If the airways and air spaces are patent to the alveolar level of the lung, the nuclear medicine ventilation image demonstrates activity in the periphery of the lung. If a proximal lesion is obstructing air space in the bronchial airways and blocking ventilation to the distal alveolar level or if the distal alveolar air spaces are consolidated with fluid, the image shows no activity in the periphery of the lungs, with the result that a ventilation defect is seen.

4. How does a pulmonary embolism typically appear on a nuclear medicine lung scan?

A pulmonary embolism causes vascular blockage in the proximal pulmonary arterial vasculature. Because the pulmonary circulation is "end-arterial" no well-developed collateral pulmonary arterial vascular channels exist. As a result of the proximal pulmonary arterial blockage, there is no pulmonary arterial circulation to distal pulmonary capillary beds. The absence of circulation causes a perfusion defect on the nuclear medicine perfusion image that is typically peripheral, wedge shaped, and subsegmental or segmental in size, corresponding to the end-arterial vascular distribution of the obstructed artery. Because there is no physiologic mechanism to divert lung ventilation away from areas of the lung that are not perfused, the nuclear medicine ventilation image demonstrates activity in the area of the nuclear medicine perfusion defect. A ventilation-perfusion (V/Q) mismatch is therefore present, and an increase in the alveolar-arterial gradient usually, but not always, results. The chest radiograph typically shows no lung infiltrates.

5. What disorders other than pulmonary embolism can produce V/Q mismatches on lung scans?

Although the most common cause of a V/Q mismatch on lung scan is pulmonary embolism, other disorders can produce a similar imaging pattern. Vasculitis in the pulmonary arterial circulation, for instance, can lead to in situ thrombosis that obstructs proximal pulmonary arteries, resulting in a V/Q mismatch. Anomalous pulmonary vessels that receive blood from the left-sided circulation (usually from branches of the aorta) can also result in a V/Q mismatch. In these conditions, pulmonary capillaries in lung regions perfused by the systemic arterial vessels do not receive radionuclide, which is injected into the systemic venous circulation. These lung regions consequently appear to have perfusion defects (absence of perfused radioactive particles) even though blood perfusion (albeit from systemic arteries) is present. Additionally, hypoplastic or atretic pulmonary arterial vessels have little pulmonary blood flow because of their small size and may not allow sufficient Tc-MAA or Tc-HAM to pass, resulting in a V/Q mismatch.

Mediastinal or hilar masses, such as neoplasms, may also generate a V/Q mismatch by extrinsically compressing pulmonary arteries without affecting the adjacent airways. Finally, any pathophysiologic process that causes pulmonary precapillary arteriovenous right-to-left shunting causes a V/Q mismatch because the injected Tc-MAA or Tc-HAM is shunted to the left-sided circulation before it can be trapped in the right-sided pulmonary capillary bed. Precapillary shunting can be present in pulmonary arterial hypertension, in severe lung disease of any cause, and within some lung neoplasms.

6. How does the presence of airway disease affect lung scan images?

Patients with acute asthmatic exacerbations, bronchiectasis, and bronchitis may have varying degrees of blockage in the proximal bronchial airways. Because airway ventilation is "end-bronchial," no well-developed collateral pulmonary airway channels exist. As a result of the proximal pulmonary bronchial blockage, there is no pulmonary ventilation to distal alveolar air spaces. This causes a ventilation defect on the nuclear medicine ventilation image that is typically peripheral, wedge shaped, and subsegmental or segmental in size, corresponding to the end-bronchial distribution of the obstructed airways. Because there is a physiologic mechanism that diverts lung perfusion away from areas of the lung that are not ventilated, in the area of the nuclear medicine ventilation defect the perfusion image demonstrates a corresponding perfusion defect that is peripheral, wedge shaped, and subsegmental to segmental in size. A V/Q match therefore results; the chest radiograph typically demonstrates no lung infiltrates.

7. What is the usual appearance of pneumonia on nuclear medicine lung scans?

Pneumonias fill alveoli and airways with inflammatory exudate, usually in a subsegmental or segmental pattern depending on the severity and extent of the infection. The resulting airway obstruction interferes with the bulk flow migration of the Tc-DPTA aerosol or the Xe gas into the distal pulmonary alveolar air spaces, causing a nuclear medicine ventilation defect corresponding to the region of air space consolidation. Because lung perfusion is diverted away from areas of the lung that are not ventilated, in these areas the nuclear medicine perfusion image demonstrates a corresponding peripheral, wedge shaped perfusion defect that is subsegmental to segmental in size. A V/Q match therefore results. The chest radiograph demonstrates a corresponding pulmonary infiltrate in the region of the V/Q match.

8. How does pulmonary embolism with infarction typically appear on nuclear medicine lung scans?

Patients who have an insufficient bronchial circulation to maintain blood flow to the lung interstitium because of large pulmonary emboli may sustain pulmonary ischemia or infarction. Resulting increases in membrane permeability and onset of vascular hemorrhage and tissue necrosis generate alveolar filling and pulmonary consolidation, which also occur in patients with pneumonia. A perfusion defect is caused by the pulmonary embolism and vascular obstruction. A ventilation defect is caused by the fluid in the airspace. A V/Q match consequently results. The chest radiograph shows a corresponding pulmonary infiltrate in the region of the V/Q matched defect.

Some patients with pulmonary embolism who experience lung ischemia or infarction may have a perfusion defect larger than the ventilation defect and the radiographic pulmonary infiltrate. This "penumbra" effect occurs when only the central portions of hypoperfused lung regions distal to an obstructing embolus are ischemic or infarcted. The larger region of hypoperfused lung appears as a perfusion defect and the more central region of ischemic or infarcted lung develops a smaller ventilation defect or pulmonary infiltrate.

9. What is the appearance of pleural effusions on nuclear medicine lung scans?

A pleural effusion of any cause typically produces a matched V/Q defect corresponding to the region of the effusion. This pattern develops because the pleural fluid overlying the lung blocks the detection of the emitted gamma rays. If the pleural effusion produces compressive atelectasis of the adjacent pulmonary parenchyma, a larger V/Q defect occurs that encompasses the region of effusion and atelectasis. This pattern is the result of a lung ventilation defect in the non-ventilated, atelectatic lung that does not receive the inhaled radionuclide. A corresponding perfusion defect develops in the same region because pulmonary blood flow is diverted away from the area of poor ventilation. The chest radiograph demonstrates the effusion and the adjacent lung atelectasis that correspond to the V/Q defect.

Pleural effusions caused by an underlying pulmonary embolus typically generate a perfusion defect associated with a smaller ventilation defect. The perfusion defect results from obstruction of the pulmonary vasculature by the pulmonary embolism. The smaller ventilation defect results from the shadowing effect of the pleural effusion that blocks the transmission of gamma rays from the underlying lung during the ventilation scan. Because the pleural effusion resulting from pulmonary embolism is typically smaller than the zone of hypoperfused lung, the perfusion defect is typically larger than the ventilation defect. Similarly, the perfusion defect is larger than the radiographically apparent pleural effusion or adjacent atelectatic lung when the effusion results from a pulmonary embolism.

10. Can pulmonary embolism appear as a V/Q match on lung scan?

Pulmonary embolism typically appears as V/Q mismatch, but matched defects can occur when lung ischemia or infarction develops or a pleural effusion is present. In these clinical settings, the perfusion defect may be larger than the ventilation defect and chest radiographic abnormality.

Other situations, however, may also be associated with V/Q matches in patients with pulmonary embolism. Experimental studies in canine models and clinical reports in humans indicate that temporary reflex bronchoconstriction lasting from minutes to hours may occur after pulmonary embolism without infarction. This bronchoconstriction may result from decreased carbon dioxide in the involved lung areas, loss of lung volume because of decreased or absent blood flow, local absorption of bronchial constrictive agents from the surface of clots and injured lung tissue, or atelectasis resulting from loss of pulmonary surfactant.

11. What is the basic nuclear medicine interpretation scheme for lung scans with respect to perfusion scans, ventilation scans, and chest radiographs?

Because pulmonary embolism can produce both lung scan V/Q mismatches and V/Q matches and nonpulmonary embolic disease can produce similar abnormalities, the nuclear medicine lung scan cannot absolutely determine the presence of pulmonary embolism. The lung scan interpretation involves assigning a percent probability of pulmonary embolism based upon the presence or absence of matched defects, the extent of mismatch defects if present, and the corresponding appearance of the chest radiograph (CXR). Since Biello published the first widely accepted interpretation scheme, various investigators have modified the basic algorithm, with the result that there are now many interpretation schemes and great confusion in lung scan interpretation.

A basic diagnostic scheme is presented below. The overall likelihood of pulmonary embolism is considered to be the highest probability of any of the described groupings that may be

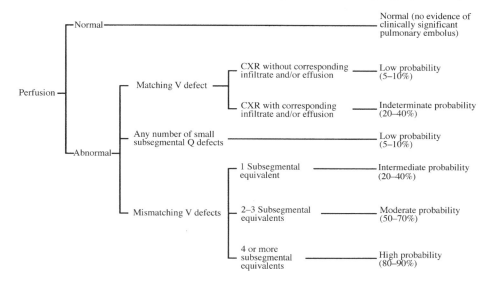

present. A *small subsegment* is less than 25% of a segment; a *subsegment* is 25–75% of a segment; a *segment* is more than 75% of a segment; 2 subsegments are equivalent to 1 segment.

12. Are nuclear medicine lung scans with V/Q defects at the location of a chest radiographic infiltrate or effusion always indeterminate probability?

No. Accumulating lung scan data indicate that in certain circumstances this indeterminate category can be subclassified as shown in this figure. CXR = chest radiograph. "Significantly" smaller or larger has never been defined precisely; as a rule of thumb, significantly is a size difference of 2 to 1.

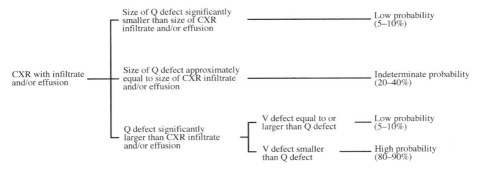

13. If there is lung consolidation-infiltrate or effusion on the chest radiograph and there is clinical suspicion of pulmonary embolism, should a lung scan be performed?

Yes. The presence of infiltrate or effusion on a chest radiograph does not predetermine that the lung scan will be indeterminate probability. The relative sizes of the corresponding perfusion defects and radiographic abnormalities may alter the indeterminate interpretation. (Please refer to question 24 for comparison of the relative sizes of perfusion defects, ventilation defects, and radiographic infiltrates and effusions.) Also, if there are V/Q mismatches in other areas of the lung, the likelihood of pulmonary embolism may be increased above the indeterminate probability range.

14. If interpretation of lung scans results in only a probability estimate, what is the value of this technique in the clinical evaluation of pulmonary embolism?

The Prospective Investigation of Pulmonary Embolism Diagnosis (PIOPED) concluded that "Clinical assessment combined with the ventilation/perfusion scan established the diagnosis or exclusion of pulmonary embolism only for a minority of patients—those with clear and concordant clinical and ventilation/perfusion scan findings."[11] That is, if the clinical assessment is a low pretest probability of pulmonary embolism and the lung scan interpretation is either normal or low probability, concordance exists and pulmonary embolism is extremely unlikely. Similarly, if the clinical assessment indicates a high pretest probability of pulmonary embolism and the lung scan interpretation is high probability, concordance exists and pulmonary embolism is extremely likely. All other permutations of pretest and test probabilities result in disconcordance, which requires a pulmonary angiogram to definitively exclude or prove pulmonary embolism.

The PIOPED data also demonstrated that abnormal lung scans have a high sensitivity (at least 98%) for detection of pulmonary embolism. A highly sensitive test is an ideal screening study for the presence of a disease. Several series that have followed patients with normal lung scans longitudinally have shown that a normal lung perfusion excludes the presence of clinically significant pulmonary embolism; other studies have shown that low probability scans are reliable relative to clinical outcomes.

15. If there are few cases of concordance and many cases of disconcordance in the PIOPED data, why not proceed immediately to pulmonary angiography?

The amount of concordance and disconcordance varies depending on the clinical thresholds for ordering a lung scan; that is, there is a greater concordance rate compared to the PIOPED data at institutions where there is a low threshold for ordering lung scans on low suspicion patients or a high threshold for ordering lung scans on high suspicion patients. The concordance and discordance rates are therefore institution specific.

A nuclear medicine study should always be performed because the lung scan is noninvasive and the radiosubstances that are used are not associated with any allergic or anaphylactoid reaction. Pulmonary angiography is an invasive procedure with risks related to intravascular catheter manipulations, passage of the intravascular catheter through the right-sided cardiac chambers, and intravascular contrast reactions. Because the nuclear medicine lung scan is a highly sensitive screening test for detection of pulmonary embolic disease, finding a normal perfusion scan essentially excludes clinically significant pulmonary embolism in most clinical settings. Also, lung scan results that are concordant with the clinical impression eliminate the need for further diagnostic evaluations. Finally, identifying the location of one or more perfusion defects can guide the radiologist in performing the pulmonary angiogram.

16. Under what circumstances is a lung ventilation scan not performed?

The lung ventilation scan is a closed system and there must not be any air leak from the nose, the mouthpiece, or the tracheostomy site in patients with an artificial airway. If a patient is unwilling or unable to cooperate, significant contamination of the scanning room, the gamma camera, and the nuclear medicine technologist can easily result. If contamination occurs, the entire scanning room cannot be used for any nuclear medicine study until the room is cleared of radioactivity. Ventilation scans, therefore, cannot be performed on all patients. A patient on a ventilator or a patient with a tracheostomy tube can undergo a ventilation scan if the trachea around the airway tube can be sealed, such as with an inflatable cuff.

17. If a lung ventilation scan is not done, how is interpretation of an abnormal perfusion scan affected?

If a ventilation scan cannot be performed, the specificity of the perfusion scan decreases markedly because it is impossible to determine if observed perfusion defects are matched or mismatched. In this setting, only a range of diagnostic probabilities can be provided to the clinician. If a ventilation scan is not done, it is more likely that a pulmonary angiogram will be necessary.

A lung perfusion scan should be performed even if a ventilation scan is not possible because a normal perfusion scan excludes clinically significant pulmonary embolism. On an abnormal perfusion scan, the location of the perfusion defect(s) guides the selection of pulmonary vasculature for angiographic evaluation. Alternatively, other studies such as lower extremity Doppler ultrasound or lower extremity impedance plethysmography can be performed for evaluation of possible deep venous thrombosis.

18. Can portable nuclear medicine perfusion and ventilation scans be performed at the patient's bedside?

According to the Standards for Radiation Protection of the Nuclear Regulatory Commission (NRC), there are no regulations forbidding the use of perfusion radiosubstance administration and scanning at the bedside as long as the radiation exposure is kept within the limits allowed for an unrestricted area (defined as an area wherein access is not limited or controlled by the radionuclide licensee). Because usually no room radiation contamination results from the use of liquid injectable radiosubstances, lung perfusion studies can be performed portable at the patient's bedside.

However, NRC regulations related to ethereal and diffusible radiosubstances make the performance of the aerosol Tc-DPTA or the gas Xe ventilation scan at the patient's bedside extremely complicated and impractical.

19. Are portable lung perfusion scans equal in quality and diagnostic value to lung perfusion scans obtained in the nuclear medicine department?

No. Portable cameras have several disadvantages compared with stationary cameras. Because the portable gamma cameras are smaller so as to be mobile, the field of view is typically significantly smaller compared with that of stationary cameras. Therefore, it is not always possible to include the entire lung in a single image obtained with portable equipment. Also, although portable cameras are mobile, they are bulky (they are much larger than the typical portable radiography equipment, for instance), making proper placement by the patient's bedside difficult. In addition, the number of projection angle images that can be obtained from a patient who is confined to bed may be limited because of the radioattenuation of the mattress and the bed paraphernalia.

20. What are the risks of radiation exposure from nuclear medicine lung scans to the patient and to the clinical personnel caring for the patient?

After a nuclear medicine lung scan, patients are radioactive until the intravenously administered or inhaled radiosubstances either decay or are eliminated from the body. For all diagnostic nuclear medicine studies the amount of radiation exposure due to the patient's being radioactive is well below the limits set by the NRC for an unrestricted area. Patient sequestration, posting of warning signs, and controlling access to a patient's room are required only when radionuclides are administered therapeutically, e.g., for thyroid gland ablation or treatment of thyroid cancer.

The typical whole body radiation dose to the patient is less than 10 millirems (mrem) for lung perfusion scans, less than 50 mrem for lung Tc-DPTA aerosol ventilation scans, and less than 10 mrem for lung Xe gas ventilation scans. In comparison, the average yearly background radiation exposure to an individual in the United States averages approximately 300 mrem. The typical dose for a standard frontal and lateral chest radiograph approximates 12 mrem to the lungs; for a standard upright and supine abdominal radiograph, it approximates 50 mrem to the trunk tissues. There have been no direct statistically confirmed effects of radiation exposure in adults at doses less than 20 rems, and the unborn fetus (which is more radiosensitive than the adult) at doses less than 1 to 5 rems. Even though there are no regulations limiting the total amount of radiation a patient can receive from medical diagnostic imaging studies, no patient should be exposed to ionizing medical imaging radiation if not medically indicated because the long-term effects of low levels of radiation are not known.

The radiation dose delivered to a health care worker who cares for a patient undergoing a radionuclide study is much less than the total dose received by the patient because the worker spends only limited time around the patient, is physically distant from the patient, and may attend the patient after the radionuclide has already undergone some interval decay.

CONTROVERSIES

21. Which agent produces better ventilation scans, Xe gas or Tc-DPTA aerosol?

Because of the physical characteristics of Xe gas, when it is used the ventilation study traditionally has been performed before the perfusion study and only one projection angle of the ventilation study can be obtained. The posterior projection is usually obtained because this angle allows the most lung segments to be visualized compared with other views. Therefore, the interpretation of V/Q matches and V/Q mismatches can be problematic, especially if a perfusion defect is located anteriorly in the lungs. Because of the physical characteristics of Tc-DPTA aerosols, ventilation scans with this radiosubstance can be performed either before or after lung perfusion scans. Furthermore, all perfusion projection angles can be obtained so that matches and mismatches can be evaluated directly, projection by projection. Unfortunately, aerosols tend to produce "hot spot" artifacts in the airways, especially in patients with airway disease, that can make interpretation difficult. The choice of radiosubstance is subjective. Some believe that the use of Xe gas versus Tc-DPTA aerosol ventilation scans in different studies has contributed to the inconsistencies reported among different interpretation schemes.

22. What are appropriate interpretation categories for describing the probability of pulmonary embolism?

The original Biello interpretation scheme employed 4 categories: normal (0% probability of pulmonary emboli), low (5–10%), intermediate-indeterminate (20–40%), and high (80–90%).

Some believe that there is sufficient statistical evidence to classify the likelihood of pulmonary embolism into 5 categories: normal (0%), low (5–10%), intermediate-indeterminate (20–40%), moderate (50–70%), and high (80–90%). It is generally agreed that the more mismatch lung equivalents that are present, the greater the likelihood of pulmonary embolism. It is debated whether there is clinical utility in describing separate "intermediate-indeterminate" and "moderate" categories; that is, because the likeihood of pulmonary embolism is neither sufficiently low nor sufficiently high to confidently rule in or rule out pulmonary embolism in both of these categories, there may be no clinical usefulness for describing an additional probability category of "moderate." (See the chapter on thromboembolic disease for a discussion of this point.)

23. Do lung scan interpretations of low probability really represent at most a 5–10% chance of pulmonary embolism?

A large amount of clinical data and published reports indicate that a low probability interpretation makes pulmonary embolism unlikely. A Canadian center, however, has consistently reported studies in which a high probability interpretation makes pulmonary embolism likely, but a low probability interpretation does not make pulmonary embolism unlikely. In these series the overall likelihood of pulmonary embolism is reported to be 25 to 40% using standard low probability matched V/Q scan appearance parameters. The recently revised and tested PIOPED data interpretation has also raised the possibility that matched defects, especially if solitary, have a greater chance of pulmonary embolism than those generally considered as "low" probability; low probability in revised PIOPED is between 0 and 20% likelihood of pulmonary embolism.

24. Should a ventilation scan be performed in areas of perfusion defects corresponding to radiographic consolidation-infiltrates or effusions in an attempt to subclassify the indeterminate category?

Virtually all published reports have used the relative size of the perfusion defect compared with the chest radiographic abnormality as a criterion for further interpretative subclassification. Biello believed that a ventilation scan was useful only if the perfusion defect was significantly larger than the chest radiographic abnormality. It is logical, based upon known respiratory pathophysiology, that comparison of the size of the ventilation defect with the size of the perfusion defect in an area of radiographic consolidation or effusion should be as accurate or more accurate than comparison of the relative sizes of the perfusion defect and radiographic abnormality—that is, the ventilation scan is more accurate than the chest x-ray for assessing ventilation abnormalities. Therefore, some centers routinely perform ventilation scans on all patients with perfusion defects and corresponding chest x-ray abnormalities, and compare the relative sizes of the perfusion and ventilation defects in the area of chest x-ray abnormality to determine the likelihood of pulmonary embolism. Such a method, although it is logical and reasonable and is being used at several institutions, has never been validated in the published literature.

25. What is the significance of small subsegmental perfusion defects if they are mismatched?

The significance of small subsegmental perfusion defects is being debated. Some believe that any mismatch regardless of size—especially in young patients or in patients without underlying lung disease—is significant and should not be reported as low probability. These investigators argue that insufficient data exist to predict the absence of thromboemboli because most of these patients do not undergo pulmonary angiography with subselective pulmonary artery contrast injection and spot magnified peripheral images. Such techniques are considered necessary to visualize these small emboli during angiography. Others believe that small subsegmental V/Q mismatches may indeed represent small emboli, but they do not affect the clinical course of patients because such small clots undergo rapid lysis and do not require anticoagulant therapy. It is generally thought that small pulmonary emboli occur intermittently physiologically and are of no clinical significance. If this conclusion is correct, there must be a pulmonary embolism threshold size that determines clinical symptoms and relevance.

26. Should the evaluation of pulmonary embolism be limited to clinical assessment, nuclear medicine lung scan, and pulmonary angiography?

Some take the point of view that pulmonary thromboembolism is merely the pulmonary manifestation of deep venous thromboembolism. Therefore, other diagnostic imaging tests such as bilateral lower extremity Doppler ultrasound and bilateral lower extremity serial impedance plethysmography should be useful. The literature has diagnostic work-up schemes that utilize additional modalities to improve diagnostic accuracy, especially when the lung scan is intermediate-indeterminate or no ventilation scan can be performed. Contrast venography and nuclear medicine fibrinogen studies have also been utilized in the past. The best and most accurate diagnostic work-up scheme has yet to be established.

BIBLIOGRAPHY

1. Biello D: Radiological (scintigraphic) evaluation of patients with suspected pulmonary thromboembolism. JAMA 257:3257–3259, 1987.
2. Biello D, Mattar A, Osei-Wusu A, et al: Interpretation of indeterminate lung scintigrams. Radiology 133:189–194, 1979.
3. Gottschalk A, Sostman H, Coleman R, et al: Ventilation-perfusion scintigraphy in the PIOPED study. Part II. Evaluation of the scintigraphic criteria and interpretations. J Nucl Med 34:1119–1126, 1993.
4. Hull R, Raskob G: Low probability lung scan findings: A need for change. Ann Intern Med 114:142–143, 1991.
5. Hull R, Raskob G, Ginsberg J, et al: A noninvasive strategy for the treatment of patients with suspected pulmonary embolism. Arch Intern Med 154:289–197, 1994.
6. Hull R, Raskob G, Coates G, et al: Clinical validity of a normal perfusion lung scan in patients with suspected pulmonary embolism. Chest 97:23–26, 1990.
7. Kotlyarov E, Reba R: The concept of using abnormal V/Q segment equivalents to refine the diagnosis of pulmonary embolism. Invest Radiol 15:383, 1981.
8. Mettler R, Guiberteau M: Essentials of Nuclear Medicine Imaging, 3rd ed. Philadelphia, W.B. Saunders, 1991.
9. Neuman R, Sostman H, Gottschalk A, et al: Current status of ventilation-perfusion imaging. Semin Nucl Med 10:198–217, 1980.
10. Palmer E, Scott J, Strauss H, et al: Practical Nuclear Medicine. Philadelphia, W.B. Saunders, 1992.
11. PIOPED Investigators: Value of the ventilation/perfusion scan in acute pulmonary embolism. Results of the prospective investigation of pulmonary embolism diagnosis (PIOPED). JAMA 263:2753–2759, 1990.
12. Smith R, Maher J, Miller R, et al: Clinical outcomes of patients with suspected pulmonary embolism and low probability aerosol-perfusion scintigrams. Radiology 164:731–733, 1987.
13. Sostman H, Coleman R, DeLong D, et al: Evaluation of revised criteria for ventilation-perfusion scintigraphy in patients with suspected pulmonary embolism. Radiology 193:103–107, 1994.
14. Strauss E, Sostman H, Gottschalk A, et al: Radiographic parenchymal opacity, matching perfusion defect, and normal ventilation: A sign of pulmonary embolism? Radiology 163:505–506, 1987.
15. Webber M, Gomes A, Roe D, et al: Comparison of Biello, McNeil, and PIOPED criteria for the diagnosis of pulmonary emboli on lung scans. Am J Roentgenol 154:975–981, 1990.

III. Laboratory Evaluation

7. ARTERIAL BLOOD GASES

Dean Hess, Ph.D., R.R.T.

1. What are arterial blood gases?

The term *arterial blood gases* refers to measurements of pH, Pco_2, and Po_2 in arterial blood. Measured values for hemoglobin saturation with oxygen (O_2Hb), carboxyhemoglobin (COHb), and methemoglobin (metHb) may be included. Many laboratories also report calculated values such as oxygen saturation, bicarbonate concentration, and base excess. Arterial blood gases reflect the condition of the blood leaving the pulmonary circulation. Thus, these measurements are the result of the ability of the lungs to oxygenate the blood (i.e., oxygenation) and to remove carbon dioxide (i.e., ventilation). The pH is determined by the ability of the lungs to remove carbon dioxide and the presence of fixed acids in the blood.

2. When is measurement of arterial blood gases indicated?

Arterial blood gas measurement is indicated to evaluate oxygenation, ventilation, and acid-base status. Typically, arterial blood gas values are obtained if the patient's clinical presentation suggests an abnormality in oxygenation, ventilation, or acid-base status. Arterial blood gas levels are also obtained to evaluate changes in therapy that might affect oxygenation, such as a change in the inspired oxygen concentration (FIO_2), applied level of positive end-expiratory pressure (PEEP), airway pressure, ventilation (ventilator rate change, tidal volume change), or acid-base balance (sodium bicarbonate administration or acetazolamide therapy). Because of its high cost and invasive nature, arterial blood gas assessment should never be considered routine.

3. What are common complications of arterial puncture?

Arterial puncture for blood gases is relatively risk-free and commonly is performed by non-physicians (e.g., respiratory therapists). Complications of arterial puncture include:

Pain   Arteriospasm
Arterial trauma   Thrombus formation
Nerve damage   Infection
Bleeding with hematoma formation

4. How can the complications of arterial puncture be avoided?

Although arterial blood may be obtained from several arteries (e.g., radial, brachial, femoral, axillary, ulnar, dorsalis pedis, temporal), the risk of complications is decreased when the radial artery is used. The radial artery is usually chosen for several reasons:

- Collateral blood flow to the hand occurs through the ulnar artery; thus, damage to the radial artery should not compromise blood flow to the hand, which is commonly assessed using the modified Allen's test.
- Unlike the brachial artery, the radial artery is far enough away from nerves (e.g, medial nerve) that damage to the nerve is unlikely.
- The radial site is generally more aseptic than the femoral site.
- The radial artery is often near the surface so it is easy to palpate, and pain from the puncture is lessened.

The risk of bleeding complications is increased in patients receiving anticoagulant therapy or thrombolytic therapy and in those with coagulopathy. If any of these risks are present, pressure must be manually applied to the puncture site until all signs of bleeding are absent (minimum of 5–10 minutes). The risk of pain and injury is decreased by use of a 22- or 23-gauge needle and performance of the procedure only by individuals with the requisite training and skill.

Infection is an issue of concern. The risk of infection is as important to the clinician performing the puncture as to the patient undergoing the procedure; thus, appropriate precautions must be observed during the collection of arterial blood.

5. When is an arterial catheter indicated?

There are two principal indications for an arterial catheter: (1) continuous monitoring of arterial blood pressure in hemodynamically unstable patients and (2) the need for frequent arterial blood gas samples or other laboratory assessment (e.g., blood chemistry, hematologic studies). Although arterial catheters are inserted in virtually every critically ill patient in some hospitals, this practice is unwarranted and has been shown to increase the number of laboratory tests obtained. These unnecessary laboratory tests increase the cost of providing care and may result in serious blood loss requiring transfusion.

6. Describe the complications associated with arterial catheters.

Complications associated with arterial catheters are rare. Serious complications include hemorrhage, vascular occlusion, and infection. Thrombus formation is avoided by use of a continuous irrigation system. Although irrigation fluid traditionally contained a dilute heparin solution, it has been shown that continuous irrigation is the important feature and heparin may not be necessary. When blood is collected from arterial catheters, the irrigation solution must be cleared from the connected tubing so that it does not contaminate the sample obtained for blood gas analysis. This can cause considerable blood loss if samples are collected frequently. Blood conservation kits are available commercially to minimize this blood loss.

7. Why are arterial blood gas samples transported on ice?

Blood is living tissue and metabolism by blood cells continues in the syringe while the sample is transported to the laboratory. As a result, Po_2 in the blood sample decreases, Pco_2 increases, and pH decreases. This effect, which results in a preanalytic error (i.e., an error due to collection and transport of the sample), can be diminished by transport and storage of the sample in ice-water slush before analysis. As a practical rule, arterial samples do not need to be iced if the sample is analyzed within 10 minutes. Prompt analysis is important because it not only reduces errors resulting from metabolic effects within the sample but also provides rapid report of results to the bedside. Delay in reporting of arterial blood gas results may have life or death consequences.

The metabolic effects on the blood sample are caused primarily by the activity of leuckocytes. In patients who are leukemic (leukocytosis > 100,000 cells/μl), the Pao_2 of the blood sample may decrease very quickly. This effect, called *leukocyte larceny*, results in a measured Pao_2 much lower than the Pao_2 that actually exists in the patient. Leukocyte larceny should be expected in patients with leukocytosis. In such patients, the arterial blood sample must be placed in ice water and analyzed immediately. It may be impossible to accurately determine the Pao_2 of patients in extreme leukocytosis, and in vivo methods (e.g., pulse oximetry) may be more reliable than arterial blood gas levels in such patients.

8. How should an arterial blood gas sample be handled if it cannot be analyzed promptly?

If the sample must be stored for a long time before analysis (e.g., more than 30 minutes), a glass rather than plastic syringe should be used. The solubility of oxygen (and carbon dioxide) is increased in ice water. With plastic syringes (unlike glass syringes), this may result in greater amounts of oxygen dissolved in the blood sample because oxygen diffuses from the ice water, across the plastic, and into the sample. When the sample is warmed to 37° C in the blood gas analyzer, oxygen comes out of solution and increases the P_{O_2} of the sample. The result is that the measured PaO_2 level is higher than the PaO_2 level in the sample originally collected from the patient.

9. Why is heparin used in blood gas syringes?

Coagulation of the blood sample must be avoided because clots interfere with the function of the blood gas analyzer. Traditionally, liquid sodium heparin was used to prevent clotting in the syringe. However, dry lyophilized lithium heparin is now used so that electrolyte measurements can be performed using the blood gas sample (if desired). Dry heparin furthermore reduces the risk of preanalytic errors caused by dilution of the sample with the volume of liquid form of heparin.

10. Can too much or too little heparin affect results of blood gas measurement?

The P_{O_2} and P_{CO_2} of liquid heparin are virtually the same as the P_{O_2} and P_{CO_2} of ambient air (about 150 mmHg and 0 mmHg, respectively, at sea level). The measured P_{O_2} and P_{CO_2} of a blood sample are, therefore, altered when liquid heparin dilutes blood in the blood gas syringe. Heparin dilution causes the measured P_{CO_2} of the sample to decrease and the P_{O_2} of the sample to move toward 150 mmHg (i.e, the measured P_{O_2} increases if the true value is less than 150 mmHg and decreases if the true value is more than 150 mmHg). High concentrations of heparin are acidic (pH less than 7) and lower the pH of the sample; however, diluted concentrations of heparin (1,000 units/ml) prevent coagulation of the specimen and have a pH similar to that of normal blood. If liquid heparin is used, its effects can be minimized by using only enough to fill the dead volume of the needle and syringe; this small volume is adequate to prevent clot formation in the sample.

11. Why must arterial blood gas samples be obtained anaerobically?

Perhaps the most common preanalytic error related to blood gases is contamination of the sample with room air. At sea level, air has a P_{O_2} of about 150 mmHg and a P_{CO_2} of about 0 mmHg. Thus, if the sample is contaminated with air, the measured P_{O_2} of the sample increases if the true value is less than 150 mmHg and decreases if the true value is more than 150 mmHg. Contamination of the sample with air lowers the P_{CO_2} of the sample, with a resultant increase in pH. Blood gas samples must be collected, transported, and analyzed using anaerobic methods; any air bubbles that accidentally enter the sample must be removed immediately.

12. Can the PaO_2 normally be less than 75 mmHg or more than 100 mmHg?

The PaO_2 can never be greater than the partial pressure of oxygen that exists in the alveolar space (alveolar P_{O_2}, abbreviated PAO_2). In normal healthy individuals breathing ambient air, the PaO_2 is about about 5–10 mmHg less than the PAO_2. This difference represents the alveolar to arterial (A-a) gradient. The modified alveolar gas equation can calculate the PAO_2:

$$PAO_2 = (EBP \cdot FIO_2) - (1.25 \cdot PaCO_2)$$

where EBP is the effective barometric pressure. Effective barometric pressure is the difference between barometric pressure and water vapor pressure at body temperature (47 mmHg at 37° C). Taking the example of an individual breathing room air ($FIO_2 = 0.21$) at sea level (barometric pressure = 760 mmHg) who has a normal $PaCO_2$ (40 mmHg), the PAO_2 is approximately 100 mmHg. Considering the normal A-a gradient of 5–10 mmHg, the measured PaO_2 would be 90–95 mmHg.

The alveolar gas equation predicts that the PAO_2 will be less than 100 mmHg if the barometric pressure is less than 760 mmHg. Thus, the normal PaO_2 is lower at higher altitudes. For example, the PaO_2 is about 75 mmHg at an altitude at which ambient barometric pressure is 650 mmHg. On the other hand, PAO_2 will be more than 100 mmHg with hyperbaric conditions, which is the therapeutic goal when patients are treated with hyperbaric oxygen. PAO_2 also increases with an increase in FIO_2. The alveolar gas equation predicts that the PAO_2 will be about 675 mmHg when

100% oxygen is breathed at sea level; thus, the Pa_{O_2} is normally more than 600 mmHg at these conditions.

13. What is the highest possible Pa_{O_2} for a normal person breathing 50% oxygen at sea level and what is the highest possible Pa_{O_2} for a normal person breathing room at an ambient pressure of 500 mmHg?

The highest possible Pa_{O_2} for a normal person breathing 50% oxygen at sea level is:

$$P_{A_{O_2}} = (713 \cdot 0.50) - (1.25 \cdot 40) = 300 \text{ mmHg}$$

In actual fact, the A-a gradient increases physiologically with increasing $F_{I_{O_2}}$, so the measured Pa_{O_2} in a person breathing 50% oxygen at sea level would be considerably less than the Pa_{O_2} of 300 mmHg.

Taking another example, the highest possible Pa_{O_2} for a normal person breathing room air at an ambient pressure of 500 mmHg (EBP = 453 mmHg) is:

$$P_{A_{O_2}} = (453 \cdot 0.21) - (1.25 \cdot 40) = 45 \text{ mmHg}$$

14. How much time should be allowed after an $F_{I_{O_2}}$ change before assessment of arterial blood gas levels?

This important clinical issue relates to the amount of time required to establish a new steady state after a change in the level of oxygen or ventilatory support. If too little time is allowed, the blood gas results will not reflect the new clinical conditions; too much time, however, could subject the patient to a long period of potentially harmful blood gas levels. The time required to reach steady state after an $F_{I_{O_2}}$ change depends on the alveolar ventilation and the functional residual capacity; lower alveolar ventilation or larger functional residual capacity requires a longer time for equilibration. Unless the patient has obstructive lung disease (which results in lower alveolar ventilation and larger functional residual capacity), 5 minutes is usually an adequate time to reach a new steady state after a change in $F_{I_{O_2}}$. For patients with obstructive lung disease, 30 minutes should be allowed to reach a new steady state after a change in $F_{I_{O_2}}$.

It is also important to know how long to wait before assessment of blood gas levels after a change in PEEP or minute ventilation. About 15 minutes is required to reach a steady state after a PEEP change, but recommendations for wait time after a change in minute ventilation are difficult to predict. For full ventilatory support, a new steady state may be reached quickly (in less than 10 minutes). However, this may not be the case when the level of ventilatory support is changed during weaning from mechanical ventilation. During weaning, changes in blood gases occur late with respiratory muscle fatigue, and clinical signs (e.g., tachypnea, use of accessory muscles, thoracoabdominal dys-synchrony) may occur earlier than hypercapnia.

15. Are blood gas levels stable in critically ill patients or are they variable in apparently stable patients?

Arterial blood gas levels may vary considerably over brief 5- to 10-minute intervals in critically ill mechanically ventilated patients who otherwise appear stable. Different measured values may reflect physiologic alterations, such as subtle changes in cardiopulmonary function or patient repositionings that alter distribution of blood flow to the lungs, or they may result from preanalytic error. Variability is greatest for Pa_{O_2} and less for Pa_{CO_2} and pH. It is important not to react too strongly to a single blood gas result that differs from previous results in an otherwise clinically stable patient. This may lead to needless ventilator adjustments for blood gas changes that reflect variability of the measurement rather than changes in the clinical status of the patient.

16. Why can't venous blood gases be used instead of arterial blood gases?

Arterial blood gases reflect lung function. Venous blood gases reflect the adequacy of tissue oxygenation and tissue carbon dioxide clearance. It is generally accepted that a low mixed venous P_{O_2} (less than 35 mmHg) reflects tissue hypoxia and may be the result of decreased oxygen delivery or increased tissue oxygen uptake. Venous P_{O_2} is typically much lower than arterial P_{O_2}, and there is often little relationship between the two. For example, the mixed venous P_{O_2} may be low and the arterial P_{O_2} may be high if cardiac output is reduced, lung function is normal, and $F_{I_{O_2}}$ is high. Normally, the mixed venous P_{CO_2} is only slightly greater than the arterial P_{CO_2}. However, venous P_{CO_2} depends on blood flow, and in cases of low blood flow (e.g., cardiac arrest), the mixed venous P_{CO_2} may be very high even though the arterial P_{CO_2} may be normal or even decreased. Because arterial and mixed venous blood gases are determined by different physiologic mechanisms, inferences about one cannot be made from the other.

17. List the causes of hypoxemia.

Hypoxemia is defined by a Pa_{O_2} of less than 80 mmHg in a person breathing room air at sea level. There are five general causes of hypoxemia. Two causes of hypoxemia are predicted from the alveolar gas equation—decreased inspired P_{O_2} (e.g., altitude) and increased P_{CO_2} (e.g., hypoventilation). The other three causes of hypoxemia are the result of lung disease—shunt, ventilation-perfusion ($\dot{V}/\dot{Q}$) mismatch, and diffusion defect. Shunt is a common cause of hypoxemia in critically ill patients and its origin may be pulmonary (e.g., atelectiasis, pneumonia, ARDS, congestive heart failure) or cardiac (e.g., patent foramen ovale). $\dot{V}/\dot{Q}$ mismatch, which results from poor distribution of ventilation relative to blood flow, produces hypoxemia with airway diseases such as emphysema, chronic bronchitis, cystic fibrosis, and asthma. Diffusion defect is less important clinically and may produce hypoxemia with a reduced Pa_{O_2} only during exercise.

Clinical Causes of Hypoxemia

CAUSE	UNDERLYING PROBLEM
Decreased inspired oxygen	Altitude
Hypoventilation	Respiratory center depression, neuromuscular disease
Shunt	Atelectasis, pneumonia, pulmonary edema, ARDS
$\dot{V}/\dot{Q}$ mismatch, poor distribution of ventilation	Airway secretions, bronchospasm
Diffusion defect	Pulmonary fibrosis, emphysema, pulmonary resection

18. How does hypoxia differ from hypoxemia?

Hypoxemia refers to decreased delivery of oxygen from the atmosphere to the blood, and *hypoxia* refers to decreased delivery of oxygen to the tissues. It is important to recognize that hypoxemia may occur without hypoxia and vice versa. There are five general causes of hypoxia.

Clinical Causes of Hypoxia

CAUSE	UNDERLYING PROBLEM
Hypoxemic hypoxia	A lower than normal Pa_{O_2} (hypoxemia)
Anemic hypoxia	Decreased red blood cell count, carboxyhemoglobin, hemoglobinopathy
Circulatory hypoxia	Decreased cardiac output, decreased local perfusion
Affinity hypoxia	Decreased release of oxygen from hemoglobin to the tissues
Histotoxic hypoxia	Cyanide poisoning

19. What determines hemoglobin oxygen saturation and how is it affected by carboxyhemoglobin and methemoglobin?

The saturation of hemoglobin is determined by the oxyhemoglobin dissociation curve, for which oxygen saturation is a function of P_{O_2}. The affinity of hemoglobin for oxygen is high at high saturations (more than 90%, P_{O_2} more than 60 mmHg) and less at lower saturations.

This effect facilitates oxygen loading in the lungs (where the P_{O_2} is high) and oxygen unloading to the tissues (where the P_{O_2} is low). The position of the oxyhemoglobin dissociation curve is not fixed. Factors that shift the curve to the left increase the affinity of hemoglobin for oxygen, and factors that shift the curve to the right decrease the affinity of hemoglobin for oxygen.

Saturation of hemoglobin is also affected by conditions such as COHb and metHb. Carbon monoxide attaches to oxygen binding sites of hemoglobin with a high affinity and decreases the ability of hemoglobin to carry oxygen. Thus, the hemoglobin oxygen saturation cannot be greater than 70% if the COHb level is 30%. Methemoglobin is produced when the iron in the hemoglobin molecule is converted from its reduced state (Fe^{++}) to its oxidized state (Fe^{+++}). Hemoglobin can carry oxygen only if the iron is in the reduced state. Thus, metHb decreases the ability of hemoglobin to transport oxygen.

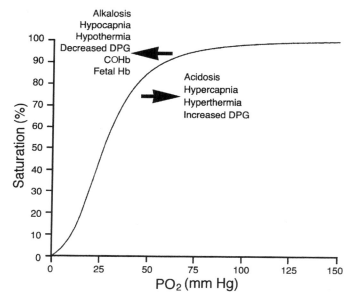

Normal oxyhemoglobin dissociation curve.

20. How is oxygen saturation measured?

Oxygen saturation is measured by CO-oximetry. The CO-oximeter measures oxygen saturation by a light absorption method. Multiple wavelength CO-oximetry can measure COHb (i.e., carbon monoxide saturation) and metHb in addition to oxyhemoglobin (i.e., oxygen saturation).

21. Why might a patient have a high Pa_{O_2} (e.g., 150 mmHg) but a low oxygen saturation (e.g., 60%)?

From the oxyhemoglobin dissociation curve, one would predict that the oxygen saturation should be nearly 100% when the Pa_{O_2} is 150 mmHg. The explanation for a low saturation with a high Pa_{O_2} is that something has decreased the ability of hemoglobin to bind oxygen. A reasonable explanation for this is the presence of COHb or metHb. This possibility should be investigated by history, physical examination, and assay for the presence of COHb or metHb using CO-oximetry. Pulse oximetry is not appropriate for this evaluation. Because pulse oximeters use only two wavelengths of light, they are unable to adequately differentiate oxyhemoglobin, COHb, and metHb.

22. What is the Henderson-Hasselbalch equation?

The Henderson-Hasselbalch equation describes the relationship between pH, HCO_3^-, and P_{CO_2}:

$$pH = 6.1 + \log \frac{[HCO_3^-]}{(0.03 \cdot P_{CO_2})}$$

23. What is the difference between a respiratory acid-base disturbance and a metabolic acid-base disturbance?

Changes in pH resulting from changes in HCO_3^- are called **metabolic acid-base disorders** and changes in pH resulting from changes in P_{CO_2} are called **respiratory acid-base disorders**. An increase in pH caused by an increase in HCO_3^- is a metabolic alkalosis and an increase in pH caused by a decrease in P_{CO_2} is a respiratory alkalosis. A decrease in pH caused by a decrease in HCO_3^- is a metabolic acidosis and a decrease in pH caused by an increase in P_{CO_2} is a respiratory acidosis.

24. What is a compensated acid-base disturbance?

Whenever the ratio HCO_3^- to $(0.03 \cdot P_{CO_2})$ is 20 to 1, the pH is normal (7.40). A compensated respiratory acid-base disorder occurs when a physiologic change in HCO_3^- occurs secondary to a P_{CO_2} change so that the HCO_3^- to $(0.03 \cdot P_{CO_2})$ is 20 to 1 and thus the pH is normal. Likewise, a physiologic change in P_{CO_2} may occur secondary to an HCO_3^- disorder so that the HCO_3^- to $(0.03 \cdot P_{CO_2})$ is 20 to 1 and thus the pH is normal (i.e., respiratory compensation for a metabolic disturbance).

25. List common acid-base disturbances.

	pH	*HCO₃⁻*	*Paco₂*
Respiratory acidosis			
Uncompensated	↓	nl	↑
Partially compensated	↓	↑	↑
Fully compensated	nl	↑	↑
Respiratory alkalosis			
Uncompensated	↑	nl	↓
Partially compensated	↑	↓	↓
Fully compensated	nl	↓	↓
Metabolic acidosis			
Uncompensated	↓	↓	nl
Partially compensated	↓	↓	↓
Fully compensated	nl	↓	↓
Metabolic alkalosis			
Uncompensated	↑	↑	nl
Partially compensated	↑	↑	↑
Fully compensated	nl	↑	↑

↓ = decreased; ↑ = increased; nl = normal.

26. Describe the acid-base disorder associated with pH = 7.54, Paco₂ = 55 mmHg, and HCO₃⁻ = 15 mmol/l.

According to the Henderson-Hasselbalch equation, it is impossible for the pH to be increased (more than 7.40) if the $Paco_2$ is increased (more than 40 mmHg) and the HCO_3^- is decreased (less than 24 mmol/l). Therefore, there must be a laboratory or transcription error; the pH, the $Paco_2$, or the HCO_3^- is incorrect. It is impossible to know which is wrong without examining the patient and repeating the blood gas analysis.

27. What are common causes of acid-base disturbances?

Clinical Causes of Common Acid-Base Disturbances

Respiratory acidosis (hypoventilation)
   Respiratory center depression: pathologic, iatrogenic
   Disruption of neural pathways affecting respiratory muscles: neuropathy, trauma
   Neuromuscular blockade: disease, paralyzing agents
   Respiratory muscle weakness: fatigue, disease

Respiratory alkalosis (hyperventilation)
   Respiratory center stimulation: hypoxia, anxiety, central nervous system pathology
   Iatrogenic: excessive mechanical ventilation

Metabolic acidosis
   Lactic acidosis (e.g., hypoxia)
   Ketoacidosis (e.g., uncontrolled diabetes)
   Uremic acidosis (e.g., renal failure)
   Loss of base from lower gastrointestinal tract (e.g., diarrhea)
   Loss of base from kidneys (e.g., acetazolamide, renal tubular acidosis)
   Poisons (e.g., methanol, ethylene glycol, aspirin)

Metabolic alkalosis
   Hypokalemia
   Loss of acid from upper gastrointestinal tract (e.g., vomiting or gastric suction)
   Bicarbonate administration

---

28. How is the anion gap useful to explain acid-base disturbances?

The anion gap is useful to differentiate causes of metabolic acidosis. Metabolic acidosis can be associated with a normal anion gap (hyperchloremic acidosis) or with an increased anion gap (normochloremic acidosis). The anion gap is calculated as:

$$\text{anion gap} = [Na^+] - ([Cl^-] + [HCO_3^-])$$

A normal anion gap is 8–12 mmol/l. Causes of metabolic acidosis with an increased anion gap include lactic acidosis, diabetic ketoacidosis, and azotemic (renal) acidosis. Causes of metabolic acidosis with a normal anion gap include loss of bicarbonate from the gastrointestinal tract (e.g., diarrhea), acetazolamine therapy, renal tubular acidosis, or excessive chloride administration (e.g., volume expansion with normal saline, HCl, NH_4Cl).

CONTROVERSIES

29. Should calculated values for SaO_2 and HCO_3^- be reported with arterial blood gas results?

Oxygen saturation (SaO_2) can be calculated from PaO_2 and pH, a function commonly available on blood gas analyzers. However, the calculated SaO_2 may differ considerably from the measured SaO_2. The calculated SaO_2 considers only the effects of PO_2 and pH and disregards other physiologic effects on the oxyhemoglobin dissociation curve. The calculated SaO_2 also does not consider the effects of COHb and metHb, resulting in an overestimation of SaO_2 when these are present. If significant levels of COHb or metHb are present, one might argue that the calculated SaO_2 is not only incorrect but also misguides appropriate clinical management.

The metabolic component of acid-base interpretation is usually given as the HCO_3^-. The HCO_3^- is usually calculated from measured $PaCO_2$ and pH using the Henderson-Hasselbalch equation. The pK in the Henderson-Hasselbalch equation is assumed to be 6.1, which might not be accurate in critically ill patients. This assumption thus introduces errors into the HCO_3^- calculation. The metabolic component can also be expressed as base excess, which requires knowledge of the hemoglobin concentration. Because hemoglobin concentration is usually not measured at the time of blood gas analysis, an assumed value for hemoglobin is used to calculate base excess. This assumption introduces errors into the calculation. Although many clinicians use HCO_3^- or base excess to evaluate the metabolic component of acid-base balance, these calculations are often not precise because of the assumptions incorporated into their calculation.

30. Should arterial blood gas results be corrected to the patient's temperature?

Blood gases and pH are measured at 37° C (normal body temperature). If the patient's temperature is abnormal, the in vivo blood gas and pH values will differ from those measured and reported by the blood gas laboratory. Using empiric equations, the blood gas analyzer can adjust the measured values to the patient's body temperature. The use of temperature-adjusted values for blood gases and pH is controversial. Although normal values are known for euthermia, normal values during hypothermia and hyperthermia are unknown. The acid-base changes that occur with hypothermia and hyperthermia may be homeostatic. The treatment of acid-base disturbances should be guided by the unadjusted values (i.e., those measured at 37° C). However, temperature adjustment of blood gases and pH is useful to follow changes in these values with changes in body temperature. Temperature adjustment also allows the clinician to differentiate temperature-related changes from physiologic changes. Temperature adjusted values should also be used to compare blood gas levels with exhaled gas values (e.g., end-tidal PCO_2) and to calculate oxygen content indices (e.g., shunt arterial) or tension indices (e.g., Pao_2/PAo_2).

BIBLIOGRAPHY

1. AARC Clinical Practice Guideline: Sampling for arterial blood gas analysis. Respir Care 37:913–917, 1992.
2. Beasley KE, Darin JM, Durbin CG: The effect of respiratory care department management of a blood gas analyzer on the appropriateness of arterial blood gas utilization. Respir Care 37:343–347, 1992.
3. Browing JA, Kaiser DL, Durbin CG: The effect of guidelines on the appropriate use of arterial blood gas analysis in the intensive care unit. Respir Care 34:269–276, 1989.
4. Bruck E, Eichorn JH, Ray-Meredith S, et al: Percutaneous collection of arterial blood for laboratory analysis. National Committee for Clinical Laboratory Standards. H11A; 5:39–59, 1985.
5. Clifton GD, Branson P, Kelly JH, et al: Comparison of normal saline and heparin solutions for maintenance of arterial catheter patency. Heart Lung 20:115–118, 1991.
6. Dennis RC, Ng R, Yeston NS, et al: Effect of sample dilutions on arterial blood gas determinations. Crit Care Med 13:1067–1068, 1985.
7. Harrison RA: Acid-base balance. Respir Care Clin North Am 1:7–22, 1995.
8. Harten A, Berg B, Inerot S, Muth L: Importance of correct handling of samples for the result of blood gas analysis. Acta Anaesthesiol Scand 32:365–368, 1988.
9. Hess D, Agarwal NN: Variability of blood gases, pulse oximeter saturation, and end-tidal carbon dioxide pressure in stable, mechanically ventilated trauma patients. J Clin Monit 8:111–115, 1992.
10. Hess D, Elser R, Agarwal N: The effect of measured versus calculated hemoglobin oxygen saturation, carboxyhemoglobin, and methemoglobin on the pulmonary shunt calculation. Respir Care 29:1001–1005, 1984.
11. Hess D, Good C, Didyoung R, et al: The validity of assessing arterial blood gases 10 minutes after an FIO_2 change in mechanically ventilated patients without chronic pulmonary disease. Respir Care 30:1037–1041, 1985.
12. Hess D, Kacmarek RM: Techniques and devices for monitoring oxygenation. Respir Care 38:646–671, 1993.
13. Kozlowski-Templin R: Blood gas analyzers. Respir Care Clin North Am 1:35–46, 1995.
14. Mahoney JJ, Harvey JA,Wong RJ, et al: Changes in oxygen measurements when whole blood is stored in iced plastic or glass syringes. Clin Chem 37:1244–1248, 1991.
15. Mahoney JJ, Vreman HJ, Stevenson DK, et al: Measurement of carboxyhemoglobin and total hemoglobin by five specialized spectrophotometers (CO-oximeters) in comparison with reference methods. Clin Chem 39:1693–1700, 1993.
16. Malley WJ: Clinical Blood Gases: Application and Noninvasive Alternatives. Philadelphia, W.B. Saunders, 1990.
17. Mandgar D, Thrush DN, Connell GR, et al: Direct or modified Seldinger guide wire-directed technique for arterial catheter insertion. Anesth Analg 76:714–717, 1993.
18. Matthews PJ: CO-oximetry. Respir Care Clin North Am 1:47–68, 1995.
19. Peruzzi WT, Martin M: Oxygen transport. Respir Care Clin North Am 1:23–35, 1995.
20. Sasse SA, Chem PA, Mahutte CK: Variability of arterial blood gas values over time in stable medical ICU patients. Chest 106:187–193, 1994.
21. Shapiro BA: Temperature correction of blood gas values. Respir Care Clin North Am 1:69–76, 1995.

22. Shapiro BA,Kozolowski-Templin R, Peruzzi WT: Clinical Application of Blood Gases, 5th ed. Chicago,
    Mosby-Year Book, 1994.
23. Siggaard-Anderson O, Fogh-Andersen N, Gothgen IH, et al: Oxygen status of arterial and mixed venous
    blood. Crit Care Med 23:1284–1293, 1995.
24. Silver MJ, Yue-Han L, Gragg LA, et al: Reduction of blood loss from diagnostic sampling in critically ill
    patients using a blood-conserving arterial line system. Chest 104:1711–1715, 1993.
25. Weibley RE, Riggs CD: Evaluation of an improved sampling method for blood gas analysis from in-
    dwelling arterial catheters. Crit Care Med 17:803–805, 1989.

8. PULSE OXIMETRY

Philip L. Goodman, R.R.T., and Robert F. Wolken, B.S., R.R.T.

1. What is pulse oximetry?

Pulse oximetry is a noninvasive method of measuring oxygen saturation of hemoglobin in pulsating blood vessels.

2. How does pulse oximetry work?

A microprocessing unit is connected to a sensor probe containing light emitting diodes (LED) and a photodetector that is positioned directly opposite the LED. Light is transmitted at 660 nm (red) and 940 nm (infrared). The oxygen saturation is determined by comparing the amount of red light absorbed to the amount of infrared light absorbed by both deoxygenated hemoglobin (Hb) and oxyhemoglobin (HbO_2).

3. What is the Beer-Lambert law of absorption?

This law is a combination of Beer's law and Lambert's law. Beer's law states that the optical density of a homogeneous absorbing substance is directly proportional to the concentration of the absorbing substance. Lambert's law states that the optical density of a homogeneous medium is directly proportional to the thickness of the medium. Spectrophotometry is based on these two principles.

4. When was the first pulse oximeter introduced?

The first oximeter was built by Carl Mathes in 1935. Glen Milliken coined the term *oximeter* in 1942 to describe a lightweight device he developed for aviation research. The first pulse oximeter combining both spectrophotometry and plethysmography was developed by Takuo Aoyagi for the Nihon Kohden Corporation. Because of its sensitivity to motion and large size, it was not widely used. The first clinically accepted pulse oximeter was developed in the late 1970s by Scott Wilbur of Boulder, Colorado.

5. How accurate are pulse oximeters?

Most manufacturers report an accuracy of plus or minus 2% for saturations that are greater than 70%. The reported accuracy drops to plus or minus 3% for saturations between 50 and 70%. These claims can be somewhat misleading, as studies have shown that pulse oximetry values (SpO_2) fall within plus or minus 4–5% of CO-oximetry values (SaO_2) 95% of the time. Therefore, a pulse oximetry measurement of 90% may correspond to a CO-oximetry measured saturation of 85–95% in 95% of patients!

6. Are there differences among various pulse oximeter models?

There may be clinically significant differences among measurements made with pulse oximeters of different manufacturers because of different calibration curves, LED variances, and quality control factors. Differences may occur even among units from the same manufacturer as new software revisions are made. Such potential variability should be kept in mind in areas where different oximeters are available for use. Changes in SpO_2 measurements during intermittent use of different pulse oximeters may reflect variances between monitors and may not be representative of an actual change in the patient's condition.

7. Does nail polish affect pulse oximetry?

The effect of nail polish on the accuracy of pulse oximeters depends on its color. Polish that absorbs light at the oximeter's transmission wavelengths (660 nm and 940 nm) will alter the SpO_2 measurements. Both green and blue polish have increased absorbance at 660 nm, which produces a lower SpO_2 reading. Black nail polish has increased absorbance at both 660 and 940 nm and also causes a lower SpO_2 reading, but to a lesser extent than does green or blue. Red nail polish does not exhibit absorbance in the oximeter's range and should not affect SpO_2 readings. In order to ensure accurate measurements, all nail polish should be removed from the nailbed to be used before the probe is placed or an alternative site should be used.

8. If the pulse oximeter reads 90% or more, does the patient have an acceptable Pao_2?

Not necessarily. It is important to remember the factors that can shift the position of the oxyhemoglobin dissociation curve and alter the relationship between a given Pao_2 and the corresponding level of hemoglobin saturation. These factors include temperature, pH, $Paco_2$, and 2,3,DPG.

Clinical example. A blood gas sample was drawn from a patient breathing room air. The values obtained were pH 7.40, $Paco_2$ 36 mmHg, and Pao_2 61 mmHg. No abnormal hemoglobin species were present and a simultaneous pulse oximetry reading measured the SpO_2 at 90%. The patient was in no distress, had a heart rate of 68 beats per minute (bpm), and was breathing at a respiratory rate of 20 breaths per minute. Two hours later the patient became acutely tachycardiac with a heart rate of 138 bpm and tachypneic with a respiratory rate of 44 breaths per minute. The pulse oximeter reading was stable at 90%. Another blood gas sample was drawn and the values obtained were: pH 7.50, $Paco_2$ 24 mmHg, and Pao_2 50 mmHg. The patient had clearly become hypoxemic even though the pulse oximeter was showing an acceptable SpO_2. The patient's hyperventilation caused an acute respiratory alkalosis, shifting the oxyhemoglobin dissociation curve to the left; the effect of the left shift would result in the same hemoglobin saturation at a significantly lower Pao_2.

9. How does dyshemoglobinemia affect pulse oximetry?

Abnormal levels of hemoglobin species such as carboxyhemoglobin (COHb) and methemoglobin (metHb) can account for variances between SpO_2 and Sao_2. Because current pulse oximeters use only two wavelengths of light, they are capable of detecting only two species of hemoglobin, Hb and HbO_2. Given that COHb and metHb absorb red and infrared light at the same wavelengths as Hb and HbO_2, their presence affects the SpO_2 measurements, but they cannot be differentiated. COHb is read as HbO_2 and any amount will falsely elevate the value of the SpO_2 reading. If a high level of metHb is present, SpO_2 is erroneously low when the Sao_2 is more than 85% and erroneously high when the Sao_2 is less than 85%. Increased metHb levels therefore can result in either overestimation or underestimation of SpO_2, depending on the actual Sao_2. The presence of fetal hemoglobin (FeHb) has not been shown to affect the accuracy of SpO_2 measurements. Although not entirely correct, saturation measurements by pulse oximetry are commonly referred to as *functional saturation*, whereas saturation measurements made by CO-oximeters are referred to as *fractional saturation*. The following equations point out the differences between these two types of saturation measurements and help to explain why SpO_2 readings can differ from Sao_2 measurements:

$$\text{Functional saturation} = \frac{HbO_2}{HbO_2 + Hb} \times 100\%$$

$$\text{Fractional saturation} = \frac{HbO_2}{HbO_2 + Hb + COHb + metHb} \times 100\%$$

10. Name some other limitations of pulse oximetry.

The accuracy of pulse oximetry can be affected by several factors that should be recognized by anyone who obtains or uses pulse oximetry data. Most errors in pulse oximetry measurement are the result of poor signal quality (e.g., low perfusion) or excessive noise (e.g., motion artifact). The accuracy of measurements can be enhanced by use of a series of measurements to verify reproducibility or by continuous monitoring of SpO_2 for several minutes to establish a steady-state reading. If the unit displays a plethysmographic waveform or signal strength monitor, this feature should be used to optimize accurate measurements. Intravascular dyes such as methylene blue have been reported to cause falsely low SpO_2 values. Severe anemia (Hb less than 5 gm/dl) may affect accuracy since oximetry depends on light absorption by hemoglobin. Despite earlier reports to the contrary, hyperbilirubinemia does not appear to affect SpO_2. Skin pigmentation may yield less accurate values because of various technical problems such as poor signal strength. Another purported explanation for measurement error in dark pigmented people is that light from the probe's LEDs may take the path of least resistance and travel subcutaneously to the photodetector, never coming in contact with the patient's pulsating vascular bed.

11. What is the "penumbra effect"?

Penumbra (from Latin *paene*, meaning *almost*, and *umbra*, meaning *shade*) refers to the partially lighted area surrounding the complete shadow of a body, as in an eclipse. Incorrectly positioned pulse oximetry probes may still provide a pulsatile signal yet prevent adequate illumination of the photodetector by the LED. Light shunted from the LED to the photodetector can theoretically cause a falsely low SpO_2 if the SaO_2 is more than 85% and a falsely high SpO_2 if the SaO_2 is less than 85%.

12. In addition to its effect on the oxyhemoglobin dissociation curve, how does body temperature affect the pulse oximeter's readings?

Body temperature above or below normal causes the sensor LEDs to shift their spectral outputs (0.2 nm/Celsius degree), which can result in an overestimation or underestimation of SpO_2. Correcting for this temperature-induced wavelength shift is not clinically relevant in most instances.

13. Is there any advantage to using a particular type of sensor or monitoring site?

Sensors are available in a variety of sizes and configurations. Fingers, toes, and earlobes are the most common locations for probe placement. Selection of a sensor site should be based on where the most stable and strongest signal can be obtained. Nondisposable "clothespin" probes are best used for spot checks or for patients who are not too active. Adhesive-backed sensors are probably better suited for long-term monitoring and for patients who are restless and therefore more likely to cause displacement of the clip-on probe.

14. What is the risk of cross-contamination with use of a nondisposable sensor?

A report on residual bacterial contamination of nondisposable sensors found that 66% of the sensors that were identified as ready for patient use were contaminated with bacteria. The sensors in this study were cleaned in between patients with 70% isopropyl alcohol, sani-cloth, and a 10% bleach solution, or were not cleaned at all. Although no published reports implicate the spread of nosocomial infections via pulse oximeter sensors, other nondisposable devices such as blood pressure cuffs, stethoscopes, and reusable ECG bulbs have been shown to serve as environmental reservoirs of infection. Although sensors intended for single patient use readily address the concerns about spreading nosocomial infection by the sharing of these devices, they can create a substantial cost outlay. The decision of whether to use disposable or nondisposable sensors should be made on an individual basis. Use of single patient probes for immunocompromised patients, for example, appears to be appropriate utilization of disposable sensors. The development of more effective cleaning protocols and the use of laminated sensors combined with disposable protective shields also decrease the risk of spreading infection while helping to control costs.

15. Are there any potential complications of pulse oximetry use?

Pulse oximetry is relatively safe. However, since the sensors contain electronic circuitry, there is the potential for malfunction causing thermal burns. In one report, three patients received burns on their fingers from a defective LED in a finger probe. Other burns have been attributed to a finger probe that was connected to a pulse oximeter of a different manufacturer, resulting in a higher voltage being sent to the probe and a measured temperature of $234°$ F. Burns have also been associated with pulse oximetry use during MRI. Pressure sores and tissue necrosis can be caused by improper probe placement or failure to monitor and change probe placement as necessary. Pressure injuries are more common with spring-loaded sensors and in patients who have impaired peripheral perfusion, are receiving vasoconstrictors, or have other conditions that make them susceptible to cutaneous tissue breakdown. Other potential complications include false-negative results for hypoxemia or false-positive results for normoxemia or hyperoxemia, leading to inappropriate treatment.

16. List some other uses for pulse oximetry.

Other less proven uses include:
• Assessment of collateral circulation before arterial cannulation
• Monitoring of vascular blood flow in transplanted digits
• Screening for desaturation while eating
• Acting as a feedback device for patients with COPD who are learning pursed-lip breathing
• During newborn resuscitation, gauging the efficacy of airway maneuvers, especially in babies with intrapartum complications such as meconium aspiration

17. What type of patients should be assessed with oximetry?

Pulse oximetry has become the standard of care in the operating and recovery rooms of most modern hospitals. In addition, the Technology Assessment Task Force of The Society of Critical Care Medicine has recently recommended continuous pulse oximetry monitoring for patients requiring mechanical ventilatory support. Pulse oximetry provides immediate feedback on ventilator oxygenation manipulations (FIO_2, PEEP) and provides early detection of desaturation events that could lead to adverse sequelae such as cardiac arrhythmias. Unrecognized hypoxemic episodes have also been documented by pulse oximetry during patient transport and procedures such as bronchoscopy, endoscopy, cardiac catheterization, and sleep apnea screening. The use of pulse oximetry in routine screening of pulmonary outpatients has not been established because unrecognized hypoxemia is uncommon in the absence of associated clinical findings. Pulse oximeters are widely used in neonatal intensive care units, where they have replaced transcutaneous oxygen monitors. The primary limitation of the pulse oximeter is its inability to accurately detect and monitor hyperoxia.

CONTROVERSIES

18. Should pulse oximetry be used in prescribing long-term oxygen therapy?

Currently, Medicare guidelines allow reimbursement for home oxygen if the PaO_2 is equal to or less than 55 mmHg or the oxygen saturation by cooximetry or pulse oximetry is equal to or less than 85%. These values can be increased to a PaO_2 of 59 mmHg or an oxygen saturation of 89% under certain conditions or diagnoses.

For: Pulse oximetry is a quick, noninvasive, and relatively inexpensive way to evaluate a patient's oxygenation status. It can provide oxygenation measurements on a continuous basis as well as during both static and dynamic conditions. In contrast, invasive arterial blood gas analysis imposes risk of infection, thrombosis, and vascular injury and provides information about a patient's oxygenation status only at the precise time the arterial blood sample was obtained.

Against: Pulse oximeters cannot distinguish between HbO_2 and abnormal Hb species such as COHb and metHb. Thus, it is possible that the actual SaO_2 may be 85% with a COHb as low as

2.1% and metHb as low as 0.6% with simultaneous SpO_2 of 88%. This situation would fail to meet the Medicare guidelines for home oxygen reimbursement if pulse oximetry were the sole determinant of HbO_2 saturation. In fact, one study performed simultaneous arterial blood gas analysis and pulse or ear oximetry on 55 patients with chronic lung disease. These investigators found that 80% of the patients with a resting Pao_2 value of equal to or less than 55 mmHg had SpO_2 values equal to or greater than 85%. Thus, these patients did not qualify for Medicare reimbursement by pulse oximetry values but did so by Pao_2 measurement criterion. A similar study of 16 patients found 5 patients (31%) would not have met Medicare reimbursement criteria by pulse oximetry measurements alone.

BIBLIOGRAPHY

1. Barker SJ, Tremper KK, Hyatt J, et al: Effects of methemoglobinemia on pulse oximetry and mixed venous oximetry. Anesthesiology 67:A171, 1987.
2. Bowton DL: A critical review of pulse oximetry. Clin Pulm Med 1:181–187, 1994.
3. Carlin BW, et al: The use of cutaneous oximetry in the prescription of long term oxygen therapy. Chest 94:239–241, 1988.
4. Chellar L, Snyder JV, et al: Accuracy of pulse oximetry in patients with hyperbilirubinemia. Respir Care 36:1383–1386, 1991.
5. Cote CJ, Golstein EA, et al: The effect of nail polish on pulse oximetry. Anesth Analg 67:638–646, 1988.
6. Garfield BR, Graybeal JM: Accuracy of laminated disposable pulse-oximeter sensors. Respir Care 40:728–733, 1995.
7. Golish JA, McCarthy: Limitation of pulse oximetry in detecting hypoxemia. Chest 94(Suppl):505, 1988 (abstract).
8. Kanal E, Shellock FG: Burns associated with clinical MR examinations. Radiology 176:585, 1990.
9. Kelleher JF, Ruff RH: The pneumbra effect: Vasomotor-dependent pulse oximeter artifact due to probe malposition. Anesthesiology 7:787–791, 1989.
10. Loggan M, Kerby GR, Pingleton SK: Is routine assessment of arterial oxygen saturation in pulmonary outpatients indicated? Chest 94:242–244, 1988.
11. McCarthy K, Decker MJ, Strohl KP, et al: Pulse oximetry. In Kacmarek KM, Hess K, Stoller JK (eds): Monitoring in Respiratory Care. St. Louis, Mosby-Year Book, 1993, pp 309–347.
12. Moore FA, Haenel JB, Moore EE, et al: Hypoxic events in the surgical intensive care unit. Am J Surg 160:647–651, 1990.
13. Murphy KG, Secunda JA, Rockoff MA: Severe burns from a pulse oximeter. Anesthesiology 73:350–352, 1990.
14. Neff T: Routine oximetry: A fifth vital sign? Chest 94:227, 1988.
15. Schnapp LM, Cohen NH: Pulse oximetry: Uses and abuses. Chest 98:1244–1250, 1990.
16. Severinghause JW, Kelleher JF: Recent development in pulse oximetry. Anesthesiology 76:198–1038, 1992.
17. Sloan T: Finger injury by an oxygen saturation monitor probe. Anesthesiology 68:936–938, 1988.
18. Tremper KK, Barker SJ: Pulse oximetry. Anesthesiology 70:98–108, 1989.
19. Welch JP, DeCesare R, Hess D: Pulse oximetry: Instrumentation and clinical application. Respir Care 35:584–601, 1990.
20. Wilkin MC: Residual bacterial contamination on reusable pulse oximetry sensors. Respir Care 38:1155–1160, 1993.

9. PULMONARY FUNCTION TESTING

Lee K. Brown, M.D., and Albert Miller, M.D.

1. What is spirometry?

Spirometry is the measurement of the volume of air that can be inhaled or exhaled. Since residual volume (RV) is defined as the volume of air that remains in the lungs after maximal exhalation, spirometry can never directly measure any volume or capacity that includes RV. Modern spirometers may measure respired volume directly, or (more commonly) they may measure flow, then electrically or digitally integrate the flow to calculate volume. In practice, the patient wears noseclips to prevent leakage of air out of the nares and breathes into the spirometer through a plastic or paper mouthpiece. The various lung volumes and capacities (a capacity is defined as the sum of two or more volumes) include expiratory reserve volume (ERV), functional residual capacity (FRC), inspiratory capacity (IC), inspiratory reserve volume (IRV), and tidal volume (TV).

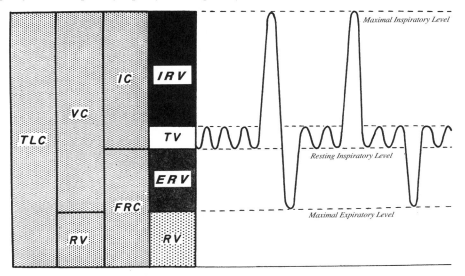

Spirogram depicting the various subdivisions of total lung capacity (TLC). (From Comroe JH, Forster RE, DuBois AB, et al: The Lung. Chicago, Year Book, 1962, p 8; with permission.)

2. What maneuvers are used in the performance of spirometry?

1. **Slow vital capacity (SVC).** The patient breathes tidally, then inhales slowly to total lung capacity (TLC) followed by a slow exhalation to RV. The total volume of air slowly exhaled is the SVC.

2. **Forced vital capacity (FVC).** The patient breathes tidally, inhales slowly to TLC, and then exhales, as hard and as fast as possible, to RV. In most cases, the patient is then instructed to inhale once more, also as hard and as fast as possible, back to TLC. The total volume of air rapidly exhaled is the FVC.

3. **Maximal voluntary ventilation (MVV).** The patient breathes in and out through the spirometer, as rapidly and deeply as possible, for either 12 or 15 seconds. The total volume of air exhaled or inhaled during that period of maximal breathing is measured, expressed in terms of liters/minute, and reported as the MVV.

3. What measurements are made using the SVC maneuver?

The SVC maneuver is used to measure slow vital capacity and is also essential in the determination of static lung volumes, which include RV, functional residual capacity (FRC), and TLC. Rather than each of these volumes and capacities being measured individually, common practice is to measure FRC, then use an SVC measure to obtain ERV and IC. TLC can be easily be obtained by adding IC to FRC, and RV is obtained by subtracting ERV from FRC (see figure in question 1).

4. What measurements are made using the FVC maneuver?

When spirometrically measured volume is plotted against time during the expiratory portion of an FVC maneuver, the result is a curve termed the *forced expiratory spirogram*. Volumes, timed volumes, and average flows are easily derived from this curve; the four most commonly used parameters thus obtained are FVC, ERV, forced expiratory volume in one second (FEV$_1$), and forced expiratory flow between 25% and 75% of FVC (FEF$_{25-75\%}$).

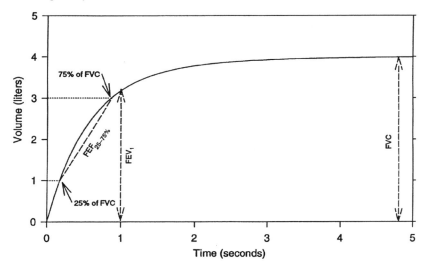

Spirogram of a forced expiratory effort from TLC to RV, depicting FVC and FEV$_1$; the average flow between 25% and 75% of vital capacity (FEF$_{25-75\%}$) is obtained from the slope of the line connecting these two points on the spirogram.

5. Does reduced FVC indicate a restrictive disorder?

FVC depends on the values of both TLC and RV; FVC declines if TLC falls or RV rises. The dependence of FVC on TLC led to its use as an indicator of restrictive impairment as a result of lung disease or chest wall disease. Lung disorders that fill or obliterate alveoli (e.g., consolidation, interstitial fibrosis) or remove alveolar volume (lung resection) reduce TLC and thus FVC. Chest wall disorders that interfere with the expansion of the lungs within the thorax (e.g., kyphoscoliosis) or weaken the inspiratory muscles (amyotrophic lateral sclerosis, myasthenia gravis, or other causes of diaphragmatic paresis) also reduce TLC and thus FVC.

FVC also declines if RV is elevated. Although increased RV can be related to weakness of the expiratory muscles (primarily the rectus and transversus abdominis and the internal and external obliques) because of neuromuscular disorders, it is much more commonly the result of obstructive airway disease and air trapping.

6. Why is ERV measured?

ERV depends on the mobility of the diaphragm and is reduced in neuromuscular disorders. It is also reduced by abdominal processes that interfere with diaphragmatic movement, such as obesity or ascites. ERV also falls immediately after abdominal surgery; this fall is frequently attributed to incisional pain, but it may have more to do with mechanical or neuromuscular interference with diaphragmatic motion.

7. What is the difference between a timed volume such as FEV$_1$ and an average flow such as FEF$_{25-75\%}$?

Even though timed volumes such as FEV$_1$ are expressed in units of volume, the fact that they are collected over a fixed span of time means that they are actually average flows, just as FEF$_{25-75\%}$ is. The most commonly used timed volume, FEV$_1$, represents the amount of air exhaled during the first second of the FVC maneuver and is really just the average flow during that first second of expiration. FEF$_{25-75\%}$ is the average flow during the "middle half" of the FVC maneuver, starting when 25% of the FVC has been exhaled and ending when 75% of the FVC has been collected in the spirometer. Both measurements are reduced when resistance to airflow increases because of airway obstruction. However, $FEF_{25-75\%}$ may more closely reflect the status of the "small airways" (those less than 2 mm in diameter), although this is controversial.

8. Why should $FEF_{25-75\%}$ reflect airflow in these small airways?

$FEF_{25-75\%}$ is measured at lower lung volumes than is FEV_1. At lung volumes less than approximately 70% of FVC, flow will not increase with additional expiratory force once a minimum threshold of effort is achieved. This "effort independence" has been attributed to the equal pressure point theory: during a forced exhalation, airway pressure progressively declines as one travels from the alveolus (upstream) to the mouth (downstream). This drop in pressure is attributable to airway resistance and exists only when airflow is present. At some point downstream in the conducting airways, intraluminal pressure falls below the pressure compressing the airway (equivalent to pleural pressure plus lung elastic recoil pressure) and the airway collapses and becomes occluded. The greater the expiratory effort (pleural pressure), the greater the tendency for this occlusion to occur. Because the occlusion interrupts airflow, intraluminal pressure rises and reopens the airway. In reality, these bronchi probably do not open and close, but reach some sort of equilibrium so that increases in expiratory force (above a minimum threshold) do not increase airflow; instead, airflow is proportional to lung elastic recoil divided by the resistance of the airways between the alveoli and the equal pressure point (the small airways). Thus, flows at lung volumes less than approximately 70% of FVC (such as $FEF_{25-75\%}$) are thought to reflect resistance in these small airways.

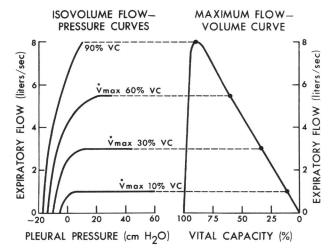

Effort independence of flow during forced expiration at lower lung volumes. **Left,** Flow versus pleural pressure curves at four different lung volumes expressed as percent of VC. **Right,** A forced expiratory flow-volume loop from a single maximal effort. (From Murray JF: The Normal Lung: The Basis for Diagnosis and Treatment of Pulmonary Disease, 2nd ed. Philadelphia, W.B. Saunders, 1986, p 100; with permission.)

9. Is reduced FEV_1 or $FEF_{25-75\%}$ always diagnostic of airway obstruction?

No. These indices of obstruction frequently decline to some extent in restrictive disorders as well. One example is a patient with severe kyphoscoliosis, such that measured FVC is 2.0 L despite a predicted FVC of 5.0 L. Predicted FEV_1 for this patient might be 3.5 L, but there is obviously no chance that the patient will achieve this since only 2.0 L can be exhaled for the entire breath. Thus, spirometric flows and volumes often decline in the presence of restrictive impairment.

To overcome this limitation in the use of spirometric indices of obstruction, the parameters FEV_1/FVC and $FET_{25-75\%}$ were developed. FEV_1/FVC defines obstruction in terms of the fraction of FVC that can be exhaled in one second, rather than an absolute volume; if FEV_1 falls to a greater degree than FVC, FEV_1/FVC declines and obstruction is present. FEV_1/FVC is somewhat age dependent. For adults aged less than 40 years, at least 75% of FVC should be exhaled in one second; between the ages of 40 and 60 years, this value should be 70% or more, and for subjects aged 60 years or older should be more than 65%. $FET_{25-75\%}$ represents the time it takes for the "middle half" of FVC to be exhaled (the time during which $FEF_{25-75\%}$ is computed). Algebraically, $FET_{25-75\%} = FVC/(2FEF_{25-75\%})$; thus, if FVC is reduced because of restriction but $FEF_{25-75\%}$ is decreased out of proportion to the fall in FVC, $FET_{25-75\%}$ is elevated. Increased $FET_{25-75\%}$ is another relatively volume-independent marker of obstruction that may be particularly indicative of small airways obstruction.

10. What is a flow-volume loop?

The flow-volume loop is another way of displaying the information collected during the forced spirogram. Instead of showing volume versus time, the flow-volume loop displays instantaneous flow vs. volume.

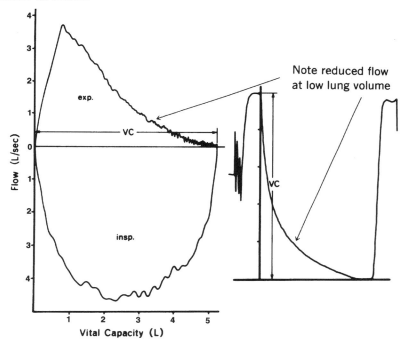

Maximal expiratory and inspiratory flow-volume loop (**left**) and spirogram from the same effort (**right**). The expiratory limb demonstrates the upwardly concave "tail" associated with small airway obstruction. (From Petty TL, Lakshminarayan S: Practical pulmonary function tests. In Petty TL (ed): Pulmonary Diagnostic Techniques. Philadelphia, Lea & Febiger, 1975, p 23; with permission.)

11. List the advantages of of the flow-volume loop.

1. Instantaneous flows are easily read from the curve, including peak flow (the maximum flow achieved, characteristically inscribed early in the effort) and the various flows at low lung volumes that may reflect obstruction in the small airways.

2. The overall shape of the curve can yield important information. For instance:
   • The adequacy of patient effort. Inadequate expiratory effort may result in a delayed upstroke to peak flow; early termination of effort is evidence by flow that drops abruptly to zero rather than gradually declining as the curve meets the volume axis at the end of the breath; coughing or extra breaths are also readily apparent.

- Small airway obstruction. An expiratory effort with a long, upwardly-concave tail indicates that much of the FVC at low lung volumes is exhaled at low flow rates, consistent with small airway obstruction.
- Upper airway obstruction. Obstruction in, and downstream from, the mainstem bronchi characteristically affects peak flow the most, resulting in flattening of the flow-volume loop. Both expiratory and inspiratory limbs of the loop are flattened when upper airway obstruction is fixed (e.g., tracheal stenosis). Nonfixed (variable) lesions in the extrathoracic airway (e.g., bilateral vocal cord paralysis) primarily affect the inspiratory limb, when the vocal cords are drawn more closely together by suction; the cords are pushed apart during exhalation, so that the expiratory limb looks relatively normal. Variable lesions in the intrathoracic airway (e.g., tracheomalacia) are relieved during inhalation (negative intrathoracic pressure pulls open intrathoracic airways), causing the inspiratory limb to appear normal while the expiratory limb flattens.
- All of the spirometric indices available from the forced expiratory spirogram can still be obtained from the flow-volume loop, as long as a "timing mark" is generated by the apparatus to indicate the one-second point to allow the computation of FEV_1.

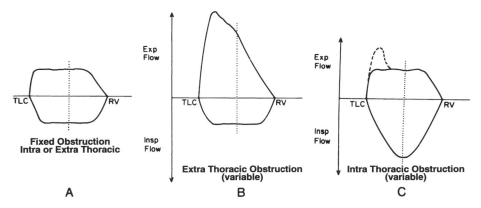

Flow-volume loops in upper airway obstruction. **A**, Fixed intrathoracic or extrathoracic obstruction. **B**, Variable extrathoracic obstruction. **C**, Variable intrathoracic obstruction. Incomplete flattening of the expiratory limb (dashed line) is occasionally observed. (Reprinted by permission of the publisher from Kryger M, Bode F, Antic R, et al: Diagnosis of obstruction of the upper and central airways. Am J Med 61:87, 1976. Copyright 1976 by Excerpta Medica, Inc.)

12. When is peak expiratory flow used?

Peak expiratory flow is inscribed early in the forced exhalation, at a high lung volume. Consequently, it reflects obstruction in the larger airways and varies greatly with effort. Peak flow is most often used as an index of the degree of airway obstruction during exacerbations of bronchial asthma, since it is easily measured in the emergency department with simple equipment. In fact, the equipment is simple enough that patients can be supplied with a peak flow meter to use in the home; this leads to its second use, anticipating an exacerbation of asthma before a significant symptomatic deterioration. Patients with "brittle" asthma, who frequently require trips to the emergency department or hospital admission for treatment, can measure their own peak flow at home on a daily basis and call a medical practitioner if peak flow declines.

13. What is the significance of an improvement in FVC or FEV_1 after bronchodilator aerosol treatment?

Such a procedure is known as an assessment of "reversibility." Patients with obstructive ventilatory impairment on initial spirometry are given a bronchodilator aerosol (most frequently, a β-adrenergic agonist such as albuterol) and spirometry is repeated. An increase in either value beyond what might be expected from the normal variability of the measurement itself indicates a response to the bronchodilator; one common guideline calls for a 12% or more improvement in FVC or FEV_1. It is thought that patients who react to bronchodilators predominantly by increasing FVC (volume responders) do so by reducing the amount of trapped air behind obstructed peripheral airways (i.e., residual volume decreases). Regardless of whether a volume or flow response is present, this finding is consistent with bronchial asthma, or at least supports the use of bronchodilator therapy in that patient. The lack of an immediate response to bronchodilator administration in an obstructed patient during a brief laboratory assessment does not necessarily prove that such medication will not be of any benefit in the long term.

14. What is bronchial challenge testing?

Bronchial challenge testing is most frequently used to diagnose occult bronchial asthma; in certain specialized centers, it can also be used to detect asthma related to specific environmental agents (e.g., occupational asthma). The test is most commonly performed using the cholinergic drug methacholine chloride (histamine may also be used), prepared as a solution in buffered normal saline and administered as an aerosol. Baseline spirometry is performed after inhalation of the diluent alone, then after inhalation of increasing concentrations of the drug. The procedure is stopped if FEV_1 declines by 20% or more below baseline or when the maximum concentration is reached. Patients with bronchial asthma or other conditions leading to airway hyperreactivity will demonstrate 20% or more decrease in FEV_1 at lower concentrations of methacholine than normal subjects. For diagnosis of environmentally induced asthma, preparations of the agent suspected of producing the asthmatic reaction may be given.

15. When is it useful to measure MVV?

The MVV maneuver integrates the activity of many different parts of the ventilatory apparatus: respiratory muscles, chest wall, pulmonary parenchyma, and airways. However, derangement in some components of the ventilatory apparatus affects MVV more than derangement in others. MVV is typically reduced when obstructive impairment is present but is usually preserved in restrictive disease (with the exception of neuromuscular disease) until the disorder is severe. It is thought that patients with most restrictive conditions are able to compensate for reduced tidal volume simply by increasing respiratory frequency. In contrast, any attempt to increase MVV in obstructive disease (by increasing tidal volume or respiratory rate) requires an increase in flow, which is the limiting factor in obstruction. This observation led to the description of the air velocity index, a variable calculated as percent predicted MVV divided by percent predicted VC. This index is usually more than 1 in restrictive lung disease but reduced in obstructive disorders. Certain obstructive disorders cause a greater fall in MVV than others; because much of the MVV maneuver takes place at high lung volumes and reflects the ability to generate high peak flows, upper airway obstruction has a particular impact on this test. Finally, MVV is a sensitive indicator of neuromuscular disorders that impair the strength and endurance of the ventilatory muscles.

It is also frequently worthwhile to examine the plot of volume versus time obtained during the MVV maneuver. A progressive increase in FRC (the volume at end-expiration for each MVV breath) is consistent with dynamic air trapping (also called *breath stacking*) and indicates obstructive airway disease. In essence, the obstructed patient is unable to completely exhale the volume of the previous breath before it is time to inhale once again.

16. Is it useful to compare SVC and FVC?

Slow vital capacity and forced vital capacity are usually similar, except in obstructive airway disease or pulmonary emphysema. In these disorders, a forced expiration often causes dynamic collapse of the airways, because they are narrowed from disease or because reduced elastic recoil of the destroyed lung parenchyma fails to hold the airways open to the usual extent. The result is air trapped behind the obstruction, elevated RV, and reduced FVC. Thus, a significant disparity between SVC and FVC (in which FVC is less than SVC) suggests obstructive disease or pulmonary emphysema.

17. How are the static lung volumes measured?

Standard practice is to measure only FRC. TLC and RV are then derived by adding IC or subtracting ERV, respectively. IC and ERV are obtained from the SVC maneuver.

Three common methods are used to determine FRC. Two of the methods (helium wash-in and nitrogen wash-out) are "gas dilution" techniques that depend upon a marker gas that is distributed throughout the lungs at FRC. The other technique (body plethysmography) encloses the patient in a sealed booth; FRC is calculated by applying Boyle's law to the changes in mouth pressure and box volume that occur when the patient pants against an occluded mouthpiece.

18. List the advantages and disadvantages of each technique.

The gas dilution methods are easier for patients to perform, because they are required only to breathe normally on a mouthpiece. However, the measurement takes longer than body plethysmography because time is required for helium to equilibrate throughout the lungs in the wash-in technique or for nitrogen to be flushed out of the lungs in the wash-out technique. The amount of time can be prolonged in a patient with obstructive airway disease. Body plethysmography requires a cooperative patient who does not mind being locked within the small booth and who can perform an adequate panting maneuver against the occluded mouthpiece. The measurement itself takes only a few seconds, especially using modern, computerized equipment. Body plethysmography also measures the volume of *any* gas-containing space in the thorax, including bullae. In some patients with chronic obstructive lung disease, it is sometimes useful to measure FRC both plethysmographically and by a gas dilution technique. The difference between the two measurements (plethysmographic FRC will be larger) reflects the volume of gas contained in bullae.

19. When is it important to measure static lung volumes?

These volumes are frequently useful when spirometry alone presents a confusing or mixed picture. The most common situation occurs when both restriction (i.e., reduced FVC) and obstruction (reduced FEV_1/FVC ratio) coexist. The question is then raised as to whether both impairments are actually present (which can occur in some diseases, such as sarcoidosis) or whether FVC is reduced simply because RV is elevated because of air trapping from obstructive airway disease. If the determination of static lung volumes demonstrates that RV is elevated and TLC normal, pure obstructive impairment is diagnosed; if TLC is reduced, both obstruction and restriction are present. Less commonly, a patient with pure restrictive impairment may have normal VC, but measurement of static lung volume reveals reduced TLC *and* RV. The difference (VC = TLC − RV) may thus be normal although restrictive impairment, shown by reduced TLC, is present nonetheless. Both of these examples serve to underline the importance of measuring TLC, an index widely accepted as the gold standard test for restrictive impairment resulting from lung or chest wall disease.

20. Is there a standardized noninvasive test for assessment of gas exchange across the lung?

Such a test does exist, and is called the *diffusing capacity* of the lung (D_L) in the United States and transfer factor (T_L) in Great Britain and Europe. The test gas contains carbon monoxide and the standard method involves a 10-second breath hold ("single breath" in pulmonary function jargon) at full inspiration, so the abbreviation is DL_{CO}^{SB}. Carbon monoxide, like oxygen, has an affinity for hemoglobin so that its uptake during the breath hold is not limited by the receiving reservoir (the pulmonary blood flow) but by the surface area and nature of the air-blood interface, the tissues and fluid that make up the alveolar-capillary membrane. Other assessments of gas exchange require arterial blood gases and are therefore invasive.

21. In what types of disease does the DL_{CO}^{SB} provide information?

Decreases in DL_{CO}^{SB} reflect loss of or damage to the gas exchanging surface of the lung, as occurs in emphysema, interstitial lung disease, or pulmonary vascular diseases. In COPD, decrease in DL_{CO}^{SB} helps distinguish emphysema from obstructive chronic bronchitis or chronic asthma, in which DL_{CO}^{SB} remains normal. In interstitial lung disease, including sarcoidosis, a decrease in DL_{CO}^{SB} often precedes an abnormality in other measurements of lung function. In pulmonary vascular disease, decrease in DL_{CO}^{SB} may be the only abnormality in standard pulmonary function tests.

22. Is there a relationship between DL_{CO}^{SB} and invasive measurements of gas exchange?

The DL_{CO}^{SB} is frequently reduced in interstitial lung disease even when invasive measurements such as resting arterial Po_2 or alveolar-arterial difference in Po_2 (PAO_2–PaO_2) are normal. Performance during exercise makes these invasive tests of gas exchange more sensitive. For instance, widening of the PAO_2–PaO_2 during exercise generally correlates with substantial reduction in DL_{CO}^{SB}.

23. Does cigarette smoking affect the DL_{CO}^{SB}?

Yes. By increasing venous carboxyhemoglobin (CoHb) cigarette smoking limits transfer of this gas across the alveolar capillary membrane. This effect is minimized by having patients refrain from smoking for 24 hours before undergoing the test. DL_{CO}^{SB} values of smokers are about 20% lower than those of nonsmokers. All of this difference cannot be explained by CoHb. Because exsmokers have values intermediate between those of continuing smokers and those of lifetime nonsmokers, some of this difference may be the result of effects on the alveolar-capillary membrane that are not clinically detectable.

24. What clinical tests of pulmonary function assess respiratory muscle strength?

Many evaluations of respiratory muscle strength are not clinical tests, e.g., diaphragmatic electromyography, transdiaphragmatic pressure. A simple measurement of respiratory muscle strength is the maximal inspiratory or expiratory pressure (PI_{max} or PE_{max}) measured by a pressure transducer at the mouth when the subject makes a maximal inspiratory effort from full expiration or a maximal expiratory effort from full inspiration.

25. What is the relationship between PI_{max} or PE_{max} and standard tests of pulmonary function?

PI_{max} and PE_{max} reflect respiratory muscle weakness, PI of the inspiratory muscles (the diaphragm) and PE of the expiratory muscles including abdominals. Depending on the type and level of muscle involvement, reduction in PI_{max} or PE_{max} is a sensitive indicator of disorders characterized by respiratory muscle involvement, such as motor neuron disease (amyotrophic lateral sclerosis) and Guillain-Barré syndrome. As the disease progresses, the IC, VC, FEV_1, and flow rates progressively fall and predict the advent of respiratory failure.

BIBLIOGRAPHY

1. Allen GW, Sabin S: Comparison of direct and indirect measurement of airway resistance. Am Rev Respir Dis 104:61–71, 1971.
2. American Thoracic Society: Lung function testing: Selection of reference values and interpretive strategies. Am Rev Respir Dis 144:1202–1218, 1991.
3. Black LF, Hyatt RE: Maximal respiratory pressures: Normal values and relationship to age and sex. Am Rev Respir Dis 99:696–702, 1969.
4. Brown LK: Static lung volumes. In Miller A (ed): Pulmonary Function Tests in Clinical and Occupational Lung Disease. Orlando, Grune & Stratton, 1986, pp 77–92.
5. Chan ED, Irvin CG: The detection of collapsible airways contributing to airflow limitation. Chest 107:856–859, 1995.
6. Crapo RO: Pulmonary-function testing. N Engl J Med 331:25–30, 1994.
7. Gilbert R, Auchincloss JH: What is a "restrictive" defect? Arch Intern Med 146:1779–1781, 1986.
8. Li JTC: Home peak expiratory flow rate monitoring in patients with asthma. Mayo Clin Proc 70:649–656, 1995.
9. Miller A (ed): Pulmonary Function Tests in Clinical and Occupational Lung Disease. Orlando, Grune & Stratton, 1986.
10. Miller A: Physiologic pulmonary diagnosis: The spectrum of impairments. Allergy Proc 14:401–407, 1993.
11. Miller A, Brown LK, Sloane MF, et al: Cardiorespiratory responses to incremental exercise in sarcoidosis patients with normal spirometry. Chest 107:323–329, 1995.

12. Miller A, Thornton JC, Warshaw R, et al: Single breath diffusing capacity in a representative sample of the population of Michigan, a large industrial state: Predicted values, lower limits of normal and frequencies of abnormality by smoking history. Am Rev Respir Dis 127:270–277, 1983.
13. Robinson DR, Chaudhary BA, Speir WA Jr: Expiratory flow limitation in large and small airways. Arch Intern Med 144:1457–1460, 1984.
14. Simonneau G, Vivien A, Sartene R, et al: Diaphragm dysfunction induced by upper abdominal surgery. Role of postoperative pain. Am Rev Respir Dis 128:899–903, 1983.
15. West JB: Respiratory Physiology—The Essentials. Baltimore, Williams & Wilkins, 1995.

10. EXERCISE TESTING

Idelle M. Weisman, M.D., and R. Jorge Zeballos, M.D., D.M.Sc.

1. What is a cardiopulmonary exercise test?

Cardiopulmonary exercise testing (CPET) involves the measurement of oxygen uptake ($\dot{V}O_2$), carbon dioxide output ($\dot{V}CO_2$), minute ventilation ($\dot{V}E$), and other variables in addition to the monitoring of 12-lead electrocardiogram (ECG), blood pressure, and pulse oximetry during a maximal symptom-limited exercise test. When appropriate, the additional measurement of arterial blood gases provides important information on pulmonary gas exchange. In contrast, during standard cardiac stress testing the focus is primarily on ECG and blood pressure measurements.

2. Why is cardiopulmonary exercise testing useful?

Dyspnea on exertion and exercise intolerance are common problems in many conditions and diseases. Increasingly, CPET is being used in the diagnostic evaluation of these disorders. Standard cardiac stress tests primarily endeavor to identify ischemia and generally cannot define underlying pathophysiology in patients with exercise intolerance of nonischemic origin. The diagnostic potential of standard exercise testing can be enhanced by the concurrent measurement of $\dot{V}O_2$, $\dot{V}CO_2$, $\dot{V}E$, etc. Furthermore, resting cardiopulmonary measurements—including pulmonary functions tests, resting ECG, and systolic performance variables (left ventricular ejection fraction)—cannot reliably predict exercise performance and functional capacity.

3. List the clinical applications of CPET.

1. Assessment of (functional) exercise capacity
   - Impairment/disability evaluation
   - Preoperative evaluation
   - Selection of patients for cardiac transplantation
   - Prognosis for heart disease, pulmonary vascular disease, cystic fibrosis
2. Diagnosis
   - Evaluation of unexplained dyspnea
   - Evaluation of exercise limitation
   - Detection of early (occult) disease
   - Documentation of exercise-induced hypoxemia
3. Measurement of response to treatment
   - Therapeutic interventions: drugs, devices, supplemental oxygen, and so forth
4. Exercise prescription
   - Pulmonary and cardiac rehabilitation
   - Health maintenance
   - Athletic training

4. Which measurements are most important?

Computer systems are able to measure several variables; however, the number of measurements obtained in an individual patient depends on the indications for CPET. The most important measurements are listed below.

Cardiopulmonary Variables Measured During Clinical Exercise Testing

NONINVASIVE		INVASIVE*
BASIC	COMPLEMENTARY	ARTERIAL BLOOD
Oxygen uptake ($\dot{V}O_2$)	Work rate (WR)	SaO_2, PaO_2, $P(A\text{-}a)O_2$
Heart rate, ECG, blood pressure	CO_2 output ($\dot{V}CO_2$)	$PaCO_2$, bicarbonate, pH
Minute ventilation ($\dot{V}E$)	Respiratory frequency (f)	Lactate
Pulse oximetry (SpO_2)	Tidal volume (V_T)	
Symptoms†	Lactate threshold	

* Optional.
† Dyspnea, leg fatigue, chest pain, lightheadedness, dizziness, and so forth.

5. How are $\dot{V}O_2$, $\dot{V}CO_2$, and ventilatory variables measured?

During CPET, while exercising on a cycle ergometer or on a treadmill the patient breathes into a mouthpiece connected to a computerized system that provides on-line breath-by-breath analysis of expired respiratory gases. The computer processes three primary signals: (1) air flow to obtain ventilatory variables, such as tidal volume, respiratory rate, and $\dot{V}E$; (2) oxygen fraction, and (3) carbon dioxide fraction (concentration). Most of the measurements are obtained from these signals.

6. Should a bicycle ergometer or treadmill be used for CPET?

Although both modalities may be used for clinical purposes, electronically braked cycle ergometry may be preferable to treadmill testing for several reasons: (1) bicycle work rate can be measured, whereas on a treadmill there is no direct quantitation of work rate; (2) there is usually less noise (artifact) on ECG; (3) it is easier to collect blood samples during exercise; (4) cycle ergometers are usually less expensive and take up less space; and (5) bicycles may be safer in certain types of patients such as the elderly. The maximum oxygen consumption ($\dot{V}O_2$max) achieved during cycle ergometry is usually 5–11% less than that achieved on a treadmill because of the incorporation of arm movement on the treadmill and non–weight-bearing effect of sitting on the bicycle. Accurate interpretation requires that the patient's data be compared with normal reference values for treadmill or bicycle ergometry.

7. What protocols are used most widely for CPET with cycle ergometry?

A symptom-limited incremental exercise test on a bicycle ergometer increases the work rate for the individual patient anywhere from 5 watts (unit of work rate) for frail patients with severe COPD to 25 watts for normal subjects every minute in a stepwise fashion. With a ramp protocol the work rate also can be increased from 5 to 25 watts/minute, but the increases are continuous, usually every second. Both incremental and ramp protocols should be programmed to achieve maximal exercise (volitional exhaustion) in 8 to 12 minutes. Both protocols provide comparable information and are widely used clinically.

8. List the most important contraindications to CPET.

- Acute ECG changes suggestive of myocardial infarction
- Unstable angina
- Uncontrolled congestive heart failure
- Uncontrolled atrial/ventricular dysrhythmia
- Third-degree atrioventricular block
- Uncontrolled hypertension (systolic blood pressure > 250 mmHg, diastolic pressure > 120 mmHg)

• Thrombophlebitis or intracardiac thrombi
• Acute myocarditis, pericarditis
• Severe aortic stenosis
• Acute febrile illness
• Oxygen saturation less than 85% on room air

9. What is the normal cardiopulmonary response to exercise?

During exercise there is an increase in oxygen demand to meet the metabolic requirements of the exercising muscles. The increased oxygen demand is accomplished by the integrated response of the cardiopulmonary system, blood redistribution, and oxygen utilization by the exercising muscles. At maximal exercise, oxygen consumption can increase up to 18-fold, heart rate two to three fold, stroke volume by twofold, cardiac output fivefold, $\dot{V}_E$ 20 to 25 times, and oxygen utilization by the muscles two to three times.

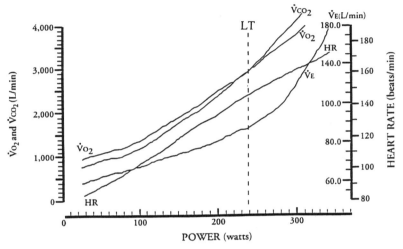

The normal response of $\dot{V}_{O_2}$, $\dot{V}_{CO_2}$, $\dot{V}_E$, and HR during a symptom-limited maximum incremental exercise is shown. These variables increase linearly with increase in work rate, until the lactate threshold (LT) is reached, at which point $\dot{V}_{CO_2}$ and $\dot{V}_E$ increase disproportionately to oxygen consumption.

10. What is the lactate threshold?

The lactate threshold, also called the *anaerobic threshold*, is an estimator of the onset of the metabolic acidosis associated with the increase in lactic acid in the blood. Although its meaning is controversial, it appears to be related to hypoxia of the exercising muscles, which occurs at approximately 50% of the $\dot{V}_{O_2}$max in normal individuals. The increase in lactic acid triggers physiologic responses, including increases in $\dot{V}_{CO_2}$ and $\dot{V}_E$ that are disproportionate to oxygen consumption. These changes allow the lactate threshold to be determined noninvasively by ventilatory variables; lactate can also be measured directly in the blood. The lactate threshold is used as an indicator of level of fitness, a monitor of the effect of physical training, and a supplementary variable in the diagnosis of exercise limitation.

11. When should arterial blood gases be measured during CPET?

The collection of arterial blood gases during exercise (by indwelling catheter) provides additional information and increases the diagnostic capabilities of the test. Arterial blood gases are recommended in patients in whom pulmonary gas exchange abnormalities are suspected, such as patients with interstitial lung disease, pulmonary vascular disease, and chronic obstructive pulmonary disease with low diffusing capacity. Also, it is advisable to collect arterial blood in patients in whom desaturation demonstrated by pulse oximetry was questionable.

12. What information is obtained from the evaluation of arterial blood?
   - Accurate diagnosis of arterial desaturation with exercise. Pulse oximetry (SpO_2) only esti-
     mates arterial oxygen saturation; actual Sao_2 could be ± 4% of the SpO_2 reading.
   - Evaluation of pulmonary gas exchange with the calculation of the alveolar arterial oxygen
     gradient $P(A-a)o_2$.
   - Determination of ventilation-perfusion mismatching (increased dead space) with the calcu-
     lation of the dead space to tidal volume ratio (VD/VT).
   Abnormalities in these measurements (SpO_2, $P(A-a)O_2$ and $VDVT$) reflect pulmonary gas ex-
change abnormalities and are usually observed in patients with pulmonary diseases.

13. What is the best index of exercise capacity?
   Measurement of the $\dot{V}o_2$max, the amount of oxygen consumed per minute at the highest
level of work that the test subject is capable of performing, remains the best available index for
the assessment of exercise capacity. Approaching or achieving maximal $\dot{V}o_2$ predicted from
normal reference values is an important criterion used for the determination of maximal aerobic
capacity. Traditionally, $\dot{V}o_2$max values have been regarded as most reliable when a $\dot{V}o_2$ plateau
(no further increase in $\dot{V}o_2$ as work rate increases) is achieved at the end of the exercise. Because
such a plateau is often not seen in patients, the highest level of $\dot{V}o_2$ achieved, or $\dot{V}o_2$ peak, is reported. Clinically, $\dot{V}o_2$ peak and $\dot{V}o_2$max are used interchangeably. A reduced $\dot{V}o_2$max response
reflects oxygen delivery (heart, lung, systemic, and pulmonary circulation) or peripheral utilization (i.e., peripheral circulation and/or muscle) abnormalities. A reformatting of the Fick equation demonstrates how dysfunction of different organ systems may affect aerobic capacity.

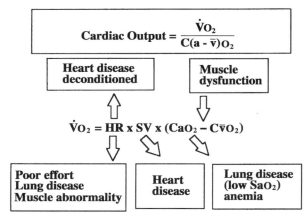

14. What mechanisms are involved in exercise limitation?
   Exercise in normal subjects is usually thought to be limited by cardiovascular factors. There
are three major categories of exercise limitation in patients with reduced $\dot{V}o_2$max:
   - **Cardiovascular limitation**, which includes the heart, pulmonary, and systemic circulation
     and blood (anemia, carboxyhemoglobin)
   - **Respiratory limitation**, which includes ventilatory (mechanical) and gas exchange
     factors
   - **Peripheral factors**, which include a broad spectrum of neuromuscular-related abnormali-
     ties that could affect oxygen utilization and mechanisms of contraction

15. How are cardiac limitation and ventilatory limitation defined?
   The human body has an enormous capacity to perform high levels of work compared to
sedentary conditions. The difference between maximal predicted values and measured values
during exercise for a variable is the reserve. CPET makes possible the evaluation of the two most

important reserves, the cardiovascular and ventilatory reserves. Since heart rate (HR) is considered a reliable indicator of cardiac capacity,

$$\text{Heart rate reserve (HRR)} = \text{predicted maximal HR} - \text{measured maximal HR}$$

The maximal voluntary ventilation of 12 seconds extrapolated to the minute (MVV) is commonly used to estimate ventilatory capacity. As such,

$$\text{Ventilatory reserve (VR)} = \text{MVV} - \dot{V}\text{Emax or } \dot{V}\text{Emax/MVV}$$

If $\dot{V}O_2$max is less than predicted:
- A **cardiovascular limitation** to exercise can be suspected if the measured HR is near or equal to the maximal HR (no HRR) and there is ventilatory reserve.
- A **ventilatory limitation** to exercise can be suspected if the $\dot{V}E$ measured at the highest level of exercise is near or equal to the ventilatory capacity (no ventilatory reserve) and there is heart rate reserve. Patients can have both cardiac and ventilatory limitation to exercise (no HRR and no VR).

16. What is the definition of a peripheral limitation?

A peripheral limitation to exercise may occur in the presence of suspected neuromuscular problems, myopathies or other muscle enzymatic deficiencies, or in severe deconditioning (e.g., heart or heart-lung transplantation). Patients with peripheral limitation have low $\dot{V}O_2$max and both HRR and VR.

17. How is CPET interpreted?

The results of CPET provide the answers to 2 basic questions:
1. Does the patient have a normal exercise capacity ($\dot{V}O_2$max)?
2. If exercise capacity is reduced, what are the probable causes?

To answer the second question, the following guidelines and helpful hints are offered:
- Examine the measurements and determine whether they are normal or abnormal compared with appropriate normal reference values.
- Evaluate abnormal response patterns and limitations to exercise; avoid excessive reliance on a single measurement (other than $\dot{V}O_2$).
- Consider what condition/clinical entities may be associated with these patterns.
- Correlate these results with the patient's clinical information, including results of other tests.

The results of CPET, like those of other physiologic tests in cardiopulmonary medicine, demonstrate only patterns of abnormality with significant overlap in the pattern of response of patients with different disorders observed. Furthermore, responses in normal individuals vary considerably. Accurate interpretation requires knowledge of such overlap and variability, including knowledge of the patient's clinical information.

18. How can CPET help distinguish between patients with heart disease and those with lung disease?

The table below demonstrates how using selected measurements CPET can help to more clearly define the physiologic basis of exercise limitation. This is a simplified table that reflects the "usual" response to exercise of patients with either cardiac or pulmonary disease.

Response to Exercise in Heart Disease and Lung Disease

	HEART DISEASE	LUNG DISEASE
$\dot{V}O_2$	Decreased	Decreased
Heart rate reserve	Variable	Increased
Ventilatory reserve	Normal	Decreased
PaO_2	Normal	Decreased
Exercise ECG	Abnormal	Normal

BIBLIOGRAPHY

1. American Association for Respiratory Care: Clinical practice guideline: Exercise testing for evaluation of hypoxemia and/or desaturation. Respir Care 37:907–912, 1992.
2. Celli BR: Exercise training in pulmonary rehabilitation. Semin Respir Med 14:132–138, 1993.
3. Gilbreth EM, Weisman IM: Role of exercise stress testing in preoperative evaluation of patients for lung resection. Clin Chest Med 15:389–403, 1994.
4. Jones NL: Clinical Exercise Testing, 3rd ed. Philadelphia, W.B. Saunders, 1988.
5. Martinez FJ, Stanopoulos I, Acero R, et al: Graded comprehensive cardiopulmonary exercise testing in the evaluation of dyspnea unexplained by routine evaluation. Chest 105:168–174, 1994.
6. Myers J, Froelicher VF: Hemodynamic determinants of exercise capacity in chronic heart failure. Ann Intern Med 115:377–386, 1991.
7. Neuberg GW, Friedman SH, Weiss MB, et al: Cardiopulmonary exercise testing: The clinical value of gas exchange data. Arch Intern Med 148:2221–2226, 1988.
8. Sue DY, Wasserman K: Impact of integrative cardiopulmonary exercise testing on clinical decision making. Chest 99:981–992, 1991.
9. Wasserman K, Hansen JE, Sue DY, et al: Principles of Exercise Testing and Interpretation, 2nd ed. Philadelphia, Lea & Febiger, 1994.
10. Weber KT, Janicki JS: Cardiopulmonary Exercise Testing. Philadelphia, W.B. Saunders, 1986.
11. Weisman IM, Connery SM, Belbel RJ, et al: The role of cardiopulmonary exercise testing in the selection of patients for cardiac transplantation. Chest 102:1871–1874, 1992.
12. Weisman IM, Zeballos RJ: An integrated approach to the interpretation of cardiopulmonary exercise testing. Clin Chest Med 15:421–445, 1994.
13. Weisman IM, Zeballos RJ: Cardiopulmonary exercise testing. Pulmonary and Critical Care Update 11:1–9, 1995.
14. Zeballos RJ, Weisman IM: Reliability of noninvasive oximetry in black subjects during exercise and hypoxia. Am Rev Respir Dis 144:1240–1244, 1991.
15. Zeballos RJ, Weisman IM: Behind the scenes of cardiopulmonary exercise testing. Clin Chest Med 15:193–213, 1994.

IV. Procedures

11. THORACENTESIS AND PERCUTANEOUS PLEURAL BIOPSY

Polly E. Parsons, M.D., and Yuan-Po Tu, M.D.

1. What are the chest x-ray findings in a pleural effusion?
Remember the axiom: **If the chest x-ray looks weird, think pleural disease.**

Any time a patient has an abnormal chest radiograph, the possibility of pleural effusion should be considered because increased densities on chest x-ray are often attributed to parenchymal disease when they actually represent pleural fluid. Classically, intrapleural fluid gives rise to relatively homogeneous opacifications, the appearance of which depends on the volume of fluid, the anatomical location, and the presence or absence of intrapleural air.

Massive effusions can cause opacification of all or most of the hemithorax with or without mediastinal shift. The major differential is drowned lung.

Moderate-sized effusions have the classic appearance of a homogenous shadow occupying the lower portion of the hemithorax, obliterating the margins of the adjacent heart and diaphragm.

Minimal or small effusions may cause a haziness of the costophrenic angle or may be completely hidden behind the dome of the diaphragm on the PA x-ray projection. Often a lateral x-ray view will be helpful because it will show blunting of the posterior gutter.

Subpulmonic effusions collect between the inferior surface of the lung and the superior surface of the diaphragm and mimic the findings of an elevated hemidiaphragm on x-ray.

Interlobular effusions have a fusiform homogeneous shadow with well-defined margins lying in the long axis of an interlobar fissure. Effusions in the minor fissures are best seen on the PA projection and those in the major fissures are best seen on the lateral projection. The x-ray findings of interlobular effusions are classically pseudotumors.

Hydropneumothorax gives a picture of a linear air fluid interface when the x-ray is taken with the patient in the upright position. The major differential diagnosis is juxtapleural intrapulmonary cavity partially filled with fluid.

2. What is the rule of thumb for estimating the amount of pleural fluid present on chest x-ray?
Blunting of the costophrenic angle: 100–150 cc
Effusion occupying 1/2 of the hemithorax: 1–1.5 L
Effusion occupying an entire hemithorax: 2.5–3 L

3. Are there any x-ray views besides PA and lateral that are helpful to evaluate a pleural effusion?
Lateral decubitus films are often helpful in determining how much fluid is present and whether it is free flowing or loculated. The lateral decubitus view ordered should correspond to the side of the effusion. Therefore, if the patient has a left-sided pleural effusion, order a left lateral decubitus chest x-ray. The film will then be taken with the patient lying on his or her left side, allowing the pleural fluid to track along the lateral pleural space where it is most easily visualized.

4. When should a diagnostic thoracentesis be considered?

Most patients with more than 10 mm of free-flowing pleural fluid demonstrated on a lateral decubitus x-ray should undergo diagnostic thoracentesis. Small effusions less than 10 mm often can be observed, but if thoracentesis is indicated, ultrasound guidance may be necessary.

The most common cause of a pleural effusion is congestive heart failure. Performing a thoracentesis on a patient with congestive heart failure usually does not add any new or helpful clinical information. However, if a patient with clinical congestive heart failure develops fever, pleuritic chest pain, or a marked discrepancy in the size of bilateral effusions, a diagnostic thoracentesis should be performed. Remember that classically the pleural effusions associated with congestive heart failure are transudates, but diuretic therapy may change the pleural effusion characteristics such that they have exudative features.

5. When should ultrasound guidance for thoracentesis be considered?

For small pleural effusions, loculated pleural fluid, pleural effusion on the side of an elevated hemidiaphragm, patient on mechanical ventilation, and bleeding diathesis.

6. What are the contraindications to a thoracentesis?

There is disagreement in the literature as to whether or not there are any absolute contraindications to performing a diagnostic thoracentesis. Some clinicians consider absolute contraindications to be be an uncooperative patient, inability to clearly palpate the rib margins, or a coagulopathy that cannot be corrected. Relative contraindications include the level of experience of the person performing the procedure, patients on mechanical ventilation (in particular those on PEEP), patients with severe COPD, patients with one lung, and patients in whom the benefit from the procedure is unlikely to outweigh the risk.

7. What are the common complications of thoracentesis?

When both major and minor complications are considered, complication rates as high as 75% have been cited. The most common complication is pneumothorax, which has been estimated to occur in 11% of patients, although only 2% will require chest tubes. The incidence of pneumothorax is greater when the thoracentesis is performed blindly and less when the thoracentesis is performed with ultrasound guidance during the procedure itself. In addition, the rate of pneumothorax varies with the size of the needle used for the procedure. Other complications include bleeding, infection, hypotension, hypoxemia, air embolism, splenic laceration, and tumor seeding of the tract. Death is a rare complication. Up to 20% of patients may complain of anxiety and pain at the site of the thoracentesis.

8. What is postthoracentesis reexpansion pulmonary edema?

Unilateral pulmonary edema may develop following a thoracentesis. This usually occurs when the pleural effusion has been present and compressing underlying lung for greater than 7 days and when more than 1.5 L of pleural fluid is removed at a time.

9. What do you do if you get bright red blood back when you doing a thoracentesis?

Although pleural effusions can be hemorrhagic, the appearance of bright red blood in the absence of chest trauma should raise concern that an intercostal artery, the spleen, or the liver has been punctured and/or lacerated. Although massive hemorrhage from a thoracentesis is rare, it is critical to carefully monitor the patient's hemodynamic status, follow the peripheral hematocrit, and correct any coagulation abnormalities. If there is any evidence of persistent blood loss, a surgeon should be consulted.

10. Which patients are at increased risk for laceration of an intercostal artery during thoracentesis?

Elderly patients. With increasing age, the tortuosity of blood vessels increases such that the amount of space between two ribs that is "safe" (i.e., free of blood vessels and nerves) is decreased.

This increase in tortuosity may start as early as age 40. Therefore, it is always important when performing a thoracentesis to insert the needle directly over the superior border of the rib to avoid puncturing a vessel.

11. I am in the middle of drawing off pleural fluid and I am drawing back air. Does this mean that I punctured the lung?

Not necessarily. Sometimes air enters the pleural space during a thoracentesis if the system (needle, stopcock, syringe) is open to air inadvertently during the procedure. Take your time and familiarize yourself with the system you are going to use prior to beginning the procedure.

12. I can't get any fluid back. Should I quit?

The inability to obtain pleural fluid (a dry tap) occurs when the thoracentesis has been performed in the wrong location or when the fluid is too viscous to be drawn through the needle. The first step is to reassess your clinical localization of the pleural fluid. If there is any question as to the location of the pleural fluid, ultrasound guidance would be appropriate for the next attempt. If you suspect that the patient has an empyema and, therefore, the fluid is very viscous, an attempt with a larger needle may be indicated. Again, assuring the location of the pleural fluid with ultrasound guidance may be prudent.

13. How much fluid do you need to obtain for a diagnostic thoracentesis?

Usually 35–50 ml are more than adequate for routine diagnostic studies, although more fluid may be helpful if cytology studies are needed.

14. What are the routine tests that should be ordered on pleural fluid?

Cell count and differential, LDH, total protein, glucose, and pH. Additional studies can be ordered depending on the differential diagnosis of the pleural effusion in the patient being evaluated. These studies include Gram stain, AFB stain, cytology, amylase, cholesterol, triglycerides, special serologies, and aerobic, anaerobic, AFB and fungal cultures.

15. Are there any gross characteristics of the pleural fluid that help make the diagnosis even while you are doing the thoracentesis?

Observation	*Diagnosis*
Grossly bloody	In absence of trauma, malignancy is most likely cause
Whitish	Chyle, cholesterol, or a large number of leukocytes
Anchovy colored	Amebic liver abscess with rupture into pleural space
Black	*Aspergillus* involvement of pleura
Fluid of same color as enteral feedings	Feeding tube placement in pleural space
Putrid odor	Empyema
Pus	Empyema
Highly viscous	Malignant mesothelioma
Yellow-green	Rheumatoid pleurisy
Food particles	Esophageal rupture
Debris	Rheumatoid pleurisy
Ammonia odor	Urinothorax

From Kennedy L, Sahn SA: Noninvasive evaluation of the patient with a pleural effusion. Chest Surg Clin North Am 4:451–464, 1994, with permission.

16. When should a percutaneous pleural biopsy be considered?

In patients with an undiagnosed exudative effusion. The majority of these patients have either tuberculosis or a malignancy. Percutaneous pleural biopsy has a diagnostic yield of greater than 75% for tuberculosis. In general, malignant pleural effusions can be diagnosed with cytology studies so a percutaneous pleural biopsy does not significantly increase the diagnostic yield in these patients.

17. What are the contraindications to a percutaneous pleural biopsy?
- Uncooperative patient—ideally patients need to be able to sit upright, follow directions, and hold their breath on command.
- Inadequate pleural fluid in the pleural space—if the pleural space is obliterated, the biopsy needle is likely to enter the lung.
- Bleeding diathesis or coagulopathy—beware of patients with renal failure who may have a prolonged bleeding time, and do not perform the procedure in patients who are anticoagulated.

18. What are the risks of a percutaneous pleural biopsy?
The risks are similar to those from thoracentesis and include pneumothorax, hypotension, hemorrhage, infection, and air embolism. To minimize the likelihood of biopsying an intercostal vessel an adage to specifically remember when doing pleural biopsies is: **Never biopsy at 12 o'clock**—meaning do not biopsy directly above the biopsy needle entry site (the equivalent of the position of the hands of the clock at 12 o'clock) because you may catch the vessel with the biopsy needle.

19. How many percutaneous pleural biopsies do I need to take?
Usually 4–6 biopsies taken at a single site are adequate for diagnosis. Despite the fact that pleural metastases and tuberculosis lesions are scattered and patchy, the few studies available suggest that performing biopises at multiple sites at the same time does not improve the diagnostic yield of the procedure.

BIBLIOGRAPHY

1. Barbers R, Patel P: Thoracentesis made safe and simple. J Respir Dis 15:841–851, 1994.
2. Canto A, Rivas J, Saumench J, et al: Points to consider when choosing a biopsy method in cases of pleurisy of unknown origin. Chest 84:176–179, 1983.
3. Carney M, Ravin CE: Intercostal artery laceration during thoracentesis. Chest 75:520–522, 1979.
4. Collins TA, Sahn SA: Thoracentesis: Clinical value, complications, technical problems, and patient experience. Chest 91:817–822, 1987.
5. Grogan DR, Irwin RS: Thoracentesis. In Rippe JM, Irwin RS, Fink MP, et al (eds): Procedures and Techniques in Intensive Care Medicine. Boston, Little, Brown, 1996.
6. Kennedy L, Sahn SA: Noninvasive evaluation of the patient with a pleural effusion. Chest Surg Clin North Am 4:451–465, 1994.
7. Kohan JM, Poe RH, Israel RH, et al: Value of chest ultrasonography versus decubitus roentgenography for thoracentesis. Am Rev Respir Dis 133:1124–1126, 1986.
8. McElvein RB: Procedures in the evaluation of chest disease. Clin Chest Med 13:1–9, 1992.
9. Quigley RL: Thoracentesis and chest tube drainage. Crit Care Clin 11:111–126, 1995.
10. Sahn SA: The pleura. Am Rev Respir Dis 138:184–234, 1988.
11. Sokolowski JW, Burgher LW, Jones FL, et al: Guidelines for thoracentesis and needle biopsy of the pleura. Am Rev Respir Dis 140:257–258, 1989.

12. BRONCHOSCOPY

Udaya B.S. Prakash, M.D.

1. What is bronchoscopy?

Perhaps the most commonly performed invasive procedure in pulmonology, bronchoscopy permits visual examination of the tracheobronchial tree, including the ability to see the fifth to seventh segmental bronchi in most adults. It also permits collection of respiratory secretions, washings from the airways, and tissue specimens from the airways and lung. Bronchoscopy also enables therapeutic removal of retained secretions, mucous plugs, clots, and obstructing tumors or other lesions by means of special techniques.

2. How is bronchoscopy performed?

The two main types of bronchoscopes employed are the flexible (fiberoptic) or rigid types. The flexible scopes can be inserted through a nostril, mouth, or tracheostomy stoma, whereas the rigid scopes can only be inserted through the mouth or tracheostomy stoma. Although topical anesthesia permits use of either instrument, general anesthesia is commonly employed for rigid bronchoscopy in adults and children and for flexible bronchoscopy in most pediatric patients. The main indications for bronchoscopy are diagnostic and therapeutic, although many patients require both indications at one sitting.

3. Is there any role for rigid bronchoscopy in the 1990s?

Yes. The indications for rigid bronchoscopy have increased since the advent of newer bronchoscopic procedures. Rigid bronchoscopy is the procedure of choice in pediatric patients with airway foreign bodies. The success rate of rigid bronchoscopy in adults with airway foreign bodies is > 90%, whereas the flexible bronchoscopy is successful in 60%. Other indications for rigid bronchoscopy include bronchoscopic laser therapy, placement of tracheobronchial prostheses (stent), and dilatation of tracheobronchial strictures. Although these procedures can be performed with flexible scopes, the rigid instrument permits the procedure to be done more quickly and allows for better management of complications.

4. What are the common diagnostic indications for bronchoscopy?

Chest roentgenographic abnormalities
Suspicion of malignancy in the airways or lungs
Hilar, paratracheal, and subcarinal lymphadenopathy
Pulmonary infections
Uncommon diffuse lung diseases
Hemoptysis
Airway foreign bodies
Refractory cough
Suspected airway trauma
Clinical suspicion of airway lesions undetectable by x-rays

5. What are the common therapeutic indications for bronchoscopy?

Retained airway secretions
Mucous plugs, clots, and foreign bodies
Obstructing neoplasms and other lesions (stenosis, stricture) of airways that require
    laser and other therapies, dilatation, and placement of airway prostheses
Treatment of hemoptysis
Placement of endotracheal tube
Management of difficult airway

6. Are there any absolute contraindications?

Absolute contraindications include totally uncooperative patient, hemodynamic instability, new myocardial infarction, unstable angina, life-threatening arrhythmias, worsening asthma or status asthmaticus, rapidly worsening hypercarbia, and lack of appropriate instruments and personnel (including an insufficiently trained bronchoscopist).

7. Is severe hypoxemia a contraindication?

No. Indeed, many bronchoscopies are indicated to detect the etiology of diffuse lung infiltrates that are responsible for severe hypoxemia. The procedure can be performed with pre- and intraoperative supplemental oxygen therapy to maintain oxygen saturation (SO_2) above 90%.

8. Is the presence of a coagulopathy a contraindication?

No. Bronchoscopy to inspect airways and obtain bronchoalveolar lavage can be safely done in patients with significant bleeding disorders, including thrombocytopenia, elevated prothrombin time, and other coagulopathies. However, biopsy of airway lesions or pulmonary parenchyma and other interventional procedures are contraindicated.

9. Is mechanical ventilation a contraindication to bronchoscopy?

No. Critically ill patients and patients on mechanical ventilation frequently require flexible bronchoscopy for the removal of retained secretions, placement or change of endotracheal tubes, diagnostic bronchoalveolar lavage, bronchoscopic lung biopsy, and assessment of hemoptysis and other pulmonary problems. The addition of positive end-expiratory pressure breathing may increase the risk of complications, such as worsening hypoxia and pneumothorax. Complications from therapeutic bronchoscopy in critically ill patients have been mild (tachycardia, cardiac arrhythmias, hypoxia, and mild degrees of aspiration) and observed in < 10% of the flexible bronchoscopies performed.

10. Should every bronchoscopy patient undergo complete blood counts, serum chemistry, prothrombin time, platelet count, and other bleeding time tests before the procedure?

No. Unless the clinical history and physical examination indicate the presence of underlying coagulopathy or diseases that predispose to excessive bleeding (such as hepatic cirrhosis), routine screening for bleeding diathesis is not indicated. Platelet counts of < 60,000 µl and a serum creatinine of > 3.0 mg/dl are associated with post-biopsy bleeding rates of 15% and 40%, respectively.

11. Should arterial blood gas analysis be performed before bronchoscopy?

No. Neither blood gas analysis nor pulmonary function tests are necessary. Most patients should be monitored with pulse oximetry and electrocardiography during the procedure. Supplemental oxygen should be delivered to maintain SaO_2 above 90%.

12. Is premedication and sedation necessary in all patients?

No. However, premedication with an antisialogogue and a sedative (glycopyrrholate, 0.3 mg IV or IM, or atropine, 0.5 mg IM; and meperidine, 50 mg IM) and intraoperative sedation (commonly with midazolam 2–5 mg IV in adults) are recommended in most patients to allay anxiety and induce antegrade amnesia. The dosages of these drugs should be titrated on the basis of the underlying clinical problem, age, and weight of the patient. Patients who are uncooperative or those who require lengthy procedures may require general anesthesia.

13. Can sedatives replace the topical anesthetic agent?

No. Almost all patients who undergo flexible bronchoscopy should receive a topical anesthetic. The commonly used anesthetic is lidocaine (usually 4% solution sprayed "as you go" through the bronchoscope). The total dose must be monitored because elderly patients, those with congestive cardiac failure, and those with liver disease may develop toxicity (seizure, arrhythmias).

Benzocaine is sometimes used initially, but its excessive use (spray duration > 6 sec) may result in the development of toxic methemoglobinemia.

14. What are the indications for bronchoalveolar lavage (BAL)?

BAL is done by wedging the flexible bronchoscope tip as far as possible into a bronchus, instilling about 100 ml of normal saline into distal areas, and then suctioning the saline back through the bronchoscope into a trap. The BAL effluent is then analyzed. BAL has a high diagnostic rate (> 95%) in lung infection caused by *Pneumocystis carinii*, excellent diagnostic rate (> 75%) in lymphangitic metastasis, and good diagnostic rate (65–80%) in mycobacterial and fungal infections. It is helpful in the diagnosis of lymphangioleiomyomatosis, pulmonary eosinophilic granuloma, and pulmonary alveolar proteinosis. BAL is not helpful in establishing the diagnosis of idiopathic pulmonary fibrosis, sarcoidosis, and other diffuse lung diseases.

15. Is protected-specimen brush better than BAL in the diagnosis of bacterial infection of the lung?

No. Most recently published studies report that BAL is as good as protected-specimen brush to identify bacterial infection of the distal respiratory tract, as long as the culture result of > 10^4/ml is used as the cutoff. It is also important to perform the BAL procedure properly to obtain optimal results.

16. Should all patients with diffuse lung disease undergo bronchoscopic lung biopsy (BLB)?

No. Presently, high-resolution CT scanning of the lung can establish the diagnosis of idiopathic pulmonary fibrosis, lymphangioleiomyomatosis, pulmonary eosinophilic granuloma, and lymphangitic metastasis, provided the clinical features are compatible with these diagnoses. However, BLB may be necessary to confirm the diagnosis in lymphangitic metastasis. BLB is nonspecific in many diffuse lung diseases, such as idiopathic pulmonary fibrosis, lung infiltrates caused by rheumatologic diseases, and many pneumoconioses.

17. How many lung biopsies are necessary?

Many recommend at least 4 biopsy specimens to obtain a 95% diagnostic rate in pulmonary sarcoidosis. In lymphangitic metastasis, 3–4 biopsies may be necessary. In lung transplantation, more than 6 biopsies may be needed to diagnose rejection. Some believe that BLB is unnecessary (because of high diagnostic yield from BAL) to diagnose infection by *Pneumocystis carinii* in patients with AIDS, but the combination of BAL and BLB will yield the diagnosis in nearly all patients with this infection. Larger biopsy forceps yield more lung tissue without increasing the risk of bleeding or pneumothorax.

18. Is fluoroscopic guidance necessary to perform BLB?

Not necessarily. In diffuse lung disease, BLB can be obtained without fluoroscopic guidance, although fluoroscopic guidance significantly reduces the risk of pneumothorax. If a localized lesion (such as a lung nodule) is to be biopsied, fluoroscopic guidance is essential.

19. Can BLB be performed in patients on mechanical ventilator?

Yes. The risk of pneumothorax, however, is slightly increased, particularly if the patient is receiving positive end-expiratory pressure (PEEP) breathing. Prior to biopsy, PEEP should be discontinued and the patient taken off the ventilator and oxygenated with "hand-bagging." Cough suppression is also important. Reinstitution of PEEP should be withheld for at least 30 minutes after BLB.

20. Can BLB be performed in a patient with thrombocytopenia?

Yes, as long as the platelet count is > 60,000/μl. If the platelet count is lower, then 4–6 units of platelets should be transfused 30–45 min before BLB. In patients taking warfarin (Coumarin),

BLB should be avoided if the INR is $\geq$ 1.5. BLB is not contraindicated if the patient is taking aspirin (< 325 mg/d). These recommendations also apply to biopsy of endobronchial lesions.

21. Is it necessary to instill epinephrine prior to BLB or endobronchial biopsy?

No. Not all endobronchial tumors bleed after biopsy, and the same observation applies to BLB. In most patients, topical application of epinephrine (usually 1:10,000 strength in 3–4 aliquots of 1.0 ml) is of minimal help. If bleeding occurs after BLB, wedging of the broncho-scope tip into the bleeding segment and slow instillation of iced normal saline (5–8 ml) usually retards the rate of bleeding. Epinephrine spray directed at the bleeding spot in a biopsied endo-bronchial lesion occasionally slows the rate of bleeding. Biopsy of suspected endobronchial car-cinoid is not contraindicated.

22. What are palliative bronchoscopic therapies?

These are treatments aimed at providing symptomatic relief in patients with advanced major airway obstruction caused by unresectable or otherwise untreatable tumors. The treatments in-clude bronchoscopic dilatation of a narrowed airway, laser ablation of the tumor, cryotherapy, electrocautery, brachytherapy (intraluminal irradiation), phototherapy, and placement of airway prostheses. Benign strictures can sometimes be treated using a dilatation technique (with balloon or rigid bronchoscope) or stent therapy.

23. Are tracheobronchial prostheses (stents) indicated in patients with airway collapse caused by chronic obstructive pulmonary disease (COPD)?

No. The collapse of the posterior membranous portion of the tracheobronchial tree including distal airways is typical in advanced COPD. Airway stents will not help patients with COPD be-cause the distal airways cannot be stented. Airway stents are indicated in patients with obstruct-ing lesions (usually tumors) of the trachea and mainstem bronchi. Stent placement into bronchi at the lobar and distal levels is difficult and impractical.

24. What are the major complications of tracheobronchial stent placement?

Migration proximally or distally; plugging of the stent lumen by thick mucous plugs result-ing in increased respiratory distress and postobstructive atelectasis or pneumonia; localized necrosis of the airway; growth of granulation tissue; and rarely, formation of fistula between the airway and esophagus or mediastinum.

25. What are the major complications of bronchoscopy?

The overall rate of complications with bronchoscopy is low; < 3% of complications involve major morbidity. Fever can develop after bronchoscopy in 10–20% of patients, but septicemia is generally absent. Other complications include severe bronchospasm, increased dyspnea, subcuta-neous or mediastinal emphysema, sinusitis, and nasal bleeding. Instillation of large volumes of saline during BAL can result in a greater decrease in oxygen saturation. Bronchoscopic lung biopsy can lead to bleeding and pneumothorax. Factors that increase the risk of hemorrhagic complications include thrombocytopenia and uremia. Immunocompromised patients with diffuse pulmonary infiltrates appear to be at high risk for bleeding.

BIBLIOGRAPHY

1. Brutinel WM, Cortese DA, Edell ES, et al: Complications of Nd:YAG laser therapy [editorial]. Chest 94:902–903, 1988.
2. Cassadori A, Di Perri G, Todescgini G, et al: Transbronchial biopsy in the diagnosis of pulmonary infil-trates in immunocompromised patients. Chest 107:101–106, 1995.
3. Greig JH, Cooper SM, Kasimbazi HJN, et al: Sedation for fibre optic bronchoscopy. Respir Med 89:53–56, 1995.

4. Hara K, Prakash UBS: Fiberoptic bronchoscopy in the evaluation of acute chest and upper airway trauma. Chest 96:627–630, 1989.

5. Kollef MH, Bock KR, Richards RD, Hearns ML: The safety and diagnostic accuracy of minibronchoalveolar lavage in patients with suspected ventilator-associated pneumonia. Ann Intern Med 122:743–748, 1995.

6. Limper AH, Prakash UBS: Tracheobronchial foreign bodies in adults. Ann Intern Med 112:604–609, 1990.

7. Matsushima Y, Jones RL, King EG, et al: Alterations in pulmonary mechanics and gas exchange during routine fiberoptic bronchoscopy. Chest 86:184–188, 1984.

8. Olopade CO, Prakash UBS: Bronchoscopy in the critical care unit. Mayo Clin Proc 64:1255–1263, 1989.

9. Prakash UBS: Does the bronchoscope propagate infection? Chest 104:552–559, 1993.

10. Prakash UBS (ed): Bronchoscopy. New York, Raven Press, 1994, pp 111–133.

11. Prakash UBS, Offord KP, Stubbs SE: Bronchoscopy in North America: The ACCP Survey. Chest 100: 1668–1675, 1991.

12. Prakash UBS, Utz JP: Bronchoscopic lung biopsy. In Wang KP, Mehta AC (eds): Flexible Bronchoscopy. Cambridge, MA, Blackwell Scientific, 1995, p 119.

13. Pue CA, Pacht ER: Complications of fiberoptic bronchoscopy at a university hospital. Chest 107: 430–432, 1995.

14. Ricou B, Grandini S, Nicod L, et al: Adult and paediatric size bronchoscopes for bronchoalveolar lavage in mechanically ventilated patients: Yield and side effects. Thorax 50:290–293, 1995.

15. Roethe RA, Fuller PB, Byrd RB, et al: Transbronchoscopic lung biopsy in sarcoidosis. Chest 77:400, 1980.

16. Tape TG, Bank LL, Wigton RS: Procedural skills of practicing pulmonologists: A national survey of 1,000 members of the American College of Physicians. Am J Respir Crit Care Med 151:282–287, 1995.

13. CHEST TUBES

David Ost, M.D., and Thomas Corbridge, M.D.

1. What are the indications for placement of a chest tube?

The main indications for chest tube placement are pneumothorax, hemothorax, symptomatic pleural effusion, empyema, complicated parapneumonic effusion, sclerosis of recurrent malignant effusions, and chylothorax. The decision to place a chest tube in a specific patient must be individualized based on the particulars of the case and a risk-benefit analysis.

2. Is a chest tube always required for pneumothorax?

No. If the pneumothorax is less than 20% of lung volume on a radiograph of the chest and the patient is hemodynamically stable, a strategy of watchful waiting may be appropriate, provided that serial radiographs can be done and that, if necessary, a chest tube can be placed in a timely fashion. If the pneumothorax is large or if the patient is unstable, requires subsequent mechanical ventilation, or is scheduled for general anesthesia, a chest tube should be placed. Similarly, if serial radiographs cannot be obtained or if it is not certain that the patient can be closely followed, chest tube placement should be considered.

3. Under what circumstances should a patient with pleural effusion have a chest tube?

Most pleural effusions can be managed with thoracentesis and treatment of the underlying problem. Often the effusion will not recur after a single thoracentesis. Chest tubes are required for effusions that cause symptomatic respiratory or hemodynamic compromise, empyemas, complicated parapneumonic effusions, and persistent malignant effusions that require sclerotherapy.

4. What size chest tube should be used?

Chest tubes size varies from 12 to 42 Fr. The choice of size is determined by the indication for chest tube placement: for drainage of pleural fluid of low viscosity, a 28-Fr tube is generally adequate; for higher viscosity fluids, such as those found in empyema, a 32-Fr or larger tube is preferred. Chest tubes for patients who have sustained trauma such as pneumothorax, hemothorax, or hemopneumothorax should be even larger (36–40 Fr). Smaller tubes, in the range of 12–22 Fr, are adequate for treatment of spontaneous pneumothorax.

5. Where should a chest tube be placed?

The site of entry is chosen by review of the chest radiograph and percussion of the level of pleural fluid if present. Usually the fifth or sixth interspace along the anterior axillary line anterior to the superior iliac crest and anterior to the latissimus dorsi muscle is a good choice. Only rarely should a chest tube be placed lower than the ninth interspace. In cases of pneumothorax, another option is the second intercostal space at the midclavicular line, but penetration of breast tissue and muscle make this approach more difficult. Care must be taken with the anterior approach to avoid injuring the internal mammary artery, which lies just medial to the proper insertion site.

6. Describe insertion of the chest tube.

Hemodynamically stable patients should be premedicated with narcotics and a sedative hypnotic. A drainage system should be ready so that the chest tube can be attached to suction as soon as it is in place. The patient is placed in the supine position with the involved side elevated, supported by pillows or towels, and the arms flexed overhead. The site of entry is sterilely prepared and draped. The skin and chest wall are infiltrated with 1–2% lidocaine, then the periosteum, subcutaneous tissue, and parietal pleura are infiltrated. As much as 30–40 ml of 1% lidocaine may be necessary. Aspiration of pleural fluid or air confirms entry into the pleural space. After adequate local anesthesia, a skin incision of approximately 3 cm is made with a scalpel over the rib extending into the subcutaneous tissues. The subcutaneous tissue over the superior aspect of the rib is bluntly dissected with a large clamp and an opening and spreading maneuver; care is taken to avoid the neurovascular bundle of the adjacent rib. Considerable force may be required to "pop through" the parietal pleura into the pleural space. Once this subcutaneous tunnel to the pleural space is established, the index finger is used to explore the pleural space and to identify the lung and any adhesions. Thin adhesions can be broken up in this way, although care must be taken not to tear visceral pleura and injure lung parenchyma. After exploration, a medium clamp is used to direct the chest tube into position. For pneumothorax the chest tube should be directed superiorly toward the apex of the lung. For drainage of fluid the tube should be directed into the posterior basilar area. The tube should be secured with 2-0 silk suture material using a mattress stitch and the insertion site should be covered with Vaseline gauze and a pressure dressing. All connections from the chest tube to the suction device should be carefully taped to avoid accidental disconnection. A chest radiograph should be obtained immediately to confirm tube position and to make sure that all side holes of the chest tube are within the pleural space.

7. What types of drainage devices are available and how do they work?

The most commonly used drainage systems are commercially available compartmentalized versions of the three-bottle chest tube system. The three compartments are a collection chamber, a water seal chamber, and a suction control chamber. The collection chamber traps pleural fluid or blood. The water seal chamber acts as a one-way valve, insuring that air does not return to the pleural space. The suction control chamber uses the height of the fluid in the chamber to control the amount of negative pressure. If the suction control chamber has water that is 20 cm high, then negative 20 cm of water pressure will be generated. By using the height of the fluid to control the amount of suction applied, a constant level of negative pressure can be generated regardless of the type and strength of the vacuum source.

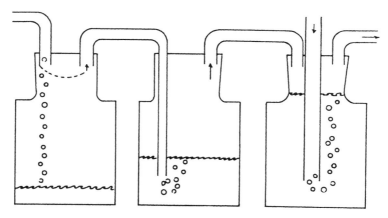

Three-bottle chest tube drainage system, consisting of (from **left to right**) collection chamber, water seal chamber, and suction control chamber. (From Iberti TJ, Stern PM: Chest tube thoracostomy. Crit Care Clin 8:883, 1992; with permission.)

8. How are function and patency of the chest tube confirmed?

In pleural effusion, collection of pleural fluid confirms proper chest tube position. In pneumothorax, condensation of air on the tube when the patient breathes helps to confirm adequate placement. After chest tube placement, the quantity and quality of drainage should be carefully documented and marked on the collection chamber. Tube function should be assessed daily by turning off the wall suction and observing the level of water in the water seal chamber. With the suction off, this level should fluctuate with patient respiration, indicating that the tube is patent and communicating with the pleural space. If the level in the water seal chamber does not fluctuate with respiration, there is an obstruction somewhere between the tube and the water seal chamber. The tube should be examined carefully to make sure that it is not twisted or kinked. Saline irrigation, tube "milking," or stripping can also be helpful if there is debris obstructing the tube. If the tube is nonfunctional (i.e., there is no variation in the water seal chamber) and cannot be cleared, it should be removed to decrease the chance of local infection.

9. What is an air leak?

When air bubbles appear through the water seal chamber, air is entering the chest tube system. It may be coming from within the body (i.e., pneumothorax) or from outside the body (i.e., a loose connection in the tubing). The site of the leak can be determined by temporarily clamping the chest tube where it enters the chest and observing the water seal chamber. If the leak continues, then the leak is located outside the body and all connections and tubing should be checked. If the leak stops upon clamping, the source of air is intrapleural, assuming the side holes are still within the pleural space and not within or outside of the chest wall, where they can suck air from outside the body.

10. How and when should a chest tube be removed?

Chest tubes should be considered for removal once drainage from the tube is minimal (less than 150 ml/24 hours). If the chest tube was placed for pneumothorax, the lung should be fully reexpanded and free of air leak for the previous 24 hours. After the decision to remove the tube is made, suction is discontinued and the tube is placed to water seal for up to 24 hours. The tube may then be clamped for several hours to ensure patient stability prior to removal. For removal of the chest tube, the patient is placed in the lateral decubitus position with the chest tube side up. The dressings and sutures around the chest tube are removed and the patient is told to take a deep inspiration. With the patient holding his or her breath or exhaling slowly from a maximal inspiration, the chest tube is rapidly pulled out in one smooth motion. The chest tube entry site is sutured and an occlusive dressing is reapplied. After the tube is removed, a follow-up chest radiograph should be obtained so that the pleural space can be evaluated. Often a small pneumothorax is present after removal of the chest tube. If the patient is stable, small pneumothoraces usually can be followed with close observation.

11. When should a chest tube be placed for sclerotherapy of malignant pleural effusion?

Approximately 50% of all pleural effusions are caused by malignancy, and the most common malignant sources of effusion are lung cancer, breast cancer, and lymphoma. Many of these patients have symptomatic effusions, leading to dyspnea, cough, and chest pain. Management consists of therapeutic thoracentesis followed by treatment of the underlying malignancy, usually with systemic chemotherapy. When malignant effusions reaccumulate despite therapy and are symptomatic, tube thoracostomy with sclerotherapy is the treatment of choice. After accumulated fluid is drained, an attempt is made to obliterate the pleural space by fusing the parietal and visceral pleurae (pleurodesis) by purposefully inducing an inflammatory response. A variety of sclerosing agents can be introduced through the chest tube to induce inflammation and pleurodesis. Of these agents, tetracycline (which is no longer available), doxycycline, talc, and bleomycin are the best studied.

12. What are the advantages and disadvantages of the various sclerosing agents?

Tetracycline was the sclerosing agent of choice for many years because of its low cost, high efficacy, and low systemic toxicity. With a dose of 15 mg per kg, success rates of up to 70% were reported for malignant effusions. The most common side effects were severe pain and fever. When tetracycline became unavailable, many physicians switched to the related drug **doxycycline**. Administration of 500 mg of doxycycline in 30 ml of saline has been shown to be effective in the treatment of malignant pleural effusions, with response rates of 61–88%.

Talc (hydrous magnesium silicate), which was first used in the 1950s for pleurodesis, must be sterilized and free of asbestos. Doses of talc for pleurodesis vary from study to study, ranging from 1 to 10 g. Talc can be instilled into the pleural space either as a slurry (through the chest tube) or poudrage (through a thoracoscope or at the time of thoracotomy). Response rates of up to 90% have been reported in the treatment of malignant effusions. The most common side effects encountered are severe pain, fever, dyspnea, granulomatous pneumonitis, and, rarely, acute respiratory distress syndrome (ARDS). ARDS has been reported to occur up to three days after talc pleurodesis, so monitoring of the patient for respiratory compromise for up to 72 hours after administration is recommended. The vigorous inflammatory response and pleural adhesions induced by talc significantly increase the risk of complications if thoracic surgical intervention later becomes necessary, perhaps making this agent less attractive than other agents (such as doxycycline) in young individuals, particularly smokers.

A variety of **cytotoxic agents** have been used as sclerosing agents. These agents are effective because they generate an inflammatory response, not because they have antineoplastic activity. Potential side effects from systemic absorption of these agents warrant consideration, since many patients receive concurrent systemic chemotherapy and are immunosuppressed. Cytotoxic agents that have been studied include nitrogen mustard (mechlorethamine), mitoxantrone, thiotepa, doxorubicin, fluorouracil (5-FU), cytarabine with cisplatin, etoposide, and bleomycin. Nitrogen mustard has a variable response rate and considerable side effects. Mitoxantrone has moderate efficacy but has been associated with leukopenia and is not widely used. Thiotepa, doxorubicin, cytarabine with cisplatin, etoposide, and 5-FU all have poor response rates and are not used clinically. The best studied and most often used agent is bleomycin. Bleomycin achieves response rates ranging from 62 to 84%. Bleomycin has been been reported to offer efficacy equal or superior to that of tetracycline. Side effects include pain, fever, and mild nausea and vomiting. Despite a 45% systemic absorption rate, bleomycin pleurodesis has not been associated with bone marrow suppression or pulmonary toxicity.

13. Which parapneumonic effusions require chest tube drainage?

The incidence of pleural effusion in pneumonia (parapneumonic effusions) varies between 36 and 57% of cases. These effusions may be uncomplicated and resolve spontaneously with antibiotics, or they may become complicated effusions, requiring chest tube placement for adequate drainage of the pleural space. Unfortunately, it is not possible to differentiate a complicated parapneumonic effusion from an uncomplicated effusion without pleural fluid analysis. Clinical criteria such as age, white blood cell count, temperature, pleuritic chest pain, and extent of pneumonia are not sufficient to separate uncomplicated from complicated parapneumonic effusions. Pleural fluid characteristics that are useful in identifying complicated effusions are pH, glucose, and lactate dehydrogenase (LDH). Generally, a parapneumonic effusion with pH of 7.30 or more, a glucose level above 60 mg/dl, and an LDH level less than 1000 U/L can be managed with antibiotics alone. If pus is aspirated at the time of thoracentesis or if the Gram stain of nonpurulent fluid reveals bacteria, prompt chest tube placement is indicated. Nonpurulent effusions with a negative Gram stain but with pH less than 7.10, a glucose level less than 40 mg per dl, or an LDH level more than 1000 U/L also should have chest tube drainage. For patients with a pleural fluid pH between 7.10 and 7.30, antibiotics, careful observation, and repeat pleural fluid analysis are indicated. If the patient fails to improve with antibiotics and repeat pleural fluid analysis reveals a decrease in pH, or if the effusion loculates, chest tube placement should be considered.

14. What is the role of thrombolytic agents in treatment of pleural space infections?

The American Thoracic Society described three stages of empyema development. In stage I, the exudative phase, thin pleural fluid with a low cellular content develops. This phase lasts briefly, as short as 24 hours, during which time the lung is readily reexpandable with chest tube drainage.

In stage II, the fibrinopurulent stage, a viscous pleural fluid with high cellular content develops, often with pus and fibrin in the pleural space. During this period there is a tendency for loculations to develop and fibrin deposition to limit reexpansion of the lung. Loculations in stage II limit adequate drainage of the pleural space, increasing the risk of persistent infection. If loculations are not adequately drained, mortality from sepsis increases, as does the need for late surgical decortication. Approaches to the problem of persistent loculated pleural effusions include early decortication, thoracoscopy, placement of additional chest tubes under CT or ultrasound guidance, and the use of intrapleural fibrinolytic agents. Streptokinase, a purified enzyme derived from group C β-hemolytic streptococci, converts plasminogen to the proteolytic enzyme plasmin. Plasmin degrades fibrin clots and fibrinogen. Urokinase is a direct activator of plasminogen, which is produced by the kidney. Both agents, when introduced into the pleural space, break down fibrin bands responsible for loculations. Various series using either streptokinase or urokinase for loculated effusions have reported success rate of 67 to 92%. Side effects with intrapleural fibrinolytics include fever, pleural pain, and development of specific immunoglobulin G antistreptokinase antibodies when streptokinase is used. A systemic fibrinolytic effect usually is not seen with intrapleural streptokinase or urokinase. Although there are no prospective studies comparing intrapleural fibrinolytic therapy with other treatment options, the excellent results reported in various series support its consideration as an effective adjunct to facilitate pleural space drainage in patients with loculated pleural effusions.

If the pleural space is not adequately drained, the patient is at risk of developing a stage III empyema characterized by a thick fibrinous membrane or "peel" that prevents complete lung expansion and may lead to a permanent restrictive defect.

15. What are the complications associated with chest tube placement?

Complications of chest tube placement include improper positioning, bleeding, nerve damage, injury to the diaphragm or lung, pain, mechanical problems, and reexpansion pulmonary edema.

When a chest tube is placed too distal within the thorax, pain or local injury from blunt trauma may result. Chest tubes improperly placed in the fissure will not adequately drain the pleural space, and a chest tube that is not inserted deeply enough may result in an air leak or sub-cutaneous emphysema if the most proximal hole of the chest tube is located outside of the pleural space.

Bleeding may occur at the incision site or from laceration of an intercostal artery or vein, or a pulmonary artery or vein. Incisional bleeding is usually easily controlled with direct pressure. Laceration of an intercostal or pulmonary blood vessel can be severe and may require surgical repair.

The chance of intercostal nerve damage is lessened by careful avoidance of the subcostal groove of the superior rib. Damage to the long thoracic nerve is also a problem; if it occurs, in-nervation of the serratus anterior may be lost, with a resultant "winged" scapula. This injury is best avoided by careful use of blunt dissection of the subcutaneous tissue. Diaphragmatic injury and injury to abdominal organs may result from chest tube placement. Conditions that result in high diaphragmatic position (including previous thoracotomy, intraabdominal injury, and supine positioning) increase the patient's risk of injury to the diaphragm or other organs. Careful prepa-ration with review of the chest radiograph and exploration of the pleural space with a finger before chest tube insertion minimize these risks.

Pain is a common problem after chest tube insertion and should be managed aggressively to avoid atelectasis and pneumonia due to splinting. Narcotics may be necessary to control pain as-sociated with chest tube insertion. Intercostal nerve blocks and intrapleural lidocaine may also be useful. Incentive spirometry helps prevent atelectasis.

Mechanical problems may occur from kinking of the chest tube or obstruction with viscous fluid or blood clots. These problems are minimized by use of an appropriately sized chest tube and careful, regular examination of the tubing and connections.

Reexpansion pulmonary edema occurs after rapid evacuation of large chronic pleural effu-sions. The risk of this complication is decreased by slow evacuation of fluid and avoidance of ex-cessively negative pleural pressure (more negative than -20 cm H_2O) during fluid evacuation. This condition is usually self-limited and responds well to conservative management with oxygen and diuresis.

BIBLIOGRAPHY

1. Klein JS, Schultz S, Heffner JE: Interventional radiology of the chest: Image-guided percutaneous drainage of pleural effusions, lung abscess, and pneumothorax. Am J Roentgenol 164:581–588, 1995.
2. Light RW: Management of spontaneous pneumothorax. Am Rev Respir Dis 148:245–248, 1993.
3. Lynch TJ: Management of malignant pleural effusions. Chest 103:385S–389S, 1993.
4. Quigley RL: Thoracentesis and chest tube drainage. Crit Care Clin 11:111–126, 1995.
5. Robinson LA, Moulton AL, Fleming WH, et al: Intrapleural fibrinolytic treatment of multiloculated tho-racic empyemas. Ann Thorac Surg 57:803–814, 1994.
6. Sahn SA: Management of complicated parapneumonic effusions. Am Rev Respir Dis 148:813–817, 1993.
7. Sahn SA: The pleura. Am Rev Respir Dis 138:184–234, 1988.
8. Seaton KG, Patz EF Jr, Goodman PC: Palliative treatment of malignant pleural effusions: Value of small bore thoracostomy and doxycycline sclerotherapy. Am J Roentgenol 164:589–591, 1995.
9. Windsor P, Como JA, Winsdor KS: Sclerotherapy for malignant pleural effusions: Alternatives to tetracy-cline. South Med J 87:709–714, 1994.

14. THE PULMONARY ARTERY CATHETER

Philip J. Fracica, M.D.

1. What are the important design characteristics of a pulmonary artery catheter?

Pulmonary artery (PA) catheters are designed for percutaneous insertion into the central vasculature to allow measurement of intravascular pressures, collection of PA blood samples, placement of temporary right ventricular pacemakers, determination of cardiac output, and continuous measurement of mixed venous hemoglobin oxygen saturation (MVO_2). The catheter is 100 cm long and 7–8 Fr in diameter with an inflatable balloon 1–2 mm from the distal end. Hash marks are placed from the catheter tip at 10-cm intervals to assist insertion.

The most commonly used PA catheter has four separate ports, each of which has a different clinical purpose. These quadruple-lumen PA catheters have a distal port at the catheter tip, a proximal port 30 cm proximal to the tip, a lumen for inflation of the distal balloon, and a lumen for the leads to a thermistor, which is located 4 cm proximal to the tip and used for determination of cardiac output. Other catheter designs have additional lumens used for infusion of fluids, cardiac pacing, and optical fiber monitoring of MVO_2. PA catheters are also available without the thermistor or proximal port.

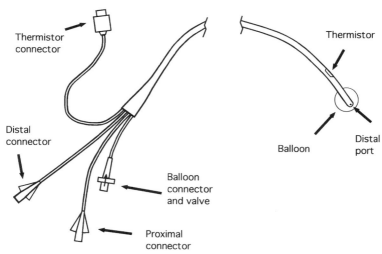

Schematic depiction of the proximal and distal ends of a PA catheter. The proximal port, which is 30 cm from the distal end, is not depicted.

2. How is a PA catheter inserted?

The PA catheter most commonly is placed percutaneously via the internal jugular, subclavian, or femoral vein by a modified Seldinger technique. The vessel is cannulated with a needle through which a flexible wire is inserted into the vein. The needle is removed and an introducer is placed over the wire. After the guide wire is withdrawn, the PA catheter is passed through the introducer approximately 15 cm into the central venous circulation.

The distal balloon is then inflated, and the PA catheter tip is "floated," i.e., carried by blood flow through the right cardiac chambers into the PA. The operator observes the characteristic pressure waveforms measured from the distal port to monitor the progress of the catheter through the right ventricle (RV) and into position within the PA. Familiarity with the appearance of right atrial (RA), RV, PA, and PA occlusion (PAO) waveforms assists catheter insertion.

While advancing the catheter, the operator should observe how much of the catheter has been inserted by noting the 10 cm hash marks at the venous puncture site. An RA waveform is usually noted when the PA catheter has been inserted 20–30 cm into the vein. An RV waveform occurs at 30–40 cm, a PA waveform at 40–50 cm, and PAO tracing at 50–60 cm. A continuous paper strip printout of the pressure tracings should be obtained while the catheter is floated to document correct placement and to record pressures within the RV as the catheter passes through the heart.

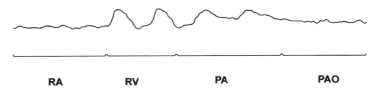

RA   **RV**   **PA**   **PAO**

Typical waveforms obtained during passage of a PA catheter.

3. What are the indications for a PA catheter?

Most clinicians consider inserting a PA catheter in patients with systemic hypotension, shock, or pulmonary edema. The PA catheter is particularly valuable when pulmonary edema is associated with oliguria. In all of these conditions, rapid optimization of intravascular volume and left ventricular preload is essential. Additional factors that influence the decision to place a PA catheter include the severity of the patient's physiologic dysfunction, the degree of uncertainty about intravascular volume, the response to initial therapy, and the risks of catheter placement in the individual patient. PA catheters are also inserted to determine the cause of unexplained lactic acidosis, pulmonary hypertension, right heart failure, and acute mitral insufficiency. Suspected cardiac tamponade and intracardiac septal defects are additional indications.

4. What intravascular pressures can be measured by a PA catheter?

PA pressure. The pressure transducer attached to the distal port allows monitoring of the PA pressure tracing, which is used to determine PA systolic (P_{PAS}), PA diastolic (P_{PAD}), and mean PA (P_{PA}) pressures. Comparison of PA pressure with PA occlusion pressure can provide insight into the mechanism of pulmonary hypertension.

Central venous pressure (P_{CV}). The pressure transducer attached to the proximal port allows monitoring of the intravascular pressure just proximal to the right atrium.

PA occlusion pressure (P_{PAO}). When the distal balloon is inflated, the catheter occludes a branch of the PA and blood flow stops beyond the catheter tip. The resulting static column of blood allows equalization of pressure from the distal lumen of the catheter to a region of the pulmonary veins referred to as the *j point*. The j point represents the anatomic junction of the pulmonary vein occluded by the PA catheter and other pulmonary veins that are not cannulated; it is the point where blood continues to flow. The pressure measured from the tip of the catheter during balloon inflation is the P_{PAO} and represents the pressure at the j point. From the j point, blood flows into the main pulmonary veins, left atrium, and left ventricle. If vascular resistance distal to the j point is low (as is normally the case), P_{PAO} will closely approximate left ventricular end diastolic pressure. Increased resistance to flow at any point distal to the j point, as occurs with mitral stenosis, will result in the P_{PAO} overestimating left ventricular end diastolic pressure.

5. What else can a PA catheter measure?

Cardiac output. The thermistor attached to some PA catheters is used to calculate cardiac output (CO) by thermodilution methods. The thermistor measures pericatheter fluid temperature and provides continuous monitoring of PA blood temperature, also termed *core temperature*. To calculate cardiac output, a bolus of fluid cooler than blood temperature is injected through the proximal port. This cool injectate causes a transient reduction in blood temperature measured at the thermistor. The duration of the temperature drop makes possible determination of a temperature-time curve. If blood flow past the catheter is brisk (high CO), the temperature rapidly returns to baseline. If blood flow is sluggish (low CO), blood temperature returns more gradually. CO can be calculated by integration of the area under the temperature-time curve and factoring in of injectate temperature and catheter callibration constants. Thermodilution CO is based on a theoretical model that assumes constant unidirectional blood flow. In patients with pulmonary or tricuspid valve regurgitation, the thermal tracer may recross the thermistor, resulting in an underestimation of true CO.

Mixed venous blood oxygen (MVO_2). MVO_2, which is a marker for adequacy of tissue oxygenation, also can be measured by PA catheter. Systemic capillary beds provide a large surface area for efficient gas exchange between circulating capillary blood and perfused tissues. By the time blood leaves a systemic capillary bed, its partial pressure of oxygen has equilibrated with the oxygen tension in pericapillary tissue. Inadequate oxygen supply results in a low pericapillary oxygen tension and increased tissue extraction of blood oxygen, leaving a low oxygen content in postcapillary venous blood. Measurement of venous oxygen saturation at a point where mixing of venous effluents from various organs has occurred theoretically provides a global marker for the adequacy of total body tissue oxygenation. Blood sampled from the pulmonary artery through the distal port of the PA catheter provides the best measure of mixed venous blood. MVO_2 can be expressed as partial pressure ($P\bar{v}O_2$), hemoglobin saturation ($S\bar{v}O_2$), or blood oxygen content ($C\bar{v}O_2$). $C\bar{v}O_2$ is a measure of the quantity of oxygen (in ml) dissolved in blood and is calculated by the following equation:

$$C\bar{v}O_2 = Hb \text{ (g/100 cc blood)} \times 1.39 \text{(ml } O_2\text{/g Hb)} \times S\bar{v}O_2 + 0.0031 \text{ (ml } O_2\text{/torr)} \times P\bar{v}O_2 \text{ (torr)}$$

where Hb = hemoglobin.

6. How can other physiologic variables be derived from measurement of MVO_2?

Arterial oxygen content (CaO_2) can be calculated by substituting PaO_2 and SaO_2 in the equation shown in question 5. Subtracting $S\bar{v}O_2$ from CaO_2 yields the amount of oxygen removed by tissues per volume of blood moving through the capillaries from the arterial to venous system. This value is the **arterial-venous oxygen content difference**, $C(a-\bar{v})O_2$. $C(a-\bar{v})O_2$ increases when the tissue is more avidly extracting oxygen. Multiplying the $C(a-\bar{v})O_2$ by the cardiac output yields the **oxygen consumption** of the body (in ml oxygen) per unit of time (minutes), abbreviated $\dot{V}O_2$. Values such as the $C(a-\bar{v})O_2$ are not directly measured by the PA catheter and are referred to as *derived* or *calculated* data. Other derived data obtained from PA catheter measurements are:

Cardiac index (CI)
Stroke volume (SV)
Stroke volume index (SVI)
Systemic vascular resistance (SVR)
Systemic vascular resistance index (SVRI)
Pulmonary vascular resistance (PVR)
Pulmonary vascular resistance index (PVRI)
Left ventricular stroke work index (LVSWI)
Right ventricular stroke work index (RVSWI)
Oxygen delivery (DO_2)
Oxygen extraction ratio (O_2ER)
Pulmonary shunt (Qs/QT)

7. What is the relationship between measured P_{PAO} and the actual pressure within the pulmonary capillaries?

Blood flow across the pulmonary vasculature is driven by the hydrostatic pressure gradient between the PA pressure and the pulmonary venous pressure, which can be measured at the j point by determination of P_{PAO}. The value for pulmonary capillary pressure, therefore should lie between the measured P_{PA} ("precapillary" pressure) and P_{PAO} ("postcapillary" pressure at the j point). The total resistance to flow across the pulmonary circulation can be calculated using the cardiac output and the P_{PA}-P_{PAO} pressure gradient. If all of the calculated resistance occurred on the arterial side of the capillaries, no pressure gradient would exist between the capillaries and j point; thus, P_{PAO} would accurately reflect capillary pressure. This is not the case, however; actual capillary pressure almost always exceeds P_{PAO}. In normal individuals approximately 40% of the drop in pressure from the PA to the j point occurs within the pulmonary veins. This allows the following estimation of pulmonary capillary pressure (P_{PC}):

$$P_{PC} = P_{PAO} + 0.4 \times (\text{mean } P_{PA}\text{-}P_{PAO})$$

Although this method is useful, the distribution of vascular resistance between the venous and arterial sides may be quite different in patients with structural and functional abnormalities of the lungs.

Pulmonary capillary pressure may be more accurately assessed based on analysis of the waveform during balloon inflation and transition of the monitored waveform from P_{PA} to P_{PAO}. This approach is based on an understanding of what happens to pressures and flows during balloon inflation. The drop in pressure is biphasic. Initially, pressures drops rapidly, probably representing rapid pressure equilibration across the arterial resistance. Pressure then falls more gradually toward the PPAO, probably representing equilibration across the venous resistance. The pressure at the inflection point between the rapid and slow phases of pressure decline after balloon inflation should equal pulmonary capillary pressure. Although this method has been shown to be accurate in careful research studies using experimental animals and humans, it is often difficult to use at the bedside.

8. Do pressures within the airways and alveoli affect measured values for P_{PAO}?

Phasic swings in alveolar and airway pressures generated during respiration are transmitted to intrathoracic vasculature causing an artifact in the pressures measured by a PA catheter. During spontaneous breathing, a phasic inspiratory decrease in intrathoracic pressure occurs that is associated with dips in P_{CV}, P_{PA}, and P_{PAO}. During positive pressure breathing in patients undergoing mechanical ventilation, inspiration is associated with phasic increases in intrathoracic pressure and PA catheter pressure. The ideal time in the respiratory cycle to measure vascular pressures is at end expiration, which is the point at which lung volumes most closely approximate functional residual capacity (FRC). FRC reflects a neutral or "rest" position of the thorax at which the contractile properties of the lungs are at equilibrium with the expansile properties of the chest wall. This equilibrium indicates that no superimposed positive or negative airway pressures exist to affect PA catheter pressure measurements.

9. Does PEEP affect the accuracy of PA catheter pressure measurements?

The application of positive end-expiratory pressure (PEEP) or the development of intrinsic PEEP increases intrathoracic pressure and artifactually raises the vascular pressures measured by a PA catheter. The artifact, however, is not clinically important until PEEP values increase above 10 cm H_2O. Measured PA catheter pressures can be adjusted toward their true values by placement of a balloon-tipped catheter into the esophagus for the determination of intraesophageal pressure. Because the esophagus is a relatively compliant structure, intraesophageal pressure approximates intrathoracic pressure, which can be used to correct measured PA catheter pressures. In actual clinical practice, however, esophageal balloons are not commonly used. A "rule of thumb" provides an estimate of true P_{PAO} adjusted for PEEP levels above 10 cm H_2O:

$$\text{Corrected } P_{PAO} = \text{measured } P_{PAO} - 0.5 \times (\text{PEEP-10})/1.36$$

The constant 1.36 converts the PEEP units of cm H_2O into mmHg, which are the units for the other terms in the equation.

10. What is the significance of West zones in measuring PA pressures?

In order for the measured P_{PAO} to equal pulmonary venous j point pressure, inflation of the PA catheter balloon must produce an unbroken column of static blood between the catheter tip and the pulmonary venous system. For such a continuous column of blood to exist, alveolar pressure must be lower than both pulmonary artery and pulmonary venous pressures. If alveolar pressures were higher than either one of these vascular pressures, alveolar walls would tamponade alveolar capillaries, interrupt the blood column, and cause measured P_{PAO} to more closely reflect alveolar rather than intravascular pressure. Vascular segments in which alveolar pressures are lower than pulmonary artery and pulmonary venous pressures are referred to as *West zone 3*. Zone 2 refers to vascular segments in which alveolar pressure exceeds pulmonary venous pressure; zone 1 segments are characterized by alveolar pressures that exceed both pulmonary artery and pulmonary venous pressures. Although there is no precise way to confirm that the PA catheter is positioned in zone 3, positioning the catheter tip below the level of the left atrium optimizes the chances of zone 3 conditions. High ventilator airway inflation pressures (marked increases in alveolar pressure) can convert portions of zone 3 regions to zone 1 or 2 conditions.

11. What is the relationship between P_{PAO} and left ventricular preload?

Preload refers to the length component of the myocardial length-tension relationship, termed the *Starling curve*. Increasing fiber length before contraction (preload) results in an increased amount and velocity of myocardial contraction until an optimal precontraction fiber length is reached, at which point myocardial contraction plateaus. The best measure of left ventricular preload would be myocardial fiber length at end diastole. Fiber length, however, cannot be measured in the clinical setting. Left ventricular end-diastolic volume (LVEDV) is directly related to fiber length and would accurately measure preload. Unfortunately, the PA catheter cannot determine vascular volumes.

The PA catheter can, however, measure P_{PAO}, which approximates left ventricular end-diastolic pressure (LVEDP). LVEDP is related to LVEDV by the ventricular pressure-volume curve (or compliance curve). If LVEDP is elevated and stroke volume is low, clinicians may infer that LVEDV (or "preload") is adequate but myocardial contractility is depressed. This inference, however, may not always be correct. Measured P_{PAO} may misrepresent LVEDV and the adequacy of preload in diastolic dysfunction, which occurs in patients who have severe left ventricular hypertrophy or a recent myocardial infarction. P_{PAO} may also underestimate preload when vascular resistance is increased between the catheter tip and the left ventricle, which can occur with mitral stenosis and obstruction of the pulmonary veins.

12. What are the causes of difficulty in placement of the PA catheter?

Inability to pass the catheter beyond the end of the introducer. This occurs when the tip of the introducer is against the vessel wall. Usually, some difficulty in blood return may be noted. Gentle traction on the introducer or withdrawal of the introducer 0.5 to 1.0 cm may result in restoration of venous return and ability to advance the catheter. Care must be taken not to withdraw too far or the introducer may be totally withdrawn from the vessel.

Resistance to advancement after insertion of 10 and 20 cm of catheter length. When the catheter can be advanced through the tip of the introducer but subsequent resistance is encountered, vascular occlusion or thrombosis should be suspected. Prior central venous cannulation, particularly of long duration, may result in subclavian or internal jugular venous thrombosis. Recent central venous puncture, particularly in coagulopathic patients, may result in formation of hematoma that can extrinsically compress the vessel. Fluoroscopy is not helpful unless performed with intravascular contrast by an operator trained in angiography. The most practical solution is contralateral central venous cannulation after it has been ascertained that no pneumothorax exists on the side of the initial attempt.

Lack of respiratory pressure variation and inability to achieve right atrial or right ventricular waveform. Respiratory pressure variation can be absent when the catheter migrates extrathoracically, usually traveling up an internal jugular vein. Withdrawal of the catheter to 10 cm and reattempted passage may be successful. Rotation of the catheter a quarter turn before advancement may help direct the catheter appropriately. Fluoroscopy should be performed if difficulties persist.

Failure to achieve a PA waveform after entering the right ventricle (RV). This is one of the most common problems with catheter placement; it usually occurs in patients with RV dilation. As a result of poor ventricular contractility associated with RV dilatation, stroke volume is not sufficient to propel the balloon into the PA; instead, the catheter coils within the RV. Significant pulmonic valve insufficiency is less commonly responsible for this problem. If the catheter is advanced 10–15 cm after an RV tracing is obtained and no PA waveform is noted, the balloon should be deflated and the catheter withdrawn until a venous tracing is obtained. The balloon should then be reinflated and advanced. Twisting the catheter quarter turns while it is advanced may be beneficial. The occurrence of premature ventricular contractions during these efforts suggests that the catheter is again coiled within the RV, causing myocardial irritability. Continued advancement of a coiled catheter can have serious consequences, including ventricular tachycardia or fibrillation, intracardiac catheter knotting, and ventricular perforation. Coiling of the catheter can be easily recognized fluoroscopically. "Torquing" or twisting the catheter while it is advanced under fluoroscopic visualization may "steer" the balloon toward the ventricular outflow tract.

13. List the risks and complications of PA catheter placement.

Complications of catheter insertion include those of venous catheterization in general as well as those specific to PA catheterization.

Complications of central venous catheters:
   Insertion site hemorrhage
   Pneumothorax
   Infection
   Venous thrombosis
   Air embolism

Complications specifically related to PA catheters:
   Cardiac perforation
   Arrhythmias, right bundle branch block
   Pulmonary infarction
   Pulmonary artery rupture
   Endocarditis
   Air embolism caused by balloon rupture
   Injury to cardiac valves, papillary muscles, or chordae tendineae

14. What can be done to minimize the risk of complications?

Insertion site hemorrhage. Systemic coaguloapthy is a major risk factor for this complication. Removal of the catheter and introducer can actually exacerbate hemorrhage. Therapy to correct coagulopathy and the avoidance of multiple venous punctures can reduce the risk of this complication. Hemorrhage from an internal jugular catheter can be more easily controlled with the application of external pressure than hemorrhage from subclavian punctures.

Pneumothorax. Pneumothorax results from puncture of the apex of the lung during attempts at internal jugular or subclavian vein cannulation. The internal jugular site may be associated with a lower risk of pneumothorax (except in patients with short necks). Care should be exercised to avoid excessively deep probing in the internal jugular approach and to avoid dorsal angulation of the needle during subclavian puncture. The presence of mechanical ventilation may increase the consequence of a puncture of the lung, making the development of a tension pneumothorax more likely and more serious.

Air embolism. During PA catheterization air embolism can develop during wire placement, improper flushing, and introducer valve dysfunction. Patients who make vigorous inspiratory efforts and generate significant negative intrathoracic pressure are at increased risk for this complication. Positioning the patient so that the insertion site is below the level of the right atrium during introducer placement can decrease the risk of air embolization. Air embolization can occasionally accompany catheter removal. Risk factors include lack of subcutaneous tissue, vigorous spontaneous respiratory efforts, and long duration of catheter placement. Use of an oc-clusive dressing immediately after catheter removal reduces the risk of this complication.

Infection. Bacteremia, septic thrombosis, infectious endocarditis, and septic emboli can de-velop subsequent to PA catheter insertion. Staphylococcus aureus, coagulase-negative staphylo-cocci, yeasts, and enteric gram-negative rods are the most frequent pathogens identified. Prolonged catheterization (more than 4 days), poor sterile technique during placement, and cuta-neous colonization at the insertion site are risk factors for catheter infection.

Cardiac trauma or arrhythmias. Operators should note the length of inserted catheter when a RV tracing is first seen. A PA waveform should be expected within the next 10 cm of catheter insertion; its appearance ensures that coiling is not occurring within the RV. The balloon should always be inflated before the RV is entered so that passage through the ventricular cham-ber will be rapid and atraumatic.

Pulmonary infarction. Most instances of pulmonary infarction related to PA catheters are caused by prolonged inflation of the balloon and catheter migration with occlusion of a distal ar-terial branch. This complication can be avoided by continuous monitoring of the PA waveform. If the PA waveform is not observed, catheter position and balloon deflation should be verified.

PA rupture. PA rupture is a rare but devastating complication of PA catheterization. Catheter-induced erosion of vascular walls or overinflation of the balloon in a small-caliber vessel con-tribute to this complication. Also, underinflation of the balloon with less than 1.5 cc of air can allow the catheter tip to project beyond the balloon, traumatizing the vessel during wedging. Other factors associated with PA rupture include pulmonary hypertension, anticoagulation, and advanced age.

15. What causes hemoptysis after pulmonary artery catheter placement?

The major causes of hemoptysis after PA catheter placement are PA rupture and pulmonary infarction.

16. What should be done if a catheter becomes knotted?

A knot can be removed from a PA catheter by passage of a wire down the catheter lumen or placement of an outer sheath to straighten the catheter. The catheter may have to be snared and removed through the inferior vena cava, or thoracotomy may be required. The assistance of an in-vasive vascular radiologist, cardiologist, or surgeon who has experience with such problems is recommended.

17. What does the physician need to know about transducers and line setup?

Physicians should be able to verify proper transducer positioning, recognize abnormal wave-forms, and understand the features of balloon malfunction.

18. What is the proper position of the transducer?

The transducer should be positioned at the level of the left atrium. Malposition of the trans-ducer above or below the appropriate position will result in measurement of falsely low or high pressures, respectively.

19. Describe abnormal waveforms.

Overwedged waveforms are characterized by a steady rise in pressure that finally goes off scale during balloon inflation. This patterns usually occurs when the distal port is occluded by impaction against the vessel wall. If an overwedged waveform occurs, the balloon should be fully deflated and the catheter pulled back 2–3 cm before reinflation.

Damped waveforms are characterized by blunted deflections and slow return of pressure to baseline after catheter flush caused by obstruction of the catheter system. Specific causes of a damped tracing include bubbles in the transducer or transducer tubing, blood clot, kinked catheter or tubing, and excessive tubing length.

Absent waveforms occur with total obstruction of the catheter or tubing, faulty calibration of the transducer, a transducer that is open to air, and extreme malpositioning of the transducer.

20. What are the indications of balloon malfunction?

When excessive resistance to balloon inflation is noted, the catheter system should be examined for catheter kinking, a closed valve to the balloon port, and catheter malposition. Excessive force should not be used to achieve inflation because it may rupture the PA or the balloon. If the valve is properly positioned, no external catheter kinking is evident, and a nondamped PA tracing is observed, the catheter should be withdrawn a few cm and reinflation attempted. If the problem persists, a chest radiograph may verify positioning and identify internal catheter kinks. Rupture of a balloon is another malfunction that must be quickly recognized. Signs of balloon rupture include loss of resistance to balloon inflation, lack of gas return into the syringe, and loss of ability to obtain a P_{PAO} tracing. Failure to recognize balloon rupture can result in repeated attempts to inflate the balloon causing venous air emboli.

21. Are there alternative methods to the PA catheter for hemodynamic monitoring?

No existing technology is superior to the PA catheter for providing continuous monitoring of both preload and cardiac output in critically ill patients. Alternative methods under investigation include the following:

Thoracic electrical bioimpedance. This technique analyzes changes in thoracic cavity electrical impedance (which is influenced by thoracic blood volume) with events in the cardiac cycle, determined by ECG analysis. This technique measures stroke volume but does not assess preload.

Echocardiography. Echocardiography can provide information on anatomy, valve function, and ventricular contractility. Estimations of cardiac output and pressures can be made with Doppler analysis. This method can be helpful when performed by a skilled operator. Limitations include the qualitative nature of the measurements, high dependence on operator ability, and limited availability for long-term monitoring.

Doppler ultrasound. This technology utilizes a continuous wave Doppler transducer to monitor aortic blood flow. The monitoring site may be transcutaneous, transesophageal, or transtracheal (transducer incorporated into an endotracheal tube). The technique provides information on aortic blood flow but is limited by dependence on precise positioning of the transducer and lack of ability to assess preload.

Radionuclide ventriculography. These methods, which include radionuclide angiography (RNA) and multiple gated acquisition (MUGA) scans, provide quantitative assessment of ejection fraction and evaluation of regional ventricular wall motion. No information on preload is provided. These techniques require use of bulky, costly gamma cameras and are unsuited for long-term monitoring.

BIBLIOGRAPHY

1. Cope DK, Grimbert F, Downey JM, et al: Pulmonary capillary pressure: A review. Crit Care Med 20:1043–1056, 1992.
2. Ermakov S, Hoyt JW: Pulmonary artery catheterization. Crit Care Med 8:773–806, 1992.
3. Ginosar Y, Sprung CL: Central venous and pulmonary artery catheter monitoring. In Levine RL, Fromm RE (eds): Critical Care Monitoring: From Pre-hospital to the ICU. St. Louis, C.V. Mosby, 1995, pp 323–342.
4. Jansen JRC: The thermodilution method for the clinical assessment of cardiac output. Intensive Care Med 21:691–697, 1995.
5. Leatherman JW, Marini J: Clinical use of the pulmonary artery catheter. In Hall JB, Schmidt GA, Wood LDH (eds): Principles of Critical Care. New York, McGraw-Hill, 1992, pp 323–342.
6. Marini JJ: Obtaining meaningful data from the Swan-Ganz catheter. Respir Care 30:572–585, 1985.
7. Matthay MA, Chatterjee K: Bedside catheterization of the pulmonary artery: Risks compared to benefits. Ann Intern Med 109:826–834, 1988.
8. Mermel LA, Maki DG: Infectious complications of Swan-Ganz pulmonary artery catheters: Pathogenesis, epidemiology, prevention and management. Am J Respir Crit Care Med 149:1020–1036, 1994.
9. Moore FA, Haenel JB, Moore EE: Alternatives to Swan-Ganz cardiac output monitoring. Surg Clin North Am 71:699–721, 1991.
10. Shephard JN, Brecker SJ, Evans TW: Bedside assessment of myocardial performance in the critically ill. Intensive Care Med 20:513–521, 1994.
11. Wiedemann HP, Matthay MA, Matthay RA: Cardiovascular pulmonary monitoring in the intensive care unit (Parts 1 & 2). Chest 85:537–549; 656–668, 1984.

15. MEDIASTINOSCOPY

Selim M. Arcasoy, M.D., and James R. Jett, M.D.

1. What are mediastinoscopy and anterior mediastinotomy?

First introduced by Carlens in 1959, mediastinoscopy, or cervical mediastinoscopy, is the *endoscopic* exploration of the superior and middle mediastinum with the use of a lighted rigid instrument, the mediastinoscope. It enables one to directly visualize and biopsy lymph nodes or other abnormal tissue present in the superior and middle mediastinum within the reach of the instrument. Anterior mediastinotomy, initially described as an alternative to cervical mediastinoscopy in 1966 by Chamberlain and McNeill, is the surgical exploration of the mediastinum. It is currently used as a complementary procedure to standard cervical mediastinoscopy for mediastinal evaluation.

2. How is mediastinoscopy performed?

Although mediastinoscopy can be performed under local anesthesia, general anesthesia is usually preferred for patient comfort, ease of surgery, and management of potential complications. It is commonly accompanied by bronchoscopy and can be done in an outpatient setting.

The patient is positioned supine on the operating table with the neck extended. A transverse incision 2 to 4 cm long between the suprasternal notch, thyroid cartilage, and medial borders of the sternocleidomastoid muscles is performed. The pretracheal fascia is entered after division and lateral traction of strap muscles. Blunt dissection is used to create a plane just anterior and lateral to the trachea. The mediastinoscope is then inserted into this plane and advanced by using the anterior tracheobronchial cartilaginous rings as reference points. The space anterior and lateral to the trachea is inspected and biopsy samples are obtained.

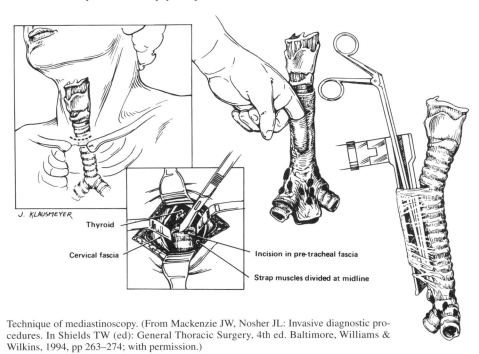

J. KLAUSMEYER

Thyroid

Cervical fascia

Incision in pre-tracheal fascia

Strap muscles divided at midline

Technique of mediastinoscopy. (From Mackenzie JW, Nosher JL: Invasive diagnostic procedures. In Shields TW (ed): General Thoracic Surgery, 4th ed. Baltimore, Williams & Wilkins, 1994, pp 263–274; with permission.)

3. How is anterior mediastinotomy performed?

Anterior mediastinotomy is done via an incision in the second intercostal space or by excision of the second or third costal cartilages (or both) immediately lateral to the sternum. The mediastinum is then entered via either a transpleural or an extrapleural approach, and biopsy samples are obtained. This procedure is usually done on the left side to gain access to the aortopulmonary and anterior mediastinal lymph nodes that cannot be reached with cervical mediastinoscopy.

4. Describe the pulmonary lymphatic drainage to the mediastinal lymph nodes.

Right paratracheal lymph nodes receive drainage directly from the right upper lobe and indirectly via subcarinal lymph nodes from the right middle and lower lobes. Aortopulmonary window, anterior mediastinal, and left paratracheal lymph nodes receive drainage primarily from the left upper and lower lobes. Lymphatic drainage from the left lung, especially the lower lobe, is commonly contralateral, involving the subcarinal and right paratracheal lymph nodes.

5. Which lymph node groups are accessible to mediastinoscopy and anterior mediastinotomy?

The following lymph node groups can be sampled during mediastinoscopy: right and left, upper and lower paratracheal lymph nodes (American Thoracic Society [ATS] stations 2R, 2L, 4R, and 4L), right tracheobronchial lymph nodes (ATS station 10R), left peribronchial lymph nodes (ATS station 10L), and anterior and superior aspects of subcarinal lymph nodes (ATS station 7). Anterior mediastinal lymph nodes (ATS station 6) and aortopulmonary window lymph nodes (ATS station 5) are not accessible by standard cervical mediastinoscopy.

A left anterior mediastonotomy provides access to the anterior mediastinal and aortopulmonary lymph nodes (ATS stations 6 and 5, respectively). The posterior aspect of subcarinal (ATS station 7), paraesophageal (ATS station 8), and inferior pulmonary ligament (ATS station 9) lymph nodes are inaccessible by either technique.

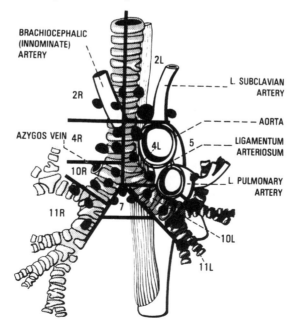

American Thoracic Society map of regional pulmonary nodes. (From American Thoracic Society, Medical Section of the American Lung Association: Clinical staging of primary lung cancer. Am Rev Respir Dis 127: 659–664, 1983; with permission.)

Proposed Definitions of Regional Nodal Stations for Prethoracotomy Staging

X	Supraclavicular nodes.
2R	Right upper paratracheal (suprainnominate) nodes: nodes to the right of the midline of the trachea between the intersection of the caudal margin of the innominate artery with the trachea, and the apex of the lung. (Includes highest R mediastinal node.) (Radiologists may use the same caudal margin as in 2L.)
2L	Left upper paratracheal (supraaortic) nodes: nodes to the left of the midline of the trachea between the top of the aortic arch and the apex of the lung. (Includes highest L mediastinal node.)
4R	Right lower paratracheal nodes: nodes to the right of the midline of the trachea between the cephalic border of the azygos vein and the intersection of the caudal margin of the brachio-cephalic artery with the right side of the trachea. (Includes some pretracheal and paracaval nodes.) (Radiologists may use the same cephalic margin as in 4L.)
4L	Left lower paratracheal nodes: nodes to the left of the midline of the trachea between the top of the aortic arch and the level of the carina, medial to the ligamentum arteriosum. (Includes some pretracheal nodes.)
5	Aortopulmonary nodes: subaortic and paraaortic nodes, lateral to the ligamentum arteriosum or the aorta or left pulmonary artery, proximal to the first branch of the LPA.
6	Anterior mediastinal nodes: nodes anterior to the ascending aorta or the innominate artery. (Includes some pretracheal and preaortic nodes.)
7	Subcarinal nodes: nodes arising caudal to the carina of the trachea but not associated with the lower lobe bronchi or arteries within the lung.
8	Paraesophageal nodes: nodes dorsal to the posterior wall of the trachea and to the right or left of the midline of the esophagus. (Includes retrotracheal, but not subcarinal nodes.)
9	Right or left pulmonary ligament nodes: nodes within the right or left pulmonary ligament.
10R	Right tracheobronchial nodes: nodes to the right of the midline of the trachea from the level of the cephalic border of the azygos vein to the origin of the right upper lobe bronchus.
10L	Left peribronchial nodes: nodes to the left of the midline of the trachea between the carina and the left upper lobe bronchus, medial to the ligamentum arteriosum.
11	Intrapulmonary nodes: nodes removed in the right or left lung specimen plus those distal to the main stem bronchi or secondary carina. (Includes interlobar, lobar, and segmental nodes.)

L = left; LPA = left pulmonary artery; R = right.
From American Thoracic Society, Medical Section of the American Lung Association: Clinical staging of primary lung cancer. Am Rev Respir Dis 127:659–664, 1983; with permission.

6. What are the indications for mediastinoscopy?

Mediastinoscopy is most commonly used for diagnosis and presurgical staging of bronchogenic carcinoma. It is also useful in the diagnosis of other causes of mediastinal lymph node enlargement, including inflammatory/granulomatous diseases (i.e., sarcoidosis, tuberculosis, and fungal infections) and neoplastic diseases (i.e., lymphoma and metastatic neoplasms). In addition, mediastinoscopy can assist in the staging of esophageal carcinoma and the drainage of mediastinal cysts.

7. What are the complications of mediastinoscopy and anterior mediastinotomy?

The average incidence of complications is 2–3%, although the incidence in different patient series varies from 0.2% to 4%. These complications include pneumothorax (usually right sided), bleeding, and recurrent laryngeal nerve injury (usually left sided). Other potential complications are injury to the phrenic nerve, esophagus, and trachea; chylothorax from thoracic duct trauma; air embolism; wound infection; cardiac dysrhythmias; and, rarely, tumor seeding. The mortality rate of mediastinoscopy is less than 1%; in several large series, no deaths were reported. Complications of anterior mediastinotomy are similar to those of standard cervical mediastinoscopy.

8. Describe the overall sensitivity and specificity of mediastinoscopy.

The overall yield of routine mediastinoscopy for documenting metastatic lymph node involvement in all patients with bronchogenic carcinoma is 30 to 35%. This is highest in small cell and lowest in squamous cell carcinoma. The yield also varies depending on the size and location of the primary tumor.

In several patient series, the reported sensitivity and specificity of mediastinoscopy in the diagnosis of metastatic spread from bronchogenic carcinoma are 80–90% and 100%, respectively. The reported sensitivity of mediastinoscopy in the diagnosis of sarcoidosis is more than 95%.

$$\text{Sensitivity} = \frac{\text{True positive}}{\text{True positive} + \text{False negative}}$$

$$\text{Specificity} = \frac{\text{True negative}}{\text{True negative} + \text{False positive}}$$

9. Name the findings at mediastinoscopy that would preclude curative surgical resection of bronchogenic carcinoma.

- Extranodal extension with invasion of vital mediastinal tissues, e.g., the great vessels or trachea
- Contralateral mediastinal spread
- Extensive mediastinal lymph node metastases or involvement of high paratracheal (ATS station 2) lymph nodes
- Small cell carcinoma with any lymph node metastases
- Firmly fixed lymphadenopathy in the aortopulmonary window or involvement of anterior mediastinal lymph nodes. (However, isolated spread to the aortopulmonary window lymph nodes that is easily resectable does not preclude an attempt at surgical resection for cure.)

10. Are there any contraindications to mediastinoscopy?

Absolute contraindications to mediastinoscopy are the presence of a tracheostomy and vascular disease at the aortic arch or innominate artery. However, mediastinoscopy can safely be performed even in the presence of superior vena cava syndrome, which was once thought to be an absolute contraindication because of the fear of excessive bleeding.

History of a previous tracheostomy, mediastinoscopy, and mediastinal radiation treatment are all considered relative contraindications to the procedure, although mediastinoscopy has occasionally been successfully performed in these settings.

11. What is extended cervical mediastinoscopy?

Also called modified mediastinoscopy, this technique was described by Ginsberg in 1987. It involves the creation of a space between the left carotid artery and the innominate artery through a standard cervical mediastinoscopy incision. It can be used to access aortopulmonary window and anterior mediastinal lymph nodes. Experience with this approach is limited, and it has not been as extensively studied or as generally accepted as standard cervical mediastinoscopy.

12. Has mediastinoscopy had an impact on the number of unnecessary thoracotomies for bronchogenic cancer?

Up to 50% of the thoracotomies for bronchogenic carcinoma performed in the middle of this century detected unresectable disease. The rate of resectability at thoracotomy currently is more than 90%. Although never studied in a randomized, prospective fashion, this improvement in resectability and the significant reduction in the number of exploratory thoracotomies or thoracotomies with partial resection are at least in part believed to be related to careful prethoracotomy mediastinal staging.

13. Does mediastinoscopy have a role in making nonsurgical treatment decisions in bronchogenic carcinoma?

The finding of mediastinal lymph node involvement not only is important in the decision about operability but also enables the physician to determine which patients are potential candidates for neoadjuvant treatment before thoracotomy. Recent studies report encouraging results after neoadjuvant therapy with combined chemotherapy and radiotherapy preceding surgery for carefully selected stage IIIA and IIIB non–small cell lung cancer. Because the role of neoadjuvant therapy for lung cancer is undergoing careful evaluation at this time, it should should not be considered the standard of care.

CONTROVERSIES

14. Should all patients with lung cancer undergo mediastinoscopy for staging?

Opinion varies concerning the need for mediastinoscopy in patients with lung cancer who are potential candidates for thoracotomy and surgical resection. Metastatic disease in mediastinal lymph nodes will be found in one third of patients, if all individuals are evaluated with mediastinoscopy. Although proponents recommend it routinely for all patients with lung cancer before thoracotomy, others consider it indicated only for select patients. Noninvasive evaluation of mediastinal lymph nodes by CT scanning may be helpful in selection of patients who require mediastinoscopy. The average sensitivity and specificity of CT scan, considering nodal size of greater than 1 cm as abnormal, are 60–85% and 62–65%, respectively. These percentages vary with the CT scan criteria used to define abnormal lymph nodes.

Based on the foregoing information, all patients with enlarged lymph nodes by CT scanning should undergo mediastinoscopy to confirm or refute malignancy, because approximately one-third of these patients will not have metastatic disease and thus may be candidates for curative resection.

The management of patients with bronchogenic carcinoma and normal-sized mediastinal lymph nodes (less than 1 cm) by CT scan criteria is more controversial. The average incidence of metastatic involvement in these lymph nodes is 25%, but it varies from 10–40% in different series.

At present, mediastinoscopy is not usually recommended in patients with peripheral pulmonary lesions smaller than 2 cm and mediastinal lymph nodes that are normal in size by CT scanning. Although the yield of mediastinoscopy in this setting is only 10%, some surgeons still perform a mediastinoscopy if the histology of the primary lesion is large cell carcinoma or adenocarcinoma. In patients with T2 or T3 primary non–small cell carcinomas, some recommend a mediastinoscopy, even if CT scan reveals normal-sized lymph nodes.

In contrast, all patients with peripheral small cell bronchogenic carcinoma should undergo mediastinoscopy because of the high incidence of metastatic spread, even if the mediastinal lymph nodes are normal in size by CT scanning.

15. What is the prognostic significance of metastatic mediastinal lymph node involvement detected at mediastinoscopy in patients with bronchogenic carcinoma?

This depends on the extent and location of lymph node involvement. N2 disease, which entails metastasis to the ipsilateral mediastinal and subcarinal lymph nodes has a better prognosis than N3 disease, which consists of metastasis to contralateral mediastinal or hilar lymph nodes, ipsilateral or contralateral scalene lymph nodes, or supraclavicular lymph nodes. The majority of patients (80–90%) who have lymph node metastasis at mediastinoscopy have unresectable disease. Only a minority of such patients (10–20%) may be candidates for curative surgical resection.

There are several reports of improved survival after complete surgical resection in a subset of patients who were found to have N2 disease at mediastinoscopy or patients who had a negative mediastinoscopy but N2 disease identified at thoracotomy. The incidence of "unexpected" mediastinal lymph node involvement at thoracotomy after a negative mediastinoscopy is 15–25%. Five-year survival rates of 15–30% have been reported in this group of patients.

16. When should anterior mediastinotomy be used in place of cervical mediastinoscopy?

Anterior mediastonotomy provides better surgical exposure and allows evaluation of hilar mobility; however, it does not permit examination and sampling of contralateral mediastinal and subcarinal lymph nodes.

Although some surgeons favor an anterior mediastinotomy for staging of left upper lobe and hilar tumors, most use the standard cervical approach first for all bronchogenic carcinomas that require mediastinal staging. If negative for metastasis, cervical mediastinoscopy is usually followed by anterior mediastonotomy, especially if there is evidence of involvement in the aortopulmonary window or anterior mediastinal lymph nodes by CT scanning. Anterior mediastinotomy is not considered an alternative but rather a supplementary procedure to standard mediastinoscopy.

BIBLIOGRAPHY

1. Albain KS, Rusch VW, Crowley JJ, et al: Concurrent cisplatin/etoposide plus chest radiotherapy followed by surgery for stages IIIA (N2) and IIIB non–small-cell lung disease: Mature results of Southwest Oncology Group Phase II Study 8805. J Clin Oncol 13:1880–1892, 1995.
2. Carlens E: Mediastinoscopy: A method for inspection and tissue biopsy in the superior mediastinum. Dis Chest 36:343–352, 1959.
3. Coughlin M, Deslauriers J, Beaulieu M: Role of mediastinoscopy in pretreatment staging of patients with primary lung cancer. Ann Thorac Surg 40:556–560, 1985.
4. Cybulsky IJ, Bennett WF: Mediastinoscopy as a routine outpatient procedure. Ann Thorac Surg 58:176–178, 1994.
5. Ginsberg RJ, Rice TW, Goldberg M, et al: Extended cervical mediastinoscopy. A single staging procedure for bronchogenic carcinoma of the left upper lobe. J Thorac Cardiovasc Surg 94:673–678, 1987.
6. Goldstraw P: Mediastinal exploration by mediastinoscopy and mediastinotomy. Br J Dis Chest 82:111–120, 1988.
7. Jahangiri M, Goldstraw P: The role of mediastinoscopy in superior vena caval obstruction. Ann Thorac Surg 59:453–455, 1995.
8. Luke WP, Pearson FG, Todd TRJ, et al: Prospective evaluation of mediastinoscopy for assessment of carcinoma of the lung. J Thorac Cardiovasc Surg 91:53–56, 1986.
9. Mackenzie JW, Nosher JL: Invasive diagnostic procedures. In Shields TW (ed): General Thoracic Surgery, 4th ed. Baltimore, Williams & Wilkins, 1994, pp 263–275.
10. Mackenzie JW, Riley DJ: Diagnostic procedures: Mediastinal evaluation-scalene lymph node biopsy, mediastinoscopy, and mediastinotomy. In Baue AE (ed): Glenn's Thoracic and Cardiovascular Surgery, 5th ed. Connecticut, Appleton & Lange, 1991, pp 159–167.
11. McCloud TC, Bourgouin PM, Greenburg RW, et al: Bronchogenic carcinoma: Analysis of staging in the mediastinum with CT by correlative lymph node mapping and sampling. Radiology 182:319–323, 1992.
12. McNeill TM, Chamberlain JM, Diagnostic anterior mediastinotomy. Ann Thorac Surg 2:532–539, 1966.
13. Patterson GA, Piazza D, Pearson FG, et al: Significance of metastatic disease in subaortic lymph nodes. Ann Thorac Surg 43:155–159, 1987.
14. Pearson GF: Staging of the mediastinum. Role of mediastinoscopy and computed tomography. Chest 103:346S–348S, 1993.
15. Shields TW: Presentation, diagnosis, and staging of bronchial carcinoma and of the asymptomatic solitary pulmonary nodule. In Shields TW (ed): General Thoracic Surgery, 4th ed. Baltimore, Williams & Wilkins, 1994, pp 1142–1143.
16. Staples CA, Muller NL, Miller RR, et al: Mediastinal nodes in bronchogenic carcinoma: Comparison between CT and mediastinoscopy. Radiology 167:367–372, 1988.

16. THORACOSCOPY

Robert J. Karman, M.D., and Praveen N. Mathur, M.B., B.S.

1. Describe the differences between medical and surgical thoracoscopy.

Medical thoracoscopy must be distinguished from video-assisted thoracic surgery (VATS). Medical thoracoscopy is used primarily for the diagnosis of pleural diseases and pleurodesis; VATS is used for minimally invasive thoracic surgery and offers the opportunity to proceed with open thoracotomy if necessary. VATS is performed in the operating room with the use of complex instruments, multiple ports of entry, double lumen intubation, and general anesthesia. In contrast, medical thoracoscopy may be performed in the endoscopy suite, with the use of local anesthesia and conscious sedation. Typically, only one or two ports of entry are required and simple, nondisposable instruments are used for medical thoracoscopy. In the appropriate clinical situations, medical thoracoscopy may be utilized instead of VATS at a substantial cost savings. In this chapter, medical thoracoscopy will be referred to hereafter as *thoracoscopy*.

2. What is medical thoracoscopy?

Medical thoracoscopy, or pleuroscopy, is the endoscopic examination of the thoracic cavity. After thorough evaluation with pleural fluid analysis and closed pleural biopsy, the cause of up to 25% of pleural abnormalities or effusions remains indeterminant. Medical thoracoscopy enhances our diagnostic capability and has become a valuable tool in diagnosing and treating pleural and parenchymal lung diseases without the morbidity, mortality, or cost of open thoracotomy.

3. What is the history of thoracoscopy?

In 1910, Jacobeus used a modified cystoscope to evaluate the pleural cavity and lyse adhesions to create pneumothoraces for the treatment of tuberculosis (TB). The use of thoracoscopy declined with the arrival of antituberculous therapy. However, recent technologic advances such as improved optical and video technology have revitalized the use of this procedure as a diagnostic and therapeutic tool.

4. What are the indications for thoracoscopy?

Thoracoscopy has both diagnostic and therapeutic indications. **Diagnostic thoracoscopy** should be considered only after careful routine evaluation of pleural abnormalities. Indications include exudative pleural effusions of unknown origin, suspected mesothelioma, cancer, TB, and benign or other pleural disorders, including empyema and spontaneous pneumothorax. Exudative pleural effusions, caused by malignancy or TB, are diagnosed only 60–70% of the time after repeated thoracentesis and closed needle pleural biopsy. Thoracoscopic evaluation, however, increases the sensitivity to 95–97%. In patients in whom adequate thoracoscopic visualization is possible, an unequivocal pathologic diagnosis of benign diseases can be made, with a specificity approaching 100%.

Therapeutic indications for thoracoscopy include lysis of adhesions and thoracoscopic talc pleurodesis for malignant pleural effusions, spontaneous pneumothorax, and recurrent nonmalignant pleural effusions.

5. What are contraindications to thoracoscopy?

Contraindications to thoracoscopy include the lack of a pleural space, respiratory insufficiency requiring ventilatory support, pulmonary arterial hypertension, and uncorrectable bleeding disorders. Relative contraindications include uncontrolled cough, unstable cardiovascular status, and hypoxemia that is not caused by a large pleural effusion.

6. How is the patient evaluated before thoracoscopy?

A comprehensive medical assessment before thoracoscopy includes:

Chest x-ray, frequently supplemented with bilateral decubitus or chest CT scan (or both) to further assess pleural and parenchymal abnormalities

Pleural fluid analysis

One or more closed biopsies of the pleura

Arterial blood gas analysis to evaluate respiratory status

Routine blood tests, including coagulation parameters

ECG

In addition, pulmonary function tests may be helpful.

7. What equipment is used for thoracoscopy?

The rigid thoracoscope, rather than the flexible thoracoscope, is currently the most common and useful instrument in thoracoscopy. It provides both excellent optical quality and maneuverability within the pleural space. Additional instruments include:

Introduction trocar	Xenon light source
Probes for palpation	Thoracostomy tray
Suction catheters	Video camera
Forceps for coagulation or biopsy	Monitor

8. How is thoracoscopy performed?

After continuous cardiac, hemodynamic, and pulse oximeter monitoring is instituted, the patient is placed in the lateral decubitus position with the hemithorax to be inspected in the superior position. The entry point, which is the fourth or fifth intercostal space, in the midaxillary line, is prepared and draped in a sterile fashion. Local anesthetic is then injected into the site. The patient is consciously sedated via intravenous administration of a narcotic and midozalam. Blunt dissection at the point of entry is performed and an artificial pneumothorax is created, allowing the lung to collapse. At this point, the trocar and thoracoscope can now be introduced safely. Pleural fluid is removed and the thoracoscope is directed to systematically evaluate the entire chest cavity. Thoracoscopy may be performed by the single puncture method, in which the instruments are introduced through the operating channel of the thoracoscope, or by the double puncture method, in which a second point of entry is made through which instruments are introduced and manipulated. Biopsy forceps may be inserted through the working channel or through the second puncture site to perform biopsy or coagulation of the pleural space. Similarly, talc can be insufflated through the working channel or through the second point of entry under direct thoracoscopic visualization to ensure that the entire pleural space is covered with talc and pleurodesis is effective.

9. What structures are visualized by thoracoscopy?

During thoracoscopy, if no adhesions are present, the entire parietal surface of the thoracic cavity can be seen with the telescope (0-degree) except for the immediate area of the hilum and the point of entry of the thoracoscope. However, with the additional use of the 50-degree telescope these areas also can be visualized. Anatomic relationships and intrathoracic structures are well recognized by location of the major parenchymal fissures. The diaphragm is identified by its anterior position and respiration-related movement. Major vascular structures are readily observed through the transparent pleura. Sometimes, however, distinguishing between pleural inflammation and malignancy may be difficult, and several biopsy samples may be needed. The surface of the normal lung is pink and soft. Atelectatic areas are purplish-red with a clear edge, whereas anthracotic areas are black and can be easily identified. Malignant nodules and emphysematous bullae may also be apparent protruding from the surface. The inability of a lobe to collapse may indicate an obstructing endobronchial lesion or tumor mass.

10. Is thoracoscopic talc pleurodesis superior to other methods of pleurodesis?

Talc pleurodesis by insufflation (poudrage) performed during thoracoscopy ensures complete drainage of fluid and distribution of talc over the entire pleural surface. Thoracoscopic talc pleurodesis is the most effective method of pleurodesis when compared with other modalities, including the administration of talc "slurry" by tube thoracostomy. Thoracoscopic talc pleurodesis has also proved to be superior to the intrapleural administration of either bleomycin or tetracycline (90% versus less than 60%, respectively).

11. When should thoracoscopic pleurodesis be considered for the treatment of malignant effusions?

Thoracoscopic pleurodesis may be considered under the following conditions:
- If malignancy is established by positive cytologic studies, biopsy, or even examination of a frozen section at the time of thoracoscopy.
- The pleural effusion rapidly reaccumulates after drainage and is the source of symptoms documented to clinically improve with thoracentesis.
- The lung is expandable after drainage of the effusion so that the visceral and parietal pleura will be in opposition for pleurodesis to occur. A trapped lung resulting from the lack of ability to expand because of an obstructing endobronchial lesion, adhesion, or a complicated pleural process, is the main reason for failure of thoracoscopic talc pleurodesis.
- The patient is in satisfactory clinical condition, able to tolerate thoracoscopy, and has a relatively good performance status and life expectancy.

12. What care is required after thoracoscopy?

A chest tube is required after every procedure. The placement and duration of the chest tube varies with the indication for thoracoscopy. During a diagnostic procedure, when biopsy samples are taken from only the parietal pleura, a chest tube may be required for only a few hours. At the conclusion of the procedure, a chest tube is placed through the same incision as the thoracoscope and is directed cranially to evacuate the pneumothorax created for the procedure. If the lung has fully expanded and there is no air leak, the chest tube may be removed within 3–4 hours. Typically, patients undergoing diagnostic thoracoscopy are discharged from the hospital within 24 hours of the procedure. After talc pleurodesis, however, a second incision is required to place a chest tube at the lowest possible interspace for maximum drainage. It may take 3–6 days for the drainage to decrease to less than 150 cc/24 hours before the chest tube may be withdrawn if no air leak exists. A daily chest radiograph is required to assess chest tube position, fluid reaccumulation, and lung reexpansion.

13. List the complications of thoracoscopy.

Thoracoscopy is a safe procedure with a relatively low morbidity and mortality rate. Complications include:

Prolonged air leak (2%)	Postoperative fever (16%)
Oxygen desaturation (2%)	Infection (2%)
Subcutaneous emphysema (2%)	Hemorrhage (2%)

No deaths were reported in one large study, whereas another review found one death to have occurred in 8000 procedures.

14. What is the role of thoracoscopy in the diagnosis and treatment of malignant mesothelioma?

Thoracoscopy has a valuable role in the diagnosis and management of malignant mesothelioma, a disease found in approximately 2000 patients per year in the United States. Thoracoscopy has also been useful in the staging of mesothelioma. In asymptomatic early stage mesothelioma, nonspecific inflammation, fine granulations, lymphangitis, and local thickening of the parietal pleura by the costovertebral gutter and on the diaphragm are among the earliest thoracoscopic findings. Large samples of pleura obtained at thoracoscopy help to differentiate mesothelioma from metastatic adenocarcinoma and to stage mesothelioma if aggressive surgical intervention is being considered. Recent studies have shown that intrapleural chemotherapy may be useful in the treatment of mesothelioma. If intrapleural chemotherapy is being considered, thoracoscopy provides access to the pleural space and a way to directly evaluate therapeutic response.

CONTROVERSY

15. Is there a role for thoracoscopy in the diagnosis and treatment of spontaneous pneumothorax?

Some authorities advocate the use of thoracoscopy in all patients with a spontaneous pneumothorax to identify the type of pneumothorax and initiate the appropriate therapy. The classification of pneumothoraces includes:

Type I	Normal lung surface
Type II	Adhesions
Type III	Bullae less than 1.5 cm
Type IV	Bullae large than 2 cm

Thoracoscopic intervention has been suggested to cauterize or seal lesions or bullae of less than 1.5 cm. In addition, thoracoscopic pleurodesis with talc has been shown to decrease the recurrence rate of spontaneous pneumothorax. In young individuals, however, talc pleurodesis is controversial because it may complicate any future thoracic procedures or surgery. Although talc is believed to be a safe agent, long-term complications are as yet unknown. In the context of uncertain recurrence rates of spontaneous pneumothoraces, unknown long-term sequelae of talc in benign disease, and relative success of conservative management of pneumothoraces without thoracoscopy, further studies are needed to define the role of thoracoscopy with or without talc pleurodesis in spontaneous pneumothoraces.

When thoracoscopically viewed bullae are larger than 2 cm, coagulation is less successful and the patient should be referred for surgical resection.

BIBLIOGRAPHY

1. Bloomberg AE: Thoracoscopy in the diagnosis of pleural effusions. NY State J Med 19:1974–1977, 1970.
2. Boutin C, Astoul P, Rey F, et al: Thoracoscopy in the diagnosis and treatment of spontaneous pneumothorax. Clin Chest Med 16:497–503, 1995.
3. Boutin C, Carginino P, Valliant PR: Thoracoscopy in the diagnosis of malignant pleural effusion. Endoscopy 12:155–160, 1980.
4. Boutin C, Rey F: Thoracoscopy in pleural malignant mesothelioma: A prospective study of 188 consecutive patients. Cancer 72:389–404, 1993.
5. Boutin C, Viallat JR, Carginino P: Thoracoscopy. In Chretien J (ed): The Pleura in Health and Disease. New York, Marcel Dekker, 1985, pp 587–621, 1985.
6. Boutin C, Viallat JR, Van Zandwijk N, et al: Activity of intrapleural recombinant gamma interferon in malignant mesothelioma. Cancer 67:2033–2037, 1991.
7. Brandt HJ, Loddenkemper R, Mai J: Atlas of Diagnostic Thoracoscopy. New York, Thieme, 1985.
8. Colt: HG: Thoracoscopic management of malignant pleural effusions. Clin Chest Med 16:505–518, 1995.
9. Dines DE, Pierre RV, Frazen SJ: The value of cells in the pleural fluid in the differential diagnosis. Mayo Clin Proc 50:571, 1975.
10. Gunnels JJ: Perplexing pleural effusion. Chest 74:390–393, 1978.
11. Hartman DL, Gaither JM, Kesler KA, et al: Comparison of insufflated talc under thoracoscopic guidance with standard tetracycline and bleomycin pleurodesis for control of malignant pleural effusions. J Thorac Cardiovasc Surg 105:743–748, 1993.
12. Light RW: Pleural Diseases. Philadelphia, Lea & Febiger, 1990.
13. Mathur PN, Loddenkemper R: Medical thoracoscopy: Role in pleural and lung diseases. Clin Chest Med 16:487–496, 1995.
14. Menzies R, Charbonneau M: Thoracoscopy for the diagnosis of pleural disease. Ann Intern Med 114:271–276, 1991.
15. Webb WR, Ozmen V, Moulder PV, et al: Iodized talc pleurodesis in the management of pleural effusions. J Thorac Cardiovasc Surg 103:881–886, 1992.

V. Airway Disease

17. ASTHMA

Elcio O. Vianna, M.D., Monica Kraft, M.D., and Richard J. Martin, M.D.

1. Is airway obstruction in asthma always reversible?

Yes. According to definition, asthma is characterized by airway obstruction that is reversible (although reversal is not complete in some patients), airway inflammation, and airway hyperreactivity. Forced expiratory volume in the first second (FEV_1) is, in most situations, the best measurement to evaluate response to a bronchodilator. At times, this response may not be evident by spirometry but may be demonstrated by a decrease in static lung volumes such as residual volume (RV), functional residual capacity (FRC), and total lung capacity (TLC). Airway resistance (Raw), airway conductance (Gaw), or specific conductance (sGaw) may occasionally be more sensitive indices. The lack of bronchodilator response may be a result of taking medications before the test, refractoriness to the drug used, or airflow obstruction from a mechanism other than bronchospasm.

2. At which age is asthma most prevalent?

The peak prevalence is in childhood. A decline occurs in the second and third decades, then an increasing prevalence is seen throughout adulthood. Boys are more often affected before adolescence and women in adulthood until age 65.

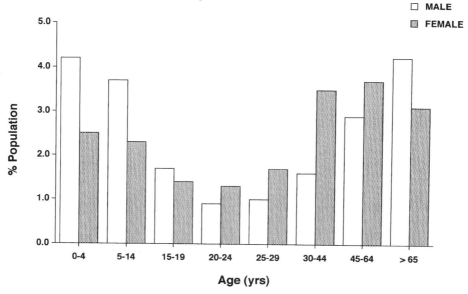

Prevalence of asthma by age and sex. (Adapted from Gerstman BB, Bosco LA, Tomita DK, et al: Prevalence and treatment of asthma in the Michigan Medicaid population younger than 45 years, 1980–1986. J Allergy Clin Immunol 83:1032–1039, 1989, and U.S. Department of Health and Human Services, PHS Resources Administration: Prevalence of Selected Chronic Respiratory Conditions in the United States, 1970. Vital Health Statistics, Series 10, No. 84. Washington, D.C., 1973.)

3. Is a positive methacholine challenge test by itself specific for the diagnosis of asthma?

No. For clinical purposes, the diagnosis of asthma is based on an impression gained by medical history, physical examination, chest radiography, and physiologic testing. Airway hyperreactivity (detected by methacholine testing), although characteristic of asthma, is not specific for diagnosis.

4. Why does the forced vital capacity (FVC) decrease in some asthmatic patients?

Because air trapping from the obstructive mechanisms limits thoracic excursions and airways blocked by inspissated plugs or bronchospasm (or both) do not conduct inspired air into the alveoli.

5. Is there any risk of late asthmatic response after methacholine challenge testing?

No. Methacholine is a nonspecific bronchoconstrictor that induces fast and easily reversible bronchospasm. Antigens used in specific bronchoprovocation testing may induce both immediate bronchospasm (early asthmatic reaction) and delayed, long-lasting bronchoconstriction (late asthmatic reaction). The latter is associated with development of airway inflammation.

6. How can airway hyperreactivity be evaluated by using peak expiratory flow rate?

In asthmatics overnight lung functions falls as much as 50%. The magnitude of this circadian variation correlates with the degree of airway reactivity and can be assessed by peak expiratory flow rate (PEFR) measurements. The PEFR variability may be calculated from at least two values (morning and night) following the formula:

$$\text{Daily variability} = \frac{\text{highest PEFR} - \text{lowest PEFR} \times 100}{\text{highest PEFR}}$$

7. Does an increased number of eosinophils in blood and sputum indicate that an asthmatic is atopic?

No. Peripheral blood and sputum eosinophilia often accompanies both atopic and nonatopic asthma. Regardless of the origin of asthma, eosinophils infiltrate airways and may be linked to the development of airway hyperreactivity through their ability to produce bronchoconstrictor, chemotactic, and vasoactive products. Eosinophils also act through their capacity to damage surrounding tissue, including epithelium, by releasing their cytotoxic granule content.

8. Why do many patients with occupational asthma continue experiencing symptoms of asthma even when they avoid the triggering factor?

Continuing asthma in these patients is a manifestation of chronic airway inflammation that, although initiated by an agent inhaled at work, persists in its absence. Airway inflammation, in either occupational or nonoccupational asthmatics, underlies the phenomenon of airway hyperreactivity that correlates with the degree of symptoms.

9. Which presentation of "asthma" is more likely to be vocal cord dysfunction?

Vocal cord dysfunction (VCD) is a cause of airway obstruction that may mimic asthma. A common but not specific patient profile is a woman between the ages of 20 and 40 years with more than a high-school education, often employed in a health-related field, and tendency to be overweight. Typically, patients with VCD are misdiagnosed as having refractory asthma and have a history of high utilization of medical resources, with several admissions and emergency room visits, including intubation and tracheostomy. Food allergies and chemical sensitivities are diagnosed in many patients. In some patients exercise may precipitate symptoms. Patients may refer to their laryngeal area as the site of airway limitation; they may not improve with a bronchodilator but will improve breathing a helium-oxygen (70%/30%) mixture or with speech therapy techniques. Definitive diagnosis depends on visualization of the vocal cords.

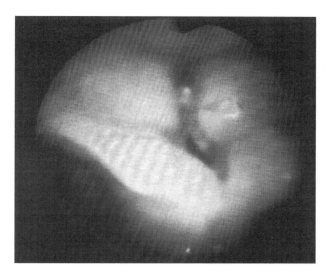

Paradoxical vocal cord motion during inspiration in a patient with vocal cord disorder. The vocal cord is bowed and only a small posterior opening is seen at total lung capacity.

10. What is the technical difference between use of a pressurized metered-dose inhaler and use of a powder inhaler?

For a metered-dose inhaler (MDI), the slower the inspiratory flow rate, the greater the quantity of drug that penetrates into the lungs. Coordination of actuation on inhalation may be difficult and often causes inadequate clinical response. For powder inhalers, coordination is not the challenge because these devices are breath actuated. Instead, the challenge is generating sufficient inspiratory flow because powder inhalers require high flow to deliver the drug to the lungs.

11. What are the indications for inhaled and systemic corticosteroids in chronic asthma?

Chronic persistent asthma is an indication for inhaled corticosteroids even if only mild asthma is present (episodes of cough, wheezing, or dyspnea more than once or twice a week).

Oral corticosteroid treatment should be used when other forms of therapy, including high doses of inhaled corticosteroids, have failed to mitigate the patient's asthma. It should be continued only if shown to reduce substantially chronic symptoms or the frequency of severe exacerbations.

12. What is the best way to use β-2 adrenergic agonists in acute and chronic asthma?

In acute asthma, a β-2 agonist is the medication of choice. Commonly, initial treatment consists of inhaled short-acting β-2 agonist use up to three times an hour for the first hour, then once an hour. Inhaled treatments can also be given continuously until an adequate clinical response is achieved or adverse side effects limit further administration (e.g., excessive tachycardia, arrhythmias, or tremor).

In chronic asthma, a short-acting inhaled β-2 agonist used on an as-needed basis is appropriate. Increased or daily use is a warning of deterioration of the disease and indicates the need to institute or to intensify the regular antiinflammatory therapy. Long-acting twice daily β-2 agonists can be beneficial in certain situations such as nocturnal problems and delayed interval between medication and exercise.

13. Should corticosteroids, theophylline, anticholinergics, and antibiotics be used routinely in status asthmaticus?

Status asthmaticus is a severe asthma attack that is refractory to initial conventional treatment and that may lead to death. Corticosteroids and β-agonists are first-line treatment in acute asthma. Theophylline and anticholinergics should be used in patients who do not respond adequately to initial therapy. Antibiotics are indicated in patients with fever and sputum containing neutrophils and those with clinical findings of pneumonia or acute sinusitis.

14. Does long-term oral corticosteroid therapy increase a patient's chance of being admitted after an emergency department visit for acute asthma?
Yes. Patients who have deteriorated despite the use of oral corticosteroids at home should be considered for admission, whereas patients who are not on oral corticosteroids may be expected to have a better outcome if they receive a course of corticosteroids.

15. When should an asthmatic be intubated?
Immediate intubation is indicated for patients who arrive in the emergency room in cardiopulmonary arrest, near cardiopulmonary arrest (e.g., patients unable to speak or gasping for air), in coma, or with significant obtundation. For patients who have received pharmacologic treatment, intubation should be considered if there is clinical deterioration. Changes in posture, alertness, speech, extent of accessory muscle use, and respiratory rate indicate worsening respiratory failure, in which case blood gas or peak flow confirmation is not needed for intubation.

16. When and how is a patient paralyzed during mechanical ventilation?
Muscle paralysis is indicated in patients who, in spite of sedation, continue to breath in a desynchronized manner during mechanical ventilation, placing themselves at greater risk of generating high airway pressures and losing airway access. The preferred paralytic agent, vecuronium, should be given intermittently by bolus injection. The interaction between high doses of corticosteroids, which are often given to asthmatic patients, and neuromuscular blockers such as vecuronium may increase the incidence of prolonged neuromuscular blockade. Monitoring of the response to electrical stimulation (train-of-four) is useful to determine the degree of blockade, and use of bolus administration rather than continuous IV drip can decrease the severity of this problem.

17. What should be done to decrease hyperinflation in an asthmatic on mechanical ventilation?
The risk of systemic hypotension and pneumothorax correlates directly with lung hyperinflation, which is minimized by allowing an adequate time for exhalation. Expiratory time should be prolonged by a decrease in respiratory rate (RR), tidal volume (V_T), and inspiratory time, the latter by increased inspiratory flow. RR and V_T should be reduced even if hypercapnia ensues. Allowing hypercapnia to ensue, or "permissive hypercapnia," is acceptable in the intubated asthmatic to reduce barotrauma. An infusion of bicarbonate should be considered if the systemic pH is less than 7.2; however, this is controversial.

18. When should heli-ox be used in asthma?
Heli-ox is a blend of helium and oxygen that has a gas density less than that of air. Reduced gas density has the potential to decrease airway resistance. Although there are trials showing the efficacy of heli-ox, further studies are indicated before this gas can be recommended in the routine management of patients with acute asthma. In the meantime, heli-ox should be used for patients with very severe exacerbations of asthma who do not respond to vigorous therapy.

CONTROVERSIES

19. What are the reasons that asthma mortality is increasing?
A number of explanations have been put forward, including:
- Shifts in diagnostic patterns, especially from bronchitis to asthma in young children and from COPD to asthma in older patients.
- An increase in the prevalence or severity of asthma, or both.
- Improvement in recognition of asthma.

- Changes in health care access, availability, and utilization.
- Drug effects. Links between frequent use of certain inhaled β-agonists and mortality from asthma have been suggested. Case-control studies in New Zealand and Saskatchewan linked mortality from asthma mainly with fenoterol. The withdrawal of fenoterol from New Zealand in 1990 was associated with a decline in morbidity and mortality.

Other authors argued that the case-control findings could have been confounded by severity, i.e., that patients who were prescribed β-agonists may have had more severe asthma and may have had a higher risk of death for that reason alone.

20. Does salmeterol (long-acting β-2 agonist) have antiinflammatory effects in asthmatics?

Studies in vitro and in animals showed that salmeterol has beneficial action on the cells and mediators considered important in asthma. Most studies using bronchoalveolar lavage and bronchial biopsies, however, were unable to show any significant effect of salmeterol on airway inflammation in asthmatics.

BIBLIOGRAPHY

1. Buist AS, Vollmer WM: Reflections on the rise in asthma morbidity and mortality. JAMA 264:1719–1720, 1990.
2. Corbridge TC, Hall JB: The assessment and management of adults with status asthmaticus. Am J Respir Crit Care Med 151:1296–1316, 1995.
3. Djukanovic R, Roche WR, Wilson JW, et al: Mucosal inflammation in asthma. Am Rev Respir Dis 142:434–457, 1990.
4. Gardiner PV, Ward C, Booth H, et al: Effect of eight weeks of treatment with salmeterol on bronchoalveolar lavage inflammatory indices in asthmatics. Am J Respir Crit Care Med 150:1006–1011, 1994.
5. Gershwin ME, Halpern GM: Bronchial Asthma: Principles of Diagnosis and Treatment. Totowa, Humana Press, 1994.
6. Gerstman BB, Bosco LA, Tomita DK, et al: Prevalence and treatment of asthma in the Michigan Medicaid patient population younger than 45 years, 1980–1986. J Allergy Clin Immunol 83:1032–1039, 1989.
7. Johnson M: Beta-2 agonists as anti-inflammatory therapies in the lungs. Agents Actions 41(Suppl): 27–45, 1993.
8. Martin RJ: Nocturnal asthma. Ann Allergy 72:5–10, 1994.
9. Martin RJ, Blager FB, Gay ML, et al: Paradoxic vocal cord motion in presumed asthmatics. Semin Respir Med 8:332–337, 1987.
10. McFadden ER Jr: Improper patient techniques with metered dose inhaler: Clinical consequences and solutions to misuse. J Allergy Clin Immunol 96:278–283, 1995.
11. National Heart, Lung, and Blood Institute: International Consensus Report on Diagnosis and Treatment of Asthma. Eur Respir J 5:601–641, 1992.
12. Pearce N, Beasley R, Crane J, et al: End of the New Zealand asthma mortality epidemic. Lancet 345:41–44, 1995.
13. Spitzer WO, Suissa S, Ernst P, et al: The use of beta-agonists and the risk of death and near death from asthma. N Engl J Med 326:501–506, 1992.
14. Staudinger HW, Hass JF: Beta-agonists and death from asthma. N Engl J Med 327:355, 1992.
15. U.S. Department of Health and Human Services, PHS Resources Administration: Prevalence of Selected Chronic Respiratory Conditions, United States, 1970. Vital Health Statistics, Series 10, No. 84. Washington, D.C., 1973.

18. CHRONIC OBSTRUCTIVE LUNG DISEASE

Jeon W. Lee, M.D., and Bartolome R. Celli, M.D.

1. How is chronic obstructive pulmonary disease defined?

Chronic obstructive pulmonary disease (COPD) is a disease state characterized by the presence of airflow obstruction caused by chronic bronchitis or emphysema; the airflow obstruction is generally persistent and progressive, may be accompanied by airway hyperreactivity, and may be partially reversible. Asthma, cystic fibrosis, bronchiectasis, and bronchiolitis should be excluded. Chronic bronchitis is defined as the presence of chronic productive cough for 3 months in each of two successive years in a patient in whom other causes of chronic cough have been excluded. Emphysema is defined as abnormal permanent enlargement of the airspaces distal to the terminal branches accompanied by destruction of their walls and without obvious fibrosis. COPD is defined in functional terms, chronic bronchitis in clinical terms, and emphysema in terms of anatomic pathology.

2. List the risk factors for COPD.

- **Tobacco smoking** accounts for an estimated 80–90% of the risk of developing COPD. In fact, many of the other risk factors simply represent modifiers of the host response to cigarette smoke. Age when smoking started, total pack-years, and current smoking status are predictive of COPD mortality.
- Both occupational and urban **pollution** are thought to play a role, but the significance of pollution remains unknown.
- **Infection of lower respiratory tract** during childhood may increase the subsequent risk of COPD by affecting lung function, lung growth, or pulmonary defense mechanisms. Respiratory infection in patients with established COPD may accelerate subsequent functional deterioration, and established COPD may increase the incidence and severity of respiratory infection.
- Asthma, atopy, and nonspecific **airway hyperresponsiveness** may play a role. Studies are under way to evaluate the importance of hyperresponsiveness.
- **Sex, race, heredity, and socioeconomic status.** Men have a higher prevalence of respiratory symptoms. Mortality rates are higher in whites than in nonwhites. Morbidity and mortality are inversely related to socioeconomic status. COPD may aggregate in families.
- α_1-**Antitrypsin (AAT) deficiency** is the only known genetic abnormality that leads to COPD. AAT deficiency accounts for less than 1% of COPD in the United States. Normal M alleles occur in about 90% of persons of European descent with normal serum AAT level; the phenotype is designated PiMM. More than 95% of persons in the severely deficient category are homozygous for the Z allele, designated PiZZ. PiMZ heterozygotes have serum AAT levels that are intermediate between PiMM normals and PiZZ homozygotes. In population studies, PiMZ heterozygotes do not appear to be a increased risk for COPD.

3. What are the clinical manifestations of COPD?
History

Cough (usually chronic and productive): hemoptysis is uncommon and its presence should stimulate a careful search for other causes such as cancer or tuberculosis.

Dyspnea (progressive) is not closely related to abnormalities of arterial blood gases.

Smoking: most patients are heavy smokers.

Wheezing is common.

Acute chest illness is also frequent.

Physical examination
- Chest
  Airway obstruction as evidenced by:
      Wheezes during auscultation on slow or forced breathing
      Prolongation of forced expiratory time
  Severe emphysema indicated by:
      Overdistension of lungs in stable state, low diaphragmatic position
      Decrease intensity of breath and heart sounds
  Severe disease suggested by (characteristic, not diagnostic):
      Pursed-lip breathing
      Use of accessory respiratory muscles
      Indrawing of lower interspaces
- Other signs and symptoms
  Unusual positions to relieve dyspnea at rest
  Digital clubbing (suggests lung cancer or bronchiectasis)
  Mild dependent edema (may be seen in absence of right heart failure)

4. What are the radiographic changes in COPD?

In **chronic bronchitis**, the chest radiograph may be normal, or tubular shadows (parallel or slightly tapering line shadows outside the boundary of hila) or prominent lung markings ("dirty lung") may be observed.

In **emphysema**, *overinflation*, a low, flat diaphragm, an increased retrosternal airspace, narrow heart shadow; *oligemia*, dimunition in the caliber of pulmonary vessels, with increased rapidity of tapering distally; and *bullae*, radiolucent areas larger than 1 cm in diameter and surrounded by hairline shadows may be observed. Bullae reflect only locally severe disease and are not necessarily indicative of widespread emphysema. With complicating pulmonary hypertension and right ventricular hypertrophy, the hilar vascular shadows are prominent, and the heart shadow encroaches on the retrosternal space as the right ventricle enlarges anteriorly. Emphysema is diagnosed on chest radiographs consistently when the disease is severe, never when the disease is mild, and in about 50% of instances when the disease is moderate. A chest radiograph is always indicated in the evaluation of patients with COPD, mainly to rule out other entities that may present with similar symptoms.

5. What are the abnormalities in pulmonary function tests in COPD?

The measurement of forced vital capacity in one second (FEV_1) is necessary for the diagnosis and assessment of the severity of COPD. It is also helpful in following its progression. Airflow obstruction is an important indicator of impairment of the whole person and the likelihood of blood gas abnormalities. FEV_1 is easily measurable, has less variability than other measurements of airway dynamics, and is more accurately predictable from age, sex, and height. Lung volume measurements show an increase in total lung capacity, functional residual capacity, and residual volume. The vital capacity may be decreased. The single breath-breath carbon monoxide diffusing capacity is decreased in proportion to the severity of emphysema because of the loss of alveolar capillary bed. The test is not specific, and it cannot detect mild emphysema. None of these tests can distinguish between chronic bronchitis and emphysema. Up to 30% of patients have an increase of 15% or more in FEV_1 after a β-agonist aerosol. The absence of a bronchodilator response during a single test never justifies withholding bronchodilator therapy. The determination of lung volumes or diffusion capacity is not routinely indicated in patients with COPD; these variables should be measured only in cases in which there is confusion about the physiologic nature of the disease causing the symptoms.

6. How is the severity of COPD staged?

The severity of COPD may be staged on the basis of the degree of airflow obstruction, using the criteria of the American Thoracic Society (ATS) statement on interpretation of lung function.

- **Stage 1** *(FEV₁ more than 50% predicted)* comprises the great majority of patients who will usually be cared for on a continuing basis by a general internist. Arterial blood gas measurements are not required. The presence of severe dyspnea warrants additional studies and evaluation by a respiratory specialist.
- **Stage 2** *(FEV₁ 35–49% of predicted)* includes a minority of patients who usually merit evaluation by a respiratory specialist and may receive continuing care by such a specialist.
- **Stage 3** *(FEV₁ less than 35% predicted)* also includes a minority of patients who are usually under the care of a respiratory specialist. These patients usually have abnormalities in arterial blood gases and may be candidates for oxygen therapy if hypoxemia (PaO_2 less than 55 mmHg) is documented.

7. **List the elements needed to diagnose COPD.**
   - A complete **history and physical examination** should be performed. If history and physical findings are consistent with or suggest the diagnosis of COPD, the following supportive laboratory tests also should be performed.
   - **Chest radiography:** diagnostic only of severe emphysema but essential to exclude other lung diseases.
   - **Spirometry** (pre- and postbronchodilator): essential to confirm presence and reversibility of airway obstruction and to quantify maximum level of ventilatory function.
   - **Arterial blood gases:** not needed in stage 1 COPD but essential in stages 2 and 3.
   The following tests may help to stage the disease, once the diagnosis is made:
   - **Lung volumes:** measurement of more than forced vital capacity is not necessary except in special circumstances (e.g., presence of giant bullae).
   - **Carbon monoxide diffusing capacity:** not necessary except in special instances (e.g., dyspnea out of proportion to severity of airflow limitation).

8. **What is the natural history of COPD?**
   The FEV_1 in nonsmokers without respiratory disease declines by 25 to 30 ml per year beginning at about age 35. The rate of decline of FEV_1 is steeper for smokers than for nonsmokers, and the heavier the smoking the steeper the rate. The decline in function occurs along a slowly accelerating curvilinear path. There is a direct relationship between initial FEV_1 level and the slope of FEV_1 decline. There is also a stronger association between a low FEV_1/forced vital capacity (FVC) and subsequent decline in FEV_1 in men but not in women. Age, the number of years of cigarette smoking, and the number of cigarettes currently smoked are the risk factors for more rapid decline of lung function. Acute chest illnesses generally decrease lung function for about 90 days in COPD patients. After cessation of smoking, a small amount of lung function is regained. Thereafter, the rate of decline in lung function approximates that seen in never-smokers of the same age. Smoking cessation improves prognosis regardless of age.

9. **What are the prognostic factors in COPD?**
   Predictors of mortality in patients with COPD are advancing age, severity of airway obstruction, as indicated by FEV_1, severity of hypoxemia, and the presence of hypercapnia and cor pulmonale. Marked reversibility of airway obstruction is a favorable prognostic factor. Persons with moderate obstruction but with FEV_1 more than 1.0 L have a slightly higher mortality at 10 years than an age- and gender-matched population. In persons with FEV_1 less than 0.75 L, the approximate mortality rate at 1 year is 30% and at 10 years it is 95%. However, some patients with severe airway obstruction may survive for as long as 15 years beyond the average. The reason appears to be that death in COPD generally occurs as a result of a medical complication such as acute respiratory failure, severe pneumonia, pneumothorax, cardiac arrhythmia, or pulmonary embolism.

10. **How should stable COPD be managed?**
    Once the diagnosis of COPD is established, the patient should be educated about the disease and encouraged to participate actively in therapy, especially in preventive care (e.g., immunization,

including pneumococcal and annual influenza vaccines), and to maintain an active lifestyle. Above all, a patient who still smokes must be encouraged and supported in an effort to quit. Airway obstruction should be managed with pharmacotherapy, which includes bronchodilators, antiinflammatory drugs, and mucokinetic agents. Hypoxia should be assessed, and supplemental oxygen must be administered if indicated. The response to therapy should be assessed periodically. A patient may benefit from a multidisciplinary rehabilitation program if severe symptoms or decreased functional capacity is observed over time, of if there are more than two hospital or emergency room visits per year.

11. What drug regimens are given for COPD?
- 1. For mild, variable symptoms:
  Selective β-2 agonist metered dose inhaler (MDI) aerosol, 1–2 puffs every 6–12 hours as needed, not to exceed 8–12 puffs per 24 hours.
- 2. For mild to moderate continuing symptoms:
  Ipratropium MDI aerosol, 2–6 puffs every 6–8 hours, not to be used more frequently, plus selective β-agonist MDI aerosol, 1–4 puffs as required four times daily for rapid relief, when needed or as regular supplement.
- 3. If response to step 2 is unsatisfactory or there is mild to moderate increase in symptoms:
  Add sustained-release theophylline, 200–400 mg twice daily or 400–800 mg at bedtime for nocturnal bronchospasm (serum theophylline level must be monitored intermittently).
  Consider use of sustained-release albuterol, 4–8 mg twice daily or at night only and/or consider use of mucokinetic agent.
- 4. If control of symptoms is suboptimal:
  Consider course of oral steroids (prednisone), up to 40 mg/day for 10–14 days
  If improvement occurs, wean to low daily or alternate-day dose.
  If no improvement occurs, stop abruptly.
  If oral steroid appears to help, consider use of aerosol steroid MDI, particularly if patient has evidence of bronchial hyperreactivity.
- 5. For severe exacerbation:
  Increase β-2 agonist dosage, e.g., MDI with spacer, 6–8 puffs every $1/2$–2 hours, or inhalant solution, unit dose every $1/2$–2 hours or subcutaneous administration of epinephrine or terbutaline, 0.1–0.5 ml.
  Increase ipratropium dosage, e.g., MDI with spacer, 6–8 puffs every 3–4 hours, or inhalant solution of ipratropium, 0.5 mg every 4–8 hours.
  Provide theophylline dosage intravenously with calculated amount to bring serum level to 10–15 μg/ml.
  Provide methylprednisone dosage intravenously giving 50–100 mg immediately, then every 6–8 hours; taper as soon as possible and add:
  An antibiotic, if indicated
  A mucokinetic agent if sputum is very viscous

12. What is the role of corticosteroids in COPD?
In contrast to their value in asthma management, the role of steroids in COPD is less clear. Steroids may merit more careful evaluation in individual patients on adequate bronchodilator therapy who fail to improve sufficiently or whose disease worsens. At present, there is no evidence that patients with COPD who are being treated with regular bronchodilator therapy require the protective effects of added steroid therapy, as used in asthma. Most studies suggest that only 20–30% of patients with COPD improve if given long-term oral steroid therapy. The dangers of steroids require careful documentation of the effectiveness of such therapy before a patient is put on prolonged dosing. It is possible that aerosol steroid can be used in place of low-dose oral steroids, but again there is insufficient documentation to support such therapy. Two large trials currently under way will evaluate the role of inhaled steroids in COPD.

13. Is the nebulized inhaler superior to the MDI?

No. Inhaled bronchodilators can be administered as a wet aerosol from a jet or ultrasonic nebulizer, or they can be administered from an MDI as a propellent-generated aerosol or as a breath-propelled dry powder. The relative efficiencies of the nebulizer and metered-dose inhaler vary with the techniques used for each. With optimal technique, approximately 12% of the drug is delivered from the MDI to the lung; the remainder is deposited in the mouth, pharynx, and larynx. In general, the dose required in a nebulizer is 6 to 10 times that used in an MDI to produce the same degree of bronchodilation. Inhaled bronchodilators delivered by MDI are as effective as those delivered by nebulizer. Even in the emergency setting, supervised adrenergic therapy delivered by MDI with a spacer device is as effective as nebulizer treatment.

14. What are the indications for long-term oxygen therapy in COPD?

Long-term oxygen therapy (LTOT) is indicated for patients whose disease is stable on full medical regimen and meet the following criteria:

Continuous oxygen therapy (24 hours/day)
- Resting PaO_2 less than 55 mmHg or SaO_2 less than 88%.
- Resting PaO_2 of 56–59 mmHg or SaO_2 of 89% in the presence of any of the following:
  Dependent edema suggesting congestive heart failure.
  P-pulmonale on ECG (p wave more than 3 mm in inferior leads) or cor pulmonale.
  Erythrocytosis (hematocrit more than 56).
- Resting PaO_2 more than 59 mmHg or SaO_2 more than 89:
  Reimbursable only with additional documentation justifying the oxygen prescription and a summary of more conservative therapy that has failed.

Noncontinuous oxygen therapy
- Oxygen flow rate and number of hours per day must be specified.
  During exercise: PaO_2 less than 55 mmHg or SaO_2 less than 88% with a low level of exercise.
  During sleep: PaO_2 less than 55 mmHg or SaO_2 less than 88% with associated complications such as pulmonary hypertension, daytime somnolence, and cardiac arrhythmias.

Adapted from O'Donohue WJ: Indications for long-term oxygen therapy and appropriate use. In O'Donohue WJ (ed): Long-Term Oxygen Therapy: Scientific Basis and Application. New York, Marcel Dekker, 1995, pp 53–68; and Tarpy SP, Celli BR: Long-term oxygen therapy. N Engl J Med 333:710–714, 1995.

15. What is the role of chest therapy with drainage and antibiotics in COPD?

The value of chest therapy with drainage in patients with COPD has not been documented. Trials of postural drainage in patients acutely ill with COPD have failed to show a positive effect on sputum volume, gas exchange, or spirometric measurements. Chest wall percussion and vibration used with postural drainage also lack scientific support. Furthermore, in patients acutely ill with COPD, chest percussion and vibration can cause a transient decrease in FEV_1 and an increase in functional residual capacity as a result of acute bronchospasm. In patients with cystic fibrosis, the benefits of postural drainage are limited to patients who expectorate at least 25 ml of sputum per day. Extrapolating from those observations, it is recommended that postural drainage, with or without chest percussion or vibration, be limited to hospitalized patients with COPD whose sputum production also exceeds 25 ml per day. Patients with or without COPD whose course is complicated by mucus plugging with lobar atelectasis benefit from chest therapy. The value of antibiotics has not been proved in the prevention or treatment of COPD exacerbation unless there is evidence of infection (e.g., fever, leukocytosis) or a change in the radiograph. In cases of recurrent infection, particularly in winter, prolonged courses of continuous or intermittent antibiotics may be useful.

16. When is intubation with mechanical ventilation indicated in acute exacerbation of COPD?

Although no objective guidelines exist for determining the ideal time for intubation with assisted ventilation, this support will benefit two classes of patients: (1) those who have experienced progressive worsening of respiratory acidosis or altered mental status despite aggressive pharmacologic and nonventilatory support, and (2) those with clinically significant hypoxemia that has developed despite the provision of supplemental oxygen by usual technique.

Intubation with mechanical support is indicated in the presence of one of the following major criteria or two minor criteria after the first hour of aggressive therapy:

Major criteria	Minor criteria
Respiratory arrest	A respiratory rate more than 35 beats per minute and above the value on admission
Respiratory pauses with loss of consciousness or gasping for air	
Psychomotor agitation making nursing care impossible and requiring sedation	Arterial pH value less than 7.30 and below the value on admission
A heart rate less than 50 beats per minute with loss of alertness	PaO_2 less than 45 mmHg despite oxygen therapy
Hemodynamic instability with systolic arterial blood pressure less than 70 mmHg	Worsening mental status (asterixis, confusion, lethargy, agitation)

17. What is the role of noninvasive ventilatory support in COPD exacerbation?

Noninvasive ventilation—using both facial and nasal masks in conjunction with volume-cycled ventilation, bilevel positive airway pressure, and pressure support mode—can reduce the need for intubation, the length of the hospital stay, and the in-hospital mortality rate in selected patients with COPD exacerbation. Patient features that should discourage noninvasive ventilation include hemodynamic instability, copious secretions, inability to defend the airway, poor cooperation with the technique, or impaired mental status. Noninvasive ventilation should be provided in settings where personnel are familiar with the techniques to be used and able to manage the complications associated with this mode of ventilation, which include hypoventilation, hyperventilation, aspiration, and local discomfort.

18. How does the physician determine if intubation/ventilation is likely to be successful in a patient with severe COPD?

Although subjective bedside judgment cannot accurately determine the likelihood of successful ventilation and survival, clinical data do indicate that outcome correlates with baseline function (the severity of underlying COPD when stable and daily activity level) and the presence of nonpulmonary comorbid conditions, such as gastrointestinal bleeding, pulmonary embolism, or coronary artery disease. Analysis of the typical clinical outcome of patients with COPD who present with acute respiratory failure can assist decision making for intubation and mechanical ventilation. Between 75 and 90% of such patients who are mechanically ventilated survive to hospital discharge. Overall, short-term prognosis after intubation/ventilation for severe COPD is favorable, and the long-term prognosis is similar to that of patients with the same degree of underlying respiratory impairment who have not required mechanical ventilation.

19. Is surgical therapy available for severe COPD?

The following procedures may be contemplated for the patient with COPD:

Bullectomy (resection of large bullae compressing normal lung) can be helpful in relieving severe dysfunction and dyspnea. Resection of bullae occupying more than one third of the hemithorax produces the best result.

Lung volume reduction surgery (pneumectomy of nonuniform emphysematous lung) has been encouraging. In selected patients, the improvements in symptoms, FEV_1, FVC, and arterial blood gases have been significant. Studies are underway to evaluate the role of this procedure in patients with COPD.

Double lung transplantation is the definitive procedure to improve COPD. Single lung transplantation can be lifesaving. The procedure is costly, hampered by lack of donor availability, and requires lifelong immunosuppression.

20. What elements are needed to evaluate preoperatively the risk for postoperative pulmonary complications?

This process depends on the indications for surgery, surgical site, experience of surgical team, type of anesthesia, and degree of respiratory impairment. When the nature and severity of a patient's lung disease are unclear, physiologic tests should be considered in addition to history and physical examination. Candidates for lung resection should have pulmonary function tests such as spirometry and diffusing capacity routinely performed. Routine preoperative spirometry in candidates for upper abdominal surgery can be useful in the preoperative evaluation of patients with symptoms of COPD, especially if the test has not been done previously. Preoperative arterial blood gas analysis in all patients with severe COPD is recommended if a recent test is not available. A preoperative chest radiograph in patients about to undergo noncardiothoracic surgery is sensible, because patients with COPD are at increased risk for pulmonary neoplasms. Quantitative lung scintigraphy and exercise testing may be helpful in determining risk of postoperative complications, particularly in patients undergoing lung resection. In addition, exercise testing may reveal previously unexpected cardiovascular dysfunction.

21. How is a patient with COPD managed perioperatively?

Preoperative period. General guidelines include preoperative risk evaluation, smoking cessation at least 8 weeks preoperatively, and aggressive treatment of lung dysfunction, using inhaled bronchodilators, theophylline, corticosteroids, and antibiotics as indicated. Patients with stage 2 or 3 COPD may be admitted to the hospital before surgery for multidisciplinary evaluation, patient education, and aggressive therapy.

Intraoperative considerations. The intraoperative period does not appear to pose major problems.

Postoperative period. In the immediate postoperative recovery period, a number of potential threats are present, including respiratory muscle dysfunction, acidemia, hypoxemia, and hypoventilation. In this delicate period close monitoring, and if necessary mechanical ventilatory support, are crucial to the patient with COPD. The inability to overcome diaphragmatic dysfunction probably explains the failure of deep breathing resulting in pulmonary complications. Intermittent positive-pressure breathing or incentive spirometry reduces postoperative complications after upper abdominal surgery. Continuation of the preoperatively prescribed antibiotics, bronchodilators, corticosteroids, and theophylline is standard therapy.

22. Is pulmonary rehabilitation useful in COPD?

The available evidence indicates that pulmonary rehabilitation benefits patients with symptomatic COPD. The effect of pulmonary rehabilitation programs on health care utilization are promising but require further investigation. In contrast, aerobic lower extremity training is of benefit in several areas of importance to patients with COPD. These areas include exercise endurance, perception of dyspnea, quality of life, and self-efficacy. The exact role of upper extremity exercise training programs requires further studies. Education and psychological support improve the awareness of patients and increase their understanding of the disease, but when used alone, education and support are of limited value. Pulmonary rehabilitation coupled with smoking cessation, optimization of blood gas levels, and medications offers the best treatment option with symptomatic airway obstruction.

BIBLIOGRAPHY

1. Brochard L, Mancebo J, Wysocki M, et al: Noninvasive ventilation for acute exacerbation of COPD. N Engl J Med 333:817–822, 1995.
2. Celli BR: Perioperative respiratory care. Clin Chest Med 14:253–261, 1993.
3. Fraser RG, Paré JAP, Paré PD, et al: Diagnosis of Diseases of the Chest, 3rd ed. 1994, pp 2087–2166, 1994.
4. Nelson HS: Beta-adrenergic bronchodilators. N Engl J Med 333:499–506, 1995.
5. Statement paper (American Thoracic Society): Standards for the diagnosis and care of patients with COPD. Am J Respir Crit Care Med 152:S77–S120, 1995.
6. Tarpy SP, Celli BR: Long-term oxygen therapy. N Engl J Med 333:710–714, 1995.
7. Wanke T, Formanek D, Lahrmann HM, et al: Effects of combined inspiratory muscle and cycle ergometer training exercise performance in patients with COPD. Eur Respir J 7:2205–2211, 1995.

19. OXYGEN THERAPY

Rebecca L. Meredith, R.R.T., and James K. Stoller, M.D.

1. When should supplemental oxygen be prescribed?

Long-standing hypoxemia can cause many adverse effects, including pulmonary hypertension, cor pulmonale, neuropsychiatric impairment, and most importantly, decreased survival. The clinical impact of long-standing hypoxemia and the benefits of supplemental oxygen have been most extensively studied in patients with COPD. For example, the combined results from the British Medical Research Council and the American Nocturnal Oxygen Therapy Trial (NOTT) studies demonstrated that the use of supplemental oxygen was associated with enhanced survival and improved neuropsychiatric well-being in hypoxic patients with COPD. Use of oxygen for 15 hours per day was associated with better survival rates than not using oxygen at all, but longer duration of daily use (i.e., approximately 19 hours per day) was associated with still better survival than 12 hours daily. On the basis of these findings, oxygen is recommended for use as close to 24 hours per day as possible for appropriate candidates. For patients with hypoxemia caused by COPD, aggressive treatment with bronchodilators and antibiotics (if needed for airway infections) has been shown to improve oxygenation and can obviate the need for supplemental oxygen in up to 40% of individuals. The need for supplemental oxygen should be reestablished and the dose of oxygen required should be assessed periodically, perhaps every 6 months.

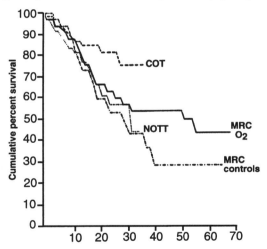

Cumulative percent survival of patients in the Nocturnal Oxygen Therapy Trial (NOTT) and Medical Research Council (MRC) controlled trials of long-term domiciliary oxygen therapy for men aged over 70. The MRC control subject ($\bullet - \bullet$) received no oxygen; the NOTT subject ($\cdots$) received oxygen for 12 hours in the 24-hour day, including the sleeping hours; MRC O_2 subjects (—) received oxygen for 15 hours in the 24-hour day, including the sleeping hours; and continuous oxygen therapy (COT) subjects ($\_ \_ \_$) received oxygen for 24 hours in the 24-hour day (on average, 19 hours). (From Flenley DC: Long-term oxygen therapy. Chest 87:99–193, 1985; with permission.)

2. List the indications for prescribing long-term oxygen therapy.

Continuous oxygen

Arterial oxygen tension (PaO_2)/arterial oxygen saturations (SaO_2)
- Resting PaO_2 less than 55 mmHg or SaO_2 less than 88%

- Resting PaO_2 56–59 mmHg or SaO_2 less than 89% in the presence of any of the following:
  Edema suggesting congestive heart failure or
  P pulmonale on ECG
- Erythrocytosis (hematocrit 56% or more)
  Resting PaO_2 more than 59 mmHg or SaO_2 more than 89% reimbursable only with additional documentation justifying the oxygen prescription and a summary that more conservative therapy has failed

Noncontinuous oxygen*
Oxygen flow rate and number of hours per day must be specified
- During exercise: PaO_2 less than 55 mmHg or SaO_2 less than 88% with low level of exertion
- During sleep: PaO_2 less than 55 mmHg or SaO_2 less than 88% with associated complications, i.e., pulmonary hypertension, daytime somnolence, cardiac arrhythmias
- More than 5% fall in saturation during sleep

* Supportive evidence less definite than that for continuous oxygen. These are criteria for Medicare reimbursement for noncontinuous oxygen.

Medicare requirements for long-term oxygen therapy
- The laboratory, **not** the oxygen supplier, must measure PaO_2 or SaO_2 (or both)
- Patient must have optimal medical management and be clinically stable before certification
- The physician must complete a medical necessity form
- Recertification and retesting in 61–90 days if the patient has an initial PaO_2 or 56–59 mmHg and saturation of 89%. All other patients need recertification after 12 months but no retesting
- Revised certification when the prescription is changed

Adapted from O'Donohue WJ: Indications for long-term oxygen therapy and appropriate use. In O'Donohue WJ (ed): Long-Term Oxygen Therapy: Scientific Basis and Application. New York, Marcel Dekker, 1995, pp 53–68; and Tarpy SP, Celli BR: Long-term oxygen therapy. N Engl J Med 333:710–714, 1995.

3. Should supplemental oxygen be prescribed during sleep?

For individuals with resting daytime hypoxemia, supplemental oxygen should be provided during sleep as part of the goal of providing oxygen for as close to 24 hours a day as possible. For COPD patients with nocturnal hypoxemia (i.e., SaO_2 less than 88%) but adequate oxygenation during wakefulness (i.e., PaO_2 more than 60 mmHg), the benefits of supplemental oxygen are less clear, but many clinicians prescribe oxygen when symptoms ascribable to hypoxemia are present (e.g., pulmonary hypertension, cardiac arrhythmias, or disrupted sleep with daytime hypersomnolence).

4. Should supplemental oxygen be prescribed during exercise?

Although hypoxemia is less frequently the cause of exercise limitation than is reaching ventilatory or cardiovascular limits, patients with hypoxemia during exercise (i.e, PaO_2 less than or equal to 55 mmHg or arterial saturation of 88% or less) may benefit from using supplemental oxygen during exercise. In this circumstance, supplemental oxygen may reduce minute ventilation, improve ventilatory muscle function, lessen dyspnea, and improve endurance. As such, many clinicians will prescribe oxygen to eligible individuals during exercise. The liter flow rates are best determined by exercise studies with intermittent blood gas sampling through an indwelling arterial line. Though less invasive, pulse oximetry measurements of oxygen saturation during exercise can be misleading, causing oxygen to be prescribed when not needed and also leading to undertreatment of hypoxemia.

5. Should supplemental oxygen be prescribed for individuals with hypoxemia due to causes other than COPD?

Yes. Although the indications and benefits of supplemental oxygen have been best studied for individuals with COPD, other hypoxemic individuals should also be considered candidates for supplemental oxygen.

6. How should an oxygen prescription be written?

Once the need for supplemental oxygen is established, a prescription can be written. It should include:

the qualifying arterial blood gas

the type of delivery system to be used (i.e., stationary system, portable or ambulatory equipment, oxygen-conserving device, and so forth)

the delivery device (i.e., nasal cannula, transtracheal catheter, mask)

the liter flow under specific conditions (i.e., sleep, rest, exercise)

the patient's diagnosis.

The physician is responsible for all forms and documentation. Medicare form 484 must be filled out for all Medicare patients and some third party payors. Oxygen prescriptions are unique in that the patient generally receives oxygen therapy before the home medical equipment (HME) company has a properly written prescription. Therefore, it is often the HME's responsibility to ensure that the patient has a proper oxygen prescription on file for reimbursement to take place.

7. Is supplemental oxygen recommended during commercial air travel?

As a result of Dalton's Law of Gases, conditions inside the cabin of a commercial airplane in flight expose travelers to conditions of hypobaric hypoxia; i.e., because the ambient pressure is decreased, the inspired oxygen tension is decreased. The specific ambient pressure within the plane depends on the altitude and properties of the plane itself, but U.S. Federal Aviation Administration rules require that the pressure inside the cabin remain below the equivalent of 8000 feet (except for brief ascents to 10,000 feet equivalent to avoid bad weather). Under conditions of hypobaric hypoxia, arterial oxygen tension falls in travelers. Because of the theoretical risks of hypoxemia, especially when arterial saturation falls below 90%, supplemental oxygen has been recommended for air travelers when their resting Pao_2 is predicted to be 50 mmHg during flight. Clinicians should attempt to predict whether an individual traveler's Pao_2 is likely to fall below 50 mmHg during air flight. For patients with normocapnic, stable COPD, several regression equations are available that help to predict the traveler's in-flight Pao_2, the most recent of which is listed below:

$$\text{Predicted } Pao_2 \text{ at } 8000 \text{ ft} = 0.294 \text{ (}Pao_2 \text{ on room air at sea level)} + 0.086 \text{ (}FEV_1\% \text{ predicted)} + 23.211$$

This calculation requires measurement of the traveler's room air resting Pao_2 and FEV_1 (without a bronchodilator). Alternative methods for predicting the traveler's in-flight Pao_2 include measurement of the Pao_2 while the traveler breathes a hypoxic gas (i.e., 15.1% oxygen) mixture meant to simulate the hypoxia during air travel, or measurement of the Pao_2 under actual hypobaric conditions (e.g., a hypobaric chamber or actual ascent to altitude). Practical constraints make the latter approaches unattractive, thereby favoring use of the regression equations. However, for patients with pulmonary diseases other than normocapnic, stable COPD (e.g., restrictive diseases, hypercapnic COPD) no predictive equations are available, and clinicians must either prescribe supplemental in-flight oxygen empirically, or determine the traveler's actual Pao_2 under hypoxic conditions (i.e., by breathing a hypoxic gas or under actual hypobaric conditions).

8. How is oxygen arranged for air travelers?

Once the decision has been made to prescribe supplemental oxygen during air flight, the traveler must arrange for in-flight oxygen to be supplied by the airline. Regulations by the U.S. Federal Aviation Administration prohibit travelers from bringing their own oxygen supplies for use in the airline cabin. Furthermore, individual airlines vary regarding the type of oxygen system they supply, the liter flow and delivery device (e.g., cannula or mask), the cost of providing oxygen (which is not covered by Medicare even if the traveler qualifies for supplemental oxygen under Medicare guidelines), and the advance time needed to arrange oxygen. As a result, it is important for the traveler to know the specific policy of the airline on which travel is planned. Notwithstanding individual variation between airlines, several general rules apply, as follows:

- Arrangements for oxygen must be made well in advance of the actual trip, usually at least 3 days for domestic trips.
- Although the specific airline may wish its medical department to speak with the traveler's physician, a written prescription for oxygen by the traveler's physician is advised. The prescription should specify the liter flow and duration of oxygen needed.
- Travelers should bring along their own nasal tubing in extra length.
- A seat near the bathroom is advised to minimize motion and time off supplemental oxygen.
- Traveling on nonstop, direct flights is advised to minimize travel time and the expense of receiving oxygen (because some air carriers charge for each leg of a connecting flight).
- Traveling during business hours is advised, especially if the traveler requires supplemental oxygen on arrival at the airport and at the travel destination. Oxygen supplied by the airline stops when the traveler leaves the plane, so that for travelers requiring supplemental oxygen at sea level (or if the travel destination is at high altitude), interaction with an oxygen vendor on arrival must be arranged separately.
- Most airlines have medical departments that can provide specific information about the carrier's oxygen policy.

9. What systems exist to provide supplemental oxygen for use at home?

Oxygen in the home is often delivered by nasal cannula at low flow rates of 2–4 L/minute. Patients often require several different systems for use at home, e.g., for use around the house (where an oxygen concentrator and a long connecting delivery tube may work well), during excursions outside the home (when a liquid oxygen portable carrier or a smaller tank such as an E-type cylinder is especially suitable), and during exercise in the home. There are three delivery systems currently available for use in the home: compressed-oxygen cylinders, liquid oxygen systems, and oxygen concentrators. Liquid oxygen systems and compressed oxygen cylinders are available for travel.

Compressed oxygen is provided in high-pressure cylinders. They are large and heavy and can cause injury because of the high pressure if the valve end of the tank is damaged. Generally, size H or G tanks are used with a duration of use at 2 L/minute of 57.5 and 39.2 hours, respectively. Several links of oxygen tubing can be attached to the tank in order to provide limited patient mobility. Smaller tanks (size D and E) are available for use when traveling; their duration of use at 2 L/minute is 2.9 and 5.1 hours, respectively. Combining the smaller units with an oxygen-conserving device may extend the duration of available oxygen to as long as 8 hours. Compressed gas systems generally require frequent visits from the home care company. If the patient is unable to change the regulator, visits may be required every other day.

Liquid oxygen systems offer several advantages over compressed oxygen cylinders, particularly for patients who are active. Stationary systems of liquid oxygen weight 240 pounds and provide 7 days of continuous oxygen at 2 L/min. Portable liquid systems can be easily refilled from the larger stationary systems; they weight less and will last four times longer than compressed oxygen cylinders at a given flow rate. The major disadvantage of liquid oxygen systems is their high cost. Oxygen itself is relatively inexpensive, but the cost of specialized home stationary units and delivery trucks dramatically increase the cost. As a result, liquid oxygen is often available only in large metropolitan areas. Liquid oxygen is stored at −183° Celsius; as the tanks warm up, the oxygen expands, requiring pressure relief valves, which waste unused oxygen. Coupling devices for the stationary and portable systems made by different manufacturers may not be compatible, which further increases the cost. An advantage of liquid systems is that patients may fill their own tanks from the stationary system, but this poses the risk of thermal burns if the liquid oxygen is accidentally poured on the skin. Therefore, as a precaution, gloves should always be worn when transfilling cylinders.

Oxygen concentrators are electrical devices that use either a molecular sieve or a semipermeable membrane. The molecular sieve separates oxygen from the air for delivery to the patient and returns nitrogen to the atmosphere. This device can deliver more than 90% oxygen at flows of up to 4 L/minutes. The membrane-type is primarily permeable to oxygen and water vapor.

These units function at a low level of efficiency, delivering oxygen concentrations of only 40%. Both types weight approximately 35 pounds and operate on wall current. Therefore, they are used as stationary sources of oxygen in the home. Periodic refilling of the device is not necessary, although periodic preventive maintenance is required. Compressed oxygen cylinders and an electric generator should be available as a backup in areas prone to frequent power failures. Delivered oxygen concentrations should be analyzed on a monthly basis.

10. List the advantages and disadvantages of the various modes of oxygen delivery.

System	Advantages	Disadvantages
Compressed gas cylinder	Provides highest flow Moderate cost Wide availability Small cylinders available for travel Low maintenance	Heavy weight Refilling difficult and required frequently Must be secured to prevent injury
Liquid oxygen	Provides moderate flow Light weight Excellent portability Ease of refilling	High cost Incompatibility of parts among vendors Waste of unused oxygen because of pressure venting Risk of thermal burns Limited availability Frequent maintenance needed
Oxygen concentrator	Unlimited gas volume Low cost Good availability Ease of use	Limited flow rates available Heavy weight Poor portability Regular maintenance needed

Adapted from Kacmarek RM: Oxygen delivery systems for long-term oxygen therapy. In O'Donohue WJ (ed): Long-Term Oxygen Therapy: Scientific Basis and Application. New York, Marcel Dekker, 1995, pp 219–234; and Tarpy SP, Celli BR: Long-term oxygen therapy. N Engl J Med 333:710–714, 1995.

11. What is the cost of supplemental oxygen?

Reimbursement to vendors of supplemental oxygen by Medicare provides a set monthly fee (approximately $300/month) regardless of the oxygen system used. As a result, the least expensive oxygen system is generally provided by the oxygen vendor unless otherwise specified by the physician's oxygen prescription. Most patients require a stationary source for use in the home, usually a concentrator. Concentrators are relatively inexpensive (approximately $2200.00 per unit) and require regular maintenance. Patients not confined to bed should have a system to supply oxygen when they are outside the home. Compressed gas or liquid oxygen systems are available as portable devices. Liquid oxygen has a higher cost (approximately $3500/unit) for a stationary system that can be the primary oxygen source and also can fill smaller cylinders for use outside the home. Compressed oxygen tanks cost approximately $350 each and require frequent refilling by the home care company.

12. What is an oxygen delivery device?

Oxygen delivery devices are the conduits through which oxygen flows from the oxygen source (e.g., tank or concentrator) to the patient. Such delivery devices can be divided into two major categories: low-flow and high-flow systems. Low-flow systems are not intended to meet the patient's total inspiratory requirements. Oxygen concentrations delivered by these devices vary with ventilatory rate and tidal volume. For example, if the tidal volume is large, the inspired FIO_2 is lower; if the tidal volume is small, the inspired FIO_2 increases. A high-flow system has a reservoir and a total gas flow that supplies the patient's inspiratory requirements. The ventilatory rate and tidal volume have no effect on inspired oxygen concentrations.

13. What oxygen delivery devices are available?

Oxygen Delivery Devices and F_{IO_2} Capabilities

DELIVERY SYSTEM	DESCRIPTION	L/MIN FLOW RATE DELIVERS F_{IO_2}	COMPLICATIONS
Nasal cannula	Flow rate of 1–6 L/min Delivers approx 4%/L Prongs insert 1 cm into each nare Comfortable and inexpensive Patient can eat and talk	1 L/min = 24% 2 L/min = 28% 3 L/min = 32% 4 L/min = 36% 5 L/min = 40% 6 L/min = 44%	Delivered F_{IO_2} depends on tidal volume and ventilatory rate Nasal passages must be patent Easily dislodged May irritate nasal passages and eyes at higher flow rates
Simple mask*	Flow rate of 5–8 L/min Clear plastic, must fit tightly on patient's face	5–8 L/min = 50–60%	Need minimum of 5 L/min to adequately flush carbon dioxide and avoid rebreathing Use cautiously on comatose patients Must fit securely to patient's face to avoid entrainment of room air and dilution of inspired F_{IO_2} Increased risk of aspiration Less comfortable than nasal cannula Easily removed
Partial rebreathing mask*	Flow rate of 6–10 L/min Clear plastic mask that incorporates reservoir bag into system to deliver oxygen concentrations > 60%	6–10 L/min = 55–70%	Flow should be sufficient to keep reservoir bag inflated on inspiration Other complications same as for simple mask
Nonrebreathing mask*	Flow rate of 10–12 L/min Clear plastic mask with reservoir bag and 2 one-way valves (1 on mask and 1 between reservoir bag and mask	10–12 L/min = 80–100%	Flow should be sufficient to keep reservoir bag inflated on inspiration Other complications same as for simple mask
Venturi mask**	Flow rates are variable Clear plastic mask with different adapters that determine F_{IO_2} Provides exact oxygen concentrations Inspired concentrations do not vary with ventilatory rate and tidal volume Delivery device of choice for COPD patients depending on hypoxic drive	2 L/min = 24% 3 L/min = 28% 4 L/min = 31% 6 L/min = 35% 8 L/min = 40% 10 L/min = 45% 12 L/min = 50% 14 L/min = 55%	Same as for simple mask

Min = minute.
* Low flow system (does not meet total patient demand).
** High flow system (meets total patient demand).
Adapted from Oakes D: Therapeutic modalities. In Clinical Practitioners' Guide to Respiratory Care. Rockville, MD, Health Educator Publications, 1988, pp 143–159; Ryerson CG, Block AJ: Oxygen as a drug: Chemical properties, benefits and hazards of administration. In Burton GG, Hodgkin JE (eds): Respiratory Care, 2nd ed. Philadelphia, J.B. Lippincott, 1984, pp 395–415; and Tarpy SP, Celli BR: Long-term oxygen therapy. N Engl J Med 333:710–714, 1995.

14. What are oxygen-conserving devices?

Delivery of oxygen to the alveoli occurs during the first sixth of the inspiratory cycle. Oxygen delivered throughout the remainder of the respiratory cycle is wasted. Oxygen-conserving devices have been developed with the intent of eliminating "wasted" oxygen flow and maximizing the efficiency of oxygen supply devices. Oxygen-conserving devices generally provide adequate oxygenation at rest, with exercise, and during sleep; conserve oxygen; are more comfortable for the patient; and generally are more economical. Three types of oxygen-conserving devices are currently available: reservoir systems, demand delivery systems, and transtracheal catheters. One type of reservoir system uses the nasal cannula as the reservoir. Such reservoir nasal cannulas have a pouch that stores 20 ml of oxygen during the expiratory phase to be delivered at the beginning of the following inspiration as a bolus. In contrast, demand delivery systems sense inspiration and deliver an inspiratory bolus of oxygen. Finally, transtracheal catheters are inserted directly into the trachea, thereby bypassing the cephalad anatomic dead space and using the upper airways as a reservoir for oxygen during end expiration. Placement of transtracheal catheters requires an office procedure that is generally performed by a pulmonologist or otolaryngologist. Oxygen-conserving devices have gained great popularity because they reduce the amount of oxygen used, decrease the cost of oxygen, and provide the patient with increased mobility and independence.

15. List the advantages and disadvantages of different oxygen-conserving devices.

Oxygen-Conserving Devices

TYPE	COST	ADVANTAGES	DISADVANTAGES
Reservoir nasal cannula	Low (approximately $23 per unit)	Reliable, easy to initiate and use 33–50% oxygen conservation	Not esthetically pleasing for patient Frequent replacement needed
Demand	High (approximately $905.00 per unit)	Greatest degree of conserving oxygen of available systems (87%)	Mechanical failure possible Complicated technology (though easy to use)
Transtracheal catheter	High (approximately $700.00 for initial placement; $98 per replacement catheter; generally every 3 months)	Esthetically pleasing for patient (i.e., hidden from sight) Decreases work of breathing Patients are more compliant with oxygen use Does not easily become dislodged during sleep	Requires special care, dexterity, and tolerance of minor annoyances and complications

Adapted from Tarpy SP, Celli BR: Long-term oxygen therapy. N Engl J Med 333:710–714, 1995; and Weill D, Make B: Oxygen-conserving devices. In O'Donohue WJ (ed): Long-Term Oxygen Therapy: Scientific Basis and Application. New York, Marcel Dekker, 1995, pp 235–256.

16. How are oxygen-conserving devices paid for or reimbursed?

Medicare reimbursement rates for home oxygen therapy are based on local costs, independent of the device used. The rate of reimbursement is set for users with liter flow rates of 1–4 liters per minute, although Medicare reimbursement is adjusted for very low or very high flow rates. For example, if the liter flow is less than 1 liter per minute, the rate of reimbursement is reduced to 50% of the base cost; whereas liter flow rates of more than 4 liters per minute raise the reimbursement rate to 150% of the base rate. Unfortunately, the new reimbursement regulations have discouraged the use of oxygen-conserving devices, particularly transtracheal oxygen, which often operates at less than 1 liter per minute. The decision to provide an oxygen-conserving service is often influenced greatly by whether or not funding can be secured; a conserving device may be deferred unless reimbursement is available.

17. How is oxygen therapy monitored and adjusted?

Oxygen therapy should be monitored and adjusted periodically, based on careful patient assessment. Oxygen therapy is best monitored by arterial blood gas or pulse oximetry measurements with target values of Pao_2 equal to or more than 60 mmHg and Spo_2 equal to or more than 90%. Readings of saturation from arterial blood gases (Sao_2) and from pulse oximetry measurement (Spo_2) generally correlate within ±2% at rest. As a way of verifying the reliability of pulse oximeter measurements, the palpated pulse or heart rate derived from the ECG and the heart rate displayed on the pulse oximeter should agree within ±5 beats. If pulse oximetry does provide accurate readings of saturation, it is preferred for titrating oxygen at rest. In this way, use of pulse oximetry can decrease the number of samples needed for arterial blood gas measurement.

18. Are there risks associated with providing supplemental oxygen?

The risks associated with oxygen use relate to the possible effects of oxygen on ventilatory control, the morbidity associated with various oxygen delivery devices, and the risks related to using a combustible substance like oxygen. With regard to effects of supplemental oxygen on ventilation, some patients with hypoxemia experience hypoventilation when supplemental oxygen is used. Two mechanisms have been proposed as the cause of hypoventilation: suppression of the hypoxic drive to breathe in individuals dependent on hypoxic drive as the major ventilatory drive and increased dead space ventilation caused by increased pulmonary perfusion after relief of alveolar hypoxia. Individuals likely to experience hypercapnia when using supplemental oxygen are those with fixed severe, airflow obstruction and preexisting hypercapnia. Other risks associated with using oxygen relate to the devices through which oxygen is delivered. A nasal cannula can cause irritation of the nasal mucosa or skin over the ears, epistaxis resulting from drying of the nasal mucosa, and psychological unease about public exposure of oxygen dependence. Complications accompanying transtracheal oxygen are frequent but usually minor. These include infection at the insertion site, catheter displacement requiring reinsertion, cough, cephalad misplacement of the catheter between the vocal cords, bleeding and tracheal obstruction related to collection of inspissated mucus on the catheter. Finally, individuals using supplemental oxygen must avoid close exposure to open flames (e.g., stove burners, cigarettes) because oxygen supports combustion and could promote fire.

19. How should patients receiving supplemental oxygen be transported within the hospital?

Transport of a patient receiving oxygen therapy within the hospital demands specific attention to patient assessment and Fio_2 requirements. Once the need for oxygen has been established by arterial blood gas analysis or pulse oximetry, transport should be planned carefully so that all necessary equipment and personnel are available. Patients receiving low flow oxygen at 1–6 liters per minute can be transported using a portable liquid vessel of oxygen, often available from the patient transportation department at larger institutions. Higher flows (more than 6 L/min) require the use of a compressed gas cylinder, usually size E. The cylinder should be checked to ensure that it is full before the transport is begun; full cylinders contain 2200 psi and will provide oxygen for 1.7 hours at a flow rate of 6 liters per minute. Clinically unstable patients ideally should have a portable pulse oximeter in place while undergoing diagnostic tests or transport to other areas of the institution. Because transporting a sick patient incurs some risk, the benefits of the diagnostic test or treatment for which transport is needed must always justify the trip.

BIBLIOGRAPHY

1. Adamo J, Mehta AC, Stelmach KA, et al: The Cleveland Clinic's initial experience with transtracheal oxygen therapy. Respir Care 35:153–160, 1990.
2. Cottrell JJ, Openbrier D, Lave JR, et al: Home oxygen therapy: A comparison of 2- vs. 6-month patient re-evaluation. Chest 107:358–361, 1995.
3. Dillard TA, Moores LK, Bilello KL, et al: The preflight evaluation: A comparison of the hypoxia inhalation test with hypobaric exposure. Chest 107:352–357, 1995.
4. Huber GL, Carter R, Mahajan VK: Transtracheal oxygen therapy. In O'Donohue WJ (ed): Long-Term Oxygen Therapy: Scientific Basis and Application. New York, Marcel Dekker, 1995, pp 257–309.
5. Kacmarek RM: Supplemental oxygen and other medical gas therapy. In Pierson DJ, Kacmarek RM (eds): Foundations of Respiratory Care. New York, Churchill Livingstone, 1992, pp 859–889.
6. Kacmarek RM: Oxygen delivery systems for long-term oxygen therapy. In O'Donohue WJ (ed): Long-Term Oxygen Therapy: Scientific Basis and Application. New York, Marcel Dekker, 1995, pp 219–234.

7. McCarthy K, Decker M, Strohl KP, et al: Pulse oximetry. In Kacmarek RM, Hess D, Stoller JK (eds): Monitoring in Respiratory Care. St. Louis, Mosby Yearbook, 1993, pp 309–347.
8. Oakes D: Therapeutic modalities. In Clinical Practitioners' Guide to Respiratory Care. Rockville, MD, Health Educator Publishers, 1988, pp 143–159.
9. O'Donohue WJ: Indications for long-term oxygen therapy and appropriate use. In O'Donohue WJ (ed): Long-Term Oxygen Therapy: Scientific Basis and Application. New York, Marcel Dekker, 1995, pp 53–68.
10. Plummer AL: The role of the home oxygen provider in education, assessment, and quality improvement. In O'Donohue WJ (ed): Long-Term Oxygen Therapy: Scientific Basis and Application. New York, Marcel Dekker, 1995, pp 197–217.
11. Ryerson GG, Block AJ: Oxygen as a drug: Chemical properties, benefits and hazards of administration. In Burton GG, Hodgkin JE (eds): Respiratory Care, 2nd ed. Philadelphia, J.B. Lippincott, 1984, pp 395–415.
12. Stoller JK: Travel for the technology-dependent individual. Respir Care 39:347–362, 1994.
13. Tarpy SP, Celli BR: Long-term oxygen therapy. N Engl J Med 333:710–714, 1995.
14. Tiep BL: Long-term home oxygen therapy. Clin Chest Med 11:505–521, 1990.
15. Tiep BL, Lewis MI: Oxygen conservation and oxygen conserving devices in chronic lung disease. Chest 92:263–272, 1987.
16. Weill D, Make B: Oxygen-conserving devices. In O'Donohue WJ (ed): Long-Term Oxygen Therapy: Scientific Basis and Application. New York, Marcel Dekker, 1995, pp 235–256.

---

20. SMOKING CESSATION

*Thomas D. MacKenzie, M.D., Carla J. Fenton, M.D.,
and Roxana Zulauf Witter, M.D., M.S.*

1. Describe the prevalence of cigarette smoking in the United States this century.

Cigarette smoking became the most popular form of tobacco consumption in the 1920s. Per capita cigarette consumption rose sharply during World War II and continued to rise until the 1950s. The first reports linking cigarette use with cancer emerged in the 1950s and were subsequently confirmed by other studies, leading to the famous *Surgeon General's Report on Smoking and Health* in 1964. Consumption eventually peaked in the late 1960s at over 4000 cigarettes per capita per year and has been declining annually ever since. The prevalence of cigarette smoking (percentage of the adult population who smoke regularly) peaked at 41% and declined annually until 1990. Of great concern to public health officials is that the prevalence has remained static since 1990, at 25% of the adult population. Moreover, some studies have suggested that the prevalence of cigarette smoking among teenagers may be rising.

2. At what age do most people start to smoke?

The average age of initiation of regular cigarette smoking has been declining since the 1920s. For persons born between 1910 and 1920, the average age of initiation was approximately 20 years. Today, the average age is 14.5 years. In 1992, 1 in 5 eighth-graders reported smoking their first cigarette in the fifth grade.

3. How do you quantify a person's smoking history?

Multiply the average number of packs smoked per day by the number of years of smoking to get the number of pack-years of smoking. For example, a 55-year-old woman who began smoking at age 15 and thinks she smoked an average of $1^{1}/_{2}$ packs (30 cigarettes)/day has a 60 pack-year smoking history (1.5 packs/day × 40 years).

4. How is nicotine dependence defined?

According to the *Diagnostic and Statistic Manual for Mental Disorders* (DSM IV), a person meets criteria for nicotine dependence if any **three** of the following behaviors occur within a 12-month period:

1. Smokes more cigarettes or smokes for a longer period of time than originally intended

2. Continuously desires to quit smoking or has made one or more unsuccessful attempts at cessation

3. Spends much time and energy getting cigarettes, smoking cigarettes, or recovering from its effects.

4. Frequently smokes or suffers from withdrawal symptoms when expected to fulfill obligations at work, school, or home

5. Gives up important social, occupational, or recreational activities because of cigarette smoking

6. Continues to smoke despite the knowledge of having persistent or recurring social, psychological, or physical problems caused or exacerbated by the use of cigarettes

7. Needs increasing amounts of nicotine to achieve the desired effect or experiences diminished effect with continued use of same amount

8. Experiences characteristic nicotine withdrawal symptoms or uses nicotine to prevent withdrawal symptoms

From the American Psychiatric Association: Diagnostic and Statistical Manual for Mental Disorders IV. Washington, DC, American Psychiatric Association, 1994, with permission.

5. What are the four A's of smoking cessation counseling?

The National Cancer Institute lists four A's for office-based interventions:

1. **Ask** about smoking at every opportunity: Tobacco exposure should be assessed at every office visit as the fifth vital sign. It raises the awareness of smokers, nonsmokers, and office staff to the importance of cessation.

2. **Advise** all smokers to stop: Physician advice is a powerful and inexpensive tool for smoking cessation, especially when given in a "teachable moment" such as an office visit for bronchitis or a tobacco-related hospitalization.

3. **Assist** patients in the cessation effort: Any health care provider can assist the patient in setting a quit date, which should be set as soon after the initial counseling session as possible. Nicotine replacement therapy should be offered to all patients except in special circumstances.

4. **Arrange** follow-up: A follow-up visit on or shortly after the quit date can improve success rates. Most relapses occur within the first 2 weeks after cessation.

In the case of children and adolescents, the NCI recommends a fifth A: **anticipatory guidance**.

6. Not all four A's are appropriate for all smokers. Which patients should receive all four A's?

The **ask** step applies to all patients who visit a health care setting. The **advise** step is for all current smokers. After the advise step, it is important to determine the willingness of the patient to make a quit attempt. If he or she is willing to set a quit date, the clinician follows the **assist** and **arrange** steps. If the patient is not willing to make a quit attempt, the clinician should make a "motivational intervention" to enhance the patient's motivation to stop.

7. What are the four R's of "motivational interventions"?

The following components of clinical interventions are designed to enhance motivation to quit smoking in patients who are not ready to make a quit attempt:

1. **Relevance:** Information should be provided that is relevant to the patient's sociodemographic characteristics, disease status, health concerns, and social situation.

2. **Risks:** Acute, long-term, and environmental risks should be discussed with the patient.

3. **Rewards:** The clinician should highlight potential rewards of stopping that seem relevant to the patient.

4. **Repetition:** The motivational intervention should be repeated every time an unmotivated smoker visits the clinic.

8. Name the typical nicotine withdrawal symptoms.

Craving for nicotine	Anger	Restlessness
Irritability	Anxiety	Increased appetite
Frustration	Difficulty concentrating	Decreased heart rate

9. What happens to pulmonary function tests with smoking? On cessation?

The FEV_1 (forced expiratory volume in 1 sec) has been used as the primary measure of pulmonary function in several studies. Among all men over the age of 45 years, the FEV_1 typically declines at a rate of 20 ml/yr as a natural consequence of aging. In the Honolulu Heart Program, men who continued to smoke showed a steeper rate of decline in FEV_1 of about 33 ml/yr. Men who were able to quit in the first 2 years of the study rapidly reduced their rate of decline to that of nonsmokers. Another study also showed that smoking intervention can significantly reduce the age-related decline in FEV_1 in middle-aged smokers with evidence of early chronic obstructive pulmonary disease.

10. How many times does a smoker typically attempt to quit before permanently giving up cigarettes?

Many times. Patients who successfully give up smoking have often made several previous attempts to quit. Therefore, if a patient relapses after a period of abstinence, the physician should not consider him or her a "treatment failure." Support, understanding, and consideration of re-enrollment in smoking cessation programs should be given.

11. What are some short-term health benefits of smoking cessation?

1. The excess risk of premature coronary heart disease falls by one-half within 1 year of abstinence.

2. Some of the toxic effects of cigarette smoking that may lead to cardiac events, such as increased platelet activation, elevated CO levels, and coronary artery spasm, are immediately reversible with cessation.

3. Pregnant women who stop during the first 3–4 months of pregnancy eliminate their risk of having a low-birth-weight baby.

12. Is inpatient smoking cessation treatment effective?

Among five well-designed studies that have been conducted on hospitalized smokers, inpatient counseling of varying intensity increased cessation rates by approximately 40%. The efficacy of the nicotine patch in hospitalized patients has not been well-studied.

13. What are some long-term benefits of smoking cessation?

1. People who stop smoking before age 50 have half the risk of dying in the next 15 years as compared to continuing smokers.

2. Overall mortality is reduced to that of nonsmokers after 10–15 years of abstinence.

3. Ten years of abstinence reduces the risk of developing lung cancer to nearly that of nonsmokers.

4. Fifteen years are required to decrease the coronary heart disease risk to that of a nonsmoker.

14. How much weight do people gain after they quit smoking?

In one large study of over 2500 smokers, the mean weight gain attributable to smoking cessation was 2.8 kg (6.2 lbs) in men and 3.8 kg (8.4 lbs) in women. Major weight gain (> 13 kg or 28.6 lbs) occurred in 10% of men and 13% of women.

15. Outline the 1996 U.S. Preventive Service Task Force recommendations for smoking cessation counseling.

The Task Force ranks its recommendations by the strength of the supporting evidence. The strongest favorable recommendation, an "A," implies that there is good evidence that the condition should be specifically considered in a periodic health examination. A "C" recommendation implies that there is insufficient evidence to recommend for or against the inclusion of the condition in a periodic health exam.

"A" recommendations

1. Cessation counseling on a regular basis for all patients who use tobacco products.

2. Pregnant women and parents with children living at home should be counseled on the potentially harmful effects of smoking on fetal and child health.

3. The prescription of nicotine patches or gum as an adjunct for selected patients.

"C" recommendations

1. The use of clonidine as an adjunct to smoking cessation counseling.

2. Clinical counseling of children, adolescents, and young adults to prevent smoking initiation (based on the lack of evidence supporting its effectiveness).

16. Is nicotine replacement therapy effective?

Two recent meta-analyses of randomized placebo-controlled trials of nicotine replacement therapy demonstrated that both nicotine polacrilex gum and transdermal nicotine are highly effective aids for smoking cessation. Both agents approximately double the smoking cessation rate at 6 months and at 1 year compared to placebo. Success rates are also influenced by the degree of nicotine dependence and by the intensity of counseling.

17. How can a clinician assess the degree of tobacco dependency in a patient?

The Fagerström tolerance questionnaire. Smokers are considered "highly dependent" if they achieve a score 8 or higher and "moderately dependent" if they score 4–7. Studies have shown that highly dependent smokers benefit more from the use of nicotine gum than less-dependent smokers. However, the data for nicotine patches are mixed. Some recent studies suggest that the benefit of the patch may be more pronounced in smokers who are less dependent on nicotine.

18. What are the indications for nicotine polacrilex gum?

- Patient is motivated to quit (ready to set a quit date).
- Patient is able to follow a complex regimen.
- Patient is medium to highly nicotine-dependent.
- Patient is able to abstain from smoking while using gum.

19. How does nicotine gum work?

The gum contains nicotine bound to an ion-exchange resin in a gum base, which allows the nicotine to be released slowly. Once the nicotine is released, it is absorbed through the buccal mucosa. The systemic nicotine alleviates withdrawal symptoms of smoking cessation.

20. How is nicotine gum prescribed?

1. Use the Fagerström scale to determine degree of dependence. Highly-dependent (> 8) smokers are given 4-mg nicotine gum for 6 weeks and then 2-mg nicotine gum until completion of therapy. Moderate (4–7) to low-dependent smokers are prescribed 2-mg nicotine gum. The mean nicotine content of a cigarette is 1.8 ± 0.4 mg.

2. Prescribe one piece of gum every hour while the patient is awake. The patient should be instructed to chew the gum until he or she senses that the nicotine has been released and then park the gum to allow absorption through the buccal mucosa. An acid environment from drinking juice, soda, or coffee will greatly impair absorption of nicotine.

3. Remove gum after 20 minutes.

4. Recommend tapering frequency of gum use after 3 months.

21. What is the length of treatment and dosing used for nicotine patches?

The maximum benefit of the nicotine patch can be gained by using a 6–8-week course of daily patches. Although some patch manufacturers initially recommended nicotine patch use for up to 3 months, recent studies have shown that end-of-treatment quit rates for 3-month patch use are essentially the same as quit rates at the end of 4 weeks and worse than quit rates after 6 weeks. Studies suggest that 6–8 weeks is enough time for nicotine withdrawal symptoms to decrease and allows the patient to develop the new skills necessary to maintain abstinence.

Many clinicians use high-dose patches uniformly in the initial 2–4 weeks and taper the dose of the patch by 2–week intervals thereafter. There is probably no significant difference in the efficacy of 24-hour versus 16-hour patches.

22. What type of counseling is needed when using nicotine patches?

In some patients the patch is effective without counseling, but counseling along with the patch uniformly increases quit rates. A meta-analysis of 17 nicotine patch studies showed that high-intensity counseling was more effective than low-intensity counseling. Furthermore, group counseling was more effective than individual counseling.

Abstinence Rates 6 Months after Smoking Cessation for Nicotine Patch Users

	ACTIVE PATCH (%)	PLACEBO PATCH (%)
All patch studies	21.8	9.4
Counseling intensity		
High	26.5	13.2
Low	19.5	7.1
Counseling format		
Group	26.3	12.6
Individual	20.0	7.7

Adapted from Fiore MC, Smith SS, Jorenby DE, Baker TB: The effectiveness of the nicotine patch for smoking cessation: A meta-analysis. JAMA 271:1940–1947, 1994.

23. Can nicotine patches be used in patients with known coronary artery disease?

It is generally believed that the patch can be used in patients with stable angina if the patient understands that the patch is a *substitute* for cigarettes and the patient is motivated to abstain totally. The patches cause no increase in cardiac symptoms or complications. Patches are contraindicated in patients who have had a recent myocardial infarction or who have poorly controlled hypertension.

24. What strategies are used to promote smoking cessation in a clinical setting?

A meta-analysis of 39 controlled trials of smoking cessation strategies showed that programs using several modes of repeated counseling and intervention are most effective for initial and long-term cessation. Interventions included physician and nonphysician individualized counseling, setting a quit date, telephone follow-up by nurses, group counseling and classes, and written materials, cassettes, and videos. Carbon monoxide monitors are often used to verify abstinence and may be useful in the initial counseling stages (demonstrating the "poison" that builds up in the blood of the smoker). The use of nicotine patches or nicotine gum should be considered in all patients.

25. Discuss the cost-effectiveness for smoking interventions.

Cost-effectiveness of a therapy can be measured in dollars spent per year of life saved (YOLS). Smoking interventions cost relatively little when compared to other medical interventions.

Estimated Cost-Effectiveness of Various Interventions

INTERVENTION	COST-EFFECTIVENESS ($ PER YOLS)
Brief physician advice	$750
Nicotine gum	$4,000–9,500
Treatment of mild to moderate hypertension	
Beta-blocker	$11,000
Angiotensin-converting enzyme inhibitor	$72,000
Papanicolaou smears every 4 yrs vs no screening	$10,000
Treatment of hypercholesterolemia	$65,000

Adapted from Tsevat J: Impact and cost-effectiveness of smoking interventions. Am J Med 93(suppl 1A): 43s–47s, 1992.

BIBLIOGRAPHY

1. Agency for Health Care Policy and Research: Smoking Cessation Clinical Practice Guideline. JAMA 275:1270–1280, 1996.
2. Bartecchi CE, MacKenzie TD, Schrier RW: The global tobacco epidemic. Sci Am May:26–33, 1995.
3. Bartecchi CE, MacKenzie TD, Schrier RW: The human costs of tobacco use (pts 1 and 2). N Engl J Med 330:907–912, 975–980, 1994.
4. Burchfiel CM, Marcus EB, Curb JD, et al: Effects of smoking and smoking cessation on longitudinal decline in pulmonary function. Am J Respir Crit Care Med 151:1778–1785, 1995.
5. Cigarette smoking among adults—United States, 1992, and changes in the definition of current cigarette smoking. MMWR 43:342–346, 1994.
6. Cigarette smoking-attributable mortality and years of potential life lost—United States, 1990. MMWR 42:230–233, 1993.
7. Fagerstrom KO: Measuring degree of physical dependence to tobacco smoking with reference to individualization of treatment. Addict Behav 3:235–241, 1978.
8. Fiore MC, Kenford SL, Jorenby DE, et al: Two studies of the clinical effectiveness of the nicotine patch with different counseling treatments. Chest 105:524–533, 1994.
9. Fiore MC, Smith SS, Jorenby DE, Baker TB: The effectiveness of the nicotine patch for smoking cessation: A meta-analysis. JAMA 271:1940–1947, 1994.
10. Surgeon General: Reducing the Health Consequences of Smoking: 25 Years of Progress: A Report of the Surgeon General: Executive Summary. Rockville, MD, Department of Health and Human Services, 1989 [DHHS publication no. (CDC) 89-8411.]
11. Surgeon General: The Health Benefits of Smoking Cessation. Rockville, MD, Department of Health and Human Services, 1990, pp 473–515. [DHHS publication no. (CDC) 90-8416.]
12. Tang JL, Law M, Wald N: How effective is nicotine replacement therapy in helping people to stop smoking? BMJ 308:21–26, 1994.
13. Tsevat J: Impact and cost-effectiveness of smoking interventions. Am J Med 93(suppl 1A):43s–47s, 1992.
14. U.S. Preventive Services Task Force: Guide to Clinical Preventive Services, 2nd ed. Baltimore, Williams & Wilkins, 1996.
15. Williamson DF, Maddans J, Anda RF, et al: Smoking cessation and severity of weight gain in a national cohort. N Engl J Med 324:739–745, 1991.

21. PULMONARY REHABILITATION

Bonnie F. Fahy, R.N., M.N., and Amy A. Silverthorn, M.D.

1. What is pulmonary rehabilitation?

In 1974, the American College of Chest Physicians' Committee on Pulmonary Rehabilitation developed a definition of pulmonary rehabilitation that was endorsed by the American Thoracic Society in 1981. According to this definition pulmonary rehabilitation is:

> An art of medical practice wherein an individually tailored, multidisciplinary program is formulated which through accurate diagnosis, therapy, emotional support and education, stabilizes or reverses both the physio- and psychopathology of pulmonary diseases and attempts to return the patient to the highest possible functional capacity allowed by his pulmonary handicap and overall life situation.

2. Who is a candidate for pulmonary rehabilitation?

Any patient with chronic lung disease who continues to be symptomatic, despite being medically stable on standard therapy, is a candidate for pulmonary rehabilitation. This includes patients with obstructive and restrictive lung diseases.

3. Is a patient with an FEV₁ of 0.5 liters who can barely walk across the room a candidate for rehabilitation?

Pulmonary function cannot be used to predict functional ability. Motivated patients who are physically able to attend outpatient pulmonary rehabilitation programs may benefit from them.

Of course, the less physically limited patients are at the time of referral, the more functional they may become after a period of rehabilitation. Many patients state that they wish they had been referred to rehabilitation earlier in the course of their disease. Pulmonary rehabilitation also can be initiated on an inpatient basis. Mentally coherent ventilator patients can benefit from instruction in breathing techniques and physical reconditioning.

4. How is the functional ability assessed?

Functional ability is assessed by an exercise tolerance test. A formal exercise study with expired gas analysis is not required to determine functional ability. Data from a simple 6- or 12-minute walk can be used to develop an exercise prescription. The expertise of a physical therapist or exercise physiologist is useful.

5. What are the essential components in a comprehensive pulmonary rehabilitation program?

The essential components can be generalized into patient instruction (the term "education" is avoided, as insurance companies tend not to reimburse "education") and exercise. Instructional topics should include:

How the normal lung works

What is wrong with the patient's lungs

Instruction in breathing retraining techniques, specifically pursed-lip and abdominal breathing

Application of breathing techniques to activities of daily living and energy conservation

Benefits of exercise

Purpose and proper use of medications and equipment, including specific instruction in the use of metered dose inhalers and oxygen therapy

Bronchial hygiene techniques, including controlled coughing. If clinically indicated, postural drainage with percussion and vibration and/or instruction in use of a positive expiratory pressure (PEP) valve.

Proper nutrition

Importance of avoiding environmental irritants, including smoking cessation

Signs of a respiratory infection and when to call the doctor

Travel tips, including oxygen requirements

Sexuality

Stress reduction and panic control

6. Of all the educational components, which is most beneficial?

Instruction in breathing techniques, particularly pursed-lip and abdominal breathing, is the most beneficial. These techniques slow respiratory rate, increase tidal volume, and improve gas exchange by preventing dynamic airway compression and improving synchrony of abdominal and thoracic musculature. Symptoms improve more frequently than physiologic parameters. Rehabilitation specialists emphasize that utilization of breathing techniques allows patients to remain "in control" of their breathing rather than having their breathing controlling them.

7. Is patient instruction (education) alone effective in improving a patient's ability to cope with his or her chronic lung disease?

Education is necessary, and alone is better than nothing, but a comprehensive pulmonary rehabilitation program should include an exercise component. In a recent study, Ries and coworkers compared education alone to a comprehensive pulmonary rehabilitation program of education and exercise.[9] They concluded that the comprehensive pulmonary rehabilitation program significantly improved exercise performance and symptoms of perceived breathlessness in patients with moderate to severe chronic obstructive pulmonary disease.

8. Is a group setting preferred over one-to-one instruction for pulmonary rehabilitation?

Yes. The major advantage of a group setting is that it brings patients with similar problems together. "Misery loves company" rings true. Patients who exhibit what is thought to be clinical depression may improve markedly when they find they are not the only ones with dyspnea or the need for supplemental oxygen. An occasional patient requires referral for in depth psychological counseling, which should be available for rehabilitation programs. Many rehabilitation programs have ongoing maintenance exercise that serves as a support group. Space should be available for family members to meet while patients are exercising, so that they, too, have a support system.

9. How do you exercise a dyspneic, scared patient?

Start slowly and offer much reassurance. The patient's current exercise ability is assessed by a simple exercise tolerance test. From that data, an exercise prescription is devised, emphasizing endurance rather than speed or strength. Although walking is the most common exercise used in pulmonary rehabilitation, an exercise prescription must be individualized and should include both upper and lower body conditioning. Upper extremity conditioning can improve upper extremity exercise tolerance and decrease the dyspnea experienced when the upper extremities are used in activities of daily living, such as lifting or combing hair.

10. Does ventilatory muscle training have a place in pulmonary rehabilitation?

Isocapnic hyperventilation, inspiratory muscle loading, and inspiratory loading have been shown to improve functioning of the inspiratory muscles in patients with pulmonary disease. Unfortunately, the improvement from ventilatory muscle training alone does not generally translate to improved exercise performance. The patient may be able to breathe through a smaller orifice on the training device but cannot walk further. Ventilatory muscle training may be appropriate for the patient who asks, "Isn't there anything else I can do?"

11. What benefits can be attributed to pulmonary rehabilitation?

• Reduced hospitalizations and emergency room visits
• Reduced respiratory symptoms (dyspnea, cough)
• Reduced anxiety and depression
• Increased exercise capacity
• Improved ability to perform activities of daily living
• Enhanced quality of life
• Increased understanding of pulmonary disease and treatment program
• Possible prolonged survival
• Possible return to employment

12. How can pulmonary rehabilitation prolong survival?

No studies directly establish that patients with chronic lung disease live longer if they participate in a pulmonary rehabilitation program. Some of the benefits of rehabilitation, however, theoretically may translate into prolonged survival in individual patients. For instance, pulmonary rehabilitation has been shown to improve patient compliance with medications, including continuous use of oxygen. Because the Nocturnal Oxygen Therapy Trial (NOTT) demonstrated that oxygen use can decrease mortality, better compliance may improve survival.

13. How do I refer a patient to pulmonary rehabilitation?

First, locate a program. If you do not know of a program at your facility, call the Respiratory Care Department. There may be a program "hiding" within your hospital. If this is unsuccessful, call the American Lung Association in your state. The American Association of Cardiovascular and Pulmonary Rehabilitation (608-831-6989) can also refer you to a program in your area.

All programs require a physician's referral. The patient documentation required for admission varies among programs. Some facilities request diagnostic studies prior to admission, whereas others complete the evaluation once the patient has enrolled. All programs should have a Medical Director who is a pulmonologist.

14. What is the referring physician's relationship to the Medical Director?

This relationship varies. Some programs have a Medical Director who is actively involved in the evaluative phase and may alter medical therapy. Other programs have a Medical Director who functions as a consultant to the other rehabilitation team members and only cares for the patient if the referring physician is unavailable.

15. What professional disciplines are included in the pulmonary rehabilitation team?

The definition of pulmonary rehabilitation states that a program is carried out by a multidisciplinary team. In some instances the team may consist of a physician and one other health care provider; in other instances the team may include a physician and any (or all) of the following:

Nurse	Social worker	Exercise physiologist
Respiratory therapist	Psychiatrist	Dietitian
Physical therapist	Psychologist	Pharmacist
Occupational therapist		

16. What is the cost and duration of a pulmonary rehabilitation program?

The cost and the duration of pulmonary rehabilitation programs vary regionally because of the differing payment allowables of Medicare intermediaries. Generally, programs are 6 to 12 weeks in duration and the cost is far less than that of one hospital admission.

BIBLIOGRAPHY

1. American Thoracic Society: Pulmonary rehabilitation. Am Rev Respir Dis 24:663–666, 1981.
2. Casaburi R, Petty TL (eds): Principles and Practice of Pulmonary Rehabilitation. Philadelphia, W.B. Saunders, 1993.
3. Celli BR: Physical reconditioning of patients with respiratory diseases: Legs, arms, and breathing retraining. Respir Care 39:482–496, 1994.
4. Connors G, Hilling L (eds): American Association of Cardiovascular and Pulmonary Rehabilitation: Guidelines for Pulmonary Rehabilitation Programs. Champaign, IL, Human Kinetics, 1993.
5. Hodgkin JE, Connors G, Bell CW (eds): Pulmonary Rehabilitation: Guidelines to Success, 2nd ed. Philadelphia, J.B. Lippincott, 1993.
6. Nocturnal Oxygen Therapy Trial Group: Continuous or nocturnal oxygen therapy in hypoxemic chronic obstructive lung disease: A clinical trial. Ann Intern Med 93:391–398, 1980.
7. Ries AL: Position paper of the American Association of Cardiovascular and Pulmonary Rehabilitation: Scientific basis of pulmonary rehabilitation. J Cardiopulmonary Rehabil 10:418–441, 1990.
8. Ries AL: What pulmonary rehab can do for your patients. J Respir Dis 16:685–704, 1995.
9. Ries AL, Kaplin RM, Limberg TM, Prewitt LM: Effects of pulmonary rehabilitation on physiological and psychosocial outcomes in patients with chronic obstructive pulmonary disease. Ann Intern Med 122:823–832, 1995.

22. CYSTIC FIBROSIS

Michael C. Iannuzzi, M.D.

1. Have the diagnostic criteria for cystic fibrosis (CF) changed since the discovery of the CF gene (cystic fibrosis transmembrane conductance regulator, or CFTR)?

The criteria for diagnosis of CF have remain unchanged. The criteria consist of elevation in sweat chloride ion concentration plus at least one of the following: (1) chronic airway disease; (2) evidence of exocrine pancreatic insufficiency (PI), or (3) diagnosis of CF in a relative (no more distant than a first cousin). These criteria continue to reliably diagnose more than 95% of children and adults with CF. Genetic testing is useful in those individuals in whom the diagnosis is entertained but who do not meet the classic diagnostic criteria.

2. What are the criteria for diagnosing pulmonary exacerbation in CF?

There are currently no universal criteria; however, a panel of experts have suggested that a pulmonary exacerbation be defined as the presence of at least three of the following:

Increased respiratory rate
Fever
Weight loss of 1 kg or more
Increased cough
Increased sputum production or change in sputum appearance
New findings on chest examination (crackles or wheezing)
New findings on chest radiograph
Decreased exercise tolerance
Decrease in FEV_1 of 10% or more from previous study obtained within 3 months
Decrease in oxygen saturation of 10% or more from baseline obtained within 3 months

3. What are the usual pathogens found in the lower airways of patients with CF?

Bacterial infection of the airways is the major cause of morbidity and mortality in patients with CF. Patients are initially colonized by *Haemophilus influenzae*, then with *Staphylococcus aureus*, and later with *Pseudomonas aeruginosa* and in some cases, *Burkholderia* (formerly *Pseudomonas*) *cepacia*. By the age of 26 years, 80% of CF patients are infected with *P. aeruginosa*. Other pathogens, including aspergillus and mycobacteria, should be considered when a patient's condition deteriorates without known cause.

4. What are the chest radiographic findings in CF?

Early in the course of the disease, the lungs are radiographically normal. As the disease progresses overinflation is seen, which represent bronchiolitis with small airway obstruction. Further progression includes bronchitis with thickened bronchial walls seen as circular lesions when the bronchi are projected in cross section and "tram lines," or parallel linear opacities, when bronchi are projected longitudinally. With further worsening, bronchiectasis develops and small cysts and rounded opacities become evident. For unknown reasons, the right upper lobe is commonly affected earlier and more severely than other lobes. Late findings are large blebs, most often in the apices.

5. Which patients are most likely to benefit from human recombinant DNase (rhDNase) and how should it be administered?

Patients with abnormal lung function (forced vital capacity less than 80% predicted) and chronic purulent sputum are most likely to benefit. Patients with normal lung function and uninfected or rarely infected sputum are unlikely to benefit. A once daily dose of 2.5 mg is standard; higher or twice daily dosing has little additional benefit. Ultrasonic nebulizers cannot be used because they cause degradation of the enzyme. A nebulizer that delivers particles in the respirable fraction (1–6 µm) should be used.

6. What is the role of bronchodilator therapy in CF?

Bronchodilator treatment is helpful in up to 30% of patients with CF, but many CF patients exhibit a paradoxical response with worsening of expiratory flow rates. Investigators have hypothesized that the paradoxical response reflects excessive loss of airway smooth muscle tone with upstream collapse, which limits effective emptying of the small airways. Since some patients may have reduced airflow in response to bronchodilators, patients should be objectively evaluated and periodically monitored for improvement while receiving bronchodilator therapy.

7. Which patients should undergo evaluation for lung transplantation?

Cystic fibrosis is the most common indication for bilateral lung transplantation; more than one third of all adult bilateral lung transplantation is carried out for CF. Patients may be considered for transplantation under the following conditions: progressive decline in weight and lung function despite adequate nutritional support and therapy; increased frequency or duration of hospitalizations; decrease in FEV_1 to 30% of predicted; and increase in $Paco_2$ requirement. Major exclusion criteria include the presence of psychosocial disorders, multiorgan failure, pan-resistant *Burkholderia cepacia*, or aspergilloma.

8. What is the significance of finding *Aspergillus* sp. on sputum culture?

Aspergillus sp. are important causes of morbidity in patients with CF; aspergillosis should be considered in patients whose lung function is rapidly deteriorating. Allergic bronchopulmonary aspergillosis (ABPA), first described in patients with asthma, occurs in 10–15% of CF patients. Cultures can be positive in the absence of significant clinical disease, but repeated isolation of the same species of *Aspergillus* is likely to be significant. Conversely, a consistent clinical picture— recurrent episodes of pulmonary infiltrates, segmental or lobar collapse, and eosinophilia—in the absence of a positive sputum culture cannot exclude ABPA. In this situation antibody tests for *Aspergillus* sp. should be obtained.

9. What is the significance of pneumothorax in patients with CF?

Up to 20% of adult CF patients eventually have pneumothorax. Pneumothorax should be suspected in patients who develop sudden onset chest pain and respiratory distress. Every patient with pneumothorax, even those without symptoms, should be hospitalized and observed for at least 24 hours. Survival after the onset of pneumothorax is about 30 months, and the chance of recurrence is 50–70%.

10. What genetic counseling should be given to couples when either partner is affected with CF?

Cystic fibrosis in either partner requires that genetic counseling be delivered to couples contemplating pregnancy. If the genetic status in the non-CF partner is unknown, the child's risk for developing CF is 1 in 50. If the non-CF partner is a heterozygous carrier, the risk is 1 in 2. Unfortunately, because there are more than a few hundred CF mutations, negative results are not definitive; it is possible that the partner with negative results could be a carrier for a rare or unidentified CF mutation. This possibility can be reduced to a 1 in 492 risk of CF in the fetus by testing for several of the common CF mutations, which detects the CF carrier state in about 90% of individuals. About 97–98% of men and about 20% of women with CF are infertile.

11. Should pregnancy be discouraged in women with CF because of potential deterioration in lung function?

Although once feared as potentially life-threatening to women with CF, pregnancy may be safe provided that the patient has excellent nutritional status and mild airway obstruction. Patients with pancreatic sufficiency and mild obstructive airway disease who were diagnosed at an older age are at lowest risk.

12. How important are airway clearance techniques in the management of CF patients?

Airway clearance techniques are critical in the management of all CF patients. There is some suggestion that exercise may be as effective as traditional chest physical therapy, but until studies are done, most experts encourage patients to incorporate both aerobic exercise and chest physical therapy in their daily routine. Recently, a handheld oral oscillator device (Flutter, VarioRaw S.A., Aubonne, Switzerland) was introduced; although the amount of sputum obtained may be the same as that from postural drainage with cough or cough alone, the Flutter is easy to use and may improve patient compliance.

13. How should CF patients with hemoptysis be managed?

Blood streaking of sputum is common; if it persists, the diagnosis of pulmonary exacerbation requiring antibiotic therapy should be considered. Major hemoptysis, defined as 240 cc in 24 hours or recurrent bleeding of more than 100 cc per day over 3 to 7 days, occurs in about 1% of all patients each year. The incidence is higher in patients more than 16 years. Patients should be admitted for close observation. Hemoptysis can often be controlled with antibiotics, bed rest, correction of coagulopathy, cough suppressants, and discontinuation of vigorous airway clearance techniques. Bronchoscopy may be necessary to localize the site of bleeding. Angiography with bronchial arterial embolization to the hypertrophied bronchial circulation may be necessary if bleeding persists.

14. What is the probable diagnosis based on the following case history?

History. A 22-year-old CF patient presents with 1 week of intermittent severe abdominal cramping, constipation, and vomiting. Physical examination reveals that the patient is afebrile. He has diffuse right lower quadrant tenderness and an easily palpable right lower quadrant mass. Rectal examination shows right-sided tenderness. The abdominal film shows a large amount of stool in the colon. Liver function tests, amylase level, urinalysis and white blood cell count are all normal.

Diagnosis. Appendicitis and intussusception should be considered; however, the most likely diagnosis is distal intestinal obstruction syndrome (DIOS) or meconium ileus equivalent.

15. How should DIOS be treated?

Nonsurgical treatment with high volumes of orally administered balanced electrolyte solutions such as Golytely (Braintree Laboratories, Inc., Braintree, MA) is usually successful. If oral balanced electrolyte is not tolerated, hydrophilic enemas, with meglumine diatrizoate (Gastrografin), for example, can be used. Oral N-acetylcysteine and cispride are useful for patients with recurrent DIOS.

16. Should antiinflammatory drugs be used to treat CF patients?

Because pulmonary inflammation occurs with infection, leading to pulmonary fibrosis and ultimately to respiratory failure, the use of antiinflammatory drugs has been investigated. A 4-year, multicenter trial of pediatric patients has shown a higher percentage of predicted FEV_1 in patients on alternative day prednisone (1 mg/kg) than on placebo. The main side effect was growth retardation. How best to administer prednisone in pediatric patients to minimize complications and whether adults would also benefit remains to be defined. In a double-blind, placebo-controlled study of 85 patients with mild lung disease, ibuprofen, 20–30 mg per kg, with close monitoring of blood levels slowed the progression of lung deterioration; patients less than 13 years of age benefited most. Many centers are treating pediatric patients with ibuprofen, but only after blood level monitoring to determine the appropriate dose of the drug for each patient. Clinical trials are warranted before ibuprofen can be advocated for adults.

BIBLIOGRAPHY

1. Aitken ML, Burke W, McDonald G, et al: Nontuberculous mycobacterial disease in adult cystic fibrosis patients. Chest 103:1096–1099, 1993.
2. Cohen AM, Doershuk CF, Stern RC: Bronchial artery embolization to control hemoptysis in cystic fibrosis. Radiology 175:401–405, 1990.
3. Davis PB (ed): Cystic Fibrosis. New York, Marcel Dekker, 1993.
4. Eigen H, Rosenstein BJ, FitzSimmons S, et al: A multicenter study of alternate-day prednisone therapy in patients with cystic fibrosis. Cystic Fibrosis Foundation Prednisone Trial Group. J Pediatr 126:515–523, 1995.
5. Figel SB, Fuchs HJ, Johnson C, et al: Comparison of three jet nebulizer aerosol delivery systems used to administer recombinant human DNase I to patients with cystic fibrosis. The Pulmozyme rhDNase Study Group. Chest 108:153–156, 1995.
6. Fuchs HJ, Borowitz DS, Christiansen DH, et al: Effect of aerosolized recombinant human DNase on exacerbations of respiratory symptoms and on pulmonary function in patients with cystic fibrosis. The Pulmozyme Study Group. N Engl J Med 331:637–642, 1994.
7. Greene KE, Takasugi JE, Godwin JD, et al: Radiographic changes in acute exacerbations of cystic fibrosis in adults: A pilot study. Am J Roentgenol 163:557–562, 1994.
8. Konstan MW, Byard PJ, Hopper CL, et al: Effect of high dose ibuprofen in patients with cystic fibrosis. N Engl J Med 332:848–854, 1995.
9. Konstan MW, Stern RC, Doershuk CF: Efficacy of the Flutter device for airway mucus clearance in patients with cystic fibrosis. Part I. J Pediatr 124:689–693, 1994.
10. Kotloff RM, FitzSimmons SC, Fiel SB: Fertility and pregnancy in patients with cystic fibrosis. Clin Chest Med 13:623–635, 1992.
11. Spector ML, Stern RC: Pneumothorax in cystic fibrosis: A 26-year experience. Ann Thorac Surg 47:204–207, 1989.
12. Taylor RF, Gaya H, Hodson ME: Pseudomonas cepacia: Pulmonary infection in patients with cystic fibrosis. Respir Med 87:187–192, 1993.

23. UPPER AIRWAY OBSTRUCTION

John L. Stauffer, M.D.

1. Discuss the terms used to describe airway obstruction.

Obstruction of the conducting airways has been classified as **upper** or **lower**, **extrathoracic** or **intrathoracic**, and **variable** or **fixed**. The use of these terms has unfortunately created some confusion. Surprisingly, there is no agreement on the meaning of the term **upper airway**. The boundary between the upper and lower airways has been variously considered to be the larynx, thoracic inlet, or tracheal carina. The term **extrathoracic** has been used both in an anatomic sense to refer to that portion of the conducting airways above the thoracic inlet and, in a physiologic sense, to refer to those airways that are unaffected by changes in pleural pressure during respiration. There is agreement that the term **variable** describes airway obstruction at any level that is affected by transmural airway pressure, while the term **fixed** describes airway obstruction at any level that is not affected by transmural airway pressure. In this chapter, we will refer to the upper airway as the air-conducting passages that are physiologically extrathoracic, i.e., not affected by changes in pleural pressure. This portion of the airway is located above the level of about the fifth or sixth tracheal ring.

2. What cardinal clinical features distinguish upper airway obstruction from lower airway obstruction?

If upper airway obstruction is defined as extrathoracic and if the obstruction is variable, it will demonstrate features of **inspiratory** airflow limitation, while lower airway obstruction demonstrates features of **expiratory** airflow limitation. In other words, variable airflow obstruction above the fifth or sixth tracheal ring produces abnormal findings on inspiration, while variable obstruction below this level produces abnormal findings on expiration. Fixed airway obstruction at any level affects both inspiration and expiration.

3. What bedside clinical findings would make an astute clinician suspect the patient has significant partial upper airway obstruction?

The features of **partial** upper airway obstruction depend upon the location of the obstruction, its severity, and whether it is variable or fixed. **Stridor** (noisy breathing) usually implies upper airway obstruction and is distinguished from wheezing and rhonchi, which are signs of lower airway obstruction. Inspiratory stridor suggests severe variable upper airway obstruction, while both inspiratory and expiratory stridor imply fixed obstruction at any level of the airway.

Dyspnea, anxiety, tachycardia, tachypnea, shallow breathing, and **cyanosis** may be observed. **Drooling** or salivation are common in cases of pharyngeal or laryngeal obstruction, such as epiglottitis. **Hoarseness** and dysphonia suggest a laryngeal source of upper airway obstruction. Significant upper airway obstruction is often accompanied by prominent use of accessory muscles of respiration. A palpable inspiratory **thrill** over the larynx is a useful clue to hypopharyngeal or laryngeal obstruction. Intercostal or supraclavicular **retractions** on inspiration may be observed as intrapleural pressures on inspiration become more negative to generate airflow through the partially obstructed upper airway segment. Auscultation will demonstrate coarse inspiratory sounds at the level of obstruction, and these may be transmitted throughout the chest.

Complete upper airway obstruction is distinguished from partial obstruction by sudden signs of severe respiratory distress or choking, aphonia, absence of stridor and breath sounds, and rapid progression to cardiac and respiratory arrest.

4. How should the head and chin of the unconscious patient be positioned to relieve upper airway obstruction?

The **head tilt–chin lift maneuver** of basic life support is used to open the airway of the unconscious patient. Remember that airway obstruction in the unconscious supine patient occurs at the levels of the base of the tongue and the epiglottis. The simple head tilt–chin lift maneuver effectively relieves upper airway obstruction at these levels. The palm of one hand is applied to the forehead to tilt the head backward, and the fingers of the other hand are used to lift the chin upward, keeping the mouth partially open.

The **jaw-thrust maneuver**, in which the mandible is lifted forward with both hands, is an alternative to the chin lift method for trained rescuers. If neck injury is suspected, the jaw-thrust maneuver is advised, as the head should not be tilted.

5. List the indications, contraindications, and complications of the Heimlich maneuver.

The Heimlich maneuver, or subdiaphragmatic abdominal thrusts, is recommended by the 1992 American Heart Association guidelines for relief of foreign-body airway obstruction in conscious or unconscious adults. The Heimlich maneuver is primarily indicated to remove solid material from the airway; its use to remove aspirated liquids is controversial. It should not be performed on healthy individuals during training in cardiopulmonary resuscitation. Chest rather than subdiaphragmatic thrusts are recommended for patients who are very obese and patients in the late stages of pregnancy.

The rare complications of the Heimlich maneuver include fractured ribs, aortic valve cusp tear, pneumomediastinum, vomiting, rupture of the esophagus, herniation of the diaphragm, rupture of the stomach, rupture of the jejunum, thrombosis of an abdominal aortic aneurysm, and chest and abdominal soreness.

6. Match the descriptions below with the correct flow-volume loops. (Answer on p. 128.)
    A. Fixed upper or lower airway obstruction
    B. Variable upper (extrathoracic) airway obstruction
    C. No upper or lower airway obstruction (normal)
    D. Variable lower (intrathoracic) airway obstruction

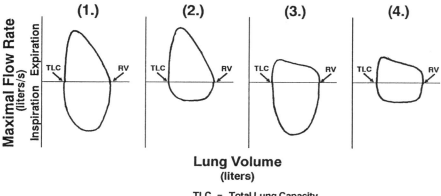

TLC = Total Lung Capacity
RV = Residual Volume

7. Is the flow-volume loop useful in identifying patients with OSA?

Patients with obstructive sleep apnea (OSA) display repeated episodes of pharyngeal occlusion during sleep as a result of reduced pharyngeal muscle tone, often accompanied by some anatomic predisposition to pharyngeal narrowing. In patients with OSA, the maximal expiratory-inspiratory flow-volume loop during wakefulness may reveal two abnormalities—the ratio of the forced expiratory flow rate to the forced inspiratory flow rate at 50% of the forced vital capacity

(FEF$_{50\%}$/FIF$_{50\%}$) in excess of 1.0, and a fluttering or "sawtooth" appearance of the expiratory and/or inspiratory portions of the loop.

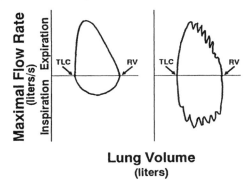

Lung Volume
(liters)

The maximal expiratory-inspiratory flow-volume loop in a patient with apnea may show the ratio of the forced expiratory flow rate to the forced inspiratory flow rate at 50% of the forced vital capacity (FEF$_{50\%}$/FIF$_{50\%}$) to be greater than 1.0 *(left)* and/or a fluttering or "sawtooth" appearance of the expiratory and inspiratory portions of the loop *(right)* (TLC = total lung capacity;RV = residual volume).

Prospective studies have revealed that these abnormalities on the flow-volume loop do not correlate with the severity of sleep-disordered breathing. In patients with OSA, the sensitivity of the FEF$_{50\%}$/FIF$_{50\%}$ ratio > 1.0 ranges from 18–67%, while the specificity ranges from 29–88% in different series. The sensitivity of the sawtooth appearance ranges from 29–85%, and the specificity from 54–100%. Parkinson's disease and neuromuscular disorders may also produce the same flow-volume loop abnormalities as are seen in OSA. Thus, the maximal expiratory-inspiratory flow-volume loop is generally not a useful test to detect OSA.

8. What causes stridor following extubation?

The commonest cause of immediate postextubation stridor is **edema of the larynx**. Less common causes include laryngeal inflammation or infection, vocal cord paresis or paralysis, laryngeal muscle dysfunction, hematomas, arytenoid dislocation, granulation tissue, and subglottic stenosis. The latter complication is particularly likely to occur in children. Retained secretions, blood clots, and foreign material may also produce stridor. Clinicians should not routinely ascribe postextubation stridor to laryngospasm, which appears to occur rarely, except after upper airway surgery. Delayed stridor following extubation should always be regarded seriously. Its differential diagnosis includes vocal cord paresis or paralysis, granulation tissue, laryngeal web, glottic and subglottic stenosis, and tracheal stenosis.

9. Name 11 strategies for managing the patient with postextubation stridor.

1. Examine the upper airway, neck, and chest carefully.
2. Suction secretions and remove any foreign material in the nose, mouth, and pharynx.
3. Observe the patient and follow vital signs and oxyhemoglobin saturation closely. Monitor arterial blood gases if needed.
4. Maintain upright posture if possible. If the patient is supine, maintain head and neck position to ensure airway patency.
5. Support ventilation with a resuscitator bag and mask, continuous positive airway pressure (CPAP) machine, or intermittent positive pressure breathing (IPPB) machine if necessary.
6. Administer topical epinephrine—5–10 ml of a 1:20 dilution of 1 ml (1 mg) of epinephrine—to the hypopharynx and glottis with an atomizer or nebulizer. (Racemic epinephrine solution—2.25%, 15 ml—is often used for this purpose but has no proven benefit compared to plain epinephrine.)
7. Treat coexisting problems such as bronchospasm if present.

8. Administer a helium-oxygen gas mixture if necessary to reduce the patient's work of breathing.

9. Avoid sedating the patient unless reintubation is imminent.

10. Be prepared to intubate the patient if necessary.

11. Consider tracheostomy if post-extubation stridor necessitates reintubation on two or more occasions.

10. When can an intubated patient with suspected laryngeal edema be safely extubated?

Perform the **cuff-leak test** by completely deflating the cuff of the endotracheal tube during positive pressure mechanical ventilation. (Be certain that the airway is adequately suctioned beforehand.) If an air leak is detected on a machine-delivered inspiration, successful extubation can be anticipated. If an air leak is not detected, laryngeal edema may be severe enough to preclude successful intubation.

Some authorities have advocated performing fiberoptic laryngoscopy to assess the degree of laryngeal edema before extubation. However, this practice cannot be supported in the absence of data that it is cost-effective.

11. A patient presents with progressive cough, dyspnea, and difficulty clearing pulmonary secretions several weeks after translaryngeal intubation for respiratory failure. What diagnosis should you always consider?

Upper airway obstruction. Laryngeal or tracheal stenosis is an important late complication of translaryngeal intubation, occurring in as many as 10% of such patients. Stenosis may occur at the level of the glottis, subglottis (cricoid ring), or at the site of the inflated endotracheal tube cuff. Stenosis rarely occurs at the previous level of the tip of the endotracheal tube. Symptoms of laryngotracheal stenosis include cough, hoarseness, inability to completely clear the airway of secretions, and dyspnea. These should not automatically be attributed to the underlying pulmonary disease or disorder for which intubation was required. If this condition is not recognized early, it may progress to respiratory failure or death from critical airway stenosis. Remember that laryngeal and tracheal injury from artificial airways is the most common cause of chronic upper airway obstruction.

12. What is the role of endoscopy in evaluating upper airway obstruction in ambulatory patients?

Indirect laryngoscopy with a light and mirror is a safe and simple procedure to evaluate the hypopharynx for tumors, laryngeal disease, and foreign bodies. Direct laryngoscopy with a fiberoptic laryngoscope is also a useful office procedure for examining patients with conditions such as unexplained hoarseness, suspected vocal cord paralysis or laryngeal cancer, or postextubation laryngeal symptoms. The fiberoptic bronchoscope is an invaluable tool for inspecting the larynx, trachea, and bronchi whenever obstruction is suspected.

When any type of upper airway endoscopy is performed, care must be taken to avoid inadvertent forcing of foreign material deeper into the airway or exacerbating airway edema. Special caution is always necessary in patients with suspected epiglottitis, but this warning is more applicable to children than to adults.

13. When should imaging studies be ordered to evaluate the patient with suspected upper airway obstruction?

The role of soft tissue views of the neck in adult patients with acute upper airway obstruction is quite limited. Soft tissue views are commonly ordered when epiglottitis is suspected, but obtaining them should not delay securing airway patency. The sensitivity and specificity of this test are not good, however. CT has replaced conventional tomography for evaluation of laryngeal and tracheal stenosis and should be considered whenever clinically significant laryngeal or tracheal obstruction is suspected. CT is especially useful in patients with suspected cancer involving the upper airway or mediastinal disease. The multiplanar capability of MRI makes it superior to CT in displaying the length of a laryngeal or tracheal stenosis.

14. What is factitious asthma? When should you suspect this diagnosis?

Factitious asthma is an important type of upper airway obstruction that may mimic bronchial asthma. This functional disorder of the larynx has also been called emotional laryngeal wheezing, hysteric croup, and Münchhausen's stridor. Cardinal features of factitious asthma include:

Repeated attacks of wheezing and dyspnea

Sudden onset and rapid resolution of symptoms

Minimal or no hypoxemia

Absence of respiratory acidosis

Lack of response to conventional therapy with bronchodilators and corticosteroids

Inspiratory as well as expiratory stridor

Abnormal flow-volume loop showing variable extrathoracic airway obstruction

Adduction of the vocal cords throughout the respiratory cycle on laryngoscopy

Normal spirometry shortly after the symptoms subside

Inconsistent effort on pulmonary function testing with variable results

Negative results of bronchial provocation tests

You should suspect this diagnosis in young or middle-aged patients with some degree of medical sophistication who have repeated emergency room visits or hospitalizations for "asthma" that has been difficult to control. A history of psychiatric illness is common. Management of factitious asthma includes psychiatric counseling and speech therapy.

15. Which connective tissue diseases may present with upper airway obstruction?

Rheumatoid arthritis, relapsing polychondritis, ankylosing spondylitis, and systemic lupus erythematosus are all known to affect the larynx or trachea.

Connective Tissue Diseases Causing Upper Airway Obstruction

CONNECTIVE TISSUE DISEASE	MECHANISM
Rheumatoid arthritis	Inflammation of cricoarytenoid joint
Relapsing polychondritis	Inflammation of laryngeal and tracheal cartilage
Ankylosing spondylitis	Inflammation of cricoarytenoid joint
Systemic lupus erythematosus	Inflammation of larynx

16. Describe the mechanism of acute pulmonary edema in upper airway obstruction.

Pulmonary edema may occur with any type of upper airway obstruction. **Laryngospasm** is a commonly reported cause. This type of noncardiogenic pulmonary edema is caused by very negative intrapleural pressure that is generated on inspiration by strong contraction of the respiratory muscles and transmitted to the perivascular interstitium. At the same time, negative intrapleural pressure increases venous return to the thorax and raises pulmonary blood volume and pulmonary microvascular hydrostatic pressure. The very negative perivascular interstitial pressure and the high microvascular hydrostatic pressure together promote the transudation of fluid into the pulmonary interstitium by Starling forces. Because this type of pulmonary edema is commonly observed at the time of relief of upper airway obstruction by intubation, it is sometimes called "postobstructive" pulmonary edema.

CONTROVERSIES

17. Is duration of translaryngeal intubation (TLI) related to severity of laryngeal injury?

Common logic would suggest that the longer an endotracheal tube is used, the more laryngeal injury would occur. However, 8 of 11 prospective studies of complications of TLI have failed to demonstrate a statistically significant association between duration of intubation and severity of laryngeal injury. This failure may be explained by the fact that such studies are difficult to perform well and that laryngeal injury complicating TLI is undoubtedly multifactorial.

Besides duration of TLI, other causes of laryngeal injury are potentially important. They include size of the endotracheal tube, geometric "fit" of the tube in the larynx, abrasion of the laryngeal surface by tube movement, capillary perfusion pressure in the laryngeal mucosa, aspiration of gastric secretions, infection of the larynx, underlying disease states, and other factors.

18. Should flow-volume loops be obtained in all patients with suspected upper airway obstruction?

No. The sensitivity and specificity of this test are low enough that its routine use is not warranted. Upper airway obstruction must be severe (tracheal diameter < 8 mm) before flow limitation becomes evident on the flow-volume loop. Furthermore, the expiratory flow-volume curve, a derivative of spirometry, is an effort-dependent test, requiring maximal patient effort to be valid. The flow-volume loop depends on the ability of the patient to generate intrathoracic pressures strong enough that the airflow rate will be limited at the site of upper airway obstruction. Patients with significant asthma or chronic obstructive pulmonary disease or those whose effort on the test is suboptimal may not display these "classic" abnormalities. Finally, the test is not feasible in patients who are acutely ill.

19. Should patients with postextubation laryngeal edema who require reintubation be given parenteral corticosteroids before the next extubation attempt?

Parenteral corticosteroids, such as dexamethasone, are given commonly in this setting. However, several prospective studies in adults and children have demonstrated no benefits from this practice.

Answers to Question 6: A (4), B (2), C (1), D (3).

BIBLIOGRAPHY

1. Aboussouan LS, Stoller JK: Diagnosis and management of upper airway obstruction. Clin Chest Med 15:35–53, 1994.
2. American Heart Association: Guidelines for cardiopulmonary resuscitation and emergency cardiac care: Part II. Adult basic life support. JAMA 268:2184–2198, 1992.
3. Darmon JY, Rauss A, Dreyfuss D, et al: Evaluation of risk factors for laryngeal edema after tracheal extubation in adults and its prevention by dexamethasone: A placebo-controlled, double-blind multicenter study. Anesthesiology 77:245–251, 1992.
4. Elliott CG, Rasmusson BY, Crapo RO: Upper airway obstruction following adult respiratory distress syndrome: An analysis of 30 survivors. Chest 94:526–530, 1988.
5. Fisher MM, Draper RF: The "cuff-leak" test for extubation. Anaesthesia 47:10–12, 1992.
6. Gropper MA, Wiener-Kronish JP, Hashimoto S: Acute cardiogenic pulmonary edema. Clin Chest Med 15:501–515, 1994.
7. Josephson GD, Josephson JS, Krespi YP, et al: Airway obstruction: New modalities in treatment. Med Clin North Am 77:539–549, 1993.
8. Krieger J, Weitzenblum E, Vandevenne A, et al: Flow-volume curve abnormalities and obstructive sleep apnea syndrome. Chest 87:163–167, 1985.
9. Lunn WW, Sheller JR: Flow volume loops in the evaluation of upper airway obstruction. Otolaryngol Clin North Am 28:721–729, 1995.
10. Mackenzie CF, Shin B, McAslan TC, et al: Severe stridor after prolonged endotracheal intubation using high-volume cuffs. Anesthesiology 50:235–239, 1979.
11. Pepin JL, Levy P, Veale D, et al: Evaluation of the upper airway in sleep apnea syndrome. Sleep 15:S50–S65, 1992.
12. Ross DA, Sasaki CT: Acute laryngeal obstruction. Lancet 344:1743–1748, 1994.
13. Stauffer JL, White DP, Zwillich CW: Pulmonary function in obstructive sleep apnea: Relationships to pharyngeal resistance and cross-sectional area. Chest 97:302–307, 1990.
14. Wiedemann HP, Matthay RA: Pulmonary manifestations of the collagen vascular diseases. Clin Chest Med 10:677–722, 1989.

24. TRACHEOSTOMY

John L. Stauffer, M.D.

1. What are the main advantages of tracheostomy compared with translaryngeal intubation for prolonged airway maintenance?
- Overall facilitation of patient care by nurses
- Ease of airway care and suctioning secretions
- Patient comfort
- Improved patient appearance
- Improved oral, nasal, and facial hygiene
- Elimination of the ongoing risks of oral, nasal, pharyngeal, and most laryngeal complications of translaryngeal intubation
- Facilitation of feeding by mouth
- Facilitation of oral communication and speech
- Reduced risk of tracheal extubation
- Ease of tube reinsertion
- Improved patient mobility
- Ease of disposition to long-term care facility

2. What are the main disadvantages of tracheostomy compared with translaryngeal intubation for prolonged airway maintenance?
- Expense (total charges in range of $2500–3500)
- Requirement for trained surgical personnel
- Requirement for anesthesia and operating room support in many cases
- Greater morbidity and mortality
- Tendency to delay decannulation and weaning from mechanical ventilation
- Greater risk of upper airway stenosis
- Potential to exacerbate injury to the larynx caused by translaryngeal intubation
- Permanent scar

3. Should tracheostomy be performed to reduce "dead-space" volume or to reduce airway resistance?
No. Compared with endotracheal tubes of the same diameter, tracheostomy tubes have less mechanical dead-space volume and impose less airway resistance. However, these difference are small enough in most clinical situations that there is no advantage in converting from translaryngeal intubation to tracheostomy for either reason.

4. When is percutaneous dilatational tracheostomy indicated?
Like conventional tracheostomy, this relatively new procedure is indicated for elective surgical access to the trachea for prolonged airway management (clearance of secretions, securing a patent airway, bypassing upper airway obstruction, and facilitation of mechanical ventilation). The main advantages compared with conventional tracheostomy are that the procedure does not require the use of the operating room and is faster, easier to perform, and less expensive. Furthermore, it creates a smaller stoma. Percutaneous dilatational tracheostomy is *not* intended to be an emergency procedure in patients with upper airway obstruction.

5. How much pressure should be maintained in the cuff of a tracheostomy tube?
The lateral pressure exerted on the tracheal wall by the tracheostomy tube cuff should ideally always be less than the capillary perfusion pressure in the tracheal mucosa in order to avoid ischemic necrosis of the mucosa. Keeping the intracuff pressure < 25 mmHg at all times should

achieve this goal. If higher cuff inflation pressures are required to seal the airway during mechanical ventilation (as in patients with high peak inflation pressures), consider using the "minimal leak" cuff inflation technique. This practices accepts a small leak of air past the cuff with each mechanical breath. Foam cuff tracheostomy tubes may also be used to reduce lateral tracheal wall pressure.

6. List the most important early and late complications of tracheostomy.

Early complications

Bleeding	Swallowing dysfunction
Pneumothorax	Aspiration
Subcutaneous or mediastinal emphysema	Pneumonia
Paratracheal tube placement	Ineffective cough
Tracheoesophageal fistula	Inadvertent decannulation
Recurrent laryngeal nerve injury	Mechanical problems with tube or cuff
Thyroid gland injury	Tracheostomy tube obstruction
Wound infection	Cardiac arrest

Late complications

Poor wound healing	Tracheomalacia
Tracheal stenosis	Chronic tracheal dilatation
Tracheoesophageal fistula	Keloid formation at stoma
Tracheoarterial fistula	Dysphagia
Granulation tissue (granuloma)	

7. Tracheostomy is often justified to avoid laryngeal injury. Can tracheostomy cause laryngeal injury?

Yes. Several studies suggest that the risk of posterior glottic stenosis from translaryngeal intubation may be increased if tracheostomy follows intubation. Infection induced by the surgical wound in the trachea and non-use of the glottic apparatus, allowing scar tissue to form, are the proposed underlying mechanisms.

8. Should tracheostomy be performed as an emergency procedure?

No. Techniques of basic life support should allow the rescuer to maintain a patent upper airway in emergency situations. In advanced life support in adults, **translaryngeal intubation** is the method of choice to establish a definitive airway. A variety of alternative airway devices, such as the laryngeal mask airway and the esophageal-tracheal double-lumen airway, are also available to provide ventilation in emergency situations. If surgical access to the trachea is required in emergency situations, such as when upper airway obstruction persists despite attempts at basic life support, cricothyroidotomy is advised and preferred to tracheostomy.

9. Should CT be performed routinely several months after tracheal decannulation to look for occult tracheal stenosis?

No. The value of this practice has not been established. Symptoms of tracheal stenosis complicating tracheostomy include dyspnea, cough, and difficulty clearing sputum. Physicians seeing patients after tracheal decannulation should be alert to the possibility of tracheal stenosis if these symptoms are present. The evaluation of such patients requires careful physical examination and pulmonary function tests, including the flow-volume loop. Fiberoptic bronchoscopy or CT is required to confirm the clinical diagnosis of tracheal stenosis.

10. How common is aspiration in critically ill patients with cuffed tracheostomy tubes?

Tracheostomy frequently impairs elevation of the larynx and glottic closure, resulting in swallowing difficulty and glottic incompetence. Almost 90% of patients with cuffed tracheostomy tubes in place aspirate pharyngeal secretions past the vocal cords and the tube cuff into the tracheal lumen, especially during swallowing. Tracheostomy tube cuffs do not prevent small amounts of fluid from entering the trachea. Aspiration during mechanical ventilation is usually silent. In one study, 50% of tracheostomy patients aspirated during swallowing.

11. Can patients talk while receiving mechanical ventilation via a cuffed tracheostomy tube?

Yes. This is one of the main advantages of tracheostomy compared with translaryngeal intubation. Deflating the tracheostomy tube cuff or lowering the cuff pressure enough to allow air to leak past the cuff during expiration may permit speech. The "electrolarynx" may also be used for this purpose. Another device is the talking tracheostomy tube, which has a separate channel for delivery of gas above the inflated cuff to permit airflow past the vocal cords. Unfortunately, none of these approaches has achieved a high success rate in patients being mechanically ventilated. After the tracheostomy patient has been weaned from the ventilator, a simple one-way valve (Passy-Muir valve) attached to the tracheostomy tube may facilitate speech if the cuff is deflated.

12. How often should patients with tracheostomy tubes be suctioned?

Tracheal suctioning abrades the tracheal and bronchial mucosa, shredding the ciliated epithelium along the tract of the suction catheter. Repeated suctioning causes impaired mucociliary clearance, hemorrhage, and mucosal inflammation as well as substantial patient discomfort. For these reasons, suctioning of the trachea should be performed only when needed, not as a routine. The best practice is to allow the nurses and respiratory therapists to suction the airway when they feel it is indicated. Standing orders for tracheal suctioning should be avoided in most cases.

13. What are the indications for tracheostomy in patients with obstructive sleep apnea (OSA) syndrome?

Tracheostomy is now employed infrequently in the management of patients with OSA syndrome. Nasal continuous positive airway pressure (nasal CPAP) has become the treatment of choice for most patients with significant symptoms caused by documented OSA. Weight loss, optimal sleep hygiene, avoidance of CNS depressants, avoidance of other risk factors, and surgical correction of nasal and pharyngeal obstruction are essential components of therapy. Dental appliances, uvulopalatopharyngoplasty, and maxillofacial surgery are indicated in selected circumstances. When all these forms of therapy have been exhausted, tracheostomy should be considered. Patients who are candidates for tracheostomy usually have life-threatening OSA complicated by advanced cor pulmonale, nocturnal cardiac arrhythmias, severe nocturnal hypoxemia, or severe respiratory acidemia often in association with obesity-hypoventilation syndrome. Rarely, a facial skeletal anomaly associated with OSA is an indication for tracheostomy.

14. What are the indications for removal (decannulation) of a tracheostomy tube? When should this be done?

A tracheostomy tube should be removed when it is no longer indicated for relief of upper airway obstruction, evacuation of lower airway secretions, airway protection, or facilitation of mechanical ventilation. Although this seems obvious, tracheal decannulation is often delayed. While extubation is usually done in a timely fashion, decannulation is frequently not accomplished with the same haste. As with extubation, decannulation should be carried out as soon as possible. If there is uncertainty about the continued need for a standard tracheostomy tube, the tracheostomy may be "downsized" by placing a tracheostomy button (Olympic or Kistner) or a size 5 or 6 metal tracheostomy tube in the stoma until decannulation is certain.

15. Discuss the main options in tracheostomy tube design and list appropriate indications for selection.

Cuffed vs. uncuffed
    Cuffed: Positive pressure ventilation, airway protection
    Uncuffed: Access to the trachea simply for suctioning secretions
Fenestrated vs. unfenestrated
    Fenestrated: Option for speech when the inner cannula is removed
    Unfenestrated: Standard
Inner cannula vs. no inner cannula
    Inner cannula: Facilitates cleaning and removal of impacted secretions
    No inner cannula: Less complicated system, temporary use

Metal vs. Nonmetal (silicone rubber, polyvinyl chloride)
  Metal: May be cleaned and used without replacement
  Nonmetal: Disposable
15-mm adapter vs. no adapter
  15-mm adapter: Permits positive pressure ventilation
  No adapter: No positive pressure ventilation is anticipated
Standard vs. alternative (tracheostomy buttons, Montgomery tube)
  Standard: Routine indications for tracheostomy
  Alternative: For special purposes, such as "downsizing" or obstructive sleep apnea

16. What should you do when the patient returns to the ICU after having elective tracheostomy in the operating room?

- Read the operation note and discuss the case with the surgeon.
- Examine the patient with special attention to the neck, chest, mediastinum, and heart. Look for bleeding, cyanosis, subcutaneous emphysema, signs of pneumothorax and pneumomediastinum, etc. Check vital signs and oxyhemoglobin saturation by pulse oximetry.
- Check the cuff pressure in the tracheostomy tube. The nitrous oxide gas used for anesthesia may diffuse into the cuff and create very high intracuff pressures.
- Obtain a portable chest radiograph. Look for subcutaneous emphysema, pneumothorax, pneumomediastinum, pneumonia, atelectasis, etc.
- Review or write the postoperative orders.

17. Who should perform tracheostomy?

A properly trained and experienced surgeon only.

CONTROVERSY

18. Should tracheostomy be performed routinely after 7–10 days of translaryngeal intubation?

No. Tracheostomy is not indicated simply because an arbitrary number of days of translaryngeal intubation have elapsed. The timing of tracheostomy depends on good clinical judgment in each case. Some patients should have tracheostomy at the time of admission, others after days or weeks of translaryngeal intubation. If a patient clearly will need an artificial airway for weeks, tracheostomy should be performed sooner rather than later, and waiting for 7, 10, or 14 days to transpire before proceeding to tracheostomy is unwise.

BIBLIOGRAPHY

1. American Heart Association: Guidelines for cardiopulmonary resuscitation and emergency cardiac care: Part III. Adult advanced cardiac life support. JAMA 268:2199–2241, 1992.
2. Anderson HL, Bartlett RH: Elective tracheostomy for mechanical ventilation by the percutaneous technique. Clin Chest Med 12:555–560, 1991.
3. Bishop MJ: The timing of tracheotomy: An evolving consensus. Chest 96:712–713, 1989.
4. Burkey B, Esclamado R, Morganroth M: The role of cricothyroidotomy in airway management. Clin Chest Med 12:561–571, 1991.
5. Elpern EH, Scott MG, Petro L, et al: Pulmonary aspiration in mechanically ventilated patients with tracheostomies. Chest 105:563–566, 1994.
6. Friedman Y, Mayer AD: Bedside percutaneous tracheostomy in critically ill patients. Chest 104:532–535, 1993.
7. Heffner JE, Casey K, Hoffman C: Care of the mechanically ventilated patient with a tracheotomy. In Tobin MJ (ed): Principles and Practice of Mechanical Ventilation. New York, McGraw-Hill, 1994.
8. Myers EN, Carrau RL: Early complications of tracheotomy: Incidence and management. Clin Chest Med 12:589–595, 1991.
9. Stauffer JL: Medical management of the airway. Clin Chest Med 12:449–482, 1991.
10. Stauffer JL, Olson DE, Petty TL: Complications and consequences of endotracheal intubation and tracheotomy: A prospective study of 150 critically ill adult patients. Am J Med 70:65–76, 1981.
11. Tolep K, Getch CL, Criner GJ: Swallowing dysfunction in patients receiving prolonged mechanical ventilation. Chest 109:167–172, 1996.
12. Wood DE, Mathisen DJ: Late complications of tracheotomy. Clin Chest Med 12:597–609, 1991.

VI. Infectious Disease

25. COMMUNITY-ACQUIRED PNEUMONIA

Hugh A. Cassiere, M.D., and Michael S. Niederman, M.D.

1. Who is at high risk for developing community-acquired pneumonia?

Patients at risk include those with coexisting medical conditions such as diabetes mellitus, chronic obstructive lung disease, and congestive heart failure; smokers; chronic alcohol abusers; and the elderly (over age 65). These factors place individuals at high risk for pneumonia by impairing the normal host defense system. Coexisting medical illness can cause several host defense defects ranging from impaired mucociliary clearance to decreased immunoglobulin production in the lower respiratory tract. Smoking can alter respiratory tract defenses by increasing mucus production and interfering with mucociliary clearance. Altered immune function can occur with advanced age, but comorbid illness is a more important influence than aging itself. The elderly, however, do have decreased bone marrow mass, decreased antibody response to vaccines, and impaired cell-mediated immunity. Chronic alcohol abuse results in cirrhosis and malnutrition that can have a detrimental effect on both humoral and cellular immunity.

2. What percentage of patients with community-acquired pneumonia have a specific causative pathogen identified?

Only 30–60% of patients have a specific causative pathogen identified, even with the use of extensive diagnostic testing, such as serologic studies, sputum culture and Gram stains, blood cultures, and microbial antigen assays. This low diagnostic yield reflects the limited sensitivity—and perhaps clinical value—of available tests, but also highlights the realization that we may not yet know all the pathogens that cause pneumonia. No differences exist, however, in clinical outcome for patients with or without an identified causative pathogen. These observations underscore the point that empiric therapy is necessary for most patients with community-acquired pneumonia.

3. What are the common pathogens that cause community-acquired pneumonia?

Streptococcus pneumoniae, Mycoplasma pneumoniae, respiratory viruses, *Legionella pneumophilia, Chlamydia pneumoniae, Haemophilus influenzae,* and occasionally *Moraxella catarrhalis* and aerobic gram-negative bacilli represent the major pathogens that cause community-acquired pneumonia. Aerobic gram-negative bacilli are becoming more prevalent as primary pathogens, possibly reflecting the changes in the population of patients who develop pneumonia. Staphylococcal pneumonia is relatively uncommon except in the setting of a postviral respiratory tract infection, such as influenza. The identity of the probable pathogens usually varies depending on patient age, comorbidity, and the severity of illness.

4. Can clinical, laboratory, or radiographic parameters predict the pathogen causing community-acquired pneumonia?

No. Most studies to date do not support the concept that the cause of pneumonia can be predicted by examination of clinical, laboratory, or radiographic data. For example, the "bulging fissure" sign of *Klebsiella pneumoniae*, the hyponatremia of *Legionella pneumophilia*, and the "atypical" presentation of mycoplasmal pneumonia are not specific enough findings to rule out other pathogens. In fact, recent studies of community-acquired pneumonia have shown that categorizing pneumonia as "atypical" versus "typical" is more of a historic exercise than one with clinical or scientific relevance. Such classification may even lead to a false sense of security and an inaccurate diagnosis that promotes inappropriate choice of antibiotic. The clearest example comes in the elderly, who may have pneumococcal pneumonia (a "typical" pathogen), with "atypical" clinical features because of age and disease-associated impairments in immune responses.

5. What factors help determine whether an individual with community-acquired pneumonia should be hospitalized?

There is no set "admission formula" to establish when a patient with community-acquired pneumonia should be hospitalized. Instead, the clinician must evaluate each patient to determine if there are several factors present that are associated with either a complicated course or an increased likelihood of mortality from pneumonia. Patients with several risk factors need to be observed and treated in the hospital. Occasionally it may be necessary to admit someone to the hospital for social reasons, such as the patient's inability to care for himself at home.

Several studies of community-acquired pneumonia have identified factors associated with a complicated course and an increased likelihood of mortality. These include:

- Advanced age (more than 65 years)
- Coexisting medical conditions
- Postsplenectomy status
- Chronic alcohol abuse
- Altered mental status
- Vital sign abnormalities: respiratory rate more than 30 breaths per minute, systolic blood pressure less than 90 mmHg, diastolic blood pressure less than 60 mmHg, or temperature more than 101° F
- Metastatic (extrapulmonary) infection
- White blood cell count less than 4,000/μl or more than 30,000/μl
- Renal dysfunction, e.g., BUN more than 20 mg/dl
- PaO_2 less than 60 mmHg or $PaCO_2$ more than 50 mmHg on room air
- Unfavorable chest radiographic patterns, such as multilobar infiltrates, effusions, cavitation, or rapidly progressive infiltrates (more than 50% increase in 48 hours)
- Evidence of severe infection, e.g., metabolic acidosis, disseminated intravascular coagulation, or other end-organ involvement
- Need for mechanical ventilation

6. What factors determine whether a patient with community-acquired pneumonia needs admission to the ICU?

Several factors have been identified that correlate with high mortality (more than 20%) in patients with community-acquired pneumonia and therefore may justify admission to the intensive care unit. In addition, certain therapies (mechanical ventilation and pressor support) are best given in the ICU. If a patient has any one of the following, severe pneumonia is present:

- Admission respiratory rate more than 35 breaths per minute
- Need for mechanical ventilation
- Chest radiograph showing either 50% increase in the infiltrate over 48 hours or bilateral or multilobar involvement
- Presence of shock
- Need for vasopressors to support blood pressure
- Severe lung injury defined by a PaO_2/FIO_2 ratio of less than 250
- Presence of acute renal failure
- Urine output less than 30 cc per hour

7. Is there a different pathogen profile in severe community-acquired pneumonia?

Yes. As in all patients with community-acquired pneumonia, *Streptococcus pneumoniae* is still the most common pathogen, but in the clinical setting of severe infection, *Legionella* sp., *H. influenzae*, and enteric gram-negative bacilli play a greater role. This concept guides the selection of the initial antibiotic treatment regimen. *Legionella pneumophilia* is more common in smokers, alcoholics, and patients presenting with multiorgan failure; it is particularly common in patients who present with acute respiratory failure requiring mechanical ventilation. Mortality from *Legionella pneumophilia* is doubled if the disease is not treated with erythromycin.

The increased incidence of gram-negative bacilli may be, in part, caused by the patient population that is predisposed to severe community-acquired pneumonia, namely the elderly and the chronically ill. The elderly and patients with severe underlying medical disease (e.g., congestive heart failure, diabetes mellitus, cirrhosis, renal failure, or carcinoma) are predisposed to oropharyngeal colonization with enteric gram-negative bacilli, which are especially virulent pathogens. The presence of gram-negative bacilli in oral secretions of chronically ill patients who are at increased risk for aspiration may account for the higher proportion of these pathogens in patients admitted with severe community-acquired pneumonia. In some studies, *Pseudomonas aeruginosa* has been identified as causing severe community-acquired pneumonia, accounting for 10–20% of all cases.

8. Once community-acquired pneumonia is suspected, what diagnostic studies are appropriate and beneficial?

A thorough history and physical examination should be performed and **standard posteroanterior and lateral chest radiographs** should be obtained. The chest radiograph is useful not only to diagnose the pneumonia but also to evaluate patients for the presence of lung cavities, pleural effusions, and other radiographic abnormalities that may predict a complicated course.

Hospitalized patients should have two samples collected for **blood cultures** in addition to blood samples for the routine chemistries and blood counts. Although blood cultures are positive only 15–30% of the time, the presence of bacteremia has a significant impact on patient management, affecting the duration of intravenous antibiotics and the length of hospital stay.

Routine chemistries and blood counts can stratify hospitalized patients with regard to risk. For example, extremes of white blood cell count, renal failure, electrolyte abnormalities, and abnormal coagulation profiles (e.g., thrombocytopenia and elevated prothrombin time/partial thromboplastin time) may influence decisions about admission to the ICU.

Diagnostic thoracentesis should be performed to evaluate for empyema in patients who have pleural effusion associated with pneumonia, because this defines a patient population that will have a complicated course and may require drainage procedures in addition to antibiotics.

9. Considering that most patients with community-acquired pneumonia have no clear pathogen identified, how is therapy initiated?

Therapy should be empiric and based upon the likelihood of certain pathogens being found in a given patient population. There are four patient categories, based upon the age of the patient, the need for hospitalization, the severity of pneumonia, and the presence of coexisting medical disease.

Empiric Therapy for Community-Acquired Pneumonia

	LIKELY PATHOGENS	THERAPY
I. Outpatient pneumonia, 60 years of age or younger, and no coexisting medical disease	*S. pneumoniae* *M. pneumoniae* Respiratory viruses *C. pneumoniae* *H. influenzae*	Macrolide (consider azithromycin or clarithromycin in smokers) **or** tetracycline
II. Outpatient pneumonia, 60 years of age or older, and/or coexisting medical disease	*S. pneumoniae* Respiratory viruses *H. influenzae* Aerobic gram-negative bacilli *S. aureus*	Second-generation cephalosporin **or** β-lactam/β-lactamase inhibitor **or** TMP/SMX **plus** consider optional macrolide

(Table continued on next page.)

Empiric Therapy for Community-Acquired Pneumonia (Continued)

	LIKELY PATHOGENS	THERAPY
III. Hospitalized patients	*S. pneumoniae* *H. influenzae* Polymicrobial Aerobic gram-negative bacilli *Legionella* sp. *S. aureus* *C. pneumoniae* Respiratory viruses	Second or third generation non- pseudomonal cephalosporin **or** β-lactam/β-lactamase inhibitor **with or without** macrolide (oral or IV)
IV. Severe illness, hospitalized patients	*S. pneumoniae* *Legionella* sp. Aerobic gram-negative bacilli (including *P. aeruginosa*) Respiratory viruses *M. pneumoniae*	Macrolide (IV) **plus** third generation antipseudomonal cephalosporin **or** ciprofloxacin **or** imipenem (Consider adding aminoglycoside or other dual antipseudomonal therapy.)

TMP/SMX = trimethoprim/sulfamethoxazole.

10. When is *S. pneumoniae* considered to be penicillin resistant?

S. pneumoniae penicillin resistance is defined on the basis of a minimal inhibitory concentration (MIC), which is the lowest antibiotic concentration that inhibits visible growth after 18–24 hours of incubation. For infections caused by *S. pneumoniae* that do not involve the meninges, an MIC of 2.0 μg per ml or more is considered to be highly resistant to penicillin G. If the MIC is 0.1 to 1.0 μg per ml, *S. pneumoniae* is intermediately resistant to penicillin G.

11. If penicillin-resistant *S. pneumoniae* is the cause of community-acquired pneumonia, how should it be treated?

Antibiotic treatment depends on the degree of penicillin resistance (intermediate versus high) and whether cephalosporin resistance is also present. If *S. pneumoniae* is only intermediately resistant to penicillin G, high-dose penicillin (150,000–200,000 U/kg/day) is considered adequate antibiotic treatment for community-acquired pneumococcal pneumonia. If the pneumococcus is highly resistant to penicillin G, its resistance patterns to the cephalosporins should be evaluated. *S. pneumoniae* is considered to be resistant to cephalosporins if the MIC to ceftriaxone or cefotaxime exceeds 2.0 μg/ml. If the pneumococcus is sensitive to cephalosporins, ceftriaxone or cefotaxime may be used to treat penicillin-resistant *S. pneumoniae* pneumonia. If *S. pneumoniae* is highly resistant to both penicillins and cephalosporins, alternative therapy with vancomycin or imipenem is warranted. The presence of penicillin resistance itself has not been shown to adversely affect outcome in community-acquired pneumonia, and outcome is equivalent whether high-dose penicillin or cephalosporins are used.

12. How are patients on empiric antibiotic therapy monitored?

Effective antibiotic therapy should improve clinical features of pneumonia in 48–72 hours. This is key to empiric therapy because antibiotics should not be changed within this time frame unless the patient has a marked clinical deterioration. Fever can continue for 2–4 days and leukocytosis may persist until day 4, even with appropriate antibiotic therapy. With these concepts in mind, the clinician must try to determine the cause of the treatment failure. Several factors cause clinical deterioration in a patient on empiric antibiotics, including:

Emergence of resistant organisms
Superinfection with nosocomial pathogens
Use of an inappropriate initial antibiotic
regimen
Infection with an unusual pathogen
(e.g, *Pneumocystis carinii*)

Disease that mimics pneumonia
(e.g., pulmonary embolus, congestive
heart failure, bronchogenic carcinoma)
Inability of host defenses to resist the
pathogen, even with adequate
antibiotic coverage

In these patients a more aggressive diagnostic work-up is necessary, including further radiologic testing and often bronchoscopic sampling of the lower respiratory tract. CT of the chest may reveal cavities, effusions, or other findings that were not detectable by the standard chest radiograph. Microbiologic studies including sputum culture and possibly bronchoscopic quantitative cultures may define the presence of resistant and unusual pathogens (e.g., tuberculosis, fungal pathogens).

13. Are invasive diagnostic tests indicated in the routine management of community-acquired pneumonia?

Not usually. Invasive diagnostic tests include transtracheal aspiration, transthoracic aspiration, bronchoscopy, and open lung biopsy. Only those patients who fail initial therapy should be considered for aggressive diagnostic testing, and more than 85% of patients respond to initial empiric therapy. Of the invasive tests mentioned, bronchoscopy with quantitative cultures is the most sensitive test. Open lung biopsy may be helpful but should be reserved for nonresponding patients, especially when a pneumonia mimic is suspected.

14. When is a patient with community-acquired pneumonia considered to have a slowly resolving pneumonia?

In the immunocompetent host, slowly resolving pneumonia is defined by two key clinical parameters, symptoms and radiographic clearing. It is characterized by a patient who is responding to therapy but in a prolonged manner. A practical definition of slowly resolving pneumonia is less than 50% radiographic clearing at 4 weeks in a patient who has symptomatically improved on therapy. This patient should be distinguished from a clinical nonresponder.

15. What is the most common cause of slowly resolving community-acquired pneumonia?

Pneumococcal pneumonia, especially if it is bacteremic, in a patient with significant coexisting medical disease may resolve slowly. In these patients, pneumonia is slow to resolve because of the impact of underlying medical illnesses on host defenses. The effects of certain medical diseases on host defenses are outlined below.

Effects of Medical Diseases on Host Defenses

COPD	Diabetes mellitus	Neoplasms
Impaired cough	Defective neutrophil function	Impaired cellular
Impaired mucocilliary clearance	Reduced cell-mediated immunity	immunity
Heart disease	**Renal failure**	Neutropenia
Impaired lymphatic drainage	Depressed humoral response	Diminished humoral
Impaired alveolar macrophage	Diminished leukocyte	response
function	chemotaxis	
Edema promotes bacterial growth	Complement depletion	

16. What are other causes of slowly resolving community-acquired pneumonia ?

Infectious
Usual infectious causes
  Pneumococcus
  Legionella sp.
  H. influenzae
  Virus

Noninfectious (pneumonia mimics)
Neoplasm
  Bronchogenic carcinoma
  Lymphoma
Immunologic and idiopathic
  Lupus pneumonitis

Unusual infectious causes	*Immunologic and idiopathic (Cont.)*
Tuberculosis	Wegener's granulomatosis
Atypical mycobacteria	Bronchiolitis obliterans organizing
Nocardia spp.	pneumonia (BOOP)
Actinomyces spp.	*Drug-induced lung injury*
Aspergillus spp.	Amiodarone toxicity
Endemic fungi	

17. List the risk factors associated with slowly resolving pneumonia.

- Age greater than 55
- Alcohol abuse
- Significant coexisting medical disease (chronic obstructive pulmonary disease, congestive heart failure, renal failure, neoplastic disease, and diabetes mellitus)
- Severe pneumonia
- Multilobar disease
- Infection with a virulent pathogen (*L. pneumophilia, S. aureus,* and gram-negative bacilli)
- History of smoking
- Persistent leukocytosis and fever
- Bacteremic infection

The issues involved in evaluating patients for resolution of pneumonia appear to be (1) underlying diseases, (2) causative pathogens (if known), (3) severity of pneumonia, (4) smoking history, and (5) advanced age. In general, 50% of patients with pneumococcal pneumonia have radiographic clearing at 5 weeks, and the majority clear in 2 to 3 months. With bacteremic disease, 50% have clear chest radiographs at 9 weeks, and most are clear by 18 weeks. It has been shown recently that radiographic resolution in community-acquired pneumonia was most influenced by the number of lobes involved and the age of the patient. Radiographic clearance decreases by 20% per decade after age 20, and disease takes longer to clear in patients with multilobar infiltrates than in those with unilobar disease.

18. How should patients with slowly resolving pneumonia be followed?

Although the most common cause of slowly resolving pneumonia is pneumococcus in the setting of abnormal host factors (smoking, alcohol, coexisting medical illness, bacteremia, and so forth), it can also be secondary to resistant organisms, atypical pathogens (*M. tuberculosis* or *P. carinii*), unusual pathogens (fungi), or underlying neoplastic disease. Because of these other diagnostic possibilities, the patient with slowly resolving pneumonia should be followed very carefully. The following diagram outlines a practical approach to this important patient population. If at any point the patient requires further diagnostic testing, CT of the chest and bronchoscopy usually provide a diagnosis.

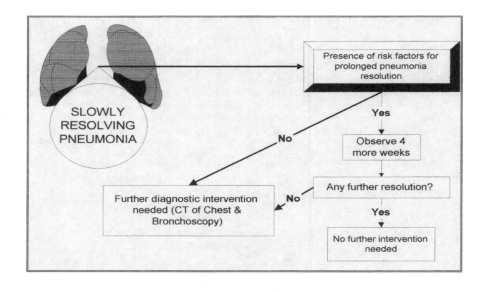

CONTROVERSY

19. Should sputum Gram stain be used routinely in the management of community-acquired pneumonia?

Pros: The sputum Gram stain is a simple diagnostic test that can be performed easily and interpreted more rapidly than any other diagnostic test used in pneumonia patients. It is relatively inexpensive and can be used to guide initial antibiotic therapy. If pneumococcus is identified on the stain, initial antibiotic therapy can be penicillin, instead of broad-spectrum antibiotics that have the theoretical ability of propagating bacterial resistance, e.g., penicillin-resistant *S. pneumoniae*. The Gram stain also can help stratify patients in regard to risk by potentially identifying pneumonia caused by high-risk pathogens, e.g., *S. aureus* and gram-negative bacilli, thereby alerting the clinician early on that the hospital course may be complicated.

Cons: Although the sputum Gram stain can yield useful information in selected patients, its routine use has several limitations. One such limitation is the fact that 40% of patients with community-acquired pneumonia cannot produce sputum. When sputum can be produced, specimens are almost always obtained by untrained individuals who collect nonpurulent samples that have little to no diagnostic usefulness. This sampling issue is further hindered by the fact that 30–45% of community-acquired pneumonia patients are already on antibiotics before hospitalization. The diagnostic yield in this patient population is reduced.

In the patient who has not been on antibiotics, another limitation to the Gram stain's usefulness is in its interpretation. Unless collected and interpreted by skilled personnel, the sputum Gram stain lacks adequate sensitivity and diagnostic usefulness. In the majority of cases the individual interpreting the sample is either inexperienced or has no clinical information to go with the sample. One study evaluated medical housestaff's ability to collect, perform, and interpret sputum Gram stain. The authors found that sputum could not be obtained in 42% of patients, and 15% of the stains were judged technically inadequate. When the test was performed properly, the positive predictive value for detecting pneumococcus was only 50%, with a false-positive rate of 50%.

BIBLIOGRAPHY

1. American Thoracic Society Guidelines for the Initial Management of Adults with Community-Acquired Pneumonia: Diagnosis, assessment of severity, and initial antimicrobial therapy. Am Rev Resp Dis 148:1418–1426, 1993.
2. British Thoracic Society and the Public Health Laboratory Service: Community-acquired pneumonia in adults in British hospitals in 1982–1983: A survey of aetiology, mortality, prognostic factors and outcome. Q J Med 239:195–220, 1987.
3. Fein AM, Feinsilver SH: Niederman MS, et al: When the pneumonia doesn't get better. Clin Chest Med 8:529–541, 1987.
4. Feinsilver SH, Fein AM, Niederman MS: Nonresolving, slowly resolving, and recurrent pneumonia. In Niederman MS, Sarosi GA, Glassroth J (eds): Respiratory Infections. Philadelphia, W.B. Saunders, 1994, pp 227–290.
5. Fine MJ, Orloff JJ, Rihs JD, et al: Evaluation of housestaff physicians' preparation and interpretation of sputum Gram stain for community-acquired pneumonia. J Gen Intern Med 6:189–198, 1991.
6. Jay S, Johanson W, Pierce A: The radiologic resolution of streptococcal pneumoniae pneumonia. N Engl J Med 293:798–801, 1975.
7. Mittl RL, Schwab RJ, Duchin JS, et al: Radiographic resolution of community-acquired pneumonia. Am J Respir Crit Care Med 149:630–635, 1994.
8. Nava JM, Bella F, Grau J, et al: Predictive factors for invasive disease due to penicillin resistant *Streptococcus pneumoniae:* Population-based study. Clin Infect Dis 19:884–890, 1994.
9. Pallares R, Linares J, Vadillo M, et al: Resistance to penicillin and cephalosporin and mortality from severe pneumococcal pneumonia in Barcelona, Spain. N Engl J Med 333:474–480, 1995.

26. NOSOCOMIAL PNEUMONIA

Susan W. Grey, M.D., and G. Umberto Meduri, M.D.

1. Define nosocomial pneumonia.
Nosocomial pneumonia (NP) is a pneumonia that develops 48 hours or more after admission to the hospital. It is the second most common hospital-acquired infection but is responsible for the highest mortality rate of all the nosocomial infections. Crude mortality rates range from 50 to 70%, and attributed mortality rates, death resulting directly from infection, ranges from 30 to 50%. Mortality is highest for bacteremic patients and those with infections caused by *Pseudomonas aeruginosa*. Most cases occur in the ICU. Ventilator-associated pneumonia (VAP) refers specifically to pneumonia that develops in patients receiving mechanical ventilation for more than 48 hours.

2. Why is it important to distinguish between nosocomial pneumonia and community-acquired pneumonia?
The pathogens responsible for NP differ from those that cause community-acquired pneumonia (CAP). *Streptococcus pneumoniae, Haemophilus influenzae, Legionella* spp., *Mycoplasma pneumoniae*, and *Chlamydia pneumoniae* are common pathogens in CAP, whereas aerobic gram-negative rods and *Staphylococcus aureus* account for most cases of NP. Therefore, antibiotic selection differs for NP and CAP.

3. Describe the pathogenesis of NP.
NP can develop through a number of different mechanisms. Direct aspiration of small volumes of colonized secretions from the upper airway is the most common. The nasopharynx and oropharynx constitute the body's first line of defense against many infections. These defenses, which include air filtration, mucociliary clearance, humoral factors, and cough reflex, are severely altered in critically ill patients and in those with an impaired level of consciousness. In intubated patients, these defenses are bypassed by the presence of the endotracheal tube (ETT). In addition, infected secretions tend to pool in the distal trachea above the inflated cuff of the ETT. All of these factors predispose patients to aspiration of infected secretions containing large numbers of bacteria.

Other, less likely mechanisms for the development of NP include bacteremic spread from another established focus of infection, inhalation of contaminated aerosols, and direct transthoracic inoculation. Factors that determine whether a patient will actually develop pneumonia include adequacy of the host immune system, bacterial burden of the inoculum, and virulence of the organism.

4. What are the risk factors associated with the development of NP?
Risk factors for the development of NP can be broadly classified into factors that alter host defenses and factors that increase exposure to bacteria. In general, risk factors include hospitalization in an ICU, use of mechanical ventilation, surgery, and previous antimicrobial therapy. The latter increases the likelihood of developing pneumonia with highly virulent, antibiotic-resistant organisms. Additional risk factors for specific subgroups have also been identified, as follows:
- **Ventilated patients:**
  Age
  COPD
  Duration of hospitalization before mechanical ventilation
  Duration of mechanical ventilation
  Use of positive end-expiratory pressure

24-hour ventilator circuit changes
Reintubation
Nasal intubation
Sinusitis
Supine head positioning
Aspiration of gastric contents
Depressed consciousness
Multiorgan dysfunction
- **Surgical patients:**
    Long preoperative stay
    Long operative procedure
    Thoracoabdominal surgery
- **Trauma patients:**
    Emergency intubation
    Head trauma
    Use of nasogastric tubes
    Pulmonary contusion
    Pulmonary laceration

5. What are the noninvasive ways to diagnose NP?

The clinical diagnosis of NP is imprecise. Signs and symptoms such as fever, leukocytosis, purulent tracheobronchial secretions, and a new or progressive infiltrate on chest radiograph are nonspecific, especially in critically ill patients. Colonization of the upper airways with gram-negative rods often provides misleading information from cultures of sputum and endotracheal aspirate (ETA). Positive blood cultures may be helpful in patients with suspected VAP, although they are neither sensitive nor specific. Some investigators have advocated quantitative cultures and graded Gram stains of ETAs to consider the concentration of polymorphonuclear neutrophils (PMN), bacteria, and intracellular organisms and the presence of elastin fibers in correlation with quantitative bacterial colony counts. In intubated patients, noninvasive methods to sample distal airways include catheters that are blindly advanced into the distal airways via the ETT to obtain lower respiratory tract secretions by simple aspiration (unprotected suctioning of respiratory secretions), protected specimen brushing (PSB), or bronchoalveolar lavage. Bronchoalveolar lavage refers to the sequential instillation and aspiration of sterile, nonbacteriostatic saline into a lung subsegment. Compared with bronchoscopic sampling nonbronchoscopic sampling is less invasive, does not require a bronchoscopist, causes less compromise in gas exchange in patients on mechanical ventilation, and has a lower cost. Potential disadvantages include sampling errors intrinsic to a blind procedure and lack of airway visualization. Results from studies evaluating nonbronchoscopic techniques have frequently shown good diagnostic agreement with bronchoscopic methods.

6. What are some of the invasive methods to diagnose NP?

Percutaneous transtracheal aspiration has been used in the past to sample proximal airway secretions; however, this methods has fallen into disfavor because of the risk of serious complications. In addition, transthoracic needle aspiration to sample distal airway secretions has been shown to be insensitive and is seldom performed.

Open lung biopsy, the gold standard for diagnosing pneumonia, is rarely indicated and should be considered only for patients who are immunocompromised, have negative bronchoscopic findings, or need a rapid and specific diagnosis.

Bronchoscopy provides direct access to the lower airways for visual inspection and sampling of bronchial and parenchymal tissues. Simple bronchoscopic aspiration of distal airways is not used for microbiologic analysis, because bacteria collecting in the suction lumen of the bronchoscope as it is advanced through the upper airways significantly compromise the results of cultures. Bronchoalveolar lavage, more sensitive, and PSB, more specific, provide more accurate information regarding the cause of pneumonia. When combined, these two procedures complement each other. Protected bronchoalveolar lavage may improve the specificity of bronchoalveolar lavage sampling. Quantitative cultures are used to discriminate infections (high concentration) from contamination (low concentration). Significant thresholds for the diagnosis of pneumonia are bacterial colony counts of 10^3 or more on PSB and 10^4 or more on bronchoalveolar lavage. Patients receiving antibiotics may have colony counts that are below the diagnostic threshold, even in the presence of pneumonia. Microscopic analysis of bronchoalveolar lavage also can be helpful in the diagnosis of pneumonia. Bronchoalveolar lavage fluid should be analyzed for Gram stain, percentage of PMNs (% PMN), and percentage of inflammatory cells (PMNs and macrophages) containing intracellular organisms (ICOs). Pneumonia is likely if the Gram stain is positive, % PMN is more than 75%, or ICO is 2% or more.

7. What are the infectious and noninfectious causes of fever in patients receiving mechanical ventilation?

Infectious causes include pneumonia, nosocomial sinusitis, catheter-related infection, and urinary tract infection, which account for most nosocomial infections in medical ICUs. Invasion by a tube (endotracheal or nasogastric) or a catheter (central line or urinary) are major risk factors for development of these infections. Fever in patients receiving mechanical ventilation is frequently multifactorial, with more than one of the previously mentioned infections present simultaneously. Localized signs of infections are difficult to elicit, and the first manifestation of infection is often fever. Abdominal infections also should be suspected in postoperative patients; those with pancreatitis, gastrointestinal carcinoma, or bleeding; or those receiving high dose corticosteroids.

Extrapulmonary noninfectious sources of fever include pancreatitis, deep venous thrombosis, and drug fever. A frequent noninfectious source of fever in patients with ARDS is pulmonary fibroproliferation. The diagnosis is suspected in patients on mechanical ventilation for 7 or more days whose lung function fails to improve and who have no other source of fever identified.

8. List some noninfectious causes of pulmonary infiltrates that may mimic NP in hospitalized patients.

Pulmonary edema
Pulmonary hemorrhage
ARDS
Atelectasis
Pleural effusion
Pulmonary embolus with and without infarction
Lung contusion
Chemical pneumonitis from aspiration
Infiltrative tumor
Radiation pneumonitis

In intubated patients, noninfectious causes of pulmonary densities can coexist with an extrapulmonary source of fever, thereby simulating pneumonia.

9. Identify the most common organisms responsible for NP and the specific risk factors associated with each pathogen.

In noncritically ill patients who develop NP and who have no specific risk factors or comorbid diseases, the most likely pathogens are *Staphylococcus aureus, Klebsiella* spp, *Enterobacteriaceae* spp., *E. coli, Proteus* spp., and *Serratia marcescens*. In addition to these organisms, patients with severe pneumonia who require admission to the ICU or who need mechanical ventilation are also at risk for *Pseudomonas aeruginosa* infection. Additional risk factors for pneumonia caused by *Pseudomonas* spp. include prolonged hospitalization, prior use of antibiotics, and sepsis. Risk factors that increase the likelihood of *Staphylococcus aureus* include coma, head injury, diabetes, renal failure, and recent influenza. Gross aspiration of acid gastric contents, especially in patients with poor dental hygiene, and recent thoracoabdominal surgery are risk factors for anaerobes. Anaerobes are uncommon pathogens in VAP; however, polymicrobial pneumonia occurs in 40% of VAP cases.

10. Name some of the atypical or unusual pathogens that cause NP.

Legionella spp. are known to cause NP. These pathogens are seen most often in patients on corticosteroids or cytotoxic chemotherapy. Patients treated previously with antibiotics who do not have an altered state of consciousness are also at increased risk. *Aspergillus* spp. are most often seen in patients treated previously with antibiotics, patients receiving corticosteroids, and patients with COPD. Viral NP may present with a clinical picture similar to that of bacterial pneumonia; as a result, the incidence is probably underestimated. The likelihood of viral pneumonia is increased in patients who fail to respond to therapy, during winter months, and when there is evidence of a viral outbreak in the hospital or community. Common viral pathogens include influenza viruses A and B and respiratory syncytial virus. Other less common viral pathogens are adenovirus, parainfluenza virus, varicella zoster virus, herpes simplex virus, cytomegalovirus, and measles virus.

11. What are appropriate empiric antibiotic regimens for NP?

For patients with mild to moderate illness and no specific risk factors or comorbid diseases, there are several therapeutic options ("standard therapy"). These options include a first-generation cephalosporin plus an aminoglycoside, a second-generation cephalosporin alone, a third-generation nonpseudomonal cephalosporin alone, a β-lactam/β-lactamase inhibitor alone, or a fluoroquinolone alone.

In patients with mild to moderate illness and specific risk factors, antibiotic therapy must be adjusted to the risk factor(s). In patients with risk factors for *Staphylococcus aureus*, vancomycin (if methicillin-resistant *Staphylococcus aureus* is suspected) should be initiated with one of the therapeutic options listed above. In patients on high-dose corticosteroids—a risk factor for *Legionella* spp.—a macrolide should be started in addition to standard therapy. In patients at risk for anaerobic infection, clindamycin or metronidazole should be started with standard therapy. Alternatively, monotherapy with a β-lactam/β-lactamase inhibitor also provides adequate coverage. In patients with severe pneumonia or other risk factors for *Pseudomonas* spp., combination therapy with two antipseudomonal antibiotics should be initiated.

12. What are the advantages of monotherapy compared with those of combination therapy?

Monotherapy minimizes antibiotic exposure and toxicities, simplifies therapy, and reduces costs. Monotherapy is adequate for most gram-positive infections except those caused by enterococci. Monotherapy in infections with gram-negative rods may be adequate in nonpseudomonal infections and in patients with mild to moderate disease.

Combination therapy has the advantages of synergy; it prevents resistance in infections with pathogens such as *Pseudomonas* and *Enterobacter* spp. and broadens coverage, because many NPs are polymicrobial. Combination therapy should be used in all pseudomonal infections and for patients with severe pneumonia who are critically ill, especially those on mechanical ventilation. Combination therapy may be necessary for nosocomial aspiration pneumonia.

13. Explain why some patients may deteriorate clinically after antibiotics are initiated.

Antibiotics kill bacteria through several different mechanisms. One is lysis of the bacterial cell wall. Lysis can result in enhanced release of endotoxin. In addition, bacterial cell wall products interact with cytokine-producing cells to promote the release of inflammatory mediators. Clinically, this can lead to the development of systemic inflammatory response syndrome and shock. Antibiotics that lyse bacterial cell walls, are bactericidal, and kill at a slower rate are more likely to produce this effect. β-Lactam antibiotics are a prime example.

14. What causes treatment failure in patients with NP?

Treatment failure of NP can result from persistence of the original organism, superinfection with a different organism, infection with an unusual pathogen, or a noninfectious cause that clinically mimics failure to respond. Persistence of the original organism may result from unrecognized resistance to initial antibiotics; development of secondary resistance during therapy (especially if monotherapy was used); and suboptimal antibiotic therapy, including wrong antibiotics, wrong combination of antibiotics, wrong dosing of antibiotics, and use of antibiotics that poorly penetrate the lungs. In addition, anatomic problems (e.g., lung abscess or empyema), poor host defenses, and infection with highly virulent organisms can result in persistent infection. Superinfection occurs in approximately 12–15% of VAPs and increases the mortality rate. Unusual pathogens such as tuberculosis, viruses, or fungi do not respond to conventional antibiotic therapy, which results in treatment failure. Apparent failure to respond clinically also may result from noninfectious causes of fever or failure to identify a concomitant extrapulmonary infection that is resistant to the administered antibiotic regimen or requires concomitant drainage.

15. How should treatment failure be approached?

Current antibiotics should be stopped, if possible, and respiratory secretions, preferably obtained by bronchoalveolar lavage and PSB, should be cultured. Potential anatomic problems should be evaluated by CT scan of the chest. An aggressive search for nonpulmonary infections should be started, with particular attention directed to the sinuses, central lines, and abdomen. Noninfectious causes of fever also should be considered. Open-lung biopsy should be done in selected patients.

16. How can NP be prevented?

Few studies regarding the prevention of NP and VAP have been designed to rigorously evaluate potential strategies. Therefore, no proven method exists, and many prophylactic strategies remain controversial. Current generally accepted recommendations include:

Infection control and surveillance

Hand washing

Isolation of patients with resistant organisms

Enteral feedings (rather than total parenteral nutrition)

Avoidance of large gastric residuals (consider using jejunal feedings)

Semierect positioning

Careful handling of respiratory therapy equipment

Lateral rotational therapy

Avoidance of unnecessary empiric antibiotics

Continuous subglottic suctioning has been evaluated and proved to decrease significantly the incidence of VAP, although its use is not widespread. Prophylactic topical tracheobronchial antibiotics and selective digestive decontamination decrease the incidence of pneumonia, but do not decrease mortality. Furthermore, they may increase antibiotic resistance, so they are not recommended for routine use in unselected populations.

BIBLIOGRAPHY

1. Centers for Disease Control and Prevention: Guidelines for prevention of nosocomial pneumonia. Respir Care 39:1191–1236, 1994.
2. Estes R, Meduri GU: Pathogenesis of ventilator-associated pneumonia: Mechanisms of bacterial colonization and airway inoculation. Intensive Care Med 21:365–383, 1995.
3. Griffin J, Meduri GU: Diagnosis of nosocomial pneumonia: New approaches. Med Clin North Am 5:1091–1122, 1994.
4. Kim JH, Galis HA: Observations on spiralling empiricism: Its cause, allure, and perils, with particular attention to antibiotic therapy. Am J Med 87:201–206, 1989.
5. Meduri GU, Eltorky M, Winer-Muram HT: Fibroproliferative phase of late ARDS. Semin Respir Infect 10:152–173, 1995.
6. Meduri GU, Maudlin GL, Wunderink RG, et al: Cases of fever and pulmonary densities in patients with clinical manifestations of ventilator-associated pneumonia. Chest 106:221–235, 1994.
7. Niederman M: An approach to empiric therapy of nosocomial pneumonia. Med Clin North Am 78:1123–1141, 1994.
8. Wunderink RG: Ventilator-associated pneumonia. Failure to respond to antibiotic therapy. Clin Chest Med 16:173–193, 1995.

27. ASPIRATION SYNDROMES

C. Hewitt McCuller, Jr., M.D., and G. Douglas Campbell, Jr., M.D.

1. What are aspiration syndromes?

Aspiration syndromes refer to the clinical and pathophysiologic effects caused by the physical introduction of foreign objects or substances into the lower respiratory tract. Aspiration syndromes may be classified according to the type of substance that enters the airways: solid materials; liquids, which may be inert (water, mineral oil) or caustic (gastric acid, hydrocarbons); or alimentary secretions, which are usually contaminated with pathogenic organisms. Aspirated materials may consist of a combination of these substances. The inflammatory response that occurs in the lungs after aspiration injury is referred to as *aspiration pneumonitis*, which results from chemical injury to lung tissue. The term *aspiration pneumonia* refers to an infectious process of the lung parenchyma resulting from introduction of pathogenic organisms into the lower respiratory tract. The two terms are often used interchangeably, but they are not necessarily synonymous.

2. What are the major risk factors for aspiration?

Aspiration into the lower respiratory tract can result from any impairment of the swallowing mechanism or lower respiratory tract defenses (e.g., cough reflex, mucociliary clearance) as well as altered consciousness, neuromuscular diseases, gastrointestinal diseases, and mechanical factors.

Risk Factors for Aspiration

Altered levels of consciousness
  Decreased gastroesophageal tone
    General anesthesia
    Narcotic and sedative drugs
  Abnormal glottic closure
    Anesthetic induction or postanesthetic recovery
    Postextubation
    Drug overdose and ethanol toxicity
    Structural lesions of the CNS (tumors,
      cerebrovascular accident, head trauma)
    Metabolic encephalopathies (electrolyte
      imbalances, liver failure, uremia, sepsis)
    Hypoxia and hypercapnia
    CNS infections
    Seizures
Gastrointestinal diseases
  Decreased gastroesophageal tone
    Alkaline gastric pH
    Gastrointestinal tract dysmotility
    Esophagitis (infectious, postradiation)
  Incompetent gastroesophageal junction
    Hiatal hernia
    Scleroderma
    Esophageal motility disorders (achalasia,
      megaesophagus)
    Tracheoesophageal fistula
  Elevated intragastric pressure or volume
    Ascites
    Gastrointestinal bleeding
    Malignancy of gastrointestinal tract
    Intestinal obstruction or ileus

Neuromuscular diseases
  Abnormal glottic closure
    Guillain-Barré syndrome
    Botulism
    Muscular dystrophy
    Parkinson's disease
    Polymyositis
    Amyotophic lateral sclerosis
    Multiple sclerosis
    Myasthenia gravis
    Poliomyelitis
Mechanical factors
  Incompetent gastroesophageal junction
    Nasogastric or enteral feeding tubes
    Upper endoscopy
  Abnormal glottic closure
    Emergency and routine airway manipulation
    Surgery to the neck and pharynx
    Trauma to the neck and pharynx
    Tumors of the upper airway
    Tracheostomy
    Endotracheal tube
Other factors
  Incompetent gastroesophageal junction (elderly)
  Elevated intragastric pressure or volume
    Diabetes (functional gastric outlet
      obstruction)
    Obesity
    Pregnancy
    Lack of molar teeth (young children)

CNS = central nervous system.

3. What factors affect pathogenesis and prognosis after the aspiration of gastric contents?

The severity of injury that occurs after gastric aspiration is directly related to the pH, volume, and particulate nature of the aspirate. An aspirate with a low pH (2.5 or less) and large volume (0.4 ml/kg or more) containing large particles has the worst prognosis, but aspiration of gastric contents at a more alkaline pH (more than 5) can also cause severe pulmonary inflammation and dysfunction, especially if particulate matter is suspended in the fluid. Clinical indicators of a less favorable prognosis may include the presence of shock, pulmonary infiltrates that encompass more than two lobes on a chest radiograph, the onset of ARDS, or secondary infection.

4. Describe the clinical findings that occur in patients with noninfectious aspiration syndromes.

The initial symptoms of foreign body aspiration vary according to the size of the aspirated object. Larger objects, such as poorly chewed food, can lodge in the larynx or trachea, leading to respiratory distress, aphonia, cyanosis, loss of consciousness, and sudden death (the "cafe coronary"). With partial tracheal obstruction, inspiratory and expiratory stridor may be present, but as the object moves distally, inspiratory stridor becomes less prominent compared with expiratory wheezing. Impaction of a foreign body in a main stem bronchus may lead to unilateral wheezing because of turbulence in both airways as well as reflex bronchospasm. Lobar or segmental impaction can result in asymmetric breath sounds, localized wheezing, or diminished air entry. Smaller objects can descend farther into the tracheobronchial tree and cause bronchial irritation, resulting in cough followed by varying degrees of dyspnea, chest pain, wheezing, fever, nausea, or vomiting. Areas of diminished breath sounds may be noted when an obstructing foreign body results in atelectasis.

Aspiration of gastric acid usually results in profound hypoxemia because of ventilation-perfusion mismatching and intrapulmonary shunt. Initially this may be due to closure of small airways and atelectasis resulting from loss of surfactant, which can be destroyed by acid or inactivated by plasma proteins. Pulmonary capillary leak and permeability edema also occur, worsening the shunt. Clinically, these changes are usually accompanied by a dramatic picture that includes the presence of gastric contents in the oropharynx, wheezing, coughing, cyanosis, fever, hypoxemia, and sometimes shock. Patients may then progress in one of three ways: (1) rapid improvement within 1 week, (2) rapid death from progressive respiratory failure, or (3) initial improvement within 1 week followed by deterioration and development of ARDS or secondary bacterial infection.

5. What are the typical radiographic findings of aspiration syndromes?

Foreign body aspiration may show several patterns of radiographic abnormalities that depend on the type of object aspirated. Typically, the more dependent areas of the lungs are involved, such as the lower lobes in the upright position, or the posterior segment of the upper lobes and the superior segment of the lower lobes when the subject is supine. In adults, aspiration more frequently involves the right side because of the acute angle of the left main stem bronchus. In children up to about age 15, the frequency of left-sided aspiration almost equals that of right sided aspiration because of bronchial symmetry. Radiopaque objects can sometimes be visualized on plain films, with or without atelectasis of the involved area. Obstruction of segmental or larger airways may lead to lobar or, more rarely, complete lung collapse. Inspiratory films may show no abnormalities, whereas expiratory films reveal air trapping on the involved side, which is demonstrated by contralateral shift of the mediastinum.

The **aspiration of large amounts of acidic material** (gastric aspiration) usually leads to general involvement of both lungs by patchy air space consolidation. The distribution is commonly bilateral and multicentric but usually favors perihilar or basal regions. Three basic patterns of disease may be seen: (1) extensive bilateral air space consolidation (confluent acinar opacities), (2) widespread but fairly discrete acinar shadows, and (3) irregular opacities that do not fit into either of these categories. This latter presentation is the most common pattern and is reported to occur in more than 40% of all cases. Radiographic findings tend to worsen initially, but usually resolve fairly rapidly. Worsening of the radiographic abnormalities after initial improvement is associated with the development of bacterial pneumonia, ARDS, or pulmonary embolism, and requires further investigation.

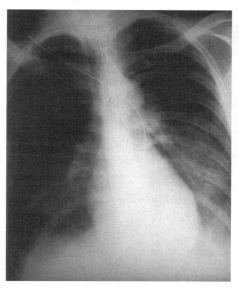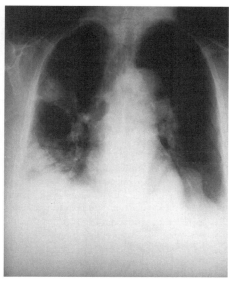

Both of these chest radiographs demonstrate basilar infiltrates; multicentric and perihilar involvement is seen on the *right*.

6. How are noninfectious aspiration syndromes treated?

Complete airway obstruction caused by foreign body aspiration must be relieved immediately. In the United States, obstruction is usually relieved by the Heimlich maneuver (subdiaphragmatic abdominal thrusts), whereas the Canadian Heart Foundation recommends a combination of abdominal thrusts and back blows. If the foreign body remains in the lower respiratory tract, the airway should be stabilized, which may require endotracheal intubation. Depending on the size of the foreign body, rigid or fiberoptic bronchoscopy should be performed to remove the object. Thoracotomy may be necessary in rare instances when bronchoscopy is unsuccessful.

In patients with massive gastric aspiration, initial therapy involves establishing and maintaining adequate oxygenation. Patients usually require intubation and mechanical ventilation with the application of positive end-expiratory pressure (PEEP) because of aspiration pneumonitis with resulting noncardiogenic pulmonary edema and an intrapulmonary shunt. In severe cases, bronchoscopy may be helpful if there is particulate matter blocking the airways, but large-volume lavage is of little benefit in minimizing the effects of gastric acid since the acid is dispersed and neutralized very rapidly.

7. Do systemic corticosteroids have a role in the treatment of aspiration syndromes?

Studies in animals and humans have shown inconsistent results regarding the benefit of corticosteroids given either before aspiration or after aspiration has already occurred. Corticosteroids predispose patients to infection and can cause fluid and electrolyte imbalance. Considering the potential risks and unproven benefit of corticosteroids in this clinical setting, their use is not recommended either parenterally or via the airway in the treatment of aspiration pneumonitis.

8. Are prophylactic antibiotics indicated in aspiration?

The routine use of prophylactic antibiotics following a witnessed aspiration is not recommended because of the risk of selecting for antibiotic-resistant organisms. Unfortunately, the clinical manifestations of secondary bacterial infection can be confused with those of chemical injury to the lung tissue. After all aspiration events, the patient should be closely observed. If clinical evidence compatible with pneumonia (i.e., new infiltrate, fever, leukocytosis) is noted, empiric antibiotics, based upon the most likely spectrum of pathogens, should be initiated for 24–48 hours and the patient closely observed. Antibiotics should be discontinued if improvement is noted in less than 24–48 hours. Clinical worsening should prompt broadening of antibiotic coverage, with strong consideration given to obtaining respiratory secretions by bronchoscopy or tracheal suctioning for microbiologic evaluation.

9. What are the infectious complications of aspiration syndromes?

Infectious complications of aspiration syndromes may present as either an acute or a chronic process. Acutely, aspiration pneumonia may be a primary event, with clinical manifestations noted within the first 24–48 hours. Although primary pneumonia is noted in only 23–30% of all cases of aspiration, its occurrence is associated with increased morbidity and mortality. The onset of aspiration pneumonia is frequently heralded by fever, leukocytosis, and development of pulmonary infiltrates; unfortunately, these findings may also occur in noninfectious aspiration pneumonitis. Many patients show initial improvement after aspiration, only to develop pneumonia 2–7 days later. These secondary pneumonias are the result of obstruction or inflammation in the lower respiratory tract that impairs the patient's host defenses. The risk of secondary infection is also increased by mechanical ventilation, hospitalization for more than 5 days, or use of H_2 blockers.

Occasionally, aspiration pneumonia presents as a chronic indolent infection. In this setting, a lung abscess may have developed. This presentation is more likely to occur in patients with particular risk factors including swallowing dysfunction, gastroesophageal reflux, poor dentition, alcoholism, and seizure activity. Lung abscesses may frequently present with fever and nonspecific findings, typically of 3 or more weeks' duration. The chest radiograph often reveals a rounded area of consolidation with or without an air-fluid level but may occasionally reveal patchy infiltrates, or even interstitial changes.

10. What pathogens cause aspiration pneumonia?

The cause of aspiration pneumonia is frequently polymicrobial, reflecting the spectrum of pathogens present in the oropharynx. The setting in which aspiration occurred (community, hospital, nursing home), recent exposure to antibiotics, and the presence of dental caries or gingival disease alter the oropharyngeal flora and the causative pathogens of aspiration pneumonia. In aspiration pneumonia occurring in the community setting, the most frequent pathogens are the aerobes *Staphylococcus aureus* and *Streptococcus pneumoniae* and anaerobic organisms such as *Bacteroides* spp., *Peptostreptococcus* spp., *Fusobacterium nucleatum*, and *Prevotella* spp. Although the same spectrum of anaerobic organisms is frequently seen in aspiration pneumonia occurring in the hospital, the spectrum of aerobic pathogens differs, especially if the patient has been hospitalized for more than 4 days, has received prior antibiotics, or is receiving mechanical ventilation. *S. aureus* (which may be methicillin resistant), enteric gram-negative bacilli (i.e., *Escherichia coli, Klebsiella* spp., *Proteus* spp.), and *Pseudomonas aeruginosa* are frequently isolated in this setting.

11. How are the infectious complications of aspiration syndrome treated?

Selection of antimicrobial agents is affected by the probable spectrum of pathogens and the likelihood of antibiotic-resistant organisms. With aspiration pneumonia occurring in the community setting, high-dose penicillin has traditionally been the drug of choice, but the presence of penicillin-resistant organisms, such as *Bacteroides* spp. and *Strep. pneumoniae*, has resulted in the increased use of clindamycin. Additionally, in one study comparing these two agents, clindamycin was reported to be more effective in resolving fever and sputum production and was associated with a lower failure rate. Aspiration in the hospital setting is more likely to involve gram-negative bacilli or *S. aureus* as well as anaerobic organisms. Empiric antibiotic therapy, in the past, has often included the use of third-generation cephalosporins. With the growing emergence of resistant organisms, however, alternative therapies (e.g., imipenem, piperacillin-tazobactam, or fluoroquinolones combined with clindamycin) are increasingly being used.

Lung abscesses usually require a prolonged course of antibiotics; when this is unsuccessful, percutaneous drainage or lobectomy may be needed. Empyemas typically require either drainage through closed thoracostomy tubes or open surgical drainage, with or without decortication.

12. How can aspiration and some of its consequences be prevented?

Aspiration of foreign bodies is the leading cause of accidental death in the home for children less than 1 year of age. Careful attention to the consistency of food, especially in very young children, as well as avoidance of small objects that could be aspirated into the tracheobronchial tree can help to prevent this problem. Adults, especially those with predisposing factors such as old age, poor nutrition, alcohol consumption, sedative drugs, and institutionalization, are at increased risk for foreign body aspiration. Correction of underlying problems where possible and attention to the consistency of food may reduce the risk of foreign body aspiration.

Small volume liquid aspiration may be prevented by elevation of the head of the bed to 30–45° in patients with swallowing disorders or gastroesophageal reflux who are at especially high risk for aspiration. Correction of reversible risk factors such as treatment of seizures, careful titration of pain medications and sedation, judicious use of nasoenteric tubes, and careful monitoring of gastric volume with nasoenteric feedings should reduce the risk of aspiration. In patients requiring long-term feeding, surgical interventions such as gastrostomy or enterostomy, often combined with an antireflux procedure such as a Nissen fundiplication, should be considered; however, many patients may still have problems with aspiration after simple gastrostomy.

Prevention may have its greatest role in massive gastric aspiration, as supportive care has not influenced overall overcome. Attention should be given to defining patients at risk. Other factors to be considered are the volume, pH, and the presence of particulate matter in the gastric contents. Patients undergoing surgery are at a significant risk, particularly at the time of anesthetic induction, especially for emergency procedures. Fasting for approximately 8–12 hours before surgery may decrease gastric volume and the amount of particulate matter and increase gastric pH. Many fasting patients, however, still have gastric volumes greater than 25 ml as well as a pH of 2.5 or less in gastric secretions. Preoperative therapy with antacids may raise gastric pH, but this benefit may be offset by the increase of gastric volume due to the antacids. H_2 antagonists such as cimetidine and ranitidine raise gastric pH and reduce gastric volume. Metoclopramide, an agent that increases gastroesophageal sphincter tone and increases antral motility and gastric emptying, is often added to further decrease gastric volume and increase gastric pH. At the time of intubation, rapid sequence induction of anesthesia will shorten the period between loss of consciousness and tracheal intubation. The application of cricoid pressure (Sellick's maneuver) during intubation may decrease the risk of aspiration. Premature postoperative extubation should be avoided because of the prolonged laryngeal incompetence that occurs after anesthesia. Obtunded patients at risk for large volume aspiration should be closely observed and placed in the head-down lateral position to reduce the volume of material aspirated in the event of aspiration.

BIBLIOGRAPHY

1. Bartlett JG: Anaerobic bacterial infections of the lung and pleural space. Clin Infect Dis 4(Suppl 16):S248, 1993.
2. Britto J, Demling RH: Aspiration lung injury. New Horizons 1:435, 1993.
3. Bynum LJ, Pierce AK: Pulmonary aspiration of gastric contents. Am Rev Respir Dis 114:1129, 1976.
4. Conrad SA, Jayr C, Peper EA: Thoracic trauma, surgery, and perioperative management. In George RB, Light RW, Matthay MA, et al (eds): Chest Medicine: Essentials of Pulmonary and Critical Care Medicine, 3rd ed. Baltimore, Williams & Wilkins, 1995, p 629.
5. DePaso WJ: Aspiration pneumonia. Clin Chest Med 12:269, 1991.
6. Downs JB, Chapman RL Jr, Modell JH, et al: An evaluation of steroid therapy in aspiration pneumonitis. Anesthesiology 40:129, 1974.
7. Dudley WR, Marshall BE: Steroid treatment for acid aspiration pneumonitis. Anesthesiology 40:136, 1974.

8. Hamelberg W, Bosomworth PP: Aspiration pneumonitis: Experimental studies and clinical observations. Anesth Analg 43:669, 1964.
9. Landay MJ, Christensen EE, Bynum LJ: Pulmonary manifestations of acute aspiration of gastric contents. AJR 131:587, 1978.
10. Levison ME, Mangura CT, Lorber B, et al: Clindamycin compared with penicillin for the treatment of anaerobic lung abscess. Ann Intern Med 98:466, 1983.
11. Limper AH, Prakash UBS: Tracheobronchial foreign bodies in adults. Ann Intern Med 112:604, 1990.
12. Niederman MS, Sarosi GA: Respiratory tract infections. In George RB, Light RW, Matthay MA, et al (eds): Chest Medicine: Essentials of Pulmonary and Critical Care Medicine, 3rd ed. Baltimore, Williams & Wilkins, 1995, p 423.
13. Pulmonary Disease Caused by Aspiration of Solid Foreign Materials and Liquids. In Diagnosis of Diseases of the Chest, 3rd ed. Philadelphia, W.B. Saunders, 1990, p 2382.
14. Schwartz DJ, Wynne JW, Gibbs CP, et al: The pulmonary consequences of aspiration of gastric contents at pH values greater than 2.5. Am Rev Respir Dis 121:119, 1980.
15. Tietjen PA, Kaner RJ, Quinn CE: Aspiration emergencies. Clin Chest Med 15:117, 1994.
16. Zucker AR, Sznajder JI: Aspiration syndromes. In Hall JB, Schmidt GA, Wood LH (eds): Principles of Critical Care. New York, McGraw-Hill, 1992, p 1727.

28. FUNGAL PNEUMONIA

Carol A. Kauffman, M.D., and Joseph P. Lynch, III, M.D.

ASPERGILLOSIS

1. What is the appropriate treatment for aspergillosis?

High dose amphotericin B (AmB), 1.0 to 1.5 mg per kg per day to a usual total dose of 2.0 gm, is the mainstay of therapy for severe, life-threatening aspergillosis. Oral itraconazole (200 mg twice daily) can be substituted for AmB after an initial favorable response. Surgical resection or debridement of necrotic or cavitary lesions may be critical as adjunctive therapy when the disease is localized (e.g., single pulmonary cavity, sinusitis, skin, bone). Itraconazole may be adequate as initial therapy for localized aspergillosis not involving the central nervous system. Itraconazole may also be used in patients failing or experiencing side effects from AmB. High doses (600 to 800 mg/day) have been recommended for central nervous system involvement. Itraconazole should be continued for at least 6–12 months, as earlier discontinuation of therapy has been associated with a high rate of relapse. A lipid formulation of AmB has recently been approved for use in patients with aspergillosis who have serious adverse effects from AmB. For fulminant aspergillosis, some investigators advocate combining flucytosine or rifampin with AmB to confer synergy. The benefit of combination therapy has not been established. Flucytosine has potential marrow toxicity and may be contraindicated in patients with limited marrow reserve. Even with aggressive antifungal therapy, mortality of aggressive aspergillosis is high (more than 70%) among patients with hematologic malignancies in relapse, bone marrow transplant, or AIDS. Mortality rates of less than 20% have been noted when the disease is localized, treatment is initiated early (within 2–4 days of onset of symptoms), underlying disease is controlled, and immune function is restored.

2. What is the role of skin or blood tests in diagnosis of invasive aspergillosis?

Skin or blood tests are of no practical value in diagnosing invasive aspergillosis. Immunodiffusion or counterimmunoelectrophoretic (CIE) techniques to detect *Aspergillus* antigens are of no clinical value. Enzyme-linked immunosorbent assays (ELISA) demonstrating Aspergillus antigen in serum or bronchoalveolar lavage (BAL) fluid are promising but not commercially available.

3. How is allergic bronchopulmonary aspergillosis diagnosed? Describe its clinical manifestations and treatment.

Both skin and blood tests may be helpful in diagnosing allergic bronchopulmonary aspergillosis (ABPA), a hypersensitivity response to *Aspergillus* spp. Clinical manifestations of ABPA include asthma, blood and tissue eosinophilia, pulmonary infiltrates, and striking elevations in levels of serum immunoglobulin E (IgE) and IgG. Both total (nonspecific) IgE and IgE antibodies directed against *A. fumigatus* are characteristic. Skin tests may allow a prompt presumptive diagnosis of ABPA. In patients with ABPA, intradermal challenge with *Aspergillus* antigen results in an immediate acute wheal and flare response (within 15–30 minutes); induration and edema at the site of inoculation usually occur 3–6 hours later. Corticosteroids (to ablate the exaggerated hypersensitivity response) are the mainstay of therapy for ABPA. Specific antimycotic therapy is not required. Favorable responses to oral itraconazole have been described. However, the course of ABPA is typically measured in years. Given the expense associated with long-term itraconazole therapy, additional long-term studies assessing outcome are required before endorsing this modality.

4. What is the significance of *Aspergillus* spp. in the sputum?

Recovery of *Aspergillus* spp. from sputum or lower respiratory tract secretions is common, particularly in patients who have received antimicrobial drugs. Isolation may reflect colonization, contamination (since *Aspergillus* spp. are ubiquitous in the environment), or invasive infection. The significance of positive cultures needs to take into account the presence or absence of risk factors for invasive pulmonary aspergillosis (IPA). Primary risk factors for IPA include severe and sustained granulocytopenia, organ transplantation, hematologic malignancy, and corticosteroid or immunosuppressive therapy. In patients with one or more of these risk factors, repetitive isolation of *Aspergillus* spp. in respiratory secretions usually reflects tissue invasion and warrants specific antifungal therapy or more aggressive diagnostic studies. Isolation of *Aspergillus* spp. in a single specimen in severely immunocompromised patients is associated with IPA in 20–40% of cases. Substantiating the diagnosis of IPA may be difficult, as sputum cultures have been positive in only 15–78% of patients with IPA in various series. Yields of bronchoscopic cultures (brushings, washings, BAL) have ranged from 40–80%. The detection of hyphae on sputum smears or in BAL fluid increases the likelihood of invasive infection. Clinical suspicion for IPA is heightened when hemoptysis; pleuritic chest pain; fever; or focal, wedge-shaped or nodular pulmonary infiltrates on chest radiographs are present. In view of the high mortality associated with IPA, an aggressive diagnostic and therapeutic approach is warranted even in asymptomatic patients who have positive cultures and recognized risk factors for IPA. In contrast, *Aspergillus* spp. frequently colonize the respiratory tract in patients with solid tumors or chronic pulmonary diseases but are rarely associated with invasive disease. Unless focal pneumonia or cavitary lesions are present, isolation of *Aspergillus* spp. in these less immunocompromised hosts does not require further evaluation or treatment.

5. What are the clinical features of mycetoma?

Mycetomas are chronic cavitary lesions that comprise a mass of fungal mycelia (typically *Aspergillus* spp.) and occur within preexisting cavities in patients with chronic pulmonary disorders. Aspergillomas may complicate pulmonary disorders such as tuberculosis, sarcoidosis, histoplasmosis, bronchial cysts, bronchiectasis, silicosis, or any chronic cavitary disease. Rarely, mycetomas develop subacutely in patients with hematologic malignancies and pulmonary aspergillosis. Mycetomas are not invasive infections; the fungi live in a saprophytic relationship with the host. Fungal mycelia grow into the walls of the cavities, but do not invade contiguous lung parenchyma or disseminate. Mycetomas are caused by *Aspergillus* spp. in more than 95% of cases; rarely mycetomas caused by Mucorales, *Candida* spp., and other fungi have been reported. Most mycetomas are asymptomatic and are discovered incidentally on chest radiographs. A rounded intracavitary mass, surrounded by a crescent of air, is characteristic. Mycetomas are predominantly located in the upper lobes. The mass may move when the patient changes position.

Ipsilateral pleural thickening is usually prominent and may antedate the development of the mycetoma. Serum precipitins against *Aspergillus* spp. (e.g., *A. fumigatus, A. niger,* or *A. flavus*) are positive in virtually all patients with aspergilloma. The natural history varies. The lesions usually grow slowly over years. Spontaneous regression has been noted in 7–10% of cases. Hemoptysis occurs in approximately 50% of patients at some time in the course of the disease. Fatal, exsanguinating hemorrhage is the most dreaded complication.

6. How is mycetoma treated?

Appropriate management of mycetoma is controversial. Treatment with intravenous AmB is ineffective; surgical resection is the only reliable cure. However, resection of mycetomas may be a formidable undertaking, since extensive pleural adhesions or parenchymal scarring is usually present. In addition, many patients with mycetomas have severe, debilitating pulmonary disease and may not tolerate a thoracotomy. Thus, surgery needs to be individualized. We believe surgical resection is reasonable for patients with mycetomas, severe hemoptysis, and no specific contraindications to surgery. Intravenous AmB or itraconazole should be given perioperatively to reduce surgical complications such as empyema or bronchopleural fistulas. Although medical therapy is rarely effective for mycetomas, anecdotal successes have been described after endobronchial or percutaneous instillation of AmB or AmB plus sodium iodide directly within the fungal cavity. Favorable responses have been cited with oral itraconazole (administered for a minimum of 6–12 months). Notwithstanding these favorable reports, medical therapy should be reserved for symptomatic patients who are not candidates for surgery.

BLASTOMYCOSIS

7. When should blastomycosis be treated and what drug should be used?

Except in rare circumstances when a patient is involved in an outbreak of blastomycosis and may have acute self-limited pulmonary blastomycosis, all patients with blastomycosis (pulmonary and other forms of infection) should be treated with an antifungal agent. Even one localized cutaneous lesion implies disseminated blastomycosis that requires therapy. The treatment of choice for non–life-threatening, nonmeningeal blastomycosis is itraconazole. Most patients respond to 200 mg daily. The dose should be increased to 200 mg twice daily for more severe infections or for patients failing to improve after receiving 200 mg daily for several weeks. Treatment should be continued until all lesions and pulmonary infiltrates have resolved. A minimum of 6 months of therapy is advised; patients with chronic cavitary pulmonary disease, chronic skin lesions, or osteoarticular disease should be treated for at least 12 months. Ketoconazole is also effective for the treatment of blastomycosis. The dosage required is 400 to 800 mg daily. At high doses (especially 800 mg daily), side effects are common and often lead to patient noncompliance. Fluconazole appears to be less effective than itraconazole or ketoconazole as therapy for blastomycosis. However, fluconazole (dose 800 mg daily) is a reasonable choice if side effects, drug-drug interactions, or poor absorption preclude use of itraconazole and ketoconazole. AmB remains the drug of choice for acute life-threatening pulmonary, meningeal, or disseminated blastomycosis. In these circumstances, a dose of 0.7–1.0 mg per kg per day is appropriate. After stabilization or improvement, itraconazole may be substituted for AmB.

8. Are skin and blood tests helpful in the diagnosis of blastomycosis?

Skin and blood testing are of little benefit in the diagnosis of blastomycosis. No skin test antigens are currently available. The standard serologic assays (e.g., complement fixation and immunodiffusion) are neither sensitive nor specific and should not be used. The Centers for Disease Control and Prevention provides an enzyme immunoassay that appears to be sensitive and specific for infection with *Blastomyces dermititidis*. This immunoassay may be useful in individual patients and in investigations of possible outbreaks. The diagnosis of blastomycosis is best made by histopathologic study (the organism has a distinctive appearance) and cultures from involved sites.

CANDIDIASIS

9. What is the significance of isolating *Candida* spp. in the sputum?

Isolation of *Candida* spp. in sputum or respiratory secretions almost always reflects colonization (particularly among patients who have received antibiotics) but rarely warrants additional diagnostic interventions and does not require specific therapy. Although primary pneumonia caused by *Candida* spp. is rare, even among immunocompromised hosts, it can occur in the context of disseminated candidiasis or in patients with profound, sustained impairment in host defenses (e.g, in patients with chronic granulomatous disease of childhood or in bone marrow transplant recipients with prolonged granulocytopenia). Repetitive isolation of *Candida* spp. in extremely debilitated patients with malignancies or impaired host defenses and pulmonary infiltrates refractory to broad-spectrum antibiotics should prompt a more aggressive diagnostic evaluation.

COCCIDIOIDOMYCOSIS

10. What is the most appropriate treatment for coccidioidomycosis?

Most patients with acute pulmonary coccidioidomycosis do not come to a physician's attention and do not require treatment with antifungal agents. Treatment is warranted for patients with persistent symptomatic pulmonary coccidioidomycosis, asymptomatic cavitary lesions on chest radiograph, or disseminated forms of the disease. Azole antifungal agents are extremely useful for treatment of non–life-threatening coccidioidomycosis. Ketoconazole, fluconazole, and itraconazole are all effective, but none has emerged as the clearly superior agent. Ketoconazole, the first azole used, is effective at doses of 400–800 mg daily. Side effects are common, especially at the higher dose. For some patients with difficult to treat disease, even higher dosages are required. The dosage of itraconazole and fluconazole used in most studies has been 400 mg daily; success rates have been similar. The choice of azole depends on side effects, absorption characteristics of the azole, drug-drug interactions, and cost. Life-threatening coccidioidomycosis mandates treatment with AmB, which is also frequently required in immunosuppressed patients (i.e., those with AIDS or organ transplant recipients), because these patient populations have a higher risk of dissemination and severe disease. The recommended dosage is 0.7–1.0 mg per kg per day. An oral azole may be substituted for AmB after the clinical condition improves. For meningeal coccidioidomycosis, fluconazole is the drug of choice. Fluconazole penetrates well into the cerebrospinal fluid and may obviate the need for intrathecal administration of AmB. Fluconazole must be continued for life, as the relapse rate for meningeal coccidioidomycosis is exceedingly high.

11. Do skin tests and serologic assays have a role in the diagnosis of coccidioidomycosis?

Two skin test antigens, coccidioidin and spherulin, are available. Skin tests are most beneficial in patients who are not from, but have recently traveled through, the endemic area and present with a clinical syndrome compatible with coccidioidomycosis. Although a positive skin test is not diagnostic of active infection, it raises the possibility of coccidioidomycosis and should prompt further work-up. Further, a negative skin test does not rule out active coccidioidomycosis, especially in immunocompromised hosts. Serologic assays are helpful in both diagnosis and assessment of prognosis. Complement fixation, immunodiffusion, and precipitin assays are available. These tests should be performed by laboratories with special expertise in fungal serologic assays (e.g., state health department laboratories or reference laboratories in endemic areas). For most cases of pulmonary or disseminated coccidioidomycosis, positive antibody titers play an adjunctive role in the diagnosis of infections because *Coccidioides immitis* is easily grown in the laboratory and the organism has a distinctive appearance in tissues. High antibody titers, especially combined with anergy to skin test antigens, usually portend a worse prognosis.

CRYPTOCOCCOSIS

12. What is the appropriate diagnostic evaluation for pulmonary cryptococcosis?

Pulmonary cryptococcosis may be difficult to diagnose because cultures and fungal smears of expectorated sputum are positive for *Cryptococcus neoformans* in less than 25% of patients. Data gleaned from immunocompromised hosts have shown that the diagnosis of pulmonary cryptococcosis can be substantiated by bronchoscopy in more than 90% of patients. Although transbronchial lung biopsies are infrequently diagnostic (less than 30% yield), cultures of BAL fluids are positive in 60–95% of patients. Cytologic studies of BAL fluid demonstrate the organism in 30–67% of cases. Recent studies have detected cryptococcal antigen (more than 1:8 titer) in BAL fluid in more than 90% of immunosuppressed patients with pulmonary cryptococcosis, even in patients without serum antigenemia. The latex agglutination assay for cryptococcal antigen is highly sensitive and may help in the prognosis of cryptococcosis.

Meningeal spread occurs in more than two thirds of patients with pulmonary cryptococcosis and may be asymptomatic. Because of the avidity of *C. neoformans* for the central nervous system (CNS) a lumbar puncture must be obtained in patients with pulmonary cryptococcosis to rule out meningeal involvement (even when no CNS symptoms are apparent). Cerebrospinal fluid (CSF) in cryptococcal meningitis characteristically has an elevated protein level, a decreased glucose level, and lymphocytic pleocytosis. However, CSF cell counts are usually normal in HIV-infected patients with cryptococcal meningitis. In AIDS patients with cryptococcal meningitis, India ink preparations are positive in 75–94% of patients; CSF antigenemia is present in more than 95%. Blood cultures are positive in more than 90% of AIDS patients with disseminated cryptococcosis, but cryptococcemia is infrequent among patients not infected with HIV who have localized pulmonary involvement.

13. What is the best treatment for cryptococcosis?

AmB combined with flucytosine is optimal therapy for cryptococcal meningitis both in patients with AIDS and patients not infected with HIV. When meningitis is present, AmB (0.7 mg/day) should be combined with flucytosine (100 mg/kg/day in four divided doses) for 2–6 weeks (or until improvement has been achieved and CSF cultures are negative). After an initial response, oral fluconazole (400 mg/day) may be substituted and continued for a minimum of 3–6 months. Severely immunocompromised patients at risk for late relapse should be maintained on low-dose fluconazole (200 mg/day) indefinitely. Although randomized trials have not been performed in patients with extrameningeal forms of cryptococcosis, we believe that this regimen is also appropriate for severe or disseminated cryptococcal infections. For localized pulmonary cryptococcosis in nonimmunocompromised patients, either AmB alone (total dose 1.5–2.0 g) or oral azoles may be used as primary therapy. Although data are limited, fluconazole (400 mg/day) or itraconazole (400 mg/day) is preferred for localized pulmonary cryptococcosis in immunocompetent hosts. These agents should not be used for severe infections or meningitis or in severely immunocompromised hosts. Higher doses of fluconazole (800 mg/day) may be effective as primary or salvage therapy in patients with severe cryptococcal meningitis. The combination of 5-flucytosine and fluconazole may be considered in lieu of AmB plus flucytosine in immunocompromised patients who do not have fulminant disease.

HISTOPLASMOSIS

14. When should histoplasmosis be treated?

Acute pulmonary histoplasmosis usually does not require treatment with an antifungal agent; however, patients who have severe or progressive pulmonary involvement after exposure to a point source of *Histoplasma capsulatum* ("epidemic histoplasmosis") should be treated. Treatment also is indicated for the following conditions:

Chronic cavitary pulmonary histoplasmosis (most affected patients have concomitant chronic obstructive pulmonary disease

Symptomatic acute disseminated histoplasmosis
Chronic progressive infection

15. What antifungal agent should be used for histoplasmosis?

Itraconazole is the preferred drug for non–life-threatening, nonmeningeal histoplasmosis. The usual dose is 200 mg daily. A dose of 200 mg twice daily may be required for the following conditions: (1) more severe disease, (2) concern about absorption of the drug, and (3) failure to respond to 200 mg daily after several weeks. Most patients with acute pulmonary or disseminated infection can be treated for a total of 6 months. Treatment should be prolonged (for 12 months or more) for patients who respond slowly to therapy. Chronic progressive disseminated infection and chronic cavitary pulmonary disease require a minimum of 12 months of therapy.

Ketoconazole is also effective for histoplasmosis. The usual dose is 400 mg per day, but 800 mg may be required in some patients. Ketoconazole is less expensive than itraconazole but is associated with more side effects. Fluconazole (800 mg daily) is modestly effective for histoplasmosis and should be reserved for patients unable or unwilling to take itraconazole or ketoconazole. AmB, approximately 0.7 gm per kg per day, is the initial treatment for life-threatening infection (especially in immunosuppressed patients). After improvement or stabilization, the patient usually can be switched to an oral azole. Histoplasmosis is a common infection in AIDS patients. Itraconazole, 200 mg twice daily, is effective for acute treatment in patients with mild to moderate disease and for lifelong maintenance therapy. AmB should be initial therapy for severe infections in AIDS patients, at least until clinical improvement is evident.

16. Do skin tests and serologic assays have a role in the diagnosis of histoplasmosis?

Skin testing with *Histoplasma* antigens is not useful in the diagnosis of histoplasmosis (except in rare circumstances) and may raise antibody titers, leading to confusion in the diagnosis. Serologic assays can be useful in diagnosing certain types of infection. Both complement fixation (CF) and immunodiffusion assays are available. Tests should be performed by laboratories proficient in fungal serologic assays. Serologic tests are most useful in patients with acute and chronic pulmonary histoplasmosis. A fourfold rise in CF titer or development of an M band in the immunodiffusion test in a patient with an acute pulmonary syndrome and a possible environmental exposure is strong evidence for acute histoplasmosis. In chronic cavitary pulmonary histoplasmosis, high titers (more than 1:32) of CF antibodies, an M band, or H and M bands in a patient with the appropriate clinical and roentgenographic picture is strong evidence for infection with *H. capsulatum*. Growth of the organism on culture is definitive but is not always possible in laboratories not familiar with *H. capsulatum*. Serologic tests may be helpful in disseminated infections, but histopathology is more sensitive and results are immediately available. For patients with disseminated infection (especially AIDS patients who have a large burden of organisms), detection of *Histoplasma* antigen by a commercially available radioimmunoassay is a sensitive and specific test.

MUCORMYCOSIS

17. Describe the clinical presentation of mucormycosis. How is it diagnosed?

Mucormycosis is an invasive infection caused by nonseptated fungi belonging to the order Mucorales (e.g., *Mucor, Rhizopus, Absidia, Cunninghamella*). Mucormycosis is rare and is confined to patients with severe impairments in host defenses. Risk factors for invasive mucormycosis include granulocytopenia, high-dose corticosteroid or immunosuppressive therapy, hematologic malignancies, diabetes mellitus with ketoacidosis, and the use of the iron chelator deferoxamine. Burns and surgical wounds may be risk factors for local or cutaneous mucormycosis. Clinical forms of mucormycosis include rhinocerebral, pulmonary, gastrointestinal, cutaneous (secondary to inoculation or hematogenous dissemination), and disseminated. *Mucorales* organisms have a predilection for invading blood vessels; hemoptysis is a well-recognized complication of pulmonary mucormycosis. It may be difficult to diagnose mucormycosis because antemortem cultures are positive in only 10–40% of cases. Isolation of *Rhizopus* spp. or *Mucor* spp.

in even a single culture requires therapy in the appropriate clinical setting. Black, necrotic debris overlying ulcers or sites of necrosis may be a clue to the diagnosis. Histologic examination is essential to rapidly substantiate the diagnosis of mucormycosis. Fungi of the order *mucorales* have broad, nonseptated hyphae that branch at right angles. Mucormycosis is highly lethal (mortality rates exceed 80% with invasive pulmonary or disseminated forms).

18. What is the best treatment for mucormycosis?

Invasive mucormycosis should be treated with high dose AmB (1.0 to 1.5 mg/kg/day to a minimum total dose of 2.0 g) combined with surgical resection or debridement of involved tissue. Control of the underlying disease or reduction in the level of immunosuppression is critical to optimize outcome. Oral antifungals have no activity against Mucorales.

DIAGNOSTIC AND TREATMENT PEARLS

19. What fungus causes pulmonary infiltrates that mimic those of invasive aspergillosis and looks like *Aspergillus* on histopathologic examination of tissues?

Pseudallescheria boydii mimics the clinical, roentgenographic, and histopathologic picture seen with invasive aspergillosis. This common environmental mold causes infection mostly in immunocompromised patients, as does *Aspergillus* spp. The most important difference between these fungi is that *P. boydii* is resistant to AmB and should be treated with azole agents. Thus, culture and not just histopathology or cytology is important in the diagnosis of invasive pulmonary fungal infections.

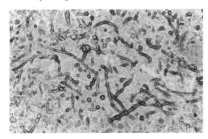

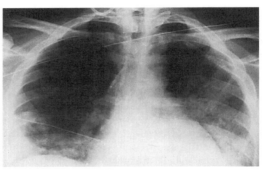

Lung biopsy specimen from patient with *Pseudallescheria boydii* infection. The histopathology of this infection mimics that of aspergillosis (acutely branching septate hyphae).

Chest radiograph shows extensive bilateral infiltrates in a liver transplant patient.

20. How should sputum be cultured when infection with an endemic mycosis is likely?

It is imperative for clinicians to alert the laboratory that diagnosis of an endemic mycosis is likely. *Coccidioides immitis* grows easily on most media within several days to weeks. Because an unsuspecting technician who opens a plate growing this organism will probably become infected, special precautions are always taken if the laboratory knows coccidioidomycosis is a possibility. *Histoplasma capsulatum* and *Blastomyces dermatitidis* grow very slowly and require special media for growth. Especially in cases of chronic cavitary pulmonary histoplasmosis, but also in blastomycosis, commensal organisms, such as *Candida*, will overgrow the culture plate before the pathogen even begins to grow. Laboratories can use special media to inhibit the growth of the commensal if they know beforehand that histoplasmosis or blastomycosis are considerations.

21. What is the best technique for administering amphotericin B?

Although AmB has been available since 1957, optimal dosage and duration of therapy remain controversial. Low dose AmB (0.4 to 0.5 mg/day, less than 500 mg total dose) may be as effective as high dose AmB (0.7 mg/day or more than 500 mg total dose) for candidemia. Higher doses (1.0–1.5 mg/kg/day) are usually required for invasive aspergillosis or mucormycosis.

Adverse effects, most of which are dose-dependent, are noted in approximately 70% of patients receiving AmB. Guidelines have been developed to lessen toxicity, but no prospective trials have assessed efficacy of the guidelines. Prolonged infusion over 3–4 hours has been advised, but side effects are not less frequent than when the drug is infused over 2 hours. Because anaphylaxis may rarely complicate the use of AmB, a test dose (1 mg) should be initiated under careful observation. Pretreatment with aspirin, diphenhydramine, hydrocortisone (20–50 mg), or heparin (500 units) is often advocated to reduce side effects; however, routine pretreatment is probably not cost-effective. These agents may be considered in patients with adverse effects or local phlebitis at the injection site. The dose of AmB can be gradually escalated over several days for non–life-threatening infections; however, dosage should escalate to the target amount within 24 hours for patients with severe invasive fungal infections.

Nephrotoxicity is the major serious side effect limiting the usefulness of AmB. Other adverse effects include fever and rigors during AmB infusion and hypokalemia, hypomagnesemia, and anemia with prolonged administration. Concomitant nephrotoxic agents should be avoided unless absolutely essential. Nephrotoxicity can be reduced by saline loading (e.g., 500 ml of 0.9% sodium chloride) before the infusion. Serum creatinine, blood urea nitrogen, electrolyte, and magnesium levels and complete blood counts should be monitored during therapy. Supplementation of magnesium or potassium may be required, according to serum levels. The dose of AmB or frequency of administration may need reduction when the serum creatinine level exceeds 2.5–3.0 mg/dl. Liposomal or AmB-lipid complexes have been developed to reduce the toxicity of AmB. Abelcet (Liposome Co., Inc., Princeton, NJ), an AmB-lipid complex, was the first of these compounds released in the United States (approved by the FDA in November 1995 to treat aspergillosis refractory to or intolerant of AmB). AmB-lipid complexes have less hematologic and renal toxicity than AmB and may be as effective. Infusion-related events such as chills, rigors, headache, nausea, and vomiting occur with a frequency similar to that seen with AmB. Other colloidal-lipid and liposomal formulations of AmB currently in use in other countries should be released soon.

22. What side effects are associated with azole antifungal agents?

The azoles have fewer side effects than AmB. Adverse effects are most common with ketoconazole, a factor that has led to decreased use of this agent for systemic mycoses. Ketoconazole may cause a dose-dependent reversible inhibition of testosterone and adrenal corticosteroid synthesis, resulting in reduced libido, gynecomastia, and impotence in males; adrenal insufficiency has rarely been described. Serious hepatotoxicity is the major serious adverse effect associated with ketoconazole; fatal hepatotoxicity occurs in fewer than 1 in 15,000 treatment courses.

Fluconazole has the fewest adverse effects. Skin rash, nausea, and elevated liver enzymes are the most common adverse effects. Alopecia may occur in 12–20% of patients receiving high dosages for more than 2 months; it reverses with cessation of the drug or a reduction in dose.

Itraconazole is generally well tolerated; its principal side effects include nausea, vomiting, abnormalities in liver function test results, hypokalemia, hypertension, and edema. Serious adverse effects requiring discontinuation of therapy occur in less than 5% of patients. Effects on the endocrine system are minimal but may occur at doses exceeding 400 mg/day.

23. Which drug-drug interactions are important to know when azole agents are used?

Because the azole antifungal agents are metabolized by the cytochrome P-450 enzyme system, drug-drug interactions can cause significant, even life-threatening, toxicities. Interactions vary with each drug, but generally itraconazole and ketoconazole have more significant interactions. Ketoconazole and itraconazole, but not fluconazole, require a low gastric pH for absorption. These drugs should not be used in patients requiring concomitant H_2 blockers, antacids, or proton pump inhibitors. In addition, one must be sure absorption is adequate in older individuals, who may be achlorhydric.

Effects of Azole Antifungal Drugs on Serum Concentrations of Concomitantly Administered Drugs

DRUG AFFECTED BY AZOLE	AZOLE ANTIFUNGAL DRUG		
	KETOCONAZOLE	ITRACONAZOLE	FLUCONAZOLE
Alterations in cytochromes P-450			
Warfarin	↑*	↑	↑*
Cyclosporine	↑*	↑*	↑*
Phenytoin	↑*	None known‡	↑*
Triazolam, alprazolam, midazolam	↑	None known	None known
Diltiazem	↑	None known	None known
Lovastatin	None known	None known	↑
Zidovudine	None known	None known	↑
Carbamazepine	None known	None known	↑*
Terfenadine	↑†	↑†	No effect§
Astemizole	↑†	↑†	None known
Loratidine	↑	None known	None known
Cisapride	↑†	↑†	↑
Oral hypoglycemics	↑	None known	↑
Isoniazid	↓*	None known	None known
Rifampin	↓*	None known	None known
Rifabutin	None known	None known	↑
FK 506	None known	None known	↑*
Quinidine	↑	None known	None known
Unknown mechanisms			
Digoxin	None known	↑*	None known

* Clinically significant interaction; serum concentrations of drug or clinical status of patient (or both) should be monitored.
† Life-threatening interaction causing arrhythmias; avoid use of combination.
‡ None known. Interaction has not been studied in human subjects; caution should be exercised when this combination is used until further information is available.
§ No effect. No clinically significant pharmacokinetic or pharmacodynamic interaction was detected when drug combination was studied in human subjects.

Effects of Concomitantly Administered Drugs on Azole Antifungal Drug Concentrations

DRUG AFFECTING AZOLE CONCENTRATION	AZOLE ANTIFUNGAL DRUG CONCENTRATION*		
	KETOCONAZOLE	ITRACONAZOLE	FLUCONAZOLE
Alterations in cytochrome P-450			
Carbamazepine	None known†	↓	None known
Phenytoin	↓	↓	None known
Isoniazid	↓	None known	None known
Rifampin	↓	↓	↓
Rifabutin	None known	↓	No effect‡
Inhibition of absorption from GI tract			
Sucralfate	↓	None known	No effect
H₂ receptor antagonists	↓	↓	No effect
Omeprazole	↓	↓	No effect
Antacids	↓	↓	No effect
Didanosine	None known	↓	None known

* Reductions in plasma azole concentrations have led to therapeutic failure for some fungal infections.
† None known. Interaction has not been studied in human subjects; caution should be exercised when this combination is used until further information is available.
‡ No effect. No clinically significant pharmacokinetic or pharmacodynamic interaction was detected when drug drug combination was studied in human subjects.

BIBLIOGRAPHY

1. Ampel NM, Dols CL, Galgiani JN: Coccidioidomycosis during human immunodeficiency virus infection: Results of a prospective study in a coccidioidal endemic area. Am J Med 94:235–240, 1993.
2. Cantanzaro A, Galgiani JN, Levine BE, et al: Fluconazole in the treatment of chronic pulmonary and nonmeningeal disseminated coccidioidomycosis. Am J Med 98:249–256, 1995.
3. Como JA, Dismukes WE: Oral azole drugs as systemic antifungal therapy. N Engl J Med 330:263–272, 1994.
4. Denning DW, Lee JY, Hostetler JS, et al: NIAID Mycoses Study Group multicenter trial of oral itraconazole therapy for invasive aspergillosis. Am J Med 97:135–144, 1994.
5. Denning DW, Stevens DA: Antifungal and surgical treatment of invasive aspergillosis: Review of 2,121 published cases. Rev Infect Dis 12:1147–1201, 1990.
6. Dismukes WE: Management of cryptococcosis. Clin Infect Dis 17(Suppl 2):S507–S512, 1993.
7. Dismukes WE, Bradsher RW Jr, Cloud GC, et al: Itraconazole therapy for blastomycosis and histoplasmosis: NIAID Mycoses Study Group. Am J Med 93:489–497, 1992.
8. Galgiani JN: Coccidioidomycosis. West J Med 159:153–171, 1993.
9. Goodwin SD, Cleary JD, Walawander CA, et al: Pretreatment regimens for adverse events related to infusion of amphotericin B. Clin Infect Dis 20:755–761, 1995.
10. Hajjeh RA: Disseminated histoplasmosis in persons infected with human immunodeficiency virus. Clin Infect Dis 21(Suppl 1):S108–S111, 1995.
11. Haron E, Vartivarian S, Anaissie E, et al: Primary *Candida* pneumonia: Experience at a large cancer center and review of the literature. Medicine (Baltimore) 72:137–142, 1993.
12. Horvath JA, Dummer S: The use of respiratory tract cultures in the diagnosis of invasive pulmonary aspergillosis. Am J Med 100:171–178, 1996.
13. Meyer RD: Current role of therapy with amphotericin B. Clin Infect Dis 14(Suppl 1):154–160, 1992.
14. Pappas P, Bradsher RW, Chapman SW, et al: Treatment of blastomycosis with fluconazole: A pilot study. Clin Infect Dis 20:267–271, 1995.
15. Rozenbaum R, Goncalves ARR: Clinical epidemiological study of 171 cases of cryptococcosis. Clin Infect Dis 18:369–380, 1994.
16. Sarosi GA, Ample N, Cohn DL, et al: Fungal infections in HIV-infected persons. Am J Respir Crit Care Med 152:816–822, 1995.
17. Sarosi GA, Davies SF: Therapy for fungal infections. Mayo Clin Proc 69:1111–1117, 1994.
18. Sharkey PK, Graybill JR, Johnson ES, et al: Amphotericin B lipid complex compared with amphotericin B in the treatment of cryptococcal meningitis in patients with AIDS. Clin Infect Dis 22:315–321, 1996.
19. Speed B, Dunt D: Clinical and host differences between infections with the two varieties of *Cryptococcus neoformans*. Clin Infect Dis 21:28–34, 1995.
20. Stevens DA: Coccidioidomycosis. N Engl J Med 332:1077–1082, 1995.
21. Tedder M, Spratt JA, Anstadt MP, et al: Pulmonary mucormycosis: Results of medical and surgical therapy. Ann Thorac Surg 57:1044–1050, 1994.
22. Wheat J, Hafner R, Korzun AH, et al: Itraconazole treatment of disseminated histoplasmosis in patients with the acquired immunodeficiency syndrome. Am J Med 98:336–342, 1995.

29. PARASITIC INFECTIONS

Om P. Sharma, M.D., and Omar Tirmizi, M.D.

1. Why is it important for health care professionals to be familiar with parasitic diseases?

Social and political upheavals, economic catastrophes, and technologic advances have blurred Nature's boundaries, and increasing travel and intercontinental migration have made our world a smaller place. Consequently, physicians and other health care workers can expect to encounter previously unfamiliar diseases and exotic medical syndromes that once occurred only in tropical and subtropical areas. Several of these diseases manifest primarily in the lungs; others involve the respiratory apparatus only in conjunction with other tissue systems. It is imperative that the modern health care worker learn to recognize, diagnose, and treat parasitic and nonparasitic illnesses heretofore unknown in the hospitals and clinics of developed countries. The possibility of a parasitic or imported illness should be considered in every visitor, tourist, political refugee, student, businessperson, or diplomat who presents with an unexplained pulmonary illness.

2. List the symptoms of pulmonary infection caused by common parasites.

Principal Symptoms of Pulmonary Parasitic Diseases

SPECIES	COUGH	WHEEZING	DYSPNEA	PNEUMONITIS	HEMOPTYSIS	CHRONIC
Ascaris	+++	+++	++	+++	+	−
Hookworm	+++	+++	++	++	−	−
Strongyloides	+++	+++	++	+++	−	−
Visceral larva migrans	+++	+++	++	++	−	−
Pneumocystis	+++	+	+++	+++	−	−
Toxoplasmosis (neonatal)	+	−	+++	+++	−	−
Entamoeba histolytica	++	−	+++	+++	−	−
Filariasis	++	++	++	++	−	−
Schistosomiasis	++	−	++	++	−	+
Paragonimiasis	++	+	++	++	+++	+++
Echinococcosis	+	−	−	−	++	+++

− + ++ +++ = Usually absent to key symptom.
Adapted from Jones JE: Signs and symptoms of parasitic diseases. Prim Care 18:153–165, 1991.

3. Which of the following parasitic diseases is caused by eating raw or undercooked freshwater crustaceans such as crabs and crayfish: (a) amebiasis, (b) melioidosis, (c) paragonimiasis, or (d) malaria?

Paragonimiasis. Paragonimiasis is a helminthic zoonosis caused by a lung fluke of the genus *Paragonimus*. Human disease is caused by ingestion of undercooked crabs and crayfish infected with metacercarial larval. Although found in Africa and Latin America, paragonimiasis is endemic in Korea, Thailand, Laos, the Philippines, China, and Japan. Amebiasis, usually considered a tropical disease, exists in every country in the world. It is transmitted from human to human and caused mainly by *Entamoeba histolytica*. Melioidosis is endemic in Vietnam, Laos, Cambodia, Thailand, the Philippines, India, and Malaysia. It is caused by *Pseudomonas pseudomallei*, a gram-negative aerobe and facultative anaerobe that is in muddy water and soil in endemic areas. Wound contamination, inhalation, and aspiration are the most likely modes of transmission. Malaria is caused predominantly by the four species of *Plasmodium: P. vivax, P. falciparum, P. ovale,* and *P. malariae*. The disease is transmitted by the bite of an *Anopheles* sp. mosquito.

4. What are the clinical features of paragonimiasis?

Paragonimiasis is a parasitic disease caused by a trematode lung fluke of the genus Paragonimus. It is mainly a disease of the young. Ninety percent of patients have blood-stained, coffee-colored, or rusty sputum. Sputum production is greatest in the morning and after brisk exercise. There are usually no constitutional symptoms, so fever or weight loss is uncommon. Physical examination is usually unremarkable; however, hemiparesis, paraplegia, or convulsions may be seen. The diagnosis is established by low-power microscopic identification of telltale operculated eggs in morning sputum specimens.

5. What are the pleuropulmonary manifestations of amebiasis?

The lung and pleura appear to be involved in 3–22% of patients with amebic abscess of the liver. The different forms of pleuropulmonary amebiasis include:
• Hematogenous pulmonary involvement without liver disease
• Independent pulmonary and hepatic involvement
• Direct extension of the liver abscess into the lung, pleural space, or pericardium

Rarely, inhalation of dust containing cysts of *E. histolytica* may cause lung disease. Most cases of thoracic involvement originate by extension of liver lesions through the diaphragm. If the abscess ruptures into a free pleural space, amebic empyema is formed. Because the most common site of an amebic abscess is the right lobe of the liver, extension is usually to the right lower lobe of the lung. The diagnosis of pleuropulmonary amebiasis should always be considered in an individual with an unexplained right lower lobe pneumonia, mass, or empyema.

6. Describe the typical clinical profile of a patient with tropical eosinophilia.

The endemic areas for tropical eosinophilia include India, Pakistan, Sri Lanka, Burma, Thailand, and Malaysia. The disease has a predilection for individuals, mostly men, from the Indian subcontinent. Symptoms include dry cough, malaise, fever, and wheezing. Typically, cough, dyspnea, and wheezing are most prominent at night. An essential feature for the diagnosis is peripheral blood eosinophilia in excess of 2000 eosinophils per ml. The chest radiograph may reveal a diffuse nodular (miliary) or an interstitial pattern. Erythrocyte sedimentation rate is almost always elevated. The presence of circulating microfilarial parasitic antigens and a prompt favorable clinical response to diethylcarbamazine are other characteristic features of the illness.

7. Which parasites cause pulmonary granulomas?

There are numerous causes of pulmonary granulomas, ranging from live replicating intracellular organisms (bacteria, mycobacteria, fungi, viruses) to nonreplicating metazoans (helminths) to inanimate substances (metals, chemical agents) and organic antigens. Parasitic causes of lung granulomas include visceral leishmaniasis (kala-azar), metazoan tissue parasites such as *Trichinella* spp., nematodes such as *Ascaris lumbricoides* and *Toxocara canis*, and trematodes such as *Schistosoma mansoni*.

8. List the pulmonary eosinophilic syndromes.

The association between pulmonary infiltrates and blood eosinophilia is recognized as *pulmonary eosinophilia*, or *pulmonary infiltration with eosinophil* (PIE). PIE appears to result from the introduction of foreign material into the human body by different routes: ingestion, infection, inhalation, skin contact, and vaginal absorption.

The parasitic causes of pulmonary eosinophilias include *Filaria* (tropical eosinophilia), *Strongyloides, Schistosoma, Ascaris, Trichinella, Ancylostoma,* and *Paragonimus* spp. The pulmonary infiltrates appear during larval migration through the lung and are usually transitory. Symptoms, which are mild and self-limited, include wheezing, coughing, hemoptysis, and dyspnea.

Pulmonary Eosinophilias

EXTRINSIC (CAUSE KNOWN)	INTRINSIC (CAUSE UNKNOWN)
Bacteria	Part of multisystem disease
Fungi	Pulmonary involvement only
Parasites	
Drugs	
Chemicals	

9. List the most common parasitic lung infections in the immunocompromised host.

Pneumonia caused by *Pneumocystis carinii* infection is common in immunodeficient persons and is a common pulmonary complication in patients with AIDS. Toxoplasmosis, though most commonly a disseminated infection, can also cause pneumonitis. *Strongyloides stercoralis* may cause life-threatening pulmonary disease. Although *Cryptosporidium* spp. have been found in the sputum, bronchoalveolar lavage fluid, and lung biopsy samples of immunodeficient patients with gastrointestinal disease, this parasite is not believed to cause lung infection.

10. Describe the manifestations of strongyloidiasis in immunocompetent and immunocompromised patients.

Strongyloides stercoralis causes infection via invasive filariform larvae that penetrate the skin and gain access to the venous system via the lymphatics. The larvae pass through the heart and into the lungs, where they break out of capillaries into the alveoli, ascend up the tracheo-bronchial tree, and are swallowed. The larvae then develop into mature adult worms in the distal duodenum and proximal jejunum. These round worms can perpetuate themselves within the host for years after the initial infection through a process of internal or external autoinfection. Uncomplicated infections in the immunocompetent patient are minimally symptomatic; however, malnutrition, malignancies, chronic renal failure, alcoholism, or hypogammaglobulinema may cause disseminated disease. In patients with AIDS, disseminated disease occurs and gastrointestinal and respiratory symptoms predominate. Pulmonary manifestations include cough, sputum production, hemoptysis, dyspnea, bronchospasm, and respiratory insufficiency. Disruption of gastrointestinal mucosal integrity by penetrating filariform larvae may facilitate the entry of gram-negative bacteria, resulting in septicemia.

11. What are the pulmonary manifestations of Chagas' disease?

American trypanosomiasis, described by Carlos Chagas (1909), is an endemic disease of rural populations, caused by a protozoan, *Trypanosoma cruzi*, which is transmitted to humans by a blood-sucking bug of the subfamily *Triatominae*. It is a widespread human infection that is reported from the southwestern United States to Argentina. Except for bronchiectasis, which results from direct infection by *T. cruzi*, lung manifestations are uncommon, and only occur secondary to infection of other organs, e.g,. the heart or esophagus. Aspiration resulting in pneumonia is a commonly encountered problem in patients with megaesophagus. In patients with congestive cardiomyopathy, pulmonary congestion or pulmonary thromboembolism may occur.

12. How are hydatid cysts of the lung managed?

Surgery is still the mainstay of management, although medical treatment is rapidly evolving. In the natural history of hydatid disease, there is a latent period of several years. Once the cyst becomes symptomatic, however, deterioration is rapid. The type of surgery depends upon the extent of lung disease and the presence or absence of symptoms. Enucleation is the procedure of choice for the simple cyst. Rupture of the cyst during enucleation is a feared complication that may lead to anaphylactic shock or result in spread of disease. Various methods of cyst sterilization are available before enucleation. Mebendazole and albendazole are anthelmintic drugs that have been found to be effective in animal and clinical trials.

13. What is the most serious pulmonary complication of schistosomiasis?

Schistosomiasis was initially seen mainly as an intestinal disease with involvement of the portal system in more severe cases. Later, lung lesions were identified that indicated the systemic character of the infection. From a clinical standpoint, chronic cor pulmonale secondary to diffuse arteriolar disease represents the most important pulmonary complication of schistosomiasis. The pulmonary disease has been reported in connection with *Schistosoma mansoni, S. haematobium*, and *S. japonicum*. Pulmonary injury may start during the invasive stage of the disease, when the circulating cercariae cause patchy congestion in the lungs; however, the more important pulmonary lesion, acute necrotizing arteriolitis, is caused by embolization of ova from the normal habitat of the worms. Hypoxemia and cyanosis are also complications of pulmonary schistosomiasis.

14. How does leishmaniasis affect the lung?

Coughing as a symptom of visceral leishmaniasis has been well documented. It appears early in the disease, persists throughout the course, and disappears with cure. Interstitial pneumonitis is also seen in some patients with visceral leishmaniasis. Cells of the reticuloendothelial system present in the lung can become infected with the flagellate *Leishmania donovani*. After the bite of an infected sandfly, *Phlebotomus ovani*, the infective amastigotes are taken up by mononuclear phagocytes, including alveolar macrophages, where they multiply. Interstitial pneumonia is thought to facilitate bacterial growth, leading to a bronchopneumonia in some patients.

BIBLIOGRAPHY

1. Chen MG, Mott KE: Progress in assessment of morbidity due to *Schistosoma japonicum* infection. Trop Dis Bull 85:R2–56, 1988.
2. Duarte MIS, Matta VLR, Corbett CEP, et al: Interstitial pneumonitis in human visceral leishmaniasis. Trans R Soc Trop Med Hyg 83:73–76, 1989.
3. Jehad Amir AK, Frdin R, Fazarad A, et al: Clinical echinococcosis. Ann Surg 182:402–408, 1975.
4. Kaul BL, Dhar SN, Chowdhary KL, et al: Pulmonary hydatid disease—abstracts. The 4th Congress of the Association of Thoracic and Cardiovascular Surgeons of Asia. 30; 1981.
5. Lung disease in the tropics. In Sharma OP (ed): Lung Biology in Health and Disease, vol 51. New York, Marcel Dekker, 1991.
6. Manson-Bahr PEC, Bell DR: Trematode infections: Schistosomiasis. In Manson's Tropical Diseases, 19th ed. London, Bailliere-Tindall, 1987.
7. Marx MB: Parasites, pets and people. Prim Care 18:153–165, 1991.
8. Morris DL: Preoperative albendazole therapy for hydatid cysts. Br J Surg 74:805–806, 1987.
9. Neva FA, Ottesen EA: Tropical (filarial) eosinophilia. N Engl J Med 298:1129–1131, 1978.
10. Rees PH, Kragere PA, Bwibo NO: Clinical aspects and treatment of visceral leishmaniasis in Kenya: A retrospective study of 71 patients. In Krager PA, Rees PH (eds): Clinical Aspects of Kala Azar in Kenya. I.C.G. Printing, Dordrecht, Netherlands, 1983.
11. Sen P, Gil C, Estrellas B, Middleton JR: Corticosteroid induced asthma: A manifestation of limited hyperinfection syndrome due to *Strongyloides stercorales*. South Med J 88:923–927, 1995.
12. Vieyra-Herrera G, Becerril-Carmana G, Padua-Gabriel A: *Strongyloides stercoralis* hyperinfection in a patient with the acquired immune deficiency syndrome. Acta Cytol 10:277–279, 1988.
13. Wyngaarden JB, Smith LH Jr, Bennett JC (eds): Cecil Textbook of Medicine, 19th ed. Philadelphia, W.B. Saunders, 1992.

30. VIRAL PNEUMONIA

Carlos E. Girod, M.D.

1. How frequently are viral pathogens identified as the cause of community-acquired pneumonia?

Viral pneumonias afflict not only immunocompromised hosts, but also immunocompetent adults and children. Viral pathogens are especially common causes of pneumonia in infants and children. In contrast, viruses are rare causes of community-acquired pneumonia in adults. The true incidence of viral pneumonia may be grossly underestimated for two reasons: first, most adults with viral pneumonia experience a self-limiting course that does not require office or hospital visits. Second, the cause of community-acquired pneumonia is uncertain in as many as 49% of all cases, probably because a proper respiratory sample cannot be obtained or a pathogen cannot be identified. In children under the age of three, viral pneumonia (caused by respiratory syncytial virus, for example) may account for as many as 50% of all cases of pneumonia. In adults, studies performed during the past three decades have identified viruses as the cause of 5–12% of all pneumonias.

2. Which patients are at risk for the development of viral pneumonia?

This question is best answered by dividing patients into two populations: immunocompetent and immunocompromised. Immunocompetent persons with viral pneumonia are usually children. Infants under the age of 6 months appear to be protected from viral pathogens. The incidence of viral pneumonia has two peaks: one in the second year of life and one during school age, after which a gradual decline occurs. In children, epidemiologic studies have identified day-care center or school attendance as a risk factor. In the immunocompetent adult, the main risk factor for the development of viral pneumonia is the presence of chronic cardiac or pulmonary disease. Increased incidence is also seen in women during childbearing years. Another risk factor for adults is contact or enclosure with a large number of people while living in military barracks, jails, nursing homes, or dormitories. Immunocompromised patients are at increased risk for viral infection with a different spectrum of pathogens than those seen in immunocompetent patients. In particular, patients undergoing organ transplantation are increased risk of viral pneumonia from pathogens such as cytomegalovirus (CMV) and herpes simplex virus (HSV). Other risk factors for development of viral pneumonia in immunocompromised hosts include cancer, radiation, chemotherapy, malnutrition, skin breakdown, or burns.

3. What clinical features suggest a viral cause of pneumonia?

There is no specific or sensitive clinical or radiologic feature that distinguishes viral from bacterial pneumonia. Nonspecific clinical symptoms and signs include cough, fever, tachypnea, and low oxygen levels. Findings on chest radiograph include unilateral or bilateral alveolar or interstitial infiltrates. Thus, the diagnosis of viral infection requires a high index of suspicion in patients at risk, such as children under the age of 3, adults with cardiopulmonary disease, or any immunocompromised host. Also, suspicion of a viral pathogen should increase when a pneumonia does not respond to antibiotic therapy or sputum cultures for bacteria are negative. A viral pathogen should be highly suspected during the winter months.

4. Name the laboratory tools available for the diagnosis of viral pneumonia.

The specimens that should be studied in patients suspected of viral pneumonia include those collected by nasal washes, nasopharyngeal swabs, throat swabs, tracheal aspirates, and sputum cultures. Respiratory samples can also be obtained by bronchoscopy or open lung biopsy. For increased yield, the specimen obtained should be immediately placed in cold viral culture or carrier medium and rapidly transported to the laboratory. Because of the usual multisystemic involvement seen in viral infection, secretions other than respiratory samples, such as urine and blood, can also be analyzed.

There are three main laboratory techniques for detecting viral pathogens in nasal swabs, respiratory samples, or serum: culture, direct detection of viral antigens by immunohistochemistry or immunofluorescence and serologic testing.

Culture of viruses is performed by inoculation of the sample into various tissue culture cell lines and direct observation of viral cytopathic activity. Viruses known to grow rapidly in culture include influenza and rhinovirus. Diagnosis by culture can be delayed, however, in slow-growing viruses such as CMV and varicella-zoster virus (VZV). Most viruses isolated from either symptomatic or asymptomatic patients are true pathogens and not representative of colonization.

Immunofluorescence and immunohistochemistry of various viral antigens in respiratory samples and nasopharyngeal epithelial cells are especially useful in diagnosing CMV, respiratory syncytial virus (RSV), adenovirus, herpes simplex, and varicella pneumonia.

Serologic testing is useful for the diagnosis of viral pneumonia. A fourfold increase in titer from acute to convalescent serum of viral-specific antibodies is consistent with a recent viral infection. Serologic studies are commonly available for the diagnosis of influenza, parainfluenza, RSV, and CMV pneumonitis.

The recent utilization of **polymerase chain reaction (PCR) and in situ hybridization** has successfully demonstrated the presence of viral pathogens in respiratory secretions, cells, and blood early in the course of infection. PCR, which was instrumental in the rapid identification of hantavirus as the pathogen in Four Corners Disease, will have an increased use in the future as a sensitive method for diagnosing viral pneumonia.

5. How successful are antiviral agents in the treatment of viral pneumonia?

The treatment of viral pneumonias has been revolutionized by the development of various agents with proven virucidal activity. Nevertheless, the cornerstone of treatment is supportive care consisting of oxygen therapy, mechanical ventilation (in severe cases), and adjunctive antimicrobial therapy to treat bacterial superinfection. Antiviral agents either block viral replication or boost the host's immune response and are very successful in vitro, but response is less encouraging in the treatment of viral pneumonia. Antiviral agents available for the treatment of viral pneumonia are shown below.

Antiviral Agents with Potential Benefit in Viral Pneumonia*

AGENT	VIRUS
Ganciclovir	CMV
Acyclovir	HSV, VZV
Interferon alpha	CMV, HSV, VZV, rhinovirus
Amantadine/rimantadine	Influenza A
Ribavirin	RSV, influenza A and B

* The only drug approved for the treatment of viral pneumonia is ribavirin for RSV. All other drugs listed are approved for nonpneumonia infections or for prophylaxis.
Adapted from Greenberg SB: Viral pneumonia. Infect Dis Clin North Am 5:615, 1991.

6. Is respiratory isolation required for patients with suspected or documented viral pneumonia?

Even when patients with viral pneumonia are being treated with antiviral therapy, evidence suggests that disease can spread to other patients or hospital personnel. It is imperative to place the patient in a respiratory isolation room and have visitors or hospital personnel wear disposable gloves, gowns, and masks. This is particularly important during the treatment of children with RSV. Cohort isolation of patients with committed hospital personnel has reduced the nosocomial transmission of RSV pneumonia from 45% to 18%. People exposed in the hospital or at home to patients with viral pneumonia—especially if it is caused by varicella, influenza, or RSV—should consider receiving immunoglobulin or pharmacologic therapy in order to avoid infection.

7. What vaccines are available for the prevention of viral pneumonia?

The most common viral vaccination program is directed to the influenza virus. The influenza vaccine has been available for 50 years and is prepared yearly based on expected or predicted major and minor mutations in viral capsular antigens. Influenza vaccine should be administered in the early fall to provide enough time for a specific antibody response. This vaccine is indicated for hospital personnel, health-related workers, adults 65 years or older, military recruits, nursing home residents, or any patient with chronic medical condition(s), especially cardiopulmonary disease. Adenoviral oral vaccines to types 3, 4, and 7 have been used effectively in military recruits, but have not yet been administered to the general population. Work is currently being done to develop vaccines directed to RSV and parainfluenza virus. Passive immunity through administration of immunoglobulin is another way of preventing viral infection. It has been limited to patients at risk for RSV, CMV, VZV, and measles viruses.

8. How effective is vaccination in preventing influenza infection?

Influenza virus types A and B account for 50% of community-acquired viral pneumonia in the adult population. Epidemics are common during the winter months, and the influenza virus can lead to several complications requiring hospitalization. Thus, yearly immunization for prevention of influenza is recommended for patients aged 65 years or older and those with high risk factors or chronic medical illness. This vaccine is also recommended for nursing home residents and health care workers. Various studies involving military recruits have demonstrated a vaccination efficacy of 70–90% in preventing laboratory-confirmed influenza infection. The main criticism of these studies is that the patient selection was limited to young patients and did not involve older patients with cardiopulmonary disease. Studies including older patients have shown much lower effectiveness rates of 45% and 31% during influenza type A and influenza type B outbreaks, respectively.

9. Are there new therapies for prophylaxis or treatment of influenza pneumonia?

The use of amantadine or rimantadine has proved to be effective in the **prophylaxis** of laboratory-confirmed influenza infection. Different studies demonstrate 71–91% efficacy of these agents in preventing clinical illness by influenza A, types H_3N_2 and H_1N_1. These medications are not free of side effects, however. Eight to 32% of patients were removed from these studies because of side effects, predominantly neurologic complaints. Nevertheless, these agents reduce the duration of clinical influenza illness by 1–2 days when administered during the first 24 hours after the onset of symptoms. For adults, amantadine is given orally, 200 mg per day, and for children under the age of 10, 4 mg per kg per day is given. The dose of amantadine should be reduced to 100 mg per day for patients over the age of 65 or with serum creatinine levels above 1.0.

Treatment of influenza pneumonia with ribavirin is still under investigation.

10. What is most common cause of upper respiratory tract infection and pneumonia in children? How is it diagnosed?

RSV is the leading cause of bronchitis and pneumonia in young children. Epidemics usually occur during the spring and winter months. Infections can be severe in children under the age of 2, sometimes requiring mechanical ventilation. The chest radiographs patterns of air-trapping or patchy consolidation are suggestive of, but not specific for, RSV infection. Some reports suggest that right upper lobe consolidation and collapse is characteristic of RSV infection. Diagnosis can be made by identification of RSV antigens using immunohistochemistry of nasopharyngeal epithelial cells obtained by swab. The test is readily available in most hospitals and outpatient clinics.

11. What therapy is available for the treatment of RSV infection?

Children hospitalized with RSV infection have been treated with ribavirin, 6 g in 300 cc of sterile water nebulized continuously for 18–22 hours per day for 3–7 days. Nebulization has to be supervised and requires a closed room to prevent aerosolation of RSV and contagious spread to hospital personnel or patients. Patients should be placed in respiratory isolation. Ribavirin has also been used in adults with severe RSV infection without prior controlled studies.

12. Which patients are at risk of CMV infection and pneumonia?

CMV is a herpesvirus. Herpesviruses are prone to attack susceptible patients, especially recipients of recent organ transplantation and patients with AIDS. CMV infection is an important complication of transplant medicine, including bone marrow, renal, heart, and lung transplants. Infection occurs from transmission by a CMV-positive transplanted organ or from reactivation in recipients with evidence of prior CMV infection. CMV is also recognized as the most common viral pathogen affecting AIDS patients. The rate of infection based on autopsy studies is as high as 49–81% of patients. In many series, CMV infection remains the leading AIDS-defining illness. CMV infection in these patients is associated with fever, weight loss, retinitis, cholangitis, esophagitis, sinusitis, colitis, gastritis, and pneumonitis. It is not uncommon for CMV to be isolated in respiratory secretions of AIDS patients **without** clear evidence of lung involvement.

13. What pretransplant work-up can predict the occurrence of subsequent CMV infection?

The pretransplant study most predictive of subsequent CMV infection is serologic evaluation of donor and recipient. The most severe and common risk factor associated with CMV infection in transplant patients is the placement of a CMV-positive organ into a seronegative recipient. This combination has a 90% risk of infection, leading to severe complications, such as rejection of the organ, pneumonitis, or death. A recent study from the Washington University Lung Transplant Group has shown that CMV infection does not develop in seronegative patients who receive a CMV-negative lung. In contrast, an independent risk factor for predicting death in lung transplant patients is the combination of a seronegative recipient receiving a seropositive organ. Patients who receive bone marrow transplants seropositive for CMV are especially at risk if the preoperative CMV titer is 1:64 or greater. Another pretransplant study that predicts the development of CMV interstitial pneumonitis in allogenic bone marrow transplant patients is the pulmonary function test. In one report, patients who developed CMV interstitial pneumonitis had an FEV_1 of less than 85% 13 days before transplant.

14. How soon after organ transplantation should CMV infection be suspected? What clinical clues suggest CMV pneumonitis?

CMV infection usually occurs 1–4 months after transplantation, which suggests that the cause is reactivation of prior infection or infection borne by the transplanted organ. Thus, pulmonary infiltrates occurring within the first month after transplantation are almost never the result of CMV, and other causes must be sought. No specific sign or symptom is associated with CMV infection. Patients usually manifest fever, malaise, cough, dyspnea, diminished exercise tolerance, and hypoxia. One third of patients may not even have a detectable radiographic infiltrate.

15. What agents are indicated for prophylaxis against CMV infection in transplant recipients?

CMV pneumonitis in transplant patients is associated with a high morbidity and mortality despite prompt institution of antiviral therapy. For this reason, CMV prophylaxis is a major component of the transplant patient's care. Its use depends on either preoperative CMV serologic studies or posttransplant CMV isolation in respiratory secretions. Transplant patients who are seronegative for CMV and receive a seronegative organ do not need CMV prophylaxis, except for the administration of CMV-negative blood products when needed. Patients who are either seronegative recipients of a CMV-positive organ or preoperatively CMV seropositive warrant prophylactic therapy. Regimens are based on the experience derived from renal transplantation, in which prophylactic use of attenuated CMV vaccine, high-dose oral acyclovir, and CMV hyperimmune globulin have demonstrated reduced severity of CMV disease. One regimen for prophylaxis in bone marrow transplant patients consists of (1) use of CMV-seronegative blood products, (2) high-dose intravenous acyclovir from 1 week before to 1 month after transplant, followed by high-dose oral acyclovir, and (3) CMV hyperimmune globulin (5 g/m²) or immune globulin (200 mg/kg) intravenously daily from 1 day before to 2 weeks after transplantation, followed by one dose every 3 weeks to 100 days after transplantation. Other regimens include the use of IV ganciclovir followed by oral acyclovir. CMV prophylaxis in lung transplant patients is not as successful. Most lung transplant centers are adopting the policy of CMV matching and avoiding donor positive/recipient negative transplants. Regimens usually include IV ganciclovir followed by oral high dose acyclovir with either polyvalent immune globulin or CMV hyperimmune globulin.

16. Is isolation of CMV in bronchoalveolar lavage or sputum sufficient to document active CMV pneumonitis?

CMV isolation in blood, urine, or bronchoalveolar lavage fluid does not necessarily suggest active CMV infection or pneumonitis. For example, viremia and CMV isolation from BAL is documented in 71–91% of high-risk transplant patients (those who receive a CMV-positive organ or are seropositive for CMV before transplantation) without evidence of active pneumonitis. Thus, most centers suggest obtaining transbronchial or open-lung biopsy samples to document the presence of tissue invasion by CMV. In lung transplant patients, bronchoscopy with BAL and transbronchial biopsy are routinely performed on days 7 and 28 after transplantation and every 3 months thereafter. Some transplant centers use direct immunofluorescent antigen detection or culture of BAL fluid for CMV and treat with ganciclovir once these tests become positive. This is a controversial topic and procedure should follow the institution's approach. Evaluation of lung tissue for the diagnosis of CMV pneumonitis remains the gold standard.

17. When and how should treatment of CMV pneumonitis be initiated in transplant patients?

In transplant patients, treatment for CMV pneumonitis is usually begun when symptoms suggestive of lung involvement occur and pulmonary infiltrates or nodules develop on chest radiograph or CT scan, or when surveillance BAL or lung biopsy samples become CMV positive. Therapy usually consists of ganciclovir with or without hyperimmune globulin. An initial response occurs in 50–70% of patients. A recent study demonstrated that the combination of ganciclovir and immunoglobulin had the lowest overall mortality. Most patients need maintenance antiviral therapy for as long as 120 days after transplantation. Prophylaxis and early treatment for presumed CMV pneumonitis in high-risk lung-transplant patients reduces mortality to 2.0–13.8%.

18. What are the clinical manifestations of CMV pneumonitis in AIDS patients?

CMV in AIDS is usually associated with retinitis, colitis, cholangitis, adrenalitis, esophagitis, and, rarely, pneumonitis. Pulmonary symptoms at the time of presentation are not specific for CMV. Findings on chest radiograph and CT scan include bilateral pulmonary nodules, ground-glass densities, true consolidation, and a true miliary pattern. Isolation of CMV in blood, BAL fluids, and urine is common without evidence of active pneumonitis. Thus, lung tissue is needed to document CMV pneumonitis. Although the mortality associated with CMV pneumonitis in AIDS patients has been difficult to estimate because diagnosis usually requires biopsy and most patients are not diagnosed before death, it is estimated to be 15–20%.

19. What recent viral outbreak with rapid respiratory failure and high fatality rate was identified in the "four corners area" of the United States?

In May 1993, a mysterious illness developed in people living in the four corners area (a region where the borders of Colorado, Utah, New Mexico, and Arizona meet). This illness attacked previously healthy persons with rapid onset of fever, muscle aches, headaches, cough, bilateral infiltrates, and respiratory failure. Most patients described a preceding prodromal period suggestive of a viral syndrome with headaches, myalgias, and gastrointestinal complaints. Patients typically were admitted to the intensive care unit with rapid respiration, tachycardia, hypotension, and hypoxia. Laboratory evaluation demonstrated leukocytosis, bandemia, and elevated hematocrit. A characteristic finding in these patients was elevated lactate dehydrogenase level and hematocrit, thrombocytopenia, hypoxia, and bilateral pulmonary infiltrates. The clinical course progressed rapidly with development of pulmonary edema, hypoxia, progressive hypotension, metabolic acidosis, and, eventually, death. Under the direction of various infectious disease centers, local physicians, and the Centers for Disease Control, aggressive evaluation with serologic testing and application of the polymerase chain reaction specific for various suspected infectious agents identified the pathogen as Hantavirus. Hantavirus is an RNA virus of the *Bunyaviridae* family. It is known to be the cause of hemorrhagic fever with renal syndrome (HFRS) in Europe and Asia. The Hantavirus pulmonary syndrome (HPS) was described and cases were identified as far away from the Four Corners region as California, Texas, and Rhode Island. Evaluation of the households for index cases demonstrated that rodents, especially the deer mouse (*Peromyscus maniculatus*), was the reservoir of the Hantavirus as demonstrated by serologic testing of captured mice. Epidemiologic studies suggest that increased rain during the spring and summer of 1993 led to an increased population of these rodents. Infection in humans occurs by inhalation of aerosolized rodent feces, urine, or saliva.

20. What agents are effective against Hantavirus infection? What preventive measures should be instituted to prevent a repeat outbreak?

Treatment for the Hantavirus pulmonary syndrome (HPS) is still uncertain. At present, there is no specific agent for Hantavirus. Therapy consists chiefly of aggressive intensive care monitoring and supportive therapy. Intravenous fluids must be administered cautiously to these patients, because a capillary leak phenomenon is suggested for development of pulmonary edema. Supportive care should include mechanical ventilation, oxygen administration, and the use of inotropic or pressor agents, if needed. Experience with the use of ribavirin in the treatment of the Asian Hantavirus syndrome (hemorrhagic fever with renal syndrome) led to its application to the HPS outbreak in the United States. In June 1993, an open label trial involving the use of IV ribavirin for HPS was approved in the United States. Case reports demonstrated successful treatment. Since the identification of Hantavirus as the cause of the Four Corners Disease, aggressive rodent control measures have been instituted in endemic areas.

21. List the diagnostic criteria for documenting Hantavirus pulmonary syndrome.

Confirmed cases must meet both clinical and laboratory criteria developed by the Centers for Disease Control as follows:

- Clinical criteria (either of the following)
  - (1) Febrile illness (more than 38.3°C) in a previously healthy person characterized by:
    - (a) unexplained ARDS; or
    - (b) bilateral pulmonary interstitial infiltrates developing within 1 week of hospitalization with respiratory compromise requiring supplemental oxygen
  - (2) Autopsy finding of noncardiogenic pulmonary edema resulting from an unexplained respiratory illness
- Laboratory criteria (any of the following)
  - (1) Positive serologic tests, either presence of Hantavirus-specific immunoglobulin M or rising titers of immunoglobulin G
  - (2) Positive immunohistochemistry for Hantavirus antigen
  - (3) Positive polymerase chain reaction for Hantavirus RNA

22. Which patients are at increased risk for developing varicella pneumonia?

Varicella is usually limited to children. Recently, however, infection is being increasingly identified in adults. Adults with varicella have a higher risk for developing pneumonia and the associated mortality rate is high. The following individuals are at risk for varicella pneumonia:

Immunocompromised patients	Newborns, especially premature newborns
AIDS patients	The elderly
Inhaled corticosteroid users	Pregnant women
Cancer patients	Smokers
Organ transplant recipients	Those with severe skin eruption
Patients with COPD	

23. Describe the typical presentation of varicella pneumonia.

Pneumonia usually develops 1 to 6 days after the onset of a characteristic rash. Symptoms include shortness of breath and cough. The chest radiograph usually shows diffuse bilateral infiltrates with some nodular pattern. Microcalcifications ranging from 2–3 mm detected in the chest radiograph can be a late sequela.

24. Is there a role for acyclovir prophylaxis in varicella infection? What is the treatment for varicella pneumonia?

Prophylaxis with oral acyclovir or VZV immune globulin (VZIG) should be considered for patients at risk for progression to varicella pneumonia. When given within 3 to 4 days of exposure to varicella, VZIG has been documented to reduce by 50% the incidence of infection and disease. Treatment for varicella pneumonia includes the administration of intravenous acyclovir, 10 mg per kg three times a day for 6–10 days. The use of adjunctive therapy with corticosteroids has been reported. With the use of acyclovir, the mortality of varicella pneumonia in the general population is 9%. In pregnant patients, the mortality has been reported to be as high as 43%.

25. Which patients are at risk of herpes simplex virus reactivation with pulmonary involvement?

Involvement of the lung by HSV was initially described by Nash and Foley in 1970. HSV infection can be reactivated in patients undergoing major surgery or suffering major burns. Clinical reviews have shown that HSV infection can involve the lower respiratory tract with findings of pulmonary infiltrates, hypoxia, and bronchospasm. A study by Tuxen and colleagues showed that HSV was isolated from respiratory secretions of some patients with ARDS. A follow-up study using acyclovir prophylaxis in ARDS failed to show improvement in clinical condition. HSV infection is treated with IV acyclovir, but success is only partial and the associated mortality is high.

BIBLIOGRAPHY

1. Bailey TC, Trulock EP, Ettinger NA, et al: Failure of prophylactic gancyclovir to prevent cytomegalovirus disease in recipients of lung transplants. J Infect Dis 165:548–552, 1992.
2. Butler JC, Peters CJ: Hantaviruses and Hantavirus pulmonary syndrome. Clin Infect Dis 19:387–395, 1994.
3. Enright H, Haake R, Weisdorf D, et al: Cytomegalovirus pneumonia after bone marrow transplantation. Risk factors and response to therapy. Transplantation 55:1339–1346, 1993.
4. Ettinger NA, Bailey TC, Trulock EP, et al: Cytomegalovirus infection and pneumonitis. Impact after isolated lung transplantation. Am Rev Respir Dis 147:1017–1023, 1993.
5. Feldman S: Varicella-zoster virus pneumonitis. Chest 106 (Suppl):22S–26S, 1994.
6. Foot ABM, Caul EO, Roome AP, et al: Cytomegalovirus pneumonitis and bone marrow transplantation: Identification of a specific high risk group. J Clin Pathol 46:415–419, 1993.
7. Gould FK, Freeman R, Taylor CE, et al: Prophylaxis and management of cytomegalovirus pneumonitis after transplantation: A review of experience in one center. J Heart Lung Transplant 12:695–699, 1993.
8. Greenberg SB: Respiratory herpesvirus infections. An overview. Chest 106(Suppl):1S–2S, 1994.
9. Greenberg SB: Viral pneumonia. Infect Dis Clin North Am 5:603–621, 1991.
10. Horak DA, Schmidt GM, Zaia A, et al: Pretransplant pulmonary function predicts cytomegalovirus-associated interstitial pneumonia following bone marrow transplantation. Chest 102:1484–1490, 1992.
11. McGuinness G, Scholes JV, Garay SM, et al: Cytomegalovirus pneumonitis: Spectrum of parenchymal CT findings with pathologic correlation in 21 AIDS patients. Radiology 192:451–459, 1994.
12. Monto AS: Viral respiratory infections in the community: Epidemiology, agents, and interventions. Am J Med 99(Suppl 6B):24S–27S, 1995.
13. Morrison YY, Rathbun RC: Hantavirus pulmonary syndrome: The four corners disease. Ann Pharmacother 29:57–65, 1995.
14. Simonsen L, Dalton MJ, Breiman RF, et al: Evaluation of the magnitude of the 1993 hantavirus outbreak in the southwestern United States. J Infect Dis 172:729–733, 1995.
15. Tuxen DV, Wilson JW, Cade JF: Prevention of lower respiratory herpes simplex virus infection with acyclovir in patients with the adult respiratory distress syndrome. Am Rev Respir Dis 136:402–405, 1987.
16. Zeitz PS, Butler JC, Cheek JE, et al: A case-control study of hantavirus pulmonary syndrome during an outbreak in the southwestern United States. J Infect Dis 171:864–870, 1995.

31. PREVENTION OF PNEUMONIA

Ann Weinacker, M.D., and Steve Nelson, M.D.

COMMUNITY-ACQUIRED PNEUMONIA

1. What vaccinations are available to prevent viral and bacterial community-acquired pneumonia?

In adults, the Centers for Disease Control (CDC) recommends vaccination against influenza and against pneumonia caused by *Streptococcus pneumoniae* in select subgroups of patients. Influenza vaccine is designed to induce immunity against the influenza viruses anticipated to cause disease in any given year, so the composition of the vaccine changes each year. The vaccine includes three virus strains, usually two influenza A and one influenza B strain. Although whole virus, subviron, and purified–surface antigen vaccines are available, the commonly used vaccine is a highly purified, inactivated virus derived from viral cultures in eggs. The currently used pneumococcal vaccine is a 23-valent vaccine, composed of purified capsular polysaccharide antigens of 23 antigenic types of *S. pneumoniae*. This vaccine, licensed for use in 1983, replaced a 14-valent vaccine in use since 1977. Of the 84 different antigenic types that have been described, the 23 types represented in the current vaccine are estimated to cause 88% of the bacteremic pneumococcal infections in the United States. There is also evidence that the antibodies induced cross-react with other antigenic types responsible for an additional 8% of bacteremic pneumococcal infections.

2. Who should receive influenza vaccine?

Influenza vaccine should be given to people at high risk for developing complications of influenza and to those who are likely to transmit influenza to these high-risk people.

Influenza Vaccine

INDICATIONS	SIDE EFFECTS	CONTRAINDICATIONS/ PRECAUTIONS
Age > 65 years	Pain at vaccination	Anaphylactic reaction
Chronically ill nursing home residents (any age)	site for 1–2 days	to eggs
Patients with:	Fever, malaise,	Acute, febrile illness
Diabetes mellitus	myalgia for	
Renal dysfunction	1–2 days	
Hemoglobinopathy	Allergic reactions	
Immunosuppression (e..g., organ transplant, HIV)	(rare)	
Chronic heart disease		
Chronic pulmonary disease		
Personnel in nursing home, hospitals, other long-term care facilities		
Visiting nurses		
Children with asthma		
Children age 6 months–18 years on long-term Aspirin therapy (they are at risk for developing Reye syndrome after a viral illness)		

3. Who should receive pneumococcal vaccine?

Adults infected with human immunodeficiency virus (HIV) are at approximately ten times greater risk for serious pneumococcal infections than uninfected individuals and should receive pneumococcal vaccine. Consideration should also be given to vaccinating hospitalized high-risk patients before discharge because most patients with serious pneumococcal infections have been hospitalized within the 5 years previous to their pneumococcal disease. Safety of the vaccine has not been established in pregnancy; women at risk should be vaccinated before they become pregnant, if possible. It has been suggested that they may also be vaccinated after the first trimester.

Pneumococcal Vaccine

INDICATIONS	SIDE EFFECTS	CONTRAINDICATIONS/ PRECAUTIONS
Age > 65 years	Pain, redness at vaccina-	Safety in pregnancy is
Patients with:	tion site	unknown
Diabetes mellitus	Fever, myalgias (< 1%)	
Chronic heart disease	Severe local reaction	
Chronic pulmonary disease	(< 1%)	
Immunosuppression (e.g., organ transplant,	Anaphylaxis (rare)	
HIV)		
Alcoholism		
Cirrhosis		
Cerebrospinal fluid leaks		
Asplenia (functional or anatomic)		
Hodgkin disease		
Lymphoma		
Multiple myeloma		
Chronic renal failure		
Nephrotic syndrome		
Hospitalized high-risk patients (before discharge)		

4. How often should the vaccines be repeated?

The **influenza vaccine** changes each year; thus, vaccination needs to be repeated annually. Vaccination should begin in September and may continue well into the influenza season (between December and March), with the recognition that it takes 2 to 3 weeks to develop antibodies. Vaccination should not be done too early, especially in high-risk settings (e.g,. nursing homes), because immunity may begin to wane within a few months.

The frequency with which **pneumococcal vaccine** should be given is less well defined. Patients who received the 14-valent vaccine and are at highest risk for serious pneumococcal disease (those with diabetes mellitus, cirrhosis, and chronic pulmonary disease) should be revaccinated using the 23-valent vaccine. Because antibody levels decrease over time, patients who have received the 23-valent vaccine and are at greatest risk for serious pneumococcal disease or who may have mounted a suboptimal response to the vaccine (e.g., patients who have had splenectomy) should be considered for revaccination after 6 years. Patients who will undergo elective splenectomy (e.g., staging of Hodgkin disease) or be immunocompromised by cancer chemotherapy or immunosuppressive drugs should receive the pneumococcal vaccine at least 2 weeks in advance of surgery or drug therapy.

5. How effective are the available vaccines?

Influenza vaccine is effective in preventing disease in up to 70% of adults younger than 65 years and in children. Estimates of effectiveness in adults older than 65 years living in the community range from 30–70%. Elderly adults living in nursing homes, however, do not mount antibody responses as effectively, and the influenza vaccine prevents illness in only 30–40%. Hospitalization and pneumonia are prevented in 50–60% of these patients, and mortality is prevented in 40–80%. **Pneumococcal vaccine** is estimated by the CDC to be 60–64% effective, although some studies suggest an efficacy as high as 81%. In those older than 65 years, the vaccine is only 44–61% effective. In spite of efficacies of up to 80% for each of these vaccines, they are severely underutilized. It has been estimated that only 20% of those in whom vaccination is recommended are actually offered vaccination by their physicians.

6. Is pneumococcal vaccine useful in patients who are functionally asplenic or splenectomized?

Pneumococcal vaccine is less effective in asplenic patients than in individuals who have spleens. The spleen helps to overcome pneumococcal infections not only by clearing poorly opsonized pneumococci but also by producing specific antibodies against *S. pneumoniae*. Asplenia, therefore, decreases the intensity of the antibody response to pneumococcal vaccine. In addition, antibody titers fall more rapidly in asplenic patients. Asplenic patients should, however, be offered the vaccine because they are at increased risk for more serious disease caused by *S. pneumoniae* and have a mortality rate of 90–95% if they develop bacteremic disease.

7. Do HIV-infected patients respond normally to the influenza and pneumococcal vaccines?

Because formation of antibodies against influenza is T-lymphocyte dependent, the response of HIV-infected persons to influenza vaccine is diminished. One study of 51 HIV-infected individuals showed that almost no influenza antibodies formed after influenza vaccine in those individuals with CD4+ lymphocyte counts less than 100×10^6/liter. Individuals with CD4+ lymphocyte counts between 100×10^6/liter and 300×10^6/liter had suboptimal levels of antibody formation, and those with CD4+ lymphocyte counts of more than 300×10^6/liter often, but not always, had protective levels of antibodies. Even in individuals with CD4+ lymphocyte counts of at least 300×10^6/liter, antibody titers were lower than those of control subjects. The response was not augmented by repeated vaccination 1 month later.

Unlike the case with influenza vaccine, antibody formation in response to pneumococcal vaccines is not dependent on T-lymphocytes. Therefore, HIV-infected individuals, even with low CD4+ lymphocyte counts, have been able to respond adequately to pneumococcal vaccine. The response is less than that of controls, however, particularly in individuals with CD4+ counts less than 500×10^6/liter.

8. What is the utility of these vaccines in patients who are on steroids or are otherwise immunosuppressed?

Chronic immunosuppression with corticosteroids alone or in conjunction with other immunosuppressive agents may diminish the antibody response to both influenza and pneumococcal vaccines. Renal transplant patients chronically immunosuppressed with prednisone, azathioprine, and cyclosporin A respond less well to influenza vaccine than normal individuals but have been shown to increase their antibody titer fourfold to influenza antigens in response to influenza vaccine. Titers decreased slightly after 2 months in this group. Responses to influenza vaccine by patients chronically immunosuppressed with prednisone alone variously have been shown to be diminished or unaffected. Chronic corticosteroid therapy may result in hypogammaglobulinemia in asthmatic patients and thereby impair the response to pneumococcal vaccine. However, a study of 14 asthmatic patients receiving daily or alternate-day therapy with 10–35 mg of prednisone showed no difference in immunoglobulin levels, pneumococcal antibody levels, or response to pneumococcal vaccine when compared with asthmatic controls who were not dependent on steroids.

9. Does vaccination alter the metabolism of any drugs?

Most interactions between influenza vaccine and other drugs have been reported in a very small proportion of patients; however, such interactions can occur. Among the reactions that have been reported are increased serum levels of phenobarbital by inhibition of hepatic enzymes, bleeding in a small number of patients taking warfarin, and alterations in phenytoin levels (increased, decreased, and unchanged levels have all been reported). Theophylline levels may also be increased, although most reports suggest that this does not occur. Carbamazepine and acetaminophen levels are unaffected.

10. Why is pneumococcal vaccine needed when antibiotics that are effective against *Streptococcus pneumoniae* are available?

Patients with bacteremic *S. pneumoniae* disease have a mortality rate of approximately 25% in spite of the use of appropriate antibiotics. This number is essentially unchanged from mortality rates in the 1950s when 24–28% of affected patients succumbed to the disease. *S. pneumoniae* currently causes 480,000–800,000 cases of pneumonia and approximately 40,000 deaths per year. Death occurs early in the course of the disease and is not affected by the use of antibiotics. The reasons for this are varied and relate to host defense mechanisms against the organism. Also, the number of penicillin-resistant isolates of *S. pneumoniae* is increasing. The high incidence of pneumococcal disease in spite of vaccination has several causes. The currently used vaccine contains antigens from the 23 capsular types estimated to cause most of the bacteremic pneumococcal infections in the United States. Other capsular types that cause pneumonia but not bacteremia may be underrepresented in the vaccine. In addition, those at highest risk for developing pneumococcal disease or its complications may be unable to mount an adequate antibody response to the vaccine. Finally, most of the patients at greatest risk never receive the vaccine.

11. If a patient receives pneumococcal vaccine but still develops pneumococcal pneumonia, what antibiotics should be used?

Vaccination against *S. pneumoniae* does not alter the choice of antibiotics to treat infections caused by that organism, should they occur. Rather, selection of an appropriate antibiotic is based on the incidence of penicillin-resistant pneumococcus in the community. Mechanisms of antibiotic resistance are unrelated to the development of immunity that occurs in response to pneumococcal vaccine.

12. When should amantadine or rimantadine be used to prevent influenza? What dosage should be used?

Amantadine and rimantadine are useful in prophylaxis or treatment of influenza type A but not type B; they are approximately 70% effective in prevention and 50% effective in treatment of influenza. The dose of amantadine is 200 mg per day in individuals younger than 65 years, and 100 mg per day in individuals older than 65 years. Rimantadine, which has fewer central nervous system side effects, is given in doses of 100 mg twice a day. The dose is reduced to 100 mg per day in elderly nursing home residents and those with severe renal or hepatic dysfunction. If used for prophylaxis, amantadine or rimantadine is given for the duration of the influenza epidemic. Either drug may also be used in individuals with influenza symptoms. To treat symptomatic influenza, the drug should be started within 24–48 hours of the onset of symptoms and continued for 5–7 days after symptoms begin. In this situation, the efficacy is greater than 50%.

There are rare reports of interactions between amantadine or rimantadine and other drugs. One patient taking amantadine was reported to have a rise in her blood pressure in response to phenelzine (a monoamine oxidase inhibitor). Hydrochlorothiazide-triamterene, cyclophenthiazide-K, and co-trimoxazole may reduce renal clearance of amantadine and predispose the patient to toxicity (ataxia, agitation, hallucinations). Quinine and quinidine also increase amantadine levels, but this may not be clinically significant. Amantadine is not recommended for patients who have convulsions or a history of gastric ulcers. Amantadine may also intensify the gastrointestinal and central nervous system side effects of anticholinergics and levodopa given to treat Parkinson's disease. Rimantadine levels are increased insignificantly by cimetidine.

Indications, Side Effects, and Contraindications to Amantadine and Rimantadine

INDICATIONS	SIDE EFFECTS	CONTRAINDICATIONS/ PRECAUTIONS
Prophylaxis or treatment of influenza type A	Nervousness, anxiety, difficulty concentrating, lightheadedness (greater incidence with amantadine)	Allergy to either drug
Immunosuppression (e.g., organ transplant, HIV)		Reduce dose for elderly, renal dysfunction (amantadine) or hepatic dysfunction (rimantadine)
Contraindications to influenza vaccine	Nausea, anorexia (3%)	
First 2 weeks after late vaccination	Delirium, hallucinations, agitation, seizures (rare)	
Unvaccinated individuals who provide care to high-risk patients		

HOSPITAL-ACQUIRED PNEUMONIA

13. Does body position affect the risk of nosocomial pneumonia?

Short-term studies have demonstrated that the supine position is associated with a greater incidence of aspiration of gastric contents and pneumonia than the sitting or semirecumbent position in who patients who require mechanical ventilation. This is true in spite of inflation of the endotracheal tube cuff. A number of studies of medical patients, trauma victims, liver transplant recipients, and stroke patients have also suggested a beneficial effect of continuously oscillating beds in preventing pneumonia in some patients. Mortality and length of intensive care unit stay have been improved in some of these studies but not in others. Other predisposing factors for nosocomial pneumonia are shown below.

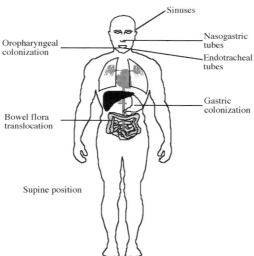

Factors predisposing patients to nosocomial pneumonia.

14. Is selective decontamination of the digestive tract effective in preventing nosocomial pneumonia?

Selective decontamination of the digestive tract is designed to decrease colonization of the oropharynx and gastrointestinal tract with potential pathogens and thus decrease nosocomial pneumonia caused by aspiration of contaminated oropharyngeal or gastric secretions. Routinely used regimens include nonabsorbable drugs active against aerobic gram-negative bacilli (an aminoglycoside plus polymyxin) and *Candida* spp. (nystatin or amphotericin B). These are applied to the mouth in an oral gel and instilled into the stomach through a nasogastric tube. Some regimens also include an intravenous antibiotic, usually a cephalosporin such as cefotaxime, intended to eradicate community-acquired pathogens without altering the normal gastrointestinal flora. Many studies of a wide variety of medical and surgical patients have shown a decrease in the incidence of pneumonia caused by gram-negative organisms, but in some cases the number of infections with gram-positive organisms increased. In spite of the decrease in the incidence of pneumonia, there has been no consistent reduction in mortality. Concern over cost and the potential for the emergence of resistant organisms have also limited the use of selective decontamination of the digestive tract.

15. In intubated patients, does the site of the tube (nasotracheal versus orotracheal) affect the risk of pneumonia?

The risk for nosocomial sinusitis and pneumonia appears to be increased in patients intubated via the nasotracheal route. In a surgical intensive care unit 162 patients requiring mechanical ventilation were evaluated with CT scans of the sinuses. Those with opacified sinuses at the beginning of the study were more likely to develop nosocomial pneumonia after 7 days of mechanical ventilation than those with normal sinuses. Patients intubated via the nasotracheal route for more than 7 days were more likely to develop opacification of their sinuses than patients intubated via the orotracheal route. Another study of 300 patients demonstrated no significant difference in the incidence of nosocomial sinusitis and pneumonia between patients who were either orally or nasotracheally intubated. There was, however, a trend toward more infections of both types (not statistically significant) in the nasotracheally intubated group.

16. Do H$_2$ blockers, antacids, and sucralfate increase susceptibility to nosocomial pneumonia?
The risk of nosocomial pneumonia appears to be increased when gastric pH is raised with H$_2$ blockers or antacids. The normally acid environment of the stomach is generally protective against bacterial colonization, and several studies have shown an increased incidence of gastric colonization in patients receiving stress ulcer prophylaxis with H$_2$ blockers or antacids. Intubated patients have a high incidence of contamination of the tracheobronchial tree with gastric contents, which may predispose them to pulmonary infection. Several studies have compared the incidence of nosocomial pneumonia in patients receiving H$_2$ blockers or antacids with the incidence in patients receiving sulcralfate. Many, but not all, of these studies have supported the use of sulcralfate instead of H$_2$ blockers or antacids to prevent stress ulceration because the risk of developing nosocomial pneumonia is lower. Sucralfate may decrease the incidence of nosocomial pneumonia not only by maintaining a low gastric pH but also by a direct bactericidal effect or by inhibiting bacterial translocation through the gut wall.

IMMUNOCOMPROMISED PATIENTS

17. What measures should be taken to prevent pneumonia in immunocompromised patients?
HIV-infected individuals and recipients of organ transplants (solid organ and bone marrow) should receive influenza and pneumococcal vaccines. HIV-infected individuals who have CD4+ lymphocyte counts of less than 200×10^6/liter or who have had previous *Pneumocystis carinii* pneumonia (PCP) should also receive prophylaxis against PCP. Transplant recipients are at risk for developing PCP and should receive prophylaxis soon after transplantation. The duration of prophylactic therapy may vary from months to 1 year postoperatively, or therapy may be restarted if the immunosuppressive regimen is increased. Other patients at risk for PCP are patients with leukemia and patients receiving corticosteroids for primary or metastatic brain cancer. The dose and duration of corticosteroid therapy that are associated with increased risk vary. In one study of 142 patients, the median maximal dose of prednisone was 80 mg per day for a median duration of 3 months. Seven of these 142 patients developed PCP within 1 month of starting prednisone. Transplant recipients who are cytomegalovirus (CMV) seropositive or receive organs from CMV-seropositive donors should receive prophylaxis against CMV infections (including CMV pneumonitis). Prophylaxis against CMV is most successful in patients who are CMV seropositive; success varies in seronegative patients. Most commonly used regimens include ganciclovir before and for a few weeks after transplantation; some include acyclovir.

18. What is the most effective agent for prophylaxis against *Pneumocystis carinii* pneumonia?
Three agents are currently in widespread use for the prevention of PCP:
• Oral trimethoprim-sulfamethoxazole (TMP-SMX), one double-strength tablet daily or one double-strength tablet three times a week (both doses appear to be equally efficacious)
• Oral dapsone, 100 mg daily
• Inhaled pentamidine, 300 mg monthly via a Respirgard II nebulizer
A recent randomized, open label trial compared the efficacy of these three drugs in 843 patients with HIV infection and less than 200×10^6 CD4+ lymphocytes per liter. In patients with more than 100×10^6 CD4+ lymphocytes per liter, there was no difference in the 36-month cumulative risk of PCP with any of the three drugs. In patients with less than 100×10^6 CD4+

lymphocytes per liter, however, the highest success rates of preventing PCP were with TMP-SMX and with high dose (100 mg/day) dapsone.

19. What drug should be used to treat a patient who develops *Pneumocystis carinii* pneumonia while on PCP prophylaxis?

There is no evidence that the choice of a drug to treat PCP should be influenced by which drug is used for prophylaxis; i.e., the use of a drug for prophylaxis in a given patient does not preclude its use for treatment of disease in that patient. The doses used for treatment of PCP are much higher than those used for prophylaxis, and there have been no reports of drug-resistant *P. carinii* as a result of prophylaxis. Choosing a treatment regimen depends more on the severity of the patient's illness and history of allergy or intolerance to any of the commonly used drugs. Currently used drugs for the treatment of PCP include TMP-SMX, trimethoprim-dapsone, clindamycin-primaquine, atovaquone, pentamidine, and trimetrexate. Corticosteroids are added in cases of severe illness caused by *P. carinii*.

MISCELLANEOUS

20. What can be done to prevent pneumonia in patients who chronically aspirate?

Chronic aspiration can be a difficult problem in patients with dysphagia resulting from strokes, severe debilitation, or head and neck surgery. Some simple techniques to help reduce aspiration are diet modification to include foods that are easily swallowed and the use of compensatory swallowing techniques. Chin tuck, multiple swallows, liquid assist, and head turn are techniques that improve swallowing efficiency in some patients. Patients who are unable to swallow often must be fed through a nasogastric or gastrostomy tube. The incidence of aspiration in these patients can be decreased if an upright position is maintained during feeding. For some patients with severe, intractable aspiration, surgical laryngotracheal separation techniques have been successful. These techniques may interfere with speech, although many patients with intractable aspiration have also lost the capacity for speech as a result of their underlying disease. Only about one third of patients are able to resume a regular diet after surgery, and more than half need to be maintained on tube feedings.

BIBLIOGRAPHY

1. Bozzette SA, Finklestein DM, Spector SA, et al: A randomized trial of three antipneumocystis agents in patients with advanced human immunodeficiency virus infection. N Engl J Med 332:693–699, 1995.
2. Cook DJ, Reeve BK, Guyatt GH, et al: Stress ulcer prophylaxis in critically ill patients. Resolving discordant meta-analyses. JAMA 275:308–314, 1996
3. deBoisblanc BP, Castro M, Everret B, et al: Effect of air-supported, continuous, postural oscillation on the risk of early ICU pneumonia in nontraumatic critical illness. Chest 103:1543–1547, 1993.
4. DePippo KL, Holas MA, Reding MJ, et al: Dysphagia therapy following stroke: A controlled trial. Neurology 44:1655–1660, 1994.
5. Duncan SR, Grgurich WF, Iacono AT, et al: A comparison of ganciclovir and acyclovir to prevent cytomegalovirus after lung transplantation. Am J Respir Crit Care Med 150:146–152, 1994.
6. Eibling DE, Snyderman CH, Eibling C: Laryngotracheal separation for intractable aspiration: A retrospective review of 34 patients. Laryngoscope 105:83–85, 1995.
7. Ferrer M, Torres A, González J, et al: Utility of selective decontamination of the digestive tract in mechanically ventilated patients. Ann Intern Med 120:389–395, 1994.
8. Fine MJ, Smith MA, Carson CA, et al: Efficacy of pneumococcal vaccination in adults. A meta-analysis of randomized controlled trials. Arch Intern Med 154:2666–2677, 1994.
9. Fink MP, Helsmoortel CM, Stein KL, et al: The efficacy of an oscillating bed in the prevention of lower respiratory tract infection in critically ill victims of blunt trauma. Chest 97:132–137, 1990.
10. Garcia-Bustos J, Tomasz A: A biological price of antibiotic resistance: Major changes in the peptidoglycan structure of penicillin-resistant pneumococci. Proc Natl Acad Sci USA 87:5415–5419, 1990.
11. Gillespie SH: Aspects of pneumococcal infection including bacterial virulence, host response and vaccination. J Med Microbiol 28:237–248, 1989.
12. Grekas D, Alivanis P, Kiriazopoulou C, et al: Influenza vaccination on renal transplant patients is safe and serologically effective. Int J Clin Pharmacol Ther Toxicol 31:553–556, 1993.

13. Hamilos DL, Young RM, Peter JB, et al: Hypogammaglobulinemia in asthmatic patients. Ann Allergy 68:472–481, 1992.
14. Hammond J, Potgieter PD, Saunders GL: Selective decontamination of the digestive tract in multiple trauma patients—is there a role? Results of a prospective, double-blind, randomized trial. Crit Care Med 22:33–39, 1994.
15. Hansten PD, Horn JR: Drug Interactions and Updates. Malvern, PA, Lea & Febiger, 1994.
16. Holzapfel L, Chevret SD, Madinier G, et al: Influence of long-term oro- or nasotracheal intubation on nosocomial maxillary sinusitis and pneumonia: Results of a prospective, randomized, clinical trial. Crit Care Med 21:1132–1138, 1993.
17. Jamin M, Damblon C, Millier S, et al: Penicillin-binding protein 2x of *Streptococcus pneumoniae*; enzymatic activities and interactions with β-lactams. Biochem J 292:735–741, 1993.
18. Johnson CC, Finegold SM: Pyogenic bacterial pneumonia, lung abscess, and empyema. In Murray JF, Nadel JA (eds): Textbook of Respiratory Medicine, Vol. 1. Philadelphia, W.B. Saunders, 1994, pp 1047–1050.
19. Kelley RE, Vibulsresth S, Bell L, et al: Evaluation of kinetic therapy in the prevention of complications of prolonged bed rest secondary to stroke. Stroke 18:638–642, 1987.
20. Kollef MH: Ventilator-associated pneumonia. A multivariate analysis. JAMA 270:1965–1970, 1993.
21. Kollef MH: The role of selective digestive tract decontamination on mortality and respiratory tract infections. A meta-analysis. Chest 105:1101–1108, 1994.
22. Korinek AM, Laisne MJ, Nicolas MH, et al: Selective decontamination of the digestive tract in neuorsur- ̄gical intensive care patients: A double-blind, randomized, placebo-controlled study. Crit Care Med 21:1466–1473, 1993.
23. Kramer MR, Stoehr C, Lewiston NJ, et al: Trimethoprim-sulfamethoxazole prophylaxis for *Pneumocystis carinii* infections in heart-lung and lung transplantation—how effective and for how long? Transplantation 53:586–589, 1992.
24. Kroon FP, van Dissel JT, De Jong JC, et al: Antibody response to influenza, tetanus and pneumococcal vaccines in HIV-seropositive individuals in relation to the number of CD+ lymphocytes. AIDS 8:469–476, 1994.
25. Lahood N, Emerson SS, Kumar P, et al: Antibody levels and response to pneumococcal vaccine in steroid-dependent asthma. Ann Allergy 70:289–294, 1993.
26. Merigan TC, Renlund DG, Keay S, et al: A controlled trial of ganciclovir to prevent cytomegalovirus disease after heart transplantation. N Engl J Med 326:1182–1186, 1992.
27. Nichol KL, Margolis KL, Wuorenma J, et al: The efficacy and cost effectiveness of vaccination against influenza among elderly persons living in the community. N Engl J Med 331:778–784, 1994.
28. Ortiz CR, La Force FM: Prevention of community-acquired pneumonia. Med Clin North Am 78:1173–1183, 1994.
29. Prevention and control of influenza. Recommendations of the Immunization Practices Advisory Committee (ACIP). MMWR 44:1–22, 1995.
30. Recommendations of the Immunization Practices Advisory Committee. Pneumococcal polysaccharide vaccine. MMWR 38:64–68; 73–76, 1989.
31. Rodrigquez-Barradas MC, Musher DM, Lahart C, et al: Antibody to capsular polysaccharides of *Streptococcus pneumoniae* after vaccination of human immunodeficiency virus-infected subjects with 23-valent penumococcal vaccine. J Infect Dis 165:553–556, 1992.
32. Rouby J-J, Laurent P, Gosnach M, et al: Risk factors and clinical relevance of nosocomial maxillary sinusitis in the critically ill. Am J Respir Crit Care Med 150:776–783, 1994.
33. Selective Decontamination of the Digest Tract Trialists' Collaborative Group: Meta-analysis of randomised controlled trials of selective decontamination of the digestive tract. BMJ 307:525–532, 1993.
34. Sepkowitz KA: *Pneumocystis carinii* pneumonia in patients without AIDS. Clin Infect Dis 17:S416–S422, 1993.
35. Sepkowitz KA, Brown AE, Telzak EE, et al: *Pneumocystis carinii* pneumonia among patients without AIDS at a cancer hospital. JAMA 267:832–837, 1992.
36. Stockley IH: Drug Interactions. A Source Book of Adverse Interactions, Their Mechanisms, Clinical Importance and Management. Oxford, Blackwell Scientific Publications, 1994.
37. Summer WR, Curry P, Haponik EF, et al: Continuous turning of intensive care unit patients shortens length of stay in some diagnostic-related groups. J Crit Care 4:45–53, 1989.
38. Torres A, Serra-Batlles J, Ros E, et al: Pulmonary aspiration of gastric contens in patients receiving mechanical ventilation: The effect of body position. Ann Intern Med 116:540–543, 1992.
39. Update on adult immunization: Recommendations of the Immunization Practices Advisory Committee (ACIP). MMWR 40:42–44, 1991.
40. Whiteman K, Nachtmann L, Kramer D, et al: Effects of continuous lateral rotation therapy on pulmonary complications in liver transplant patients. Am J Crit Care 4:133–139, 1995.
41. Winston DJ, Ho WG, Bartoni K, et al: Ganciclovir prophylaxis of cytomegalovirus infection and disease in allogeneic bone marrow transplant recipients. Ann Intern Med 118:179–184, 1993.

32. EMPYEMA AND LUNG ABSCESS

Jamie Marie Bigelow, M.D., and V. Courtney Broaddus, M.D.

1. What is a parapneumonic effusion?

A parapneumonic effusion is a neutrophilic exudative effusion adjacent to a lung with pneumonia. It can resolve either with antibiotics alone or can require drainage in addition to antibiotics. As a pneumonia progresses, inflammatory pulmonary liquid leaks into the pleural space, first appearing as an uncomplicated effusion. At this point, the effusion could presumably resolve with antibiotic therapy alone. As bacteria and inflammatory cells follow, the inflammatory process is marked by anaerobic metabolism, cytokine production, intrapleural fibrin deposition, and thickening of the pleural membranes. The later stages are generally referred to as a *complicated effusion* or *empyema*. Antibiotics may not be sufficient for resolution, and drainage of the highly inflammatory liquid may be necessary. Empyema may be parapneumonic (associated with pneumonia) or caused by spread of infection to the pleural space from other locations such as the intraabdominal or mediastinal spaces.

2. Define empyema.

There is no universally accepted definition of empyema. Operationally, the term can be used to identify highly inflammatory pleural fluids that require drainage in addition to antibiotics for resolution. Frank pus (thick, purulent liquid) in the pleural space is an empyema and this, in fact, constitutes the original and literal meaning of the term. However, most clinicians include in the term *empyema* all pleural effusions that are not grossly purulent but contain microorganisms as identified by a positive Gram stain or culture. In addition, there are many highly inflammatory parapneumonic effusions that behave as if they are infected although microorganisms are never identified. These have been described as "complicated" parapneumonic effusions and are identified clinically by a pH of less than 7.1 and a glucose level of less than 40 mg per dl. We extend the definition of empyema to these effusions as well because they behave as if they are infected and generally require drainage as well as antibiotic therapy.

3. Why are a low glucose level and a low pH clinically relevant variables for identifying empyema?

A low glucose and pH are indicators of both increased anaerobic cellular metabolism within the pleural liquid and a block to diffusion across the pleura. As bacteria invade the pleural space, they and the polymorphonuclear leukocytes that accompany them metabolize the glucose to lactic acid and carbon dioxide, which together lower the pH. The infection also results in fibrin deposition and organization of the pleural space into a thick peel. This peel prevents normalization of the pH and glucose level by blocking the diffusion of carbon dioxide out of and glucose into the pleural space.

4. What pathogens are likely to be found in lung abscesses and empyema? What are the risk factors that predict the presence of these pathogens?

In the preantibiotic era, pneumococcal infection was the most common cause of lung abscess and empyema. Currently, however, because patients with pneumococcal infection often present early with intense symptoms, they tend to be given antibiotics before empyema or lung abscess has time to develop. The most common cause of empyema and lung abscess today is a more indolent, polymicrobial infection, usually involving both aerobes and anaerobes.

The major risk factor for the development of lung abscess or empyema is aspiration. Conditions predisposing patients to aspiration, such as alcoholism, seizures, or stroke, are associated with an increased incidence of lung abscess and empyema. The presence of poor dentition increases the anaerobic bacterial load in the mouth and thus, the likelihood of infection after an aspiration event. Other conditions that predispose the lung to polymicrobic or anaerobic infections include obstruction by foreign body or tumor, bronchiectasis, and pulmonary infarction. A large number of these infections may be prevented by measures that reduce the incidence of aspiration.

The changing nature of medicine over the last century has also led to an increase in infections caused by nosocomial pathogens. The movement of the medical practice from the home to the hospital is a factor in this change. Iatrogenic immunosuppression by steroids or chemotherapy and prolonged antibiotic use also increase patients' predisposition to these infections. The incidence of postprocedure empyema and abscess has increased with the advent of thoracic surgical procedures ranging from thoracentesis to thoracotomy. Pathogens to be considered in this situation include gram-negative rods, staphylococci, and antibiotic-resistant organisms.

5. What antibiotics are recommended for empiric coverage of empyema or lung abscess?

Initial antibiotic coverage in empyema and lung abscess should be empiric, based on the patient's predisposition for particular organisms.

Lung abscess. For aspiration-related infection, the antibiotic chosen should reflect the predominance of anaerobes. In trials of empiric therapy for lung abscess, clindamycin showed superiority over penicillin, probably because the incidence of penicillin-resistant anaerobes in lung abscesses is 15–20%. Infections from an abdominal source should be treated with metronidazole, which better covers the clindamycin-resistant anaerobes frequently found in the bowel. Metronidazole alone, however, is not sufficient for aspiration because it does not treat the microaerophilic and aerobic streptococci found in mouth flora. Other drugs that have excellent in vitro activity against anaerobes include imipenem, chloramphenicol and combinations of the β-lactam/β-lactamase inhibitors, although they have not yet been subjected to clinical trials for the treatment of lung abscess.

If the patient is at risk for infection with nosocomial organisms, the antibiotic should be broadened to cover gram-negative bacteria, staphylococci, and perhaps antibiotic-resistant organisms. Second- or third-generation cephalosporins have good activity against most gram-negative bacteria, as does aztreonam or combinations of β-lactam/β-lactamase inhibitors. Methicillin-sensitive staphylococcus is well covered by clindamycin, the synthetic penicillins, and most cephalosporins. Antibiotic coverage of resistant organisms should be tailored to the particular organisms prevalent in the institution where the patient was exposed.

Empyema. The treatment of empyema has not undergone comparative antibiotic trials. Because the pathogens are similar to those causing lung abscess, the antibiotic choice can be similar. In most cases, a reasonable choice for initial empiric therapy would include clindamycin combined with a third-generation cephalosporin or, for single-agent therapy, imipenem or ticarcillin-clavulanic acid. Aminoglycosides are not effective in the treatment of empyema; their penetration into the pleural space is poor, and their activity in the pleural space is reduced as a result of the low pH and oxygen tension of that environment. If cultures are obtained, specific antibiotics can be aimed at the recovered pathogen, although other pathogens, particularly anaerobes, that may not have been cultured should nonetheless be considered for coverage.

6. How are accurate specimens obtained for culture in lung abscess and empyema?

Expectorated sputum is not accurate for diagnosis in lung abscess and empyema because it is frequently contaminated with oral flora and anaerobes cannot be recovered from it. Bronchoscopic specimens have limited value for the same reasons. Protected brush and quantitative culture techniques have been developed to overcome these obstacles but have not been validated in this situation. Transtracheal aspiration is a reliable technique for the collection of accurate specimens, particularly for the culture of anaerobes, but it is no longer taught in most training programs. Pleural fluid obtained via thoracentesis or thoracostomy tube or abscess contents obtained via transthoracic aspiration are valid specimens for anaerobic culture.

7. Can a lung abscess be distinguished from an empyema on chest radiograph?

The distinction between a lung abscess and an empyema is important because percutaneous drainage is recommended for empyema but not necessarily for lung abscess. Often the chest radiograph shows a peripheral density that may represent a fluid collection in either the lung or the pleural space. Frequently loculated, an empyema may not move on decubitus views, further confusing its distinction from a lung abscess. One radiographic clue to a pleural origin of the lesion is that the width of the density, or particularly of an air-fluid level within the density, is unequal in the frontal and lateral views. Unequal dimensions point to an oblong shape and probable location in the pleural space; equal dimensions point to a spherical shape and probable location in the lung parenchyma (Fig. 1).

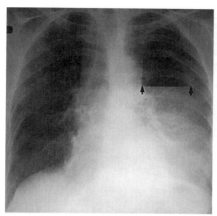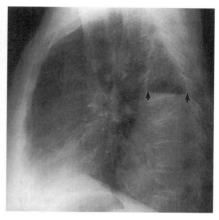

FIGURE 1.   Posteroanterior and lateral chest radiographic views of a large air-fluid level several days after an esophageal dilatation procedure in a 66-year-old woman with achalasia. The difference in length of the meniscus in the two projections *(arrows)* suggests a pleural, rather than parenchymal, location.

Nevertheless, a CT scan is often necessary to distinguish a peripheral lung abscess from an empyema. An empyema on CT scan appears as an oval and forms an obtuse angle with the chest wall. The wall of the empyema, formed by the visceral and parietal pleural membranes, is seen as two contrast-enhancing lines that separate to surround the inflammatory pleural fluid. This finding is called the "split pleura" sign (Fig. 2). In contrast, lung abscess appears as a rounded intrapulmonary mass that contacts the chest wall at an acute angle and contains central cavitation or necrosis (Fig. 3). Typically, the wall of the abscess is thick with an irregular inner margin. The CT scan can also reveal more extensive pleural involvement than suspected on the plain film, compression of adjacent lung, underlying pathology such as obstructing lung tumors or bronchiectasis, malposition of chest tubes, or complications such as bronchopleural fistula or mediastinal involvement. Thus, a CT scan can provide additional information for diagnostic and therapeutic decision-making, particularly when the initial diagnosis is unclear on chest radiograph or when the patient has not responded to initial therapy.

8. When should a parapneumonic pleural effusion or empyema be drained?

Purulent fluid must be drained immediately. It is more difficult to predict which nonpurulent effusions will require surgical drainage and which will resolve with antibiotics alone. Neither the pleural fluid neutrophil count nor the protein concentration has proved to be predictive of the need for drainage. Chemical analysis of the fluid provides more valuable information. A pleural fluid pH of 7.30 or more or a glucose level of 60 mg per dl or more is generally predictive of a good outcome with antibiotics alone, whereas a pH of less than 7.10 or a glucose level of less than 40 mg per dl indicates that drainage of the pleural space will probably be necessary. Patients with an intermediate pleural fluid pH or glucose concentration need to be evaluated either for

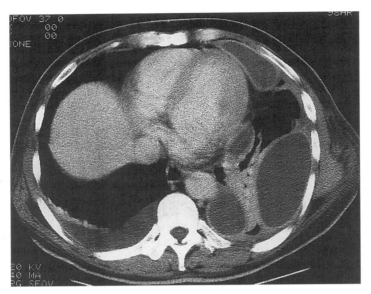

FIGURE 2. Contrast-enhanced CT scan of a patient with empyema shows apparent loculation with at least four separate collections. Pleural enhancement is evident and demonstrates the finding known as the "split pleura sign." At a more caudal level, some of these collections were seen to communicate. The empyema was successfully drained with a single pigtail catheter placed by interventional radiologists.

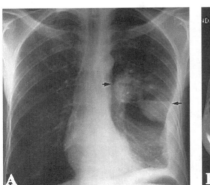 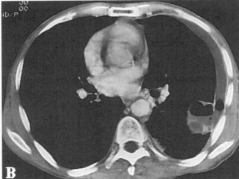

FIGURE 3. **A,** Chest radiograph of a 50-year-old man with a productive cough, fever, and chest pain. Mass-like densities with air-fluid levels are seen *(arrows)* in association with a widened pleural stripe. **B,** CT scan of the chest (at the level of the lower arrow in **A**) shows that the abnormalities consist of fluid collections in both the pleural space and the lung. Thoracentesis revealed pleural empyema (and introduced the air seen in the pleural space); blood cultures later grew *Streptococcus pneumoniae*.

their clinical response to antibiotics or by repeat thoracentesis to determine whether drainage is necessary. Although proposed as the more accurate predictor, pH readings are subject to errors in handling; exposing the fluid to air can lead to a rapid rise in pH as the volatile acid, carbon dioxide, escapes. For that reason, glucose values may be more reliable.

More recently, these criteria have come under some question. Empyema caused by *Streptococcus pneumoniae* frequently resolves with antibiotics alone. In addition, patients with parapneumonic effusions meeting the criteria for tube thoracostomy have been reported to recover with antibiotic therapy alone and patients with parapneumonic effusions not meeting the criteria for tube thoracostomy have been reported to require drainage eventually. Nonetheless, glucose level and pH are the best predictors of clinical course available and are useful guides for therapeutic decisions.

9. How is an empyema drained? What are the factors that determine success?

The standard choice for drainage has been via tube thoracostomy, usually with at least a 32-French tube. If the effusion is free flowing, as demonstrated on a lateral decubitus chest radiograph, chest tube placement usually obtains complete drainage with reexpansion of the lung. If the effusion is not free flowing, however, a single tube is not likely to drain an empyema completely. The decision to place additional chest tubes rests mainly on the clinical course of the patient. A patient may not need complete drainage to respond to therapy. If clinical improvement is not noted, however, it is likely that drainage has not been adequate. Drainage may be inadequate because of obstruction or malposition of the chest tube or the presence of multiple loculations. Ultrasound or CT scan can be useful for assessing tube position in relation to pleural fluid loculations and for directing placement of additional tubes.

10. Do fibrinolytics have a role in the treatment of empyema?

When tube thoracostomy fails to drain a loculated empyema, fibrinolytics may have a role, although there are many questions about their utility. Fibrinolytic agents may improve drainage by lysing fibrin and thus breaking down loculations and reducing the viscosity of the fluid. Theoretically, fibrinolytics should have the greatest benefit early in the course of empyema when fibrin strands have not yet become organized and when there are fewer loculations. Controlled trials of fibrinolytic therapy are needed, however, not only to evaluate its efficacy but also to determine the incidence of complications. For example, the safety profile of fibrinolytics is still an issue. In case reports, acute lung injury and bleeding diathesis have been associated with intrapleural fibrinolytic therapy.

11. When is surgery considered for treatment of empyema?

For the patient who fails to respond to thoracostomy tube drainage, surgery may be considered. If a thick, organized pleural peel or multiple loculations are associated with persistent infection, surgical drainage or decortication, or both, may be necessary. At the time of thoracotomy, the pleural space can be drained completely, adhesions can be removed, and multiple thoracostomy tubes can be placed. A thoracoscopic approach is generally limited by the poor visibility and access because of the extensive pleural disease present in empyema. In patients who are too ill to undergo thoracotomy or for whom the lung cannot be reexpanded to fill the pleural space, rib resection with prolonged open drainage (Eloesser flap) is a viable alternative.

12. What is the clinical course of the patient after successful treatment of empyema?

At the time of discharge from the hospital, the patient frequently has a thickened pleura and restrictive lung function on pulmonary function testing. In most cases, however, the peel resolves within 3 to 6 months, so that decortication of a pleural peel is rarely needed (Fig. 4). Pleural decortication may be considered in symptomatic patients with pleural thickening and lung restriction that persists for more than 6 months after empyema.

13. In addition to antibiotics, what treatment is indicated for a lung abscess?

Before the advent of antibiotics, bronchoscopic drainage or surgical resection was the mainstay of treatment. Now, antibiotics alone are sufficient to treat 80–90% of patients with lung abscess. Drainage can be aided by noninvasive measures such as expectoration with postural drainage or nasotracheal suctioning.

14. When is bronchoscopy considered in a patient with a lung abscess?

Before the advent of antibiotics, bronchoscopy was recommended by many physicians to drain the abscess cavity. In modern times, however, bronchoscopic drainage has shown little advantage over medical therapy alone in the treatment of simple lung abscess. Bronchoscopy also may increase the risk of spillage of abscess contents into normal lung or of hemorrhage.

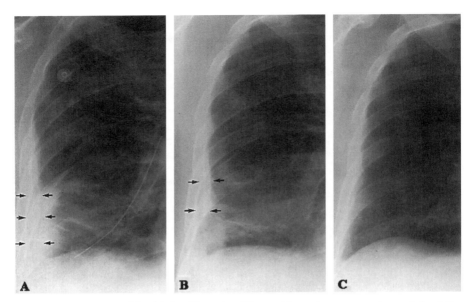

FIGURE 4. Coned view of the right hemithorax in a 57-year-old man shows progressive resolution follow-ing a streptococcal empyema. **A,** Chest thoracostomy tube is in place after 6 days of drainage immediately before its removal preceding the patient's discharge from the hospital. Pleural disease blunts the costophrenic angle and extends up the lateral chest wall. **B,** Four weeks later, on a follow-up visit, pleural thickening is still evident. At this time his vital capacity was 65% of predicted. **C,** Four months later, on a routine visit, the pleura appears nearly normal. His vital capacity also improved to 85% of predicted.

Bronchoscopy is useful diagnostically in patients with lung abscess caused by an obstructing for-eign body or neoplasm.

Careful selection of patients likely to have an obstructing lesion can therefore increase the diagnostic yield of bronchoscopy in this setting. Foreign body aspiration is often suggested by the clinical history. An obstructing neoplasm should be considered in patients without a risk of aspiration who are cigarette smokers over the age of 45. Patients with a lung abscess caused by an obstructing lesion may also have fewer systemic symptoms and less chest pain than those without obstruction. The value of the chest radiograph is limited in this situation. Neither the presence of ipsilateral lymphadenopathy nor the size or wall thickness of the abscess has been found to predict an underlying neoplasm.

15. What are the indications for surgery in the treatment of lung abscess?

There are no clinical trials that assess the indications for surgical resection versus prolonged antibiotic therapy in the treatment of lung abscess. Most of the data addressing this question come from case series. As a result, the indications for surgery have not been standardized. Massive hemoptysis is an indication for immediate surgery or bronchial artery embolization. Other indications for surgical intervention include the presence of an obstructing lesion, contin-ued fever and toxicity for more than 2 weeks, or the persistence of symptoms such as cough, weight loss or hemoptysis despite prolonged antibiotic therapy. Poor clinical status may be an ex-clusion criterion because the risk of surgery in this population is high; the mortality in this setting as reported in various series (and depending on patient selection) ranges from 9 to nearly 30%.

16. What are the alternative approaches to surgical treatment of a lung abscess? When would they be considered?

Catheter drainage has been used as an alternative to surgery in the treatment of lung abscess. There are two basic approaches to this drainage technique, transthoracic or transbronchial. The transthoracic approach involves the percutaneous placement of a catheter across the pleural space and lung parenchyma into the abscess cavity. This procedure is usually guided by ultrasound, fluoroscopy, or CT. The transbronchial approach is less well delineated in the literature. It involves either suction of the abscess contents via the bronchoscope or, because the orifice of the bronchus is often narrowed, bronchoscopic placement of a catheter into the cavity. Although typically this catheter is removed immediately, the literature has descriptions of increased success in abscess resolution when the catheter is maintained over a period of days, allowing for irrigation and continued removal of abscess contents.

These procedures can result in quick resolution of symptoms and decreased hospital stay, leading some physicians to suggest it as a primary therapy in selected patients. However, these procedures are usually considered only after antibiotic therapy has failed to resolve symptoms. Catheter and surgical drainage have not been compared in controlled trials, but comparable success rates are suggested by case reports. The potential advantages of catheter drainage include the sparing of normal lung parenchyma and the avoidance of general operative mortality in this usually debilitated population. Both percutaneous catheter drainage and surgery increase the risk of hemorrhage, of spillage of abscess contents into the pleural space or normal lung, and bronchopleural fistula.

17. What are the possible complications of a lung abscess after the primary infection has resolved?

After the infection clears, a residual abscess cavity may remain and serve as a source of persistent symptoms. Cavities may be prone to recurrent bacterial infection, especially if the predisposing factor, such as aspiration, still exists, or may become colonized by fungi, such as aspergillus. Lung adjacent to the abscess cavity is often bronchiectatic and a site of recurrent infection. Evidence of infection may include productive or nonproductive cough, hemoptysis, or systemic signs such as fever, weight loss, or malaise. When cavities are associated with evidence of persistent infection, surgical resection should be considered.

18. What is the duration of therapy for an empyema or lung abscess? What are the criteria for judging resolution?

The duration of antibiotic therapy for both empyema and lung abscess is several weeks. Antibiotics can be stopped once the patient has improved clinically, as evidenced by an absence of fever, an improved sense of well-being, and a decrease in productive cough. At the time antibiotics are stopped, both chest radiographic and pulmonary function test results still may be abnormal. These often improve over a period of months after the infection is treated.

BIBLIOGRAPHY

1. Bartlett JG: Bacterial infections of the pleural space. Semin Respir Infect 3:308–321, 1988.
2. Bartlett JG: Anaerobic bacterial infections of the lung and pleural space. Clin Infect Dis 16(Suppl 4):S248–S255, 1993.
3. Berger HA, Morganroth ML: Immediate drainage is not required for all patients with complicated parapneumonic effusions. Chest 97:731–735, 1990.
4. Broaddus VC: Infections in the pleural space: An update on pathogenesis and management. Semin Respir Crit Care Med 16:303–314, 1995.
5. Klein JS, Schultz S, Heffner JE: Interventional radiology of the chest: Image-guided percutaneous drainage of pleural effusions, lung abscess, and pneumothorax. Am J Roentgenol 164:581–588, 1995.
6. LeMense GP, Strange C, Sahn SA: Empyema thoracis: Therapeutic management and outcome. Chest 107:1532–1537, 1995.
7. Light RW, Girard WM, Jenkinson SG, et al: Parapneumonic effusions. Am J Med 69:507–512, 1980.
8. McLoud TC, Flower CDR: Imaging the pleura: Songography, CT and MR imaging. Am J Roentgenol 156:1145–1153, 1991.
9. Poe RH, Marin MG, Israel RH, et al: Utility of pleural fluid analysis in predicting tube thoracostomy/decortication in parapneumonic effusions. Chest 100:963–967, 1991.
10. Sahn SA: Management of complicated parapneumonic effusions. Am Rev Respir Dis 148:813–817, 1993.
11. Sosenko A, Glassroth J: Fiberoptic bronchoscopy in the evaluation of lung abscesses. Chest 87:489–494, 1985.

33. PNEUMONIA IN IMMUNOCOMPROMISED PATIENTS

Elizabeth L. Aronsen, M.D.

1. Who are immunocompromised patients?

An immunocompromised patient is anyone who has an altered immune system resulting in an increased risk of infections, such as pneumonia. Excluding AIDS, there are four major (and sometimes overlapping) groups of immunocompromised patients. These groups include patients with the following disorders:

1. Malignancy
2. Solid organ or bone marrow transplant
3. Congenital or acquired primary immunodeficiency
    Humoral immunodeficiencies; examples include:
        Multiple myeloma
        Common variable (acquired) hypogammaglobulinemia
        Thymoma with hypogammaglobulinemia
        Selective IgA or IgG subclass deficiencies
    Cell-mediated immunodeficiencies (CMI); examples include:
        Hairy cell leukemia
        Acute lymphocytic leukemia
        Cartilage hair hypoplasia syndrome
        Human immunodeficiency virus (HIV) syndrome
4. Chronic systemic states or conditions; examples include:
    Collagen vascular disease
    Chronic obstructive pulmonary disease
    Diabetes
    Asplenia
    Uremia
    Hepatic failure
    Malnutrition
    Alcoholism
    Steroid therapy
    Pregnancy
    Aging

2. What are the normal pulmonary defenses against disease?

- **Upper airway.** Nasal ciliated epithelia filter and humidify air.
- **Normal oral flora.** Pathogens cannot colonize patients who have normal oral flora of low virulence.
- **Cough reflexes.** Neural and chemoreceptors of the trachea are activated by noxious stimuli resulting in significant forces of air powered past an intact epiglottis, expelling particulate matter, including infectious organisms. The closed epiglottis itself provides protection against aspiration of oral flora.
- **Mucociliary escalator.** The trachea, bronchi, and membranous bronchioles have specialized mucus-producing secretory cells as well as ciliated cells. These cells act in concert to trap organisms and transport them toward the proximal airway so that the patient can expectorate them in sputum, thus keeping the lower airways and alveoli sterile.
- **Local antimicrobial factors.** Immunoglobulins (Ig) A and G, complement components, surfactant, and alveolar macrophages provide nonspecific antimicrobial defenses for the lung.

- **Specific systemic host responses.** Mechanisms of humoral and cell-mediated immunity (CMI) provide defenses against specific pathogens.

3. How do host defenses become abnormal in immunocompromised patients?

Various host defenses become impaired in different immunodeficiency states. Knowledge of what impairments are most likely to be associated with a specific immunodeficiency state allows the clinician to better predict the most likely infectious or noninfectious pulmonary pathology for a given patient. For example:

- **Upper airway.** Endotracheal tubes, tracheostomy tubes, and tracheoesophageal fistulae (such as might be seen in esophageal cancer) completely bypass the upper airway and its defenses.
- **Oral flora.** Drugs (especially antibiotics), uremia, and alcoholism result in alterations in normal oral flora.
- **Cough.** An altered mental status caused by drug or alcohol sedation, encephalopathy, or coma decreases the cough reflex and increases the risk of aspiration.
- **Mucociliary escalator.** The mucociliary escalator can be altered by abnormalities of either the secretory or the ciliated cells of the system. Abnormal mucus secretion is characteristic of cystic fibrosis. Coordinated ciliary movement is disrupted in primary ciliary dyskinesia syndromes. Mucociliary clearance is also reduced by aspirin therapy, dehydration, or toxic inhalation, as is seen in tobacco abuse.
- **Local antimicrobial factors.** Immunocompromised patients have a variety of impairments in nonspecific local antimicrobial factors. Secretory IgA and complement levels are decreased in malnutrition. Collagen vascular diseases, uremia, and alcoholism also demonstrate hypocomplementemia. Calcium channel blockers inhibit phagocytic properties of alveolar macrophages. Cancer chemotherapeutic agents, but also nonsteroidal antiinflammatory agents (NSAIDs), can result in neutropenia.
- **Specific systemic host responses**

  Humoral immunodeficiencies. In an adult population, the congenital or acquired defects in humoral immunity commonly encountered include multiple myeloma, common variable (acquired) hypogammaglobulinemia, thymoma with hypogammoglobulinemia, and selective IgA or IgG subclass deficiencies. Defects in humoral immunity are associated with recurrent pneumonias and bronchiectasis.

  Cell-mediated immunodeficiencies (CMI). Diseases in adults in which deficiency of CMI predominates include hairy cell leukemia, acute lymphocytic leukemia (ALL), cartilage hair hypoplasia syndrome, malnutrition, and alcoholism. Drug therapy with corticosteroids or cyclosporine also specifically suppress CMI.

  Combined immunodeficiency. Chronic lymphocytic leukemia and Hodgkin's disease are associated with defects in both CMI and humoral immunity. After solid organ or bone marrow transplantation, the result of specific cytotoxic therapy with drugs such as azathioprine or cyclophosphamide. Both CMI and humoral immunity are significantly affected by age and uremia and as a part of Job's syndrome (hypergammaglobulinemia E).

4. What are the causes of infectious pneumonias in immunocompromised patients?

Streptococcus pneumoniae is the most common organism that causes pneumonia in immunocompromised patients. *Haemophilus influenzae, Legionella* spp., *Staphylococcus aureus*, protozoans, fungi, viruses (especially the herpesviruses), and mycobacteria are frequently implicated. *Mycoplasma, Legionella* spp. and *Chlamydia* spp., the causative agents in the so-called atypical pneumonias, may actually represent 20–30% of community-acquired pneumonias. Organisms of low virulence and zoonoses must now be included in the differential diagnosis of infection in the immunocompromised patient. Mortality from *Pneumocystis carinii* pneumonia is up to four times higher in HIV-negative patients immunocompromised as a result of long-term steroid use (e.g., in renal or liver transplants, Wegener's granulomatosis, or malignancies) than in HIV-positive patients. Long-term steroid use also greatly increases the risk of infection caused by *Nocardia* spp. In the elderly, *S. pneumoniae, H. influenzae*, and the influenza viruses are common causes of community-acquired pneumonia. *Mycoplasma pneumoniae* pneumonia is almost never a pathogen in an elderly patient with pneumonia.

5. What is the differential diagnosis of noninfectious causes of pulmonary infiltrates in immunocompromised patients?

Infectious and noninfectious causes of pulmonary infiltrates often present with similar signs and symptoms, including cough, dyspnea, tachycardia, and fever. Noninfectious causes include:

Cardiac and noncardiac pulmonary edema
Pulmonary embolism
Pulmonary hemorrhage
Lymphangitic spread of malignancy
Primary intrathoracic malignancy
Bronchiolitis obliterans organizing pneumonia (BOOP)
Chemical (aspiration) pneumonitis
Cytotoxic or radiation pneumonitis

6. Outline the noninvasive techniques used to diagnose the cause of a pulmonary infiltrate in an immunocompromised patient.

History. Important clues to the cause of pneumonia in the immunocompromised patient are provided by the history, which should include:

Time course of the illness
Associated symptoms
Comorbid disease
Occupational, travel, or other exposure history
Current and recent medications (pulmonary effects of some medications can be delayed 6 months or more.)

Physical examination and radiologic tests. The physical examination is often nonspecific but may include high fever or signs of consolidation. Findings on chest radiograph also are often nonspecific. Pulmonary infiltrates can be primarily alveolar or interstitial or some combination of both. Both physical and radiographic findings can be helpful in prioritizing the differential diagnosis and should not be neglected. CT of the chest, with or without high resolution cuts, may provide additional clues to the diagnosis as well as suggestions for biopsy location.

Laboratory examination and cultures. Laboratory analysis of blood rarely immediately narrows the differential diagnosis but can help in patient care and prognosis. Thrombocytopenia or an abnormal coagulation profile may suggest pulmonary hemorrhage or disseminated intravascular coagulopathy (DIC). Elevated C-reactive protein may suggest bacterial infection. Acute and convalescent antibody titers are used to confirm the diagnosis of infection made by other means. Respiratory samples an be cultured for routine bacterial, viral, mycobacterial, and fungal pathogens. Ideally, samples should be collected before antibiotic therapy is started. Laboratory personnel should be alerted to suspicious organisms and to the clinical picture. Cultures should be kept for an extended period before fastidious organisms such as *Nocardia* spp. are ruled out. Induced sputum can be examined by Gram staining for bacteria, Gomori methenamine silver staining for fungus and *Pneumocystis* spp., and acid-fast staining for *Nocardia* and mycobacteria. Immunocytochemical techniques, if available, provide rapid diagnosis of particular organisms. Finally, the polymerase chain reaction nucleic acid amplification technique is increasingly used to provide rapid early diagnosis of specific viral, fungal, or mycobacterial disease that ordinarily may take weeks to culture, thus eliminating the need for empirical therapy.

7. What invasive techniques are used to determine the cause of a pulmonary infiltrate in an immunocompromised patient?

Often acutely and seriously ill patients require invasive diagnostic techniques. Data must be provided that demonstrate survival advantage before expensive and invasive diagnostic procedures, such as those listed below, are recommended.

Transtracheal or transthoracic fine needle aspiration (FNA). Transtracheal or transthoracic FNA is rarely used anymore because of the unacceptably high associated morbidity.

Fiberoptic bronchoscopy. Fiberoptic bronchoscopy with bronchoalveolar lavage (BAL) or transbronchial biopsy (TBBx) is a common approach because it can be performed rapidly, has minimum morbidity, and provides significant samples for analysis. When viral cultures are performed on BAL samples, more than 90% yield cytomegalovirus (CMV). Other viruses such as herpes, influenza, parainfluenza, rhinovirus, adenovirus, enterovirus, and respiratory syncytial virus (RSV) can also be recovered. BAL neutrophil counts of more than 20% suggest a bacterial cause in the non-neutropenic patient. TBBx yields a diagnosis more than 70% of the time, especially if the pulmonary opacities are centrally located. The benefit of TBBx appears to clearly outweigh the risk in selected patients with renal transplants or hematologic malignancies.

Video-assisted thoracoscopic (VATS) or open-lung biopsy. Lung tissue is often required for definitive diagnosis, and VATS or open-lung biopsy virtually guarantees sufficient tissue to make a diagnosis if a diagnosis is possible. However, since most immunocompromised patients experience recurrent lung disease and do not tolerate repeated surgical procedures, an open or thorascopic biopsy may be an overly aggressive approach. It is important to weigh the benefit of an invasive procedure such as open lung biopsy against the risks, especially because mortality is as high as 25% in patients with acute pulmonary infiltrates and progressive respiratory failure. The VATS approach may significantly reduce this mortality when done by an experienced surgeon.

8. What therapy should be initiated in an immunocompromised patient with pneumonia?
- Assess the severity of the patient's illness, with appropriate triage to ICU if necessary. ICU monitoring should be considered for severe pneumonia, defined as:

Tachypnea (more than 30 breaths/min)	Shock (systolic blood pressure
Arterial hypoxemia	less than 90 mmHG)
(Pao_2/Fio_2 less than 250 mmHg)	Oliguria
Multilobar involvement	Need for mechanical ventilation or vasopressors

- Provide sufficient respiratory support, including mechanical ventilation if required.
- Institute early antimicrobial therapy. In general, the more acutely and seriously ill the patient is, the broader the spectrum of antibiotics used initially. Combination therapy with an acylaminopenicillin and either an aminoglycoside or a third-generation cephalosporin is often recommended initially. Ciprofloxacin in combination with an antipseudomonal penicillin or third-generation cephalosporin will cover *Legionella* spp. and most gram-positive and gram-negative organisms (including double pseudomonal coverage); this combination provides excellent anaerobic coverage as well. Antiviral, antifungal, antiprozoal, or antimycobacterial agents should be considered early in high-risk individuals in the appropriate clinical setting. In neutropenic patients, colony-stimulating factors are often added to promote early bone marrow recovery, although current data are insufficient to prove that they positively affect outcome.
- Tailor antibiotics to the specific patient circumstances whenever possible.
- Provide adequate monitoring. A pulmonary arterial catheter may assist in fluid management and support a diagnosis of cardiovascular dysfunction versus sepsis. In intubated, mechanically ventilated patients, peripheral arterial catheterization for blood pressure monitoring and frequent blood gas sampling may be necessary. Despite the latest technologic advances and broad-spectrum antibiotics, mortality ranges still from 60–80%.

9. What pathogens should be considered in specific immunosuppressed conditions?
- **Congenital or acquired primary immunodeficiency.** Asplenia or defects in humoral immunity increase the risk of encapsulated bacteria. Abnormal CMI increases the risk of viral, fungal, and protozoal infection.
- **Solid organ or bone marrow transplant.** The timing of the acute illness with respect to transplantation increases the likelihood of specific diagnoses. After transplantation up to one-third of patients will experience an infectious complication within the first 8 months.

Early pulmonary infections are more likely to be bacterial or fungal; viral (especially CMV) or protozoal infections occur later (about 8 weeks after transplantation). The transplanted organ itself can be a repository of infectious disease.

- **Recent immunosuppressive medications.** Neutropenia after chemotherapy predisposes the immunocompromised patient to bacterial infection, antithymocyte globulin therapy to CMV infection, and long-term high-dose steroid therapy to pneumonia from *Pneumocystis carinii* or *Nocardia asteroides*.
- **Recent hospitalization** increases the risk of gram-negative organisms and *Staphylococcus aureus*.
- **Travel history and associated nonpulmonary symptoms.** Certain fungi are endemic to various areas of the country (e.g., *Histoplasma* spp. in the Midwest or *Cryptococcus* spp. in the Southwest United States). Diarrhea is more commonly associated with atypical (20%) than typical (4%) pneumonias.
- **Indwelling catheters** increase the risk of colonization and infection by coagulase-negative staphylococci.

10. How can pneumonia be avoided in the immunocompromised patient?

Influenza and pneumococcal vaccines provide prophylaxis against these diseases and should be given to all immunocompromised patients without contraindications. Resolution of the chronic systemic illness, treatment of malignancy, and support of the immunodeficient states with exogenous immunoglobulin are additional methods of reducing serious pulmonary infections. Prophylactic antibiotic and antiviral agents are routinely used in periods of predictable risk, such as immediately after transplantation or during defined neutropenic episodes after chemotherapy.

BIBLIOGRAPHY

 1. Bove P, Ranger W, Pursel S, et al: Evaluation of outcome following open lung biopsy. Am Surg 60:564–570, 1994.
 2. Brown MJ, Miller RR, Muller NL: Acute lung disease in the immunocompromised host: CT and pathologic examination findings. Radiology 190:247–254, 1994.
 3. Brown JS, Cohen J: Bacterial and viral infections in the critically ill immunocompromised host, excluding AIDS. Curr Opin Crit Care 1:358–363, 1995.
 4. Delvenne P, Arrese JE, Thiry A, et al: Detection of cytomegalovirus, *Pneumocystis carinii*, and aspergillus species in bronchoalveolar lavage fluid. Am J Clin Pathol 100:414–418, 1993.
 5. Freifeld AG: Infectious complications in the immunocompromised host. The antimicrobial armamentarium. Hematol Oncol Clin North Am 7:813–839, 1993.
 6. Grossman J, Kahn F: Noninfectious pulmonary disease in the immunocompromised host. Semin Respir Med 10:78–88, 1989.
 7. Janzen DL, Adler BD, Padley SP, Muller NL: Diagnostic success of bronchoscopic biopsy in immunocompromised patients with acute pulmonary disease: Predictive value of disease distribution as shown on CT. AJR 160:21–24, 1993.
 8. Krowka MJ, Rosenow EC III, Hoagland HC: Pulmonary complications of bone marrow transplantation. Chest 87:237–246, 1985.
 9. Leeper KV Jr, Torres A: Community-acquired pneumonia in the intensive care unit. Clin Chest Med 16:155–171, 1995.
10. Marcy TW, Reynolds HY: Pulmonary consequences of congenital and acquired immunodeficiency states. Clin Chest Med 10:503–519, 1989.
11. Primack SL, Muller NL: High-resolution computed tomography in acute diffuse lung disease in the immunocompromised patient. Radiol Clin North Am 32:731–744, 1994.
12. Skerrett SJ, Niederman MS, Fein AM: Respiratory infections and acute lung injury in systemic illness. Clin Chest Med 10: 469–502, 1989.
13. Stover DE: Diagnosis of pulmonary disease in the immunocompromised host. Semin Respir Med 10:89–100, 1989.
14. Woodhead M: Pneumonia in the elderly. J Antimicrob Chemother 34(Suppl AP):85–92, 1994.

34. TUBERCULOSIS

Neil W. Schluger, M.D.

1. What is a positive tuberculin test?

A properly administered tuberculin test, consisting of 5 tuberculin units (TU) of new tuberculin injected intradermally (usually on the volar forearm), should be read 48–72 hours after placement, and the amount of induration (not erythema) should be recorded. Reactions that consist solely of erythema usually reflect an IgE response and do not indicate a true delayed hypersensitivity response. The American Thoracic Society's guidelines for the amount of induration that should be considered positive are as follows:

- **5 mm.** Persons with HIV infection, close contacts of patients with infectious disease, and those with fibrotic lesions on chest radiograph.
- **10 mm.** Other high-risk persons, including infants and children under age 4, health care workers, recent immigrants from countries with a high prevalence of tuberculosis, recent converters (persons whose skin tests were negative within the past 2 years), medically underserved low-income populations, residents of long-term care facilities (nursing homes, mental institutions, and correctional facilities), persons with medical conditions known to increase risk of reactivation of tuberculosis (end-stage renal disease, silicosis, diabetes mellitus, injection drug use, malnutrition, prolonged immunosuppressive therapy), and persons with certain hematologic or reticuloendothelial cell malignancies.
- **15 mm.** All other persons.

The American Thoracic Society recommends that "persons who are not likely to be infected with *Mycobacterium tuberculosis* should generally not be skin tested because the predicted value of a skin test in low risk populations is poor." (See reference 1 in Bibliography.)

2. When is skin testing with second-strength tuberculin indicated?

The standard tuberculin test contains 5 TU of purified protein derivative (PPD). This dose of tuberculin has been shown to have a dose-response relationship to prior exposure to tuberculosis, so that the majority of persons with no prior history of tuberculosis exposure will have a negative test. Furthermore, radiographic evidence of previous tuberculosis correlates with a positive skin test using the 5-TU dose. For these reasons, the 5-TU dose has replaced the 1-TU dose (so-called first-strength) dose in routine testing.

If a second-strength tuberculin dose of 250 TU is used for skin testing, the frequency of positive reactions seems unrelated to prior tuberculosis exposure, and there is no correlation between radiographic evidence of prior tuberculosis and skin test results. Additionally, there is significant cross-reactivity between *M. tuberculosis* and other mycobacterial species. For these reasons, the 250-TU second-strength tuberculin should no longer be used.

3. How should a positive tuberculin test be interpreted in a person who has received vaccination with bacille Calmette-Guérin ?

Vaccination with *Mycobacterium bovis*, strain bacille Calmette-Guérin (BCG), is used to prevent tuberculosis in many countries, despite long-standing controversy about its efficacy. A recent meta-analysis concluded that the vaccine has 50% efficacy in preventing mortality from tuberculosis, and also may reduce the number of cases of miliary disease and meningitis. Because of the frequent immigration to the United States of persons from countries where immunization with BCG is practiced, it is likely that many health care providers will see patients with positive tuberculin tests who have also received BCG.

Both protective immunity and the cutaneous delayed hypersensitivity response associated with BCG vaccination disappear 10–15 years after immunization. For persons vaccinated in childhood, therefore, a positive tuberculin skin test as an adult is overwhelmingly likely to represent true tuberculosis infection rather than an effect of BCG. Thus, current recommendations are to ignore any prior history of BCG administration in the interpretation of a tuberculin skin test. This is certainly the case for persons known to be close contacts with those of active disease and persons with a large area of induration. Such patients should receive preventive isoniazid therapy. If a person has been recently vaccinated and has no recent tuberculosis contacts, a positive tuberculin skin test of 5–10 mm of induration may reflect BCG administration.

4. Who should receive preventive therapy for tuberculosis infection?

Persons with tuberculosis infection (a positive tuberculin test but no clinical or radiographic evidence of tuberculosis) are candidates for preventive therapy. All persons under 35 years of age who have tuberculosis infection should receive preventive therapy. Because of the increased risk of serious hepatotoxicity in persons over age 35, therapy in that age group should be reserved for those at increased risk of developing tuberculosis disease: persons who are HIV-seropositive, recent skin test converters, close contacts of those with active disease, recent immigrants from high-prevalence countries, and those with medical conditions that increase the risk of developing active disease (e.g., prolonged immunosuppression, end-stage renal disease, malnutrition, diabetes mellitus, silicosis, rapid unexplained weight loss, postgastrectomy states). Therapy consists of 6–12 months of isoniazid, either daily or twice weekly.

5. What is the initial diagnostic approach in a patient with suspected tuberculosis?

Clinical symptoms, chest radiography, and sputum smear examination are the mainstays of rapid diagnosis. Ultimate diagnosis rests on identification of *M. tuberculosis* in culture or demonstration of a definite clinical response to therapy. Promising diagnostic techniques such as those employing DNA amplification may have substantial impact on tuberculosis diagnosis in the future but are not currently in wide use. In most reported series, sputum smear examination is positive in 50–75% of patients with tuberculosis. Smears are more often positive in patients with cavitary disease and less often positive in patients with HIV infection who often present with manifestations of primary tuberculosis. Thus, when managing a patients with suspected tuberculosis whose sputum examination is negative, the clinician has two choices: institute therapy empirically and wait either for sputum culture results (which take 2–12 weeks) or clinical improvement (also 2–12 weeks) or pursue further testing. The test most commonly employed next is flexible bronchoscopy.

6. Should bronchoscopy be performed in patients with suspected tuberculosis who have negative sputum smears?

Bronchoscopy seems to be able to diagnose tuberculosis immediately in 35–50% of cases of smear-negative tuberculosis. The highest yield during bronchoscopy appears to come not from bronchoalveolar lavage, which infrequently shows acid-fast bacilli, but from transbronchial biopsy specimens, which show acid-fast bacilli or necrotizing granulomata.

The benefits of bronchoscopy must be weighed against its risks, which include bleeding and pneumothorax for the patient and possible nosocomial transmission of tuberculosis for the bronchoscopist. In view of the these risks, a prudent approach to the diagnosis of sputum smear negative patients with suspected tuberculosis is as follows: if expectorated sputum smears are negative, induced sputum samples should be obtained. If those are negative, empiric therapy should be instituted, and clinical response assessed while cultures are awaited. Bronchoscopy should be reserved for patients in whom the risks of empiric therapy are significant or in whom the differential diagnosis is wide and includes entities requiring early and specific treatment. Many patients with HIV infection fall into the latter group. When bronchoscopy is performed, it should be done in a setting with proper environmental and personal respiratory controls.

7. Which patients with tuberculosis should be admitted to the hospital?

The decision to admit a patient with tuberculosis to the hospital is more often based on social factors than medical ones. Most patients with tuberculosis are not physically sick enough to require hospitalization, although patients with hemoptysis, meningitis, pericarditis, severe malnutrition, or impending respiratory failure should be admitted to the hospital for evaluation and treatment. In the absence of these features, the decision to admit a patient with tuberculosis usually rests with a judgment about in which setting, in or out of the hospital, the patient is likely to pose a greater infectious hazard. Admission may be beneficial for patients who would otherwise expose large numbers of vulnerable individuals, such as children or persons with illness or immunosuppression. Admission may also be justified to initiate a course of therapy if there is concern about adherence or adverse effects from medication. If a decision not to admit a patient with tuberculosis is made, the treating physician must take steps to insure adherence to therapy and have a strategy of monitoring that adherence.

8. For how long should patients with tuberculosis be isolated?

Patients are kept in isolation until they are no longer infectious. Although infectiousness of a tuberculosis patient is difficult to quantify, several clinical characteristics are correlated with a high degree of infectiousness. These include a positive sputum smear showing acid-fast bacilli, cavitary lesions on chest radiograph, coughing, and no treatment. Patients with laryngeal tuberculosis are believed to be highly infectious. Prompt institution of therapy is certainly the mainstay of reducing infectiousness; after 2 weeks of effective chemotherapy, most patients will no longer be infectious to any great degree, particularly if cough has subsided and clinical improvement is evident. Conversion to sputum smear negativity as documented by 3 consecutive days of no demonstrable organisms on smear also provides evidence of a low infectious risk and should be a minimum criterion for discontinuing isolation. It may be prudent to isolate patients with multidrug-resistant tuberculosis for longer periods, such as the time needed for sputum cultures to become negative.

9. Should patients with extrapulmonary tuberculosis be isolated?

Patients with extrapulmonary tuberculosis are not infectious and do not require isolation. On rare occasions, certain of these patients pose an infectious risk and infection control procedures become important. For example, patients with tuberculous septic arthritis who require open irrigation of the joint space may present an infectious risk because of aerosolization of organisms. Additionally, a few patients with tuberculosis lymphadenitis will have spontaneous drainage and infectious material also may become aerosolized. Covering the wound with a dressing is important in such cases.

10. What is the infectious risk to health care providers caring for patients with tuberculosis?

The risk to health care providers of infection with *M. tuberculosis* depends on the intensity and duration of exposure to infectious patients. Those performing procedures during which respiratory droplet nuclei are likely to be created (i.e., bronchoscopy, endotracheal intubation and suctioning, or sputum induction) have the highest risk. Several recent studies have indicated that in hospitals with up-to-date infection control procedures, the annual rate of skin test conversion among employees overall is about 1%. However, earlier studies indicated that up to 11% of pulmonary fellows in training become tuberculin skin test–positive during their training, as compared with 1% of infectious disease trainees, the disparity caused partly by exposure during bronchoscopy.

Occupational risk of tuberculosis infection can be reduced by using a hierarchy of control measures. Administrative controls aimed at prompt isolation of tuberculosis suspects and prompt institution of therapy for known cases are undoubtedly the most important measures. Environmental controls, such as the use of germicidal ultraviolet irradiation, high efficiency air filters, and proper ventilation, constitute the next level of control. Finally, proper use of personal particulate respirators (standard surgical masks provide no real protection when worn by health care workers) may provide additional benefit, particularly for those at highest risk of exposure.

11. How should patients with tuberculosis be transported through the hospital?

Most exposures during transport through the hospital are likely to be brief and not associated with an increased risk of tuberculosis transmission. However, several precautions that are prudent and easy to carry out should be used. First, the patient should not leave the room except for tests and procedures that are absolutely necessary, and the patient should wear a mask whenever outside the room. The area to which the patient is to be transported should be notified in advance so that exposure to other patients and personnel can be minimized. Whenever possible, tuberculosis patients should be scheduled at the end of the day. A private elevator should be used for transport. If the patient being transported wears a mask continually, it is probably not necessary for the personnel transporting the patient or performing a test to wear particulate respirators. Finally, if certain tests or procedures are being performed commonly on tuberculosis patients (e.g, sputum induction), those locations should be renovated to ensure adequate ventilation and filtration of air, and an ultraviolet germicidal irradiation device should be installed.

12. What type of contact investigation should be done when a case of tuberculosis is detected?

Contact investigations are important public health measures because they can identify those persons at greatest risk for developing active tuberculosis after infection, and they can lead to the institution of effective chemopreventive therapy. Contact investigation should follow the concentric circle model; i.e., initial investigation should focus on those persons with the closest and most intense exposure to the index case, and the investigation should be expanded until a level of contact is reached that has no persons with evidence of recent infection. The concentric circle model applies to a contact investigation either inside or outside the hospital. All persons being investigated should have a tuberculin test, and if a test is negative, it should be repeated 12 weeks after the contact was known to have occurred. Contacts should also be questioned closely for symptoms, and any person with a positive tuberculin test or symptoms suggestive of tuberculosis should be evaluated clinically and with a chest radiograph. Persons known to have had a positive tuberculin skin test before exposure to the index case do not need chest radiographs unless they have symptoms suggestive of active tuberculosis.

13. What is the standard therapy for pulmonary tuberculosis?

Current therapy for pulmonary tuberculosis is based on several short-course regimens developed in the 1970s and 1980s. The induction phase of chemotherapy consists of 2 months of isoniazid, rifampin, and pyrazinamide followed by 4 months of continuation therapy with isoniazid and rifampin. In areas where isoniazid resistance is found in more than 4% of isolates, ethambutol or streptomycin should be added to the initial regimen until drug susceptibility results are known. Strong consideration should be given to treating all patients with programs of directly observed therapy (DOT), and this approach is mandatory if intermittent therapy is to be used. Use of this regimen to treat drug-susceptible pulmonary disease should be associated with a 100% cure rate and a relapse rate of no more than 3.5%.

14. How should antituberculosis therapy be monitored?

Properly administered, antituberculosis therapy should be extremely effective. A bacteriologic response (conversion of sputum cultures to negative) can be expected in essentially 100% of patients with tuberculosis caused by susceptible strains of *M. tuberculosis*. The most common reason for treatment failure is lack of adherence to the prescribed regimen. The following steps are critical for monitoring therapy:

- At the initiation of therapy, efforts should be made to insure that the mycobacteriology laboratory has received an adequate specimen for culture and sensitivity testing, particularly in regions where drug resistance has been noted.
- Once therapy has begun, sputum smears should be followed until negative, and the clinical response (fever, weight change) should also be noted.
- After discharge, patients should be seen at least monthly by the treating physician. The following should be done at each visit:
  Careful symptom review
  Record of the patient's weight

Sputum collected for smear and culture

Blood count, serum electrolyte levels, and liver function tests obtained to monitor for adverse effects of medications

• Chest radiographs need not be obtained frequently; a chest radiograph at the 3-month mark can be considered optional if the patient's clinical and bacteriologic response have been good, and a chest radiograph should be obtained at the completion of therapy.

Failure to respond to what should be an adequate drug regimen is overwhelmingly likely to be the result of poor patient adherence to the medical regimen.

15. Should serum levels of antituberculous drug be obtained routinely?

Dosing of antituberculous medications is usually based on body weight; none of the major chemotherapy trials relied on serum levels to adjust dosages. Therefore, in routine cases of tuberculosis, there is no reason to obtain serum levels. Under certain circumstances serum drug levels may be helpful, e.g., if a patient has been prescribed an adequate regimen but fails to have a clinical response and malabsorption of drugs is suspected. Malabsorption rarely occurs, but might be more common in patients with HIV infection. The most common reason for treatment failure in patients with tuberculosis caused by susceptible organisms is lack of adherence to the prescribed regimen.

A second scenario in which drug levels may be helpful is in managing patients with multidrug-resistant tuberculosis. In this circumstance, experts advocate obtaining drug levels and using high doses so that patients are kept at the upper end of the therapeutic range. This requires extremely close monitoring for side effects, particularly when aminoglycosides are used and ototoxicity is a major concern.

16. How should patients be monitored after completion of therapy?

Standard short-course (6 month) chemotherapy regimens are associated with low relapse rates. Most relapses occur in the first 2 years after completion of therapy. Patients who have a prompt and complete response to therapy (i.e., sputum cultures become negative within the first 2 months of therapy) do not need routine follow-up when treatment is completed. Patients whose response to therapy was slower or in whom radiographic abnormalities persist after completion of therapy should be evaluated at 6-month intervals and encouraged to report promptly any symptoms of recurrent cough, fever, or weight loss. Follow-up should be closer and more routine in patients who completed treatment for drug-resistant tuberculosis.

17. What steps should be taken with patients who do not adhere to their treatment regimens?

Adherence to medical regimens is a complex and poorly understood phenomenon; it is likely that only about 50% of patients take medications exactly according to physician instructions. In relation to tuberculosis, individual noncompliance or erratic self-administration of drugs can lead to spread of infection and the development of drug-resistant strains of mycobacteria.

The chief causes of nonadherence to antituberculous regimens are the fact that treatment continues for a long time after symptomatic improvement occurs, the side effects caused by the polypharmacy required for tuberculosis treatment, and several social factors and comorbid conditions common among tuberculosis patients. Patient counseling and education are crucial first steps in ensuring adherence. Attention to other factors such as substance abuse, mental illness, and housing, is also critical. DOT programs are the best venues in which to address these issues, and DOT should be the standard approach to tuberculosis therapy in the United States. Such programs promote adherence in a wide variety of patient groups and reduce the incidence of drug-resistant tuberculosis.

If patients fail to adhere to a regimen of DOT, more restrictive steps are required to protect the public health. Long-term enforced detention in tuberculosis wards is an option available in many states in the United States, although good DOT programs will obviate the need for detention in all but a few persons with tuberculosis.

18. Do patients with HIV infection require a longer duration of therapy?

It is recommended that patients with HIV infection receive 12 months of isoniazid preventive therapy when being treated for latent tuberculosis infection. The current American Thoracic Society/Centers for Disease Control guidelines state that patients with active tuberculosis may receive standard short-course therapy if their infection is caused by a susceptible organism and clinical response is prompt, as manifested by rapid improvement in symptoms and sputum culture conversion within the first 2 months of therapy. For HIV-infected patients who are slow to respond to therapy, a prudent approach would be to continue therapy for at least 6 months after the last positive sputum culture, then to monitor very closely for relapse after termination of therapy.

19. How should a pregnant woman with a positive tuberculin (PPD) skin test be managed?

Pregnant women with positive tuberculin skin tests should be evaluated in exactly the same manner as any other patient, i.e., with a thorough symptom review, physical examination, and a chest radiograph. Done with adequate abdominal shielding, a standard single chest radiograph in pregnancy poses no risk to the developing fetus. Delaying a chest radiograph to the postpartum period is a serious error that can result in exposure of the newborn to active tuberculosis, which may have disastrous consequences. When active tuberculosis is detected in a pregnant woman, therapy should be instituted promptly with isoniazid, rifampin, and ethambutol, none of which poses a danger to the developing fetus. Aminoglycosides and quinolones should be avoided. Few data are available regarding the safety of pyrazinamide in pregnancy, although it is used in Europe in this situation.

For pregnant women with only tuberculosis infection, isoniazid preventive therapy is recommended only if the woman is HIV seropositive, known to be a recent skin test converter, or a close contact of an individual with active tuberculosis. In all other situations, therapy can be postponed until after delivery. Because of concern about a possible higher incidence of isoniazid hepatotoxicity in the peripartum period, preventive therapy should begin 8–12 weeks after delivery.

20. When are steroids indicated in the treatment of tuberculosis?

Under certain circumstances adjunct therapy with corticosteroids may be indicated to decrease morbidity in patients with tuberculosis. Steroids should be used only in conjunction with an adequate antituberculous drug regimen; otherwise, disastrous results may occur. The two most common indications for steroids in patients with tuberculosis are tuberculous meningitis and pericarditis. Although most patients with extrapulmonary tuberculosis recover without incident, patients with meningitis may develop cerebrospinal fluid block and focal findings, such as hearing loss, which can be permanent. For these reasons, patients with central nervous system tuberculosis or tuberculous meningitis with focal findings should receive corticosteroids as adjunctive therapy.

Patients with tuberculous pericarditis are at risk for development of constrictive pericarditis and sudden death early in their course. Although steroids have long been used in the treatment of tuberculous pericarditis, exact indications for their use remain unclear. Creation of a pericardial window through a subxiphoid approach and complete pericardial stripping are probably more important therapeutic maneuvers than steroid administration. If these maneuvers are not used, steroids should be given. Some physicians use steroids even if the pericardium has been stripped.

A rare indication for steroids in tuberculosis is the patient who presents with tuberculosis and hypoxic respiratory failure mimicking ARDS. In this case steroids may decrease the inflammatory response and improve gas exchange, allowing clinical improvement before antibiotics would be expected to have an effect.

21. How should patients receiving isoniazid preventive therapy be monitored?

The most feared complication of isoniazid preventive therapy is fulminant hepatitis and hepatic failure, which may result in death. Fortunately, this is a rare complication. Isoniazid-induced hepatitis seems related to age and coexisting liver injury. Patients older than 35 years are at increased risk for this complication and should be monitored closely, with monthly symptom review and liver function tests. For persons under age 35 who have normal liver function tests at baseline and no history of prior liver disease, a monthly symptom review alone, without liver function testing, is adequate. Patients should be educated about the symptoms of hepatitis and instructed to discontinue isoniazid immediately and seek medical attention if such symptoms occur. Patients must be counseled to avoid alcohol completely, and no more than 1 month's supply of isoniazid should be dispensed to any patient. If symptomatic hepatitis results from isoniazid preventive therapy, the drug should be stopped and not reinstituted.

Transient small increases in transaminase levels are common in patients receiving isoniazid; abnormalities are observed in 15–20% of patients. These elevations in transaminase level usually resolve without discontinuation of isoniazid, and the drug need not be stopped in asymptomatic patients whose transaminase levels are within 3–5 times the normal limit. Such patients should be followed closely, however.

22. What type of preventive therapy should be given to persons exposed to cases of drug-resistant tuberculosis?

Few data exist about the efficacy of preventive regimens other than the commonly used 6–12 month course of isoniazid for latent tuberculosis infection. Persons exposed to isoniazid-resistant tuberculosis should receive 6 months' therapy with rifampin, in the usual daily dose. This approach should have a high degree of efficacy. Some advocate adding a second drug, such as ethambutol, to the preventive regimen, although there are no data on which to base this decision.

No data are available about the efficacy of any preventive regimen for patients exposed to tuberculosis resistant to isoniazid and rifampin. Many advocate observation alone in this setting, but therapy seems prudent in persons at high risk for developing active tuberculosis (children, those with HIV infection, and so forth). In such cases, a combination of ethambutol and pyrazinamide may be used, or a combination of pyrazinamide and a quinolone may seem logical. (Most authorities consider quinolones to be contraindicated in children because of potential arthropathy.) These regimens may be given for 6 months, and careful attention should be paid to excluding active disease before these preventive regimens are employed. If a person has been exposed to multidrug-resistant tuberculosis and no adequate regimen can be constructed for preventive therapy, vaccination with BCG should be considered if the patient is at high risk for development of active disease. BCG vaccine should not be given to persons with HIV infection, as it has been reported to cause disseminated disease in such cases.

CONTROVERSY

23. Should anergy testing be performed in patients with a negative tuberculin skin test and HIV infection?

Patients with coexisting HIV and tuberculosis infection are at high risk of developing active tuberculosis. For this reason, identification and treatment of persons with HIV and tuberculosis co-infection is a public health priority. However, the standard tuberculin skin test may be less helpful in HIV-infected persons, as the ability to mount a delayed hypersensitivity response depends upon intact cellular immunity, which is precisely the part of the immune system most affected by advanced HIV infection. Some have advocated that patients with HIV infection and negative tuberculin tests receive anergy testing to further assess the integrity of their cell-mediated immunity. If patients do not respond to the anergy panel, the negative tuberculin test would be considered a false-negative test, and isoniazid preventive therapy would be given.

This approach presents several problems. First, anergy is a complex and poorly understood phenomenon, and methods for assessing it are poorly standardized and often not reproducible. It is well known that many healthy individuals do not develop a reaction to one or more of the commonly used skin-test antigens (tetanus, mumps, trichophyton, or *Candida* spp.); also, positive reactions may become negative when repeated and vice versa. Second, although it is generally true that persons with advanced HIV infection are more likely to display cutaneous anergy to common antigens, this is not always the case. Third, the risk of tuberculosis is not the same among all HIV subgroups, and not every tuberculin-negative, anergic patient with HIV can be assumed to have tuberculosis infection. For example, the recently concluded Pulmonary Complications of HIV Infection Study found that cases of tuberculosis in AIDS patients varied greatly with geographic distribution. For these reasons, the case to perform anergy testing on all tuberculin-negative HIV-infected patients is not a compelling one.

A recently performed decision analysis suggested that all HIV-infected patients receive 12 months of isoniazid preventive therapy, regardless of skin tuberculin skin test status. However, this approach has not been empirically verified. At present, decisions to institute isoniazid preventive therapy in tuberculin skin test–negative patients should be made on an individual basis after careful assessment of the patient's risk for tuberculosis infection.

BIBLIOGRAPHY

1. American Thoracic Society: Treatment of tuberculosis and tuberculosis infection in adults and children. Am J Respir Crit Care Med 149:1359–1374, 1994.
2. Centers for Disease Control: Management of persons exposed to multidrug-resistant tuberculosis. MMWR 41:61–70, 1992.
3. Huebner RE, Schein MF, Bass JB: The tuberculin skin test. Clin Infect Dis 17:968–975, 1993.
4. Iseman MD: Treatment of multidrug-resistant tuberculosis. N Engl J Med 329:784–790, 1993.
5. McGowan JE: Nosocomial tuberculosis: New progress in control and prevention. Clin Infect Dis 21:489–505, 1995.
6. Menzies R, Vissandjee B, Amyot D: Factors associated with tuberculin reactivity among the foreign-born in Montreal. Am Rev Respir Dis 146:752–756, 1992.
7. Rom WN, Garay SM (eds): Tuberculosis. Boston, Little, Brown, 1996.
8. Schluger N, Ciotili C, Cohen D, et al: Comprehensive tuberculosis control for patients at high risk for non-compliance. Am J Respir Crit Care Med 151:1486–1490, 1995.
9. Schluger NW, Rom WN: Current approaches to the diagnosis of active pulmonary tuberculosis. Am J Respir Crit Care Med 149:264–267, 1994.

35. ATYPICAL MYCOBACTERIA

Michael E. Hanley, M.D., and Tony N. Hodges, M.D.

1. What are atypical mycobacteria?

These are mycobacteria that are biologically distinct from *Mycobacterium tuberculosis, M. bovis,* and *M. leprae*. Traditionally, these acid-fast bacilli were thought to be primarily saprophytic organisms that were not pathologic in humans. However, it is now recognized that these mycobacteria are occasional human pathogens, especially in immunosuppressed patients.

2. How are atypical mycobacteria classified?

The **Runyon Classification System** categorizes these organisms into four basic groups based on growth characteristics, colonial morphology, and pigmentation:

Group I—Photochromogens
Group II—Scotochromogens
Group III—Nonchromogens
Group IV—Rapid growers

Although the Runyon system has significant laboratory utility, it is of limited clinical usefulness. The **Bailey system** is an alternative schema that classifies the organisms by their response to therapy:

Easy to Treat	Difficult to Treat
M. kansasii	*M. avium-intracellulare*
M. xenopi	*M. scrofulaceum*
M. szulgai	*M. simiae*
M. marinum	*M. chelonei*
M. ulcerans	*M. fortuitum*

3. Which atypical mycobacteria are clinically significant in humans?

Group I (photochromogenic)	Group III (nonchromogenic)
M. kansasii	*M. avium-intracellulare*
M. marinum	*M. ulcerans*
M. simiae	*M. xenopi*
Group II (scotochromogenic)	Group IV (rapid-growing)
M. szulgai	*M. chelonei*
M. scrofulaceum	*M. fortuitum*

Reports of human disease due to most of the atypical organisms are unusual, generally consisting of isolated cases or, rarely, small epidemics. When human disease does occur, it most commonly results from infection with either *M. avium-intracellulare* or *M. kansasii*. One review of the frequency of mycobacteria isolated in state public health laboratories demonstrated that 65% were *M. tuberculosis*, 21% *M. avium-intracellulare*, 6.5% *M. fortuitum-chelonei*, 3.5% *M. kansasii*, and 2.3% *M. scrofulaceum*. However, many of the isolates in this review may have reflected colonization as opposed to true disease, and this review was published before the HIV epidemic.

4. What are the most common sites of infection from atypical mycobacteria?

Atypical mycobacteria have the potential to cause disease in almost any organ. Most patients develop only localized disease, although dissemination can occur in severely immunosuppressed conditions. The most common sites of infection include the lungs, skin, lymph nodes, bones, joints, urinary tract, and meninges. Cutaneous disease usually results from infection with either *M. marinum, M. ulcerans,* or *M. fortuitum. M. scrofulaceum* is the most common atypical mycobacteria associated with lymphadenitis.

5. Discuss the epidemiology of atypical mycobacteria.

Atypical mycobacteria are dispersed widely throughout the environment, although in the United States, infections from *M. avium-intracellulare* tend to be more frequent in the southeast while those due to *M. kansasii* occur more commonly in the midwest, Texas, Louisiana, and Florida. These organisms are common saprophytes that can be readily isolated from soil, water, and milk. The route of entry is likely inhalational (except for *M. marinum*) with acquisition directly from environmental reservoirs. Although atypical mycobacteria cause disease in many animals, animal–human and human–human transmission has not been proven and probably does not occur. Routine isolation of patients with pulmonary infections is therefore not warranted.

6. What conditions predispose patients to pulmonary disease from atypical mycobacteria?

Pulmonary infection from atypical mycobacteria is more common in the immune suppressed and in patients with preexisting pulmonary disorders, including bronchiectasis, chronic obstructive pulmonary disease, lung cancer, and silicosis. It may also occur in patients with no previous history of lung disease.

7. Which atypical mycobacteria cause pulmonary disease?

The lungs are the most frequent site of infection by atypical mycobacteria. Although pulmonary disease may result from infection with *M. scrofulaceum, M. szulgai, M. xenopi, M. fortuitum,* or *M. chelonei,* it most commonly occurs from infection with either *M. avium–intracellulare* or *M. kansasii.*

8. Are pulmonary infections with atypical mycobacteria more common in specific demographic patient groups?

Immunocompetent patients who develop pulmonary infections from either *M. avium-intracellulare* or *M. kansasii* tend to be middle-aged to older white males. Although underlying structural lung disease predisposes patients to infection with either organism, up to 40% of patients infected with *M. kansasii* have no other lung disease. Disseminated *M. avium-intracellulare* (but not *M. kansasii*) is often associated with HIV infection, occurring in up to 50% of HIV-seropositive patients in some autopsy series.

9. How do the clinical manifestations of pulmonary disease from atypical mycobacteria compare to those of tuberculosis?

Pulmonary disease from atypical mycobacteria is clinically, radiographically, and histologically similar to that caused by *M. tuberculosis*. Constitutional symptoms, however, tend to be less prominent, the course is frequently more indolent, and pulmonary symptoms are more subtle.

10. How is the diagnosis of pulmonary infection with atypical mycobacteria established?

The diagnosis can be very difficult to confirm. Because the organisms are common saprophytes, a positive sputum culture is nonspecific. Furthermore, skin testing for cell-mediated immunity is of limited use because appropriate antigens for most atypical mycobacteria are not available and there is significant cross-reactivity between species. Diagnosis generally requires demonstrating several criteria:

1. There should be radiographically apparent and clinically compatible lung disease without another evident cause. This diagnostic criterion is strengthened if there is evidence of progressive radiographic changes or clinical deterioration.

2. The suspected organism should be isolated from pulmonary secretions (sputum, bronchial wash, bronchoalveolar lavage) on *multiple* occasions. This criterion is likely less important in diagnosing pulmonary infection from *M. kansasii*, as this organism is rarely a saprophyte.

3. Sputum cultures should remain positive despite several months of bronchial hygiene with aerosolized saline or bronchodilators.

The diagnosis is also established if the organism is isolated from tissue having appropriate histopathologic changes.

11. How does pulmonary infection from *M. kansasii* differ clinically from that due to *M. tuberculosis*?

Lung disease from *M. kansasii* closely resembles that from *M. tuberculosis*, but *M. kansasii* tends to result in **thin-walled cavities** and a **paucity of pleural disease or effusions**. In addition, extrapulmonary disease rarely complicates infection with *M. kansasii*, usually occurring only in immunocompromised hosts.

12. How are pulmonary infections from *M. kansasii* managed?

The treatment is very similar to that for tuberculosis. *M. kansasii* is susceptible to most standard antituberculous drugs, although some resistance to isoniazid exists. A cornerstone to therapy is rifampin. Inclusion of this drug in a multidrug regimen is associated with more rapid conversion of sputum and with lower relapse rates. Standard treatment recommendations include the use of isoniazid, rifampin, and ethambutol. In some circumstances, streptomycin may be added or substituted for ethambutol for the first 2 months. Although the optimal duration of therapy is unknown, most regimens are continued for 18–24 months. In some studies, this approach has resulted in response rates nearing 100% with virtually no relapses.

13. What are the common presenting findings in patients with pulmonary *M. avium-intracellulare* (MAI) infection?

Four distinct clinical patterns have been described:
1. Solitary pulmonary nodule

2. Cavitary bronchitis or bronchiectasis with granuloma on biopsy and/or sputum repeatedly positive for MAI
3. Cavitary lung disease with scattered pulmonary nodules
4. Diffuse pulmonary infiltrates in immunocompromised patients

14. Do all patients in whom MAI is isolated from sputum require treatment?

No. Because MAI frequently colonizes the lungs of patients with structural lung disease, universal treatment of all patients with positive sputum cultures is not required. Patients with progressive lung disease or evidence of systemic dissemination should be treated promptly. However, asymptomatic patients or those in whom the diagnosis is in doubt may be observed without therapy. Therapy should be initiated at any suggestion of disease progression. It should be emphasized that patients with MAI infection may experience prolonged periods of stable lung function punctuated with periods of sudden, significant decline.

15. How is pulmonary disease from MAI managed?

Successful management involves both medical and surgical strategies. Unfortunately, MAI is resistant in vitro to most traditional antituberculous drugs. Although the initial sputum conversion rate with multidrug therapy is good, relapses are common.

Current recommendations include three to five drugs continued for 18–24 months. Isoniazid, rifampin, ethambutol, and streptomycin are used in most standard regimens. Cycloserine and ethionamide should be added in patients with extensive, aggressive disease, those with immunosuppressed states, or those who fail a more limited drug regimen. Chemotherapy followed by surgical resection should be considered in patients with limited disease who are good surgical candidates. Although it is preferable that sputum conversion occur prior to resection, some authors have advocated resection after 3–4 months of therapy regardless of sputum status.

16. Which new agents may be valuable in treating pulmonary infection from MAI?

Ciprofloxacin, rifabutin, azithromycin, clarithromycin, and clofazamine all hold significant promise in treating MAI infection. Ciprofloxacin is a fluoroquinolone that is very active in vitro against MAI and is well-tolerated with few side effects. Rifabutin is an analog of rifampin that is significantly more active against MAI than rifampin. It is approved for prophylaxis of MAI in HIV-seropositive patients. Azithromycin and clarithromycin are new macrolide antibiotics that have significant in vitro activity against MAI and achieve very high tissue levels. In addition, these latter two agents readily enter macrophages, preventing replication of intracellular organisms.

17. What are the clinical manifestations of disseminated MAI infection in HIV-seropositive patients?

The clinical manifestations of disseminated MAI infection in HIV-seropositive patients are poorly characterized because this complication usually develops late in HIV infection when other HIV-related complications exist. Although it is difficult to determine which symptoms are specific to MAI, five specific symptom complexes have been described:
1. A wasting syndrome characterized by fever, weight loss, and cachexia
2. Progressive anemia
3. Chronic abdominal pain and diarrhea
4. Chronic malabsorption
5. Extrabiliary obstructive jaundice

18. How is the diagnosis of disseminated MAI infection established in HIV-seropositive patients?

This diagnosis can be difficult to establish. Demonstration of organisms in pulmonary secretions alone rarely confirms the diagnosis because MAI frequently colonizes the lungs of HIV-seropositive patients. The diagnosis generally requires either an appropriate clinical picture in conjunction with identification of the organism from multiple body fluids or the isolation of the organism from a systemic site, such as blood, bone marrow, urine, liver, spleen, or lymph nodes.

BIBLIOGRAPHY

1. Ahn CH, McLarty JW, Ahn S, et al: Diagnostic criteria for pulmonary disease caused by *Mycobacterium kansasii* and *Mycobacterium intracellulare*. Am Rev Respir Dis 125:388–391, 1982.
2. Davidson PT: The diagnosis and management of disease caused by *Mycobacterium avium* complex, *Mycobacterium kansasii* and other mycobacteria. Clin Chest Med 10:431–443, 1989.
3. Huebner RE, Schein MF, Cauthen GM, et al: Evaluation of the clinical usefulness of mycobacterial skin test antigens in adults with pulmonary mycobacterioses. Am Rev Respir Dis 145:1160–1166, 1992.
4. Iseman MD, Corpe RF, O'Brien RJ, et al: Disease due to *Mycobacterium avium-intracellulare*: National consensus conference on tuberculosis. Chest 87:139S–149S, 1985.
5. Kotloff RM: Infections caused by nontuberculous mycobacteria: Clinical aspects. Semin Rotengenol 28:131–138, 1993.
6. O'Brien RJ: The epidemiology of nontuberculous mycobacterial disease. Clin Chest Med 10:407–418, 1989.
7. Prince DS, Peterson DD, Steiner RM, et al: Infection with *Mycobacterium avium* complex in patients without predisposing conditions. N Engl J Med 321:863–868, 1989.
8. Reich JM, Johnson JE: *Mycobacterium avium* complex pulmonary disease: Incidence, presentation, and response to therapy in a community setting. Am Rev Respir Dis 143:1381–1385, 1991.
9. Teirstein AS, Damsker B, Kirschner PA, et al: Pulmonary infection with *Mycobacterium avium intracellulare*: Diagnosis, clinical patterns, and treatment. Mt Sinai J Med 57:209–215, 1990.
10. Wolinsky E: Nontuberculous mycobacteria and associated diseases. Am Rev Respir Dis 119:107–159, 1979.

VII. Pulmonary Complications of AIDS

36. INFECTIOUS PULMONARY COMPLICATIONS OF AIDS

Dorothy A. White, M.D., and Rafael Barrera, M.D.

1. What pulmonary infections are commonly seen in patients infected with the human immunodeficiency virus (HIV)?

As with other groups of immunosuppressed patients, a large number of organisms can cause respiratory problems. Experience over the past decade of the AIDS epidemic has shown, however, that the majority of pneumonias are caused by a few organisms. At present the three most common causes of respiratory infection are *Pneumocystis carinii*, pyogenic bacteria, and *Mycobacterium tuberculosis*. *P. carinii* pneumonia (PCP) was the first infection clearly identified as HIV related and initially was the most common cause of pneumonia. More than 75% of HIV-infected patients developed PCP and it often recurred. It is now known that PCP develops at the late stages of HIV infection, when the immune impairment is profound. The best marker of immunosuppression in HIV-infected patients is the number of T lymphocytes of the helper phenotype, which are known as CD4 cells. PCP usually occurs when the CD4 count in adults is less than 200 cells per mm³. PCP is still a common cause of pneumonia in HIV-infected patients, but its frequency has decreased over the past few years as a result of the use of primary and secondary prophylaxis.

Bacterial bronchitis and pneumonia are now the most common causes of lower respiratory tract infection; they occur at frequencies greater than expected for the general population and at a wide range of CD4 counts. Bacterial pneumonia is most common at low CD4 counts. Bacterial infections were not initially considered related to HIV because they are so common in the general population. Bronchitis and pneumonia are also often recurrent, and secondary bronchiectasis has been reported. Intravenous drug abusers appear to be particularly susceptible to bacterial respiratory tract infections; cigarette smokers may also have an increased incidence.

In areas where *M. tuberculosis* is endemic, tuberculosis has become a common cause of pneumonia in HIV-infected patients.

2. Name some less common pulmonary infections.

Some of the organisms that cause respiratory problems less commonly are listed below. With the exception of the bacteria, pulmonary involvement caused by these organisms is often secondary to disseminated disease. All of these infections occur in patients with very low CD4 counts.

Bacteria	*Nocardia* spp., *Rhodococcus equi, Legionella* spp. (nosocomial)
Mycobacteria	*M. avium-intracellulare, M. kansasii*
Fungus	*Coccidioides immitis, Histoplasma capsulatum* (patients with endemic exposure), *Cryptococcus neoformans*
Virus	Cytomegalovirus, herpes simplex
Parasites	*Toxoplasma gondii, Strongyloides stercoralis*

3. What information should be obtained in the assessment of an HIV-infected patient with suspected pulmonary infection?

- Degree of immune dysfunction: CD4 level or evidence of impaired immunity, such as a history of weight loss, thrush, or previous opportunistic infections.

- Risk group for HIV: some groups such as intravenous drug users are at high risk for tuberculosis and bacterial pneumonia; others such as gay or bisexual men are at increased risk for pulmonary Kaposi's sarcoma (KS).
- Use of prophylactic drugs: for PCP and tuberculosis and compliance with these regimens.
- Exposure to or history of tuberculosis or a positive skin test.
- Residence in areas endemic for fungus or parasites.
- Acuteness of presentation.
- Oxygen saturation/Po_2: determines urgency of evaluation and treatment for PCP.
- Serum lactate dehydrogenase (LDH): may be helpful for the diagnosis of PCP.
- Radiographic pattern.

4. Which organisms cause bacterial pneumonia in the HIV-infected population?

The most commonly reported pathogens in community-acquired pneumonia are *Streptococcus pneumoniae* and *Haemophilus influenzae*; initial empiric therapy is usually directed against these bacteria. *Staphylococcus aureus* and gram-negative organisms also should be considered in seriously ill patients. Gram-negative organisms, particularly *Pseudomonas aeruginosa*, cause nosocomial pneumonia and are found particularly when the CD4 count is less than 50–100 per mm³. Unusual causes of pneumonia are *Rhodococcus equi*, *Nocardia asteroides*, group B streptococcus, *Moraxella catarrhalis*, and *Legionella pneumoniae*.

5. What antibiotics are commonly given for presumed bacterial pneumonia?

Ampicillin and cefuroxime are frequently given; in some centers a significant percentage of *H. influenzae* organisms are resistant to ampicillin and it is not used. Trimethoprim-sulfamethoxazole (TMP-SMX) is also a good choice if it can be tolerated. More expanded coverage is given in selected cases.

6. How does bacterial pneumonia present?

Presentation is similar to that in patients who are not HIV infected, namely, rapid onset (over hours to days), fever, productive cough, and dyspnea. Leukocytosis is common and the serum LDH is usually normal. Chest radiographs show segmental or lobar infiltrates (most common with *S. pneumoniae*) or reticulonodular infiltrates (frequently seen with *H. influenzae*). Cavitation may occur with *S. aureus*. Bacteremia is more common than in non–HIV-infected patients, occurring in 33% of cases caused by pneumococci and 12% of cases caused by *H. influenzae*.

7. What is the prognosis for bacterial pneumonia?

Success rates of 80–100% have been reported in community-acquired pneumonia. Response is lower in patients with advanced HIV disease, bacteremia, and nosocomial pneumonia. High mortality rates have been seen with unusual organisms such as *R. equi*.

8. Can prophylaxis be given for bacterial pneumonia?

Pneumococcal vaccine is recommended. The conjugated hemophilus vaccine should also be considered, particularly if there has been one episode of *H. influenzae*. The efficacy of these vaccines in HIV-infected patients is unproved, although they are theoretically more likely to be helpful when given early. Prevention of PCP with TMP-SMX leads to a lower incidence of bacterial infection; other prophylactic antibiotics may be helpful if TMP-SMX cannot be tolerated. In HIV-infected children with more than 200 CD4 cells per mm³, regular use of intravenous immunoglobulin has decreased the incidence of serious bacterial infections, particularly if TMP-SMX is not being given, but it has not improved survival.

9. Describe the presentation of PCP.

The onset is usually subacute or insidious (over days to weeks). Occasionally presentation is fulminant. Symptoms are fever, nonproductive cough (although some patients will have sputum), and dyspnea. A few patients are asymptomatic and the pneumonia is evident only radiographically.

The classic chest radiographic pattern is bilateral interstitial or alveolar infiltrates. Less common presentations are thin-walled cysts, upper lobe or apical infiltrates, focal infiltrates, and nodules. Pneumothorax without an iatrogenic cause also may signal the appearance of PCP. Leukocytosis is not expected, but the serum LDH is elevated in more than 90% of cases. The Po_2 is usually low and decreases further with exercise.

10. How is PCP diagnosed?

Diagnosis depends on visualization of the organism (usually the cyst form) in respiratory secretions or in lung tissue using special stains. The organism cannot be cultured in the clinical laboratory. Specimens of induced sputum, bronchoalveolar lavage, or transbronchial biopsies from bronchoscopy have the highest yield. *P. carinii* organisms are routinely visualized with Gram-Weigert, methenamine silver, and toluidine blue stains.

11. What is sputum induction? How effective is it for the diagnosis of PCP?

Expectorated sputum has a low yield because it usually does not contain material from the alveoli, where *P. carinii* organisms are located. Sputum is induced by having a patient breathe an aerosolized 3% saline solution for 10 minutes. After that time the patient is encouraged to take a series of deep coughs expectorating all sputum. If no sputum can be obtained, a second aerosolized treatment may be given. If tuberculosis is also suspected, the procedure is done in a chamber with high ventilation and high efficiency particulate air (HEPA) filters to avoid spreading infection. The sputum obtained is liquified by the addition of a mucolytic agent and the specimen is reduced by spinning. Smears or slides are made of the cellular pellet. Many patients find sputum induction unpleasant. The procedure works best if the patient is cooperative and not debilitated, nauseated, severely dyspneic, or confused. Yield is improved by the constant attention and encouragement of a trained professional. Induced sputum samples are positive in 50–90% of PCP cases, depending on the population studied and the institution's expertise.

12. What is the yield of bronchoscopy for PCP?

The usual specimens sent from bronchoscopy for PCP are bronchoalveolar lavage (BAL) and transbronchial biopsies (TBBx). BAL is performed by wedging the bronchoscope in a subsegmental bronchus. Saline (usually in 30- to 50-cc fractions) is forced out of the bronchus into the alveolar spaces, then manually aspirated. The fluid obtained is foamy and contains alveolar material. The procedure is safe and does not risk bleeding, although oxygen saturation may temporarily drop. The yield of BAL in detecting PCP in HIV-infected patients who are not using prophylaxis is close to 100%. In those using prophylaxis, some groups have noted a considerable decrease in sensitivity. TBBx has a high yield (85–100%) even when prophylaxis is being used but carries a small risk of pneumothorax and bleeding.

13. Is there a role for gallium scans and pulmonary function tests in the diagnosis of PCP?

Gallium scans usually show intense uptake in the lungs of HIV-infected patients with PCP. A positive scan is suggestive but not specific for PCP. Gallium scans are used predominantly to detect subclinical disease when the radiographic findings are minimal or normal and in patients with known pulmonary KS and worsening radiographs or symptoms. KS does not take up gallium whereas PCP does. Pulmonary function tests are also used to detect pulmonary disease when other findings are subtle. Patients with PCP tend to have a low diffusing capacity (which measures the ability of the lungs to transfer gas from the alveolar space into the pulmonary capillary blood) and commonly show significant arterial desaturation with exercise.

14. How is PCP treated?

PCP is treated either with TMP-SMX, 15 mg per kg per day orally or IV in divided doses, or pentamidine isoethionate, 4 mg per kg per day IV for 21 days. In mild cases, oral antibiotic therapy can be given on an outpatient basis and a course as short as 14 days may be adequate. In moderate to severe cases, hospitalization and IV antibiotics are needed and adjunct corticosteroid therapy is given. The drugs used for PCP have a high incidence of toxicity, and a switch to an alternative agent is often necessary. The most common side effects of TMP-SMX are rash, leukopenia, elevated transaminase levels, hepatic dysfunction, fever, and nausea and vomiting. Pentamidine causes hypoglycemia, hypertension, nephrotoxicity, hepatic dysfunction, and leukopenia. If neither drug can be tolerated, available alternatives include atovaquone, trimethoprim plus dapsone, primaquine plus clindamycin, trimetrexate plus leucovorin, or difluoromethylornithine (DFMO). Desensitization to TMP-SMX has been successful in some patients allergic to the drug.

15. Why are corticosteroids used in treatment of PCP?

Corticosteroids are recommended to reduce mortality in moderate to severe cases of PCP (Po_2 70 mm or less or A-a gradient 35 mg or more on room air). The clinical deterioration that often takes place in the first few days of treatment of PCP may be ameliorated by steroids. Prednisone—40 mg twice daily for 5 days, 40 mg daily for 5 days, and 20 mg for 11 days—is generally used.

16. What is the prognosis for PCP?

Survival of patients with a first episode is 90%; survival declines with further episodes. If respiratory failure requiring mechanical ventilation occurs, survival ranges from 14–40%.

17. Can PCP be prevented?

Prophylaxis is effective in decreasing the frequency of but not entirely eliminating PCP. Primary prophylaxis to prevent the first episode of PCP should be given to all patients with CD4 counts of 200 cells per mm³ or less or 2 weeks of unexplained fever (temperature above 37.8° C), malaise, or thrush. Secondary prophylaxis should be given to anyone with a prior episode of PCP. The current drug of choice is TMP-SMX, 1 double strength orally daily or 1 single strength daily or 1 double strength orally three times per week. Alternative drugs are dapsone, 100 mg daily; dapsone plus pyrimethamine in combinations; or aerosolized pentamidine (AP), 300 mg per month by Respirgard II Nebulizer (Marquest, Englewood, CO). Because side effects are common with TMP-SMX and dapsone, these drugs are often not tolerated over long periods of time. AP is well tolerated, although cough and bronchospasm are seen; unfortunately, however, it is not effective as systemic therapy, particularly as the CD4 count drops.

18. Are there problems for health care workers administering AP?

The safety of administration of AP by health care workers has been questioned because the worker is exposed and the drug can be detected in the urine of health care givers. Increases in asthma and decreases in diffusing capacity have been noted in respiratory therapists, although they have not clearly been proved to be related to AP. A theoretical risk of teratogenicity also exists, and pregnant women or those trying to conceive should not administer the drug. The risk of spread of tuberculosis by this procedure when cough is induced is also of concern. AP should be given in an environment that fulfills the Centers for Disease Control requirement for prevention of tuberculosis, i.e., in a chamber that has adequate gas exchange and ability to filter the drug. Respiratory barrier devices should also be worn by the health care worker.

19. What is the relationship of tuberculosis to HIV infection?

The reduction in cell-mediated immunity induced by HIV infection predisposes patients previously infected with tuberculosis to reactivation of disease. Tuberculosis may present up to many months before other opportunistic infections. Patients from countries or areas of the United States where tuberculosis is endemic, those in lower socioeconomic groups, and intravenous drug users are at high risk. Additionally, rapidly progressive tuberculosis may develop in HIV-infected patients with very low CD4 counts who are newly exposed or reexposed to *M. tuberculosis*. Those at risk are profoundly immunosuppressed HIV-infected patients, particularly in settings such as homeless shelters or hospital units where they may be exposed to the organism. Additionally, it is believed by some that development of tuberculosis may accelerate the course of HIV infection.

20. Describe the presentation of tuberculosis.

The most common presenting symptoms are fever, cough, and weight loss. Pulmonary tuberculosis occurs in 75% of patients, but the incidence of extrapulmonary tuberculosis increases as the CD4 count drops. The most common extrapulmonary disease is lymphadenitis, but brain abscesses, meningitis, pericardial disease, and gastric and bone tuberculosis are also seen. Disseminated disease is present in approximately 10% of cases and bacteremia is not uncommon.

When tuberculosis occurs relatively early in the course of HIV, chest radiographic features are similar to those of non–HIV-infected patients. Upper lobe infiltrates, which may cavitate, occur. As CD4 count drops to less than 200 cells per mm^3, focal or diffuse infiltrates, reticulonodular or miliary patterns, pleural effusions, and intrathoracic adenopathy are commonly seen. Normal radiographs are also found in up to 20% of cases of active tuberculosis in this setting.

21. Is the tuberculin skin test helpful in the diagnosis of tuberculosis?

A purified protein derivative (PPD) skin test in an HIV-infected patient is considered positive if there is 5 mm or more of induration. Anergy, which develops secondary to HIV infection, leads to false-negative results in some patients with active disease, but the PPD is often helpful and should be performed. More than 90% of HIV-infected patients with active tuberculosis have positive skin tests if the CD4 count is more than 500 cells per mm^3, but fewer than 50% have positive tests when CD4 counts are 200 per mm^3 or less.

22. How is tuberculosis diagnosed?

Clinical and radiographic features are not generally diagnostic. CT of the chest, in patients with intrathoracic adenopathy, is, however, highly suggestive of this diagnosis. Tuberculosis nodes have central low density areas presumed to be caused by caseation or necrosis with associated rim enhancement. This finding is uncommon with other causes of intrathoracic adenopathy in HIV-infected patients.

Examination of sputum is usually the first and best test for diagnosis. Cultures are positive in 85–100% of patients but take 3–6 weeks for results. Smears are positive in 30–90% of patients. A major problem in diagnosing tuberculosis is failure to consider the diagnosis and send adequate sputum specimens (three to five samples). Studies are underway using polymerase chain reaction (PCR) techniques to rapidly diagnose tuberculosis. Bronchoscopy is used if sputum smears are negative, an immediate result is needed, or if diagnoses other than tuberculosis are being considered. TBBx shows granulomas in a small percent of cases of tuberculosis, which leads to a rapid diagnosis. Culture of BAL, washing, and TBBx may also increase the yield for tuberculosis over sputum in a few cases.

When pleural fluid is present, cultures are positive in approximately 90% of cases and smears in 15%. Granulomatous changes on pleural biopsy are reported in many cases. Blood cultures may be useful and are positive in up to 40% of cases of tuberculosis in advanced HIV infection. Cultures of urine, stool, bone marrow, and sites such as liver, pericardium, and central nervous system also may be helpful in some patients.

23. How is tuberculosis treated?

Treatment is usually started with isoniazid (INH), rifampin (RIF), and pyrazinamide (PZA); if a drug-resistant organism is suspected, ethambutol (ETH) also is given for 2 months. If the organism is sensitive to all drugs, INH and RIF are continued for an additional 6 months. If the organism is resistant to either INH or RIF, treatment is longer and usually with three sensitive drugs. Directly observed therapy (DOT), which consists of supervised therapy several times a week, should be used if the patient is not compliant. There is some controversy about the length of treatment, and many clinicians treat for longer periods than indicated above.

24. What is multidrug-resistant tuberculosis? How is it treated?

Multidrug resistance (MDR) refers to organisms that are resistant to two or more drugs, including INH and RIF. Outbreaks of MDR tuberculosis have occurred in New York and other cities, and organisms have been resistant to five or six of the first-line antituberculous drugs. Treatment is difficult and requires use of other drugs based on patterns of sensitivity in a given community.

25. What is the prognosis for tuberculosis?

Prognosis with drug-sensitive organisms is good if there is compliance with regimens or DOT is used. There is a 10% failure rate and a low rate of long-term relapse. The prognosis is poor with MDR tuberculosis, which has a median survival of only several months.

26. Can reactivation of tuberculosis be prevented?

Yes, by identification and treatment of those with latent infection. Prophylaxis is indicated, after active disease is excluded, for all HIV-infected patients who are PPD positive and for those who are close contacts of patients with infectious tuberculosis. INH is usually given daily for 1 year; other drugs should be considered in areas where INH resistance is frequent. Prophylaxis is also considered in skin test–negative patients from risk groups or geographic areas with a high prevalence of *M. tuberculosis* infection, particularly if patients are anergic. The PPD should be repeated annually in skin–test negative HIV-infected patients.

27. Can primary tuberculosis be prevented?

Primary exposure to tuberculosis is prevented by good environmental precautions such as adequate ventilation, filters, ultraviolet lights, masks, and so forth in areas where patients with tuberculosis are likely to be present. Patients should be advised to avoid activities that may increase their likelihood of exposure.

CONTROVERSY

28. Does a diagnosis of PCP need to be made in all cases or can empiric therapy be given?

Some physicians treat patients with a classic presentation of PCP empirically and perform bronchoscopy only if the patient fails to respond after several days of therapy (usually 5 days). Advocates of this position believe that it saves many patients from undergoing an expensive, invasive procedure that has side effects. This position holds that even if bacterial infection was missed, it is likely to be adequately treated by TMP-SMX. Patients with most other causes of infiltrates, such as pulmonary KS, will not be harmed by a delay in diagnosis of several days. At least one randomized study supports the view that the outcome is the same at the end of 1 month whether a diagnosis was made or empiric treatment given.

Those opposing this position believe that bronchoscopy is generally well tolerated and allows specific therapy to be given early and unnecessary treatment to be avoided. TMP-SMX is not well tolerated by many HIV-infected patients, and they should not be exposed to it needlessly for conditions other than PCP. If pentamidine is given for treatment of PCP instead of TMP-SMX, patients are at risk of not being covered for bacterial pneumonia, which is potentially life threatening. Empiric therapy may delay diagnosis of tuberculosis, increasing the risk of spread of infection to health care workers and other patients. Those who do not respond will be subjected to a bronchoscopy when they may be more severely ill. Advocates of a definite diagnosis believe that the incidence of PCP is decreasing with more widespread prophylaxis and many atypical presentations of PCP occur making an empiric approach less successful.

Both empiric therapy and aggressive diagnostic approaches are both used currently. Their success depends on spectrum of disease seen (specifically the prevalence of PCP versus other entities), the resources available, and in all cases careful clinical judgment.

BIBLIOGRAPHY

1. Burack JH, Hahn JA, Saint-Maurice D, et al: Microbiology of community-acquired bacterial pneumonia in persons with and at risk for human immunodeficiency virus type 1 infection: Implications for rational empiric antibiotic therapy. Arch Intern Med 154:2589–2596, 1994.
2. Daley CL, Small PM, Schechter GF, et al: An outbreak of tuberculosis with accelerated progression among persons infected with the human immunodeficiency virus. N Engl J Med 226:231–235, 1992.
3. Hirschtick R, Glassroth J, Jordan M, et al and the Pulmonary Complications of HIV Infection Study Group: Bacterial pneumonia in persons infected with the human immunodeficiency virus. N Engl J Med 333:845–851, 1995.
4. Jones BE, Young SMM, Antoniskis D, et al: Relationship of the manifestations of tuberculosis to CD4 counts in patients with human immunodeficiency virus infection. Am Rev Respir Dis 148:1292–1297, 1993.
5. Kaplan JE, Masur K, Holmes KK, et al: USPHS/IDSA Guidelines for the prevention of opportunistic infections in persons infected with the human immunodeficiency virus: An overview. Clin Infect Dis 21 (Suppl 1):S12–S31, 1995.
6. Miller RF, Mitchell DM: *Pneumocystis carinii* pneumonia. Thorax 50:191–200, 1995.
7. Mitchel DM, Miller RF: New developments in the pulmonary diseases affecting HIV-infected individuals. Thorax 50:294–302, 1995.
8. Official statement of the American Thoracic Society and Centers for Disease Control: Treatment of tuberculosis and tuberculosis infection in adults and children. Am J Respir Crit Care Med 149:1359–1374, 1994.
9. Tietjen PA, Stover DE: *Pneumocystis carinii* pneumonia. Semin Respir Crit Care 16:173–186, 1995.
10. Tu J, Biem J, Detsky A: Bronchoscopy versus empirical therapy in HIV-infected patients with presumptive *Pneumocystis carinii* pneumonia: A decision analysis. Am Rev Respir Dis 148:370–377, 1993.
11. Vander Els NJ: Approach to the patient with pulmonary disease. Semin Respir Crit Care Med 16:240–250, 1995.
12. Walker BA, White DA: Management of the HIV-infected patient: Pulmonary disease. Med Clin North Am 80:1996.

37. NONINFECTIOUS PULMONARY COMPLICATIONS OF AIDS

Allan R. Tunkel, M.D., Ph.D., and Jeffrey Glassroth, M.D.

1. What is the incidence of pulmonary Kaposi's sarcoma in patients with AIDS?

Clinical studies have reported an incidence of pulmonary Kaposi's sarcoma in up to one-third of patients with cutaneous disease; the incidence is 50% in autopsy series. Cutaneous manifestations usually precede visceral disease, in some cases by years.

2. Do all patients with pulmonary Kaposi's sarcoma have cutaneous involvement?

Patients with pulmonary Kaposi's sarcoma almost always have cutaneous disease, although there have been occasional reports of lung involvement in the absence of other evidence of disease. In fact, many patients (27–100%) with pulmonary Kaposi's sarcoma have oropharyngeal or tracheobronchial evidence of Kaposi's sarcoma, which may facilitate the diagnosis.

3. What is the chest radiographic pattern of pulmonary Kaposi's sarcoma?

Two chest radiographic patterns are most commonly seen in patients with pulmonary Kaposi's sarcoma. The first pattern (noted in 57–83% of patients) is the radiographic appearance of interstitial infiltrates that usually follow septal lines; these infiltrates may be localized with focal areas of consolidation and have a perihilar predominance. A second major pattern (reported in 15–33% of patients) is a predominance of nodular infiltrates that are ill defined and of various sizes; coalescence may occur with areas of patchy consolidation. Pleural effusions are very common (in up to 60% of patients), may be unilateral or bilateral, and are usually, although not always, associated with concomitant parenchymal disease. Chest CT, particularly high resolution (HRCT), may be useful diagnostically in patients with Kaposi's sarcoma. In one series, 92% of patients with histologically documented parenchymal or endobronchial Kaposi's sarcoma had abnormal, ill-defined hilar densities extending into the adjacent pulmonary parenchyma along distinctly perivascular and peribronchial pathways. This pattern is similar to that of other types of lymphangitic carcinomatosis.

4. How is the diagnosis of pulmonary Kaposi's sarcoma best made?

The diagnosis of pulmonary Kaposi's sarcoma is often difficult to confirm histologically and is, therefore, often made presumptively based on clinical and radiographic findings and exclusion of other entities. Definitive diagnosis can be made only on biopsy. Cytology of sputum, bronchial washes, and examination of bronchoalveolar lavage or pleural fluid (or both) are not helpful. The yield of transbronchial biopsy ranges from 0–18%. The low yield results from the deep submucosal location of the endobronchial lesions and the patchy nature with which the tumor infiltrates lung parenchyma. It is necessary to see the architecture of spindle cells in association with vascular slits to make a histologic diagnosis. Endoscopic visualization of typical Kaposi's lesions is acceptable for diagnosis, especially in patients with biopsy-proven disease from other sites (e.g., skin or mucous membranes) and a typical chest radiographic pattern. One autopsy study confirmed the presence of parenchymal disease in 100% of patients with known endobronchial disease, although endobronchial disease may be absent in many cases of parenchymal disease. Open lung biopsy has the highest yield but is rarely performed because bronchoscopy is usually adequate to visualize airway lesions and rule out the possibility of infection.

5. Is it risky to biopsy pulmonary lesions in patients with Kaposi's sarcoma?

Some investigators consider transbronchial biopsy of Kaposi's sarcoma lesions to be high risk for potential bleeding (given their vascular nature), although others have not found this to be true. In a recent study from Brazil, 11 of 25 patients who underwent such biopsies had no complications. Transbronchial biopsies appear to be safe, and excessive bleeding is rare in patients with parenchymal pulmonary disease. Less information is available concerning biopsy of endobronchial lesions.

6. Why isn't a transthoracic pleural biopsy helpful for the diagnosis of Kaposi's sarcoma?

Pleural involvement is a frequent finding in the late stages of Kaposi's sarcoma and is manifested by a rapid accumulation of pleural fluid, which is often bilateral and of moderate size. Chemical analysis of pleural fluid almost always demonstrates an exudate, although there have been rare reports of transudates and chylous effusions, probably caused by lymphatic obstruction. The results of cytologic and histologic analysis of pleural fluid and pleural biopsy specimens have been uniformly negative because of the visceral subpleural location of Kaposi's sarcoma in the lung and the lack of a pathognomonic cytologic abnormality to aid in the diagnosis. Although several cytokines have been proposed as markers of Kaposi's sarcoma, none has proved useful thus far for diagnosis.

7. Is there a role for radionuclide scanning in the diagnosis of pulmonary Kaposi's sarcoma?

Sequential nuclear scanning with gallium and thallium may have a role in noninvasively distinguishing intrathoracic Kaposi's sarcoma from other malignancies and infections involving the chest. Gallium uptake rarely occurs in patients with Kaposi's sarcoma (in contrast to those with other malignancies, such as lymphoma, and infections). Thallium is taken up by both patients with Kaposi's sarcoma and those with lymphoma, but not in patients with *Pneumocystis carinii* pneumonia. Therefore, negative gallium and positive thallium uptake may be useful for the diagnosis of Kaposi's sarcoma, although further large-scale studies are needed to confirm these findings.

8. Does pulmonary Kaposi's sarcoma respond to therapy?

Therapeutic modalities to treat Kaposi's sarcoma include biologic modifiers (e.g., interferon-α), radiotherapy, and chemotherapy. Once pulmonary disease occurs, chemotherapy is almost always indicated because of the rapid progression of the disease and the need for a rapid response. Kaposi's sarcoma responds to single-agent therapy with drugs such as vincristine, vinblastine, bleomycin, doxorubicin, and possibly epirubicin, although higher response rates are achieved with combination chemotherapy. One retrospective review of patients with disseminated pulmonary Kaposi's sarcoma treated with adriamycin, bleomycin, and vincristine reported that 80% had complete or partial remission with a median survival of 10 months (versus 6 months for nonresponders). The most active regimens contain doxorubicin; the combination of doxorubicin, bleomycin, and vincristine is relatively well tolerated and frequently used. Recent data have shown that liposomes specifically target Kaposi's sarcoma lesions, and some studies suggest that liposomal daunorubicin is an effective and less toxic modality when given as conventional chemotherapy.

9. What is the prognosis for Kaposi's sarcoma in patients with pulmonary involvement?

The median survival of HIV-infected patients with extensive pulmonary disease as a result of Kaposi's sarcoma is 2–6 months, although one study reported an average survival of 15 months, and survival up to several years has occasionally been reported. Features predictive of shortened survival include the presence of a pleural effusion, severe shortness of breath, and an absolute CD4 lymphocyte count of less than 100 per mm^3.

10. What are the complications of pulmonary Kaposi's sarcoma?

Complications include upper airway obstruction from laryngeal involvement; pulmonary hemorrhage; and respiratory failure caused by massive parenchymal involvement, massive pleural effusion, or pulmonary edema from lymphangitic obstruction. Hypoxemia and progressive pulmonary infiltrates can result in respiratory failure exclusively because of Kaposi's sarcoma in the lungs. Survival to extubation when mechanical ventilation is initiated in such cases is uncommon.

11. What is the frequency of chest involvement in AIDS patients with non-Hodgkin's lymphoma?

Thoracic involvement with non-Hodgkin's lymphoma has been reported to range from 6–31% of AIDS patients in most large series, although pulmonary complaints are not usually the major presenting features. More commonly, pulmonary involvement is noted at initial presentation in association with other clinical manifestations or is discovered during the staging process. The lung can be the initial or the only site of involvement, however.

12. What are the characteristic radiographic findings in AIDS patients with pulmonary non-Hodgkin's lymphoma?

Chest radiographs most commonly show parenchymal infiltrates (including interstitial and air space disease) and single or multiple nodules. Pleural effusions (unilateral or bilateral) are often noted in the absence of parenchymal disease. In contrast to non-AIDS patients, few mediastinal and hilar nodes are present. Pulmonary nodules may grow at very rapid rates, doubling in days to weeks in some cases.

13. What is the yield of bronchoscopy for the diagnosis of pulmonary non-Hodgkin's lymphoma?

Bronchoscopy with transbronchial biopsy has a poor yield for the diagnosis of pulmonary non-Hodgkin's lymphoma (nondiagnostic in each of four patients in one report), although there are rare reports of positive biopsies. Needle aspiration of focal lesions has been useful, although experience is limited. Generally, open lung biopsy is required. For patients with pleural effusion, thoracentesis and pleural biopsy has some utility; in one study this modality was diagnostic in five of eight patients.

14. What is the prognosis for HIV-infected patients with non-Hodgkin's lymphoma?

For all HIV-infected patients with non-Hodgkin's lymphoma, median survival is only 6.5 months. However, only occasionally do the respiratory effects of these lymphomas result in significant morbidity or mortality. Factors associated with a poor response to therapy for non-Hodgkin's lymphoma include a history of an AIDS-defining illness before the diagnosis of lymphoma, bone marrow involvement, and a low Karnofsky performance status. In the absence of these factors, prognosis is more favorable; complete remission is attained after therapy in up to 75% of patients and median survival is 11.3 months.

15. What is the frequency of lymphocytic interstitial pneumonitis in HIV-infected patients?

Lymphocytic interstitial pneumonitis (LIP) has been observed in the adult and pediatric HIV-infected population. The incidence in infants and children is quite high (up to 40%); LIP ranks second only to *Pneumocystis carinii* as a cause of pulmonary disease in pediatric AIDS patients. The incidence in adults appears much lower, perhaps 1% of patients. A nonspecific interstitial pneumonitis, usually of low grade, seems more common among adults.

16. What is the prognosis for LIP in children?

The natural history of LIP varies. Typically, untreated LIP is characterized by progressive hypoxemia and worsening infiltrates on chest radiographs; corticosteroids can be considered for patients with progressive pulmonary deterioration once an infectious cause has been excluded. Dramatic improvement with steroid therapy has been observed.

17. Is it helpful to screen asymptomatic HIV-infected persons for pulmonary complications?

No. Studies have shown that pulmonary function and radiographic screening are not useful for this purpose and are more likely to produce falsely positive results than to identify actual disease processes. However, these and other studies are clearly helpful in evaluating patients with symptoms of pulmonary disease. Likewise, testing to establish a baseline, especially in intravenous drug users, who often have radiographic and diffusing capacity (DLCO) abnormalities related to drug use, may be helpful.

CONTROVERSIES

18. Is the incidence of lung cancer increased in HIV-infected patients?

Several reports have concluded that the incidence of lung cancer (and other solid tumors) may be increased in HIV-infected patients. Reasons for this increase in incidence are unclear because this tumor is not increased in frequency in other immunosuppressed patients. It has been postulated that immune surveillance might play a role, but there is little correlation between absolute CD4 lymphocyte count and time of lung cancer diagnosis. In one review, six cases of bronchogenic carcinoma were documented in 500 HIV seropositive patients (a 14-fold increased incidence compared with the general population). Other studies have failed to confirm this association, however. These data may represent coexistence of a common illness (i.e., lung cancer) with the recent epidemic of HIV infection. In most series, almost all patients had a history of cigarette smoking and were relatively young at the time of diagnosis (median age of 43 years); adenocarcinoma was the histologic subtype in 44–100% of cases.

19. What is the clinical course in HIV-infected patients with lung cancer?

Some studies have suggested that HIV-infected patients with an advanced stage of disease have a more fulminant, rapidly declining course resulting from lung cancer when compared with a control population. In one retrospective review of 23 HIV-infected patients with lung cancer, the median survival from the time of lung cancer diagnosis was 3 months; advanced stages of both HIV infection and lung cancer may have accounted for the poor survival. Data on survival in published series are somewhat limited by the failure to account for concomitant illnesses, the relative ability of each group to tolerate various therapeutic modalities, and poor documentation of the cause of death.

20. Is the incidence of pulmonary embolism increased in HIV-infected patients?

Pulmonary embolism has been described in patients with AIDS, although it remains unclear whether AIDS can lead to a hypercoagulable state. Some AIDS patients have prothrombotic abnormalities, such as increased anticardiolipin IgG activity and low protein S and protein C concentrations. Low free protein S concentrations were noted in two patients with AIDS and deep venous thrombosis; low concentrations were also noted in 22 of 71 AIDS patients tested prospectively. Although the lupus anticoagulant is common in AIDS patients (prevalence estimated to be 45%), thrombotic complications of this phenomenon appear to be rare. The frequency of primary pulmonary hypertension is probably increased among HIV-infected persons. This entity also should be considered in the evaluation of possible pulmonary vascular disease in such patients.

21. Is bronchial asthma more common among HIV-seropositive persons?

No definitive answer can be provided on this point. Several small studies have proposed that reversible airflow obstruction and increased bronchial reactivity (e.g., to methacholine) occur more commonly among HIV-seropositive persons. However, other investigators have been unable to confirm those observations.

BIBLIOGRAPHY

1. Aaron SD, Warner E, Edelson JD: Bronchogenic carcinoma in patients seropositive for human immunodeficiency virus. Chest 106:640–642, 1994.
2. Becker DM, Saunders TJ, Wispelwey B, et al: Case report: Venous thromboembolism in AIDS. Am J Med Sci 303:395–397, 1992.
3. Cadranel J, Mayaud C: Intrathoracic Kaposi's sarcoma in patients with AIDS. Thorax 50:407–414, 1995.
4. Coblentz C: The chest radiograph in the acquired immunodeficiency syndrome. Semin Respir Med 13:275–292, 1992.
5. Flores MR, Sridhar KS, Thurer RJ, et al: Lung cancer in patients with human immunodeficiency virus infection. Am J Clin Oncol 18:59–66, 1995.
6. Kuhlman JE: Pulmonary manifestations of acquired immunodeficiency syndrome. Semin Roentgenol 29:242–274, 1994.
7. Meduri GU, Stein DS: Pulmonary manifestations of acquired immunodeficiency syndrome. Clin Infect Dis 14:98–113, 1992.
8. Ognibene FP: Nonspecific and lymphocytic interstitial pneumonitis in HIV-infected individuals. Semin Respir Crit Care Med 16:227–230, 1995.
9. Rosen MJ, Lou Y, Kvale PA, et al: Pulmonary function tests in HIV-infected patients without AIDS. Am J Respir Crit Care Med 152:738–745, 1995.
10. Schattner G, White DA: Pulmonary manifestations of malignancies associated with HIV infection. Semin Respir Crit Care Med 16:216–226, 1995.
11. Schneider RF, Hansen NI, Rosen MJ, et al: Lack of usefulness of radiographic screening for pulmonary disease in asymptomatic HIV-infected adults. Arch Intern Med 156:191–195, 1996.
12. Tenholder MF, Jackson HD: Bronchogenic carcinoma in patients seropositive for human immunodeficiency virus. Chest 104:1049–1053, 1993.
13. Vander Els NJ: Approach to the patient with pulmonary disease. Semin Respir Crit Care Med 16:240–250, 1995.
14. Wallace JM, Rao AV, Glassroth J, et al: Respiratory illness in persons with human immunodeficiency virus infection. Am Rev Respir Dis 148:1523–1529, 1993.
15. White DA, Matthay RA: Noninfectious pulmonary complications of infection with the human immunodeficiency virus. Am Rev Respir Dis 140:1763–1787, 1989.

VIII. Pulmonary Vascular Diseases

38. THROMBOEMBOLIC DISEASE

Gideon Besson, M.D., and Harold I. Palevsky, M.D.

1. What are the signs and symptoms of pulmonary embolism?

The clinical presentation of pulmonary embolism varies with the size of the embolus and the patient's underlying cardiopulmonary functional status. Large pulmonary emboli that occlude the main pulmonary artery may present as an acute, fatal event. Somewhat smaller clots may present as a syncopal event. Very small pulmonary emboli that occlude the distal pulmonary vasculature may cause only transient dyspnea with pleuritic pain. The extent of hemodynamic and gas exchange abnormalities observed may be disproportionate to the size of the clot as a result of the release of humoral factors, possibly largely serotonin, occurring after clots interrupt flow in the pulmonary vascular bed.

In the Urokinase–Streptokinase Pulmonary Embolism Trials (USPET) and Prospective Investigation of Pulmonary Embolism Diagnosis (PIOPED) studies, the most common complaint regardless of clot size was dyspnea (82–85%). Pleuritic chest pain was the second most common complaint, then cough (50% of patients), hemoptysis, and syncope. Hemoptysis was more commonly observed in patients in the USPET study and was most often associated with smaller clots.

Frequency of Signs and Symptoms of Pulmonary Embolism in Women versus Men and Massive versus Submassive Pulmonary Embolism

SYMPTOM/SIGN	PIOPED DATA		USPET DATA	
	WOMEN	MEN	MASSIVE	SUBMASSIVE
Dyspnea	80%	78%	85%	82%
Pleuritic chest pain	60%	57%	64%	85%
Cough	41%	40%	53%	52%
Hemoptysis	10%	21%	23%	40%
Leg pain	23%	30%		
Leg swelling	24%	36%		
Pleural rub	2%	7%		
Crackles	60%	57%		
Mean heart rate ± SD (beats/min)	98 ± 19	93 ± 18		
Mean respiratory rate ± SD (breaths/min)	24 ± 8	23 ± 7		
Syncope	—	—	20%	4%

SD = standard deviation from the mean.

2. How does pulmonary embolism present in patients undergoing mechanical ventilation?

The ventilated critically ill patient is at greatly increased risk for pulmonary emboli because of immobilization, long-term intravenous lines, infections, and recent trauma or surgery. Unfortunately, the presentation and evaluation of thromboembolic disease may be hampered by a lack of suggestive complaints from a sedated and possibly paralyzed patient. Tachycardia often may be the only immediate manifestation of distress available to prompt a clinical evaluation of primary thromboembolic disease.

Other signs result from the physiologic changes that occur when a pulmonary embolism obstructs blood flow to pulmonary segments distal to a clot. In these lung regions, perfusion decreases but ventilation remains unchanged. The resulting increase in dead space ventilation causes an increase in P_{CO_2}, which results in an increase in minute ventilation. An unexplained rise in minute ventilation, therefore, may suggest the presence of a pulmonary embolism. In weak or paralyzed patients who cannot trigger the ventilator, the respiratory rate and tidal volume are fixed at the level of the ventilator settings. An increase in dead space ventilation, therefore, may cause an increase in P_{CO_2} and possibly a decrease in P_{O_2} without a change in lung compliance. The combination of tachycardia, an increase in P_{CO_2}, a decrease in P_{O_2}, and an unchanged lung compliance may warrant further investigation. The diagnostic accuracy for pulmonary embolism of a drop in P_{O_2} with an unchanged lung compliance has been examined in ventilated trauma patients. Of 583 ventilated patients cared for in a trauma service, 48 developed a decrease in P_{O_2} without a change in lung compliance. Forty-four percent of these patients had positive pulmonary angiograms for pulmonary emboli. No other instances of pulmonary emboli were identified in this population of patients who had the diagnosis pursued off of the study protocol. This study may overestimate the utility of this clinical presentation for the diagnosis of pulmonary embolism because patients who did not have a change in lung compliance did not undergo pulmonary angiography.

3. What is the significance of arm vein deep venous thrombosis?

More than 90% of pulmonary emboli arise from the deep venous system of the lower extremities. Occasionally, however, patients with upper extremity deep venous thrombosis experience thromboembolic events. Deep venous thrombosis of the axillary or subclavian veins occurs in three clinical settings: (1) spontaneous thromboses that may be idiopathic or associated with strenuous upper arm work or athletic-related effort, (2) thromboses associated with central venous cannulation, and (3) miscellaneous occurrences related to trauma, intravenous drug use, and intrathoracic tumors. A recent review of 71 case reports and 17 patient series indicates that up to 10% of these patients may experience an associated pulmonary embolism. Embolic phenomena associated with upper extremity deep venous thrombosis have a clinical importance similar to that of pulmonary emboli from lower extremity sources; 10% of patients with pulmonary emboli related to upper extremity deep venous thrombosis die from their thromboembolic event.

4. What are the typical chest radiographic findings in patients with pulmonary emboli?

The standard chest radiograph may be helpful in the diagnostic evaluation of patients with suspected pulmonary embolism. However, a normal chest radiograph does not eliminate the possibility of pulmonary embolism and the radiographic findings associated with the disease are nonspecific.

Of the associated findings, decreased vascularity in one lung causing a unilateral increase in radiographic lucency (Westermark's sign) suggests the presence of a large pulmonary embolus. This finding may be associated with prominence of the central pulmonary artery shadows. A wedge-shaped peripheral infiltrate (Hampton's hump) may be seen after a pulmonary embolus that occludes distal vessels in the pulmonary arterial tree. Most wedge-shaped pulmonary infiltrates resolve over time and, although historically the infiltrate has been ascribed to a pulmonary infarction, it probably represents hemorrhagic edema. The most frequently seen radiographic pattern in patients with pulmonary embolism, however, is a combination of nonspecific parenchymal infiltrates, atelectasis, and pleural effusions.

The presence of radiographic abnormalities does not obviate the value of the ventilation-perfusion lung scan. Finding unmatched perfusion defects, especially in areas where the chest radiograph is relatively normal, warrants further consideration of pulmonary embolism. Also, the lung scan retains its diagnostic accuracy in patients with diffuse, relatively symmetrical radiographic abnormalities, such as those seen in interstitial lung disease, congestive heart failure, and obstructive pulmonary disease.

5. **Do patients with pulmonary embolism always have hypoxemia or an increased alveolar-arterial gradient?**

Patients with pulmonary emboli frequently have tachypnea and may present with hyperventilation and a resulting respiratory alkalosis. The P_{O_2} may be variably elevated, normal, or low, but the alveolar-arterial (A-a) gradient is most often increased. No absolute value of P_{O_2} or A-a gradient, however, can reliably exclude the diagnosis of pulmonary embolism in a patient with a clinical presentation suggestive of the disease. Furthermore, it was recently shown in a group of 64 patients with angiographically proven pulmonary embolism that A-a gradients ranged from 11.6–83.9 mmHg. Three patients who had strongly suggestive histories of pulmonary embolism and confirmed disease presented with a P_{O_2} of less than 85 and a normal A-a gradient. Although normal A-a gradient and P_{O_2} may reassure the clinician that the thromboemboli are not severe or extensive, these findings do not obviate a further work-up in a patient with clinical presentation suggestive of the disease.

6. **What is the significance of severe hypoxemia in a patient with pulmonary embolism?**

Large or multiple pulmonary emboli can lead to obstruction in a substantial portion of the pulmonary vascular bed, resulting in an increase in dead space ventilation, an increase in pulmonary artery pressures, and an increase in the A-a gradient. This is associated with decreased P_{O_2} and evidence of right heart failure (peripheral edema, distended neck veins, tricuspid regurgitation, a right sided S4, and a loud P2). In patients who have a patent foramen ovale, atrial septal defect, or ventricular septal defect, however, increases in pulmonary artery pressure may result in unloading of the right ventricle by shunting blood flow to the left side of the heart, bypassing the pulmonary bed. When this extrapulmonary shunt occurs signs of right heart failure are absent and arterial P_{O_2} is low, typically less than 60 mmHg, and fails to improve with the patient breathing supplemental 100% oxygen. Activation of a right-to-left shunt in patients with pulmonary emboli may promote paradoxical embolization and resulting embolic strokes or occlusion of other systemic arterial vascular beds.

Patients with suspected pulmonary emboli who present with very low P_{O_2} should undergo ventilation-perfusion lung scans with additional images obtained over the brain and kidneys. Normally, the technetium-labeled microaggregated albumin used for the perfusion scan is trapped in the lungs and never enters the systemic circulation. In the setting of an extrapulmonary shunt, however, the radiolabeled particles cross directly to the left side of the heart and are trapped in systemic capillary beds. Images taken over the brain or kidneys, therefore, show radioactivity. Additionally, the shunt fraction can be calculated from the ratio of counts measured systematically to total counts.

7. **How are lung scans used to diagnose pulmonary emboli?**

The ventilation-perfusion lung scan is the initial study for the specific diagnosis of pulmonary embolism in patients with suggestive clinical findings. A normal perfusion lung scan excludes the diagnosis with more than 98% confidence. A high probability lung scan (multiple segmental defects that ventilate but do not perfuse) in the setting of high clinical suspicion (estimated likelihood of pulmonary embolism more than 80%) has a 96% positive predictive value. Unfortunately, the PIOPED study showed that 59% of patients with angiographically documented pulmonary embolism have an abnormal lung scan that is not high probability. These "intermediate," indeterminate," and "low" probability lung scans offer less diagnostic accuracy compared with normal or high-probability scans. Some investigators pool these results into the category of "nondiagnostic."

A low-probability lung scan associated with a low clinical suspicion (estimated likelihood of pulmonary embolism less than 20%) has a 96% negative predictive value. An intermediate probability scan (which represent 42% of all lung scans results in the PIOPED study) requires further diagnostic evaluation. Further evaluation is also indicated for patients who have a lung scan result that does not agree with the physician's clinical impression. In unstable patients who require urgent diagnosis or in those with underlying cardiopulmonary disease, a pulmonary angiogram may be indicated. Conversely, in stable patients, evaluation of the lower extremities may detect venous thrombosis and establish an indication for anticoagulation or placement of an inferior vena caval filter. However, 50% of patients with proven pulmonary emboli may have normal non-invasive studies of the lower extremity.

8. Can the predictive accuracy of lung scans be improved?

The PIOPED study provides data and a method of reasoning that allow clinicians to improve the predictive value of a ventilation-perfusion lung scan by taking into account the patient's clinical presentation. The combination of a high index of suspicion (more than 80% likelihood of pulmonary embolism on clinical grounds) and high-probability lung scan has a 96% positive predictive value for pulmonary embolism. Conversely, a low (less than 20%) clinical suspicion combined with a high-probability lung scan drops the positive predictive value to 56%. This means that almost 50% of patients with this clinical presentations will have a false-positive lung scan. Furthermore, the PIOPED study indicates that the diagnostic accuracy of a high-probability lung scan is reduced to 74% in patients with prior thromboembolic disease. Lung scan abnormalities in this setting probably represent unresolved defects from a previous embolic event. Lungs scans represent the cornerstone study in the diagnostic algorithm for pulmonary embolism but should not be interpreted in isolation. If the index of suspicion is low but the scan is high probability, confirmation of the diagnosis with further diagnostic studies is needed. Three major disease categories other than thromboembolism that can cause defects on perfusion scans are listed below.

- Prior pulmonary embolism (residual organized thrombotic material, not acute clot).
- Compression or entrapment of pulmonary vasculature.
  Mass lesion (i.e., malignancy, especially lung cancer)
  Adenopathy (i.e., malignancy, sarcoid, tuberculosis, broncholithiasis)
  Mediastinal fibrosis (i.e., idiopathic, post–radiation therapy)
  Compression by adjacent vascular structure (i.e., aortic aneurysm)
- Intraluminal obstruction of pulmonary vasculature
  Congenital vascular anomaly
    1. Agenesis
    2. Hypoplasia
    3. Coarctation
    4. Stenosis/branch stenosis
  Malignancy
    1. Metastatic (i.e., renal cell, myxoma, cardiac sarcoma)
    2. Primary tumor of pulmonary artery (i.e., sarcoma)
  Arteritis (i.e, Takayasu's disease, schistosomiasis)

9. What diagnostic modalities other than lung scans and pulmonary angiograms can assist with the diagnosis of venous thromboembolic disease?

The performance of lung scans coupled with impedance plethysmography, venous Doppler studies, and pulmonary angiograms has provided a highly sensitive and specific approach for diagnosing pulmonary embolism. Impedance plethysmography and duplex ultrasonographic studies can detect the presence of deep venous thrombosis in the lower extremity noninvasively. Implementation of these diagnostic studies, however, often presents a time-consuming challenge, requiring performance of studies sequentially. Noninvasive lower extremity tests may be negative initially in 50% of patients with pulmonary embolism and may require serial studies. Furthermore, pulmonary angiography is an invasive study that entails patient morbidity and a small but important risk of mortality. It is hoped that the newer diagnostic studies based on CT and MRI technology that are now undergoing clinical trials will simplify the approach to diagnosis.

10. Describe the new diagnostic studies based on CT and MRI technology.

Helical (spiral) CT and electron beam CT (EBCT) have increased image acquisition speed and resolution compared with conventional CT and have been reported to detect central to segmental pulmonary emboli with 95% sensitivity and 80% specificity. In one recent study, EBCT was compared with lung scanning in patients with angiographically proven pulmonary emboli. The study results indicated that EBCT was more sensitive and specific than lung scans in 38 of the 60 patients. CT scanning has an added advantage in that it may reveal pathology other than or in addition to embolic disease to explain clinical symptoms.

MRI scanning technology can demonstrate interruptions in flow across the pulmonary arterial bed in patients with pulmonary embolism and at the same time obtain images of the deep veins of the pelvis and lower extremities. These studies were previously limited by cardiac and respiratory motion artifact. Scan times are decreasing, however, and computer assistance allows for "respiratory gating" of scans so that imaging is not limited to patients who can hold their breath. MRI has the advantage of not needing iodinated contrast, and the time saved by imaging lower extremity veins and pulmonary bed simultaneously may make this modality a cost-effective means of diagnosing clinically significant thromboembolic disease.

These new technologies, however, remain investigational and require larger clinical studies to determine their role in patients with suspected pulmonary emboli.

11. Should impedance plethysmography or duplex ultrasonographic studies of the lower extremities be used for the initial diagnostic evaluation of patients with pulmonary embolism?

No. In the initial evaluation of a patient with a suspected pulmonary embolism, it is critically important to establish the presence of pulmonary emboli with a lung scan to determine prognosis, need for thrombolytic therapy, and explanation for respiratory systems. Lung scans, therefore, remain as the initial and pivotal diagnostic test for patients with cardiopulmonary symptoms compatible with pulmonary embolism. Noninvasive studies of the lower extremity serve to establish the diagnosis of deep venous thrombosis in patients with nondiagnostic lung scans. They also evaluate the likelihood of recurrent pulmonary emboli by demonstrating the presence of remaining lower extremity clot in patients who have already experienced a thromboembolic event.

12. How can the available tests be used to make a diagnosis of pulmonary embolism?

The following algorithm outlines an evidence-based approach to the diagnosis of pulmonary embolism based on recent data. A normal lung scan effectively excludes the possibility

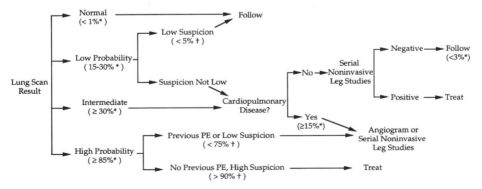

Diagnostic algorithm for pulmonary embolism. PE = pulmonary embolism. * Strongly supported by clinical studies; † Suggested by clinical studies. Percentages in parentheses indicate likelihood of pulmonary embolism. (From Kelley MA, Carson JL, Palevsky HI, et al: Diagnosing pulmonary embolism. New facts and strategies. Ann Intern Med 114:300–306, 1991, with permission.)

of pulmonary embolism. A high-probability scan strongly supports the diagnosis of pulmonary embolism and justifies the initiation of therapy unless the patient has had a previous pulmonary embolism or clinical suspicion of pulmonary embolism is low. A low-probability lung scan combined with low clinical suspicion has less than a 5% likelihood of pulmonary embolism, so observation without therapy is warranted with this combination of results. Positive noninvasive studies of the lower extremities can identify the presence of deep venous thrombosis and establish the need for anticoagulation. Patients with negative results of leg studies and nondiagnostic lung scans can then be followed with serial leg studies in the absence of cardiopulmonary disease or proceed to pulmonary angiography if they have sufficiently severe cardiopulmonary disease that a recurrent pulmonary embolism would be life-threatening.

13. Can patients with hemoptysis caused by pulmonary embolism be treated with full dose heparin?

Although no studies have specifically addressed this question, our practice has been to anticoagulate patients with a confirmed diagnosis of pulmonary embolism despite the presence of hemoptysis. Hemoptysis, however, may warrant additional diagnostic studies, such as bronchoscopy, to rule out accompanying lesions, such as endobronchial malignancies, because significant hemoptysis as a presenting manifestation of pulmonary embolism is unusual.

14. Which patients with pulmonary embolism should be treated with thrombolytic agents?

Thrombolytic therapy should be used in the treatment of patients with pulmonary emboli that obstruct a substantial portion of the pulmonary vascular bed. It is generally accepted that occlusion of more than 50% of the pulmonary vascular bed warrants thrombolysis, although some clinicians consider thrombolytic therapy in younger patients who have obstruction of 25–33% of the pulmonary circulation. Regardless of the degree of pulmonary obstruction, thrombolytic therapy should be considered whenever pulmonary emboli result in hemodynamic instability or respiratory compromise. In addition, some investigators have proposed evaluating stable patients with large pulmonary emboli by echocardiography; any evidence of right ventricular dysfunction or dilation is used as a rationale for treating with thrombolytic agents. This approach is currently being evaluated in a randomized trial.

15. What thrombolytic agents are available? What are their therapeutic and pharmacologic differences?

The U.S. Food and Drug Administration has approved three thrombolytic agents for the treatment of pulmonary embolism: streptokinase, urokinase, and recombinant tissue type plasminogen activator (rt-PA.) Only streptokinase has been approved for the treatment of deep venous thrombosis. When administered systemically, all of the agents lower fibrinogen, plasminogen, and α-2 antiplasmin levels and generate a systemic lytic state. In clinical practice, the theoretic fibrin selectivity of rt-PA has not proved to be of clinical importance in distinguishing among the available agents and it has not been associated with a lower rate of bleeding complications.

According to the standard protocols for treatment of venous thromboembolism, streptokinase and urokinase are administered by continuous peripheral IV infusion for 12–72 hours whereas tissue plasminogen activator is given as a 100-mg dose over 2 hours. These standard dosing protocols for pulmonary embolism or deep venous thrombosis (or both) do not include the concurrent use of antithrombotic medications such aspirin or heparin. Only after the completion of a course of thrombolytic therapy is standard anticoagulation instituted.

We question whether the standard, time-based dosing protocols for thrombolytic therapy are optimal. In our practice, once thrombolytic therapy is initiated, we continue treating until all of the thrombus is lysed or until serial imaging shows that the remaining thrombus is resistant to further lysis. Often this requires treatment for longer than the recommended period.

Approved Thrombolytic Therapy for Venous Thromboembolism

AGENT	PLASMA CLEARANCE	LOADING DOSE	HOURLY DOSE	RECOMMENDED DURATION
Streptokinase	12–18 min	250,000 IU over 30 min	100,000 IU	PE: 24 h DVT: 48–72 h
Urokinase	15–20 min	4,400 IU/kg over 10 min	4,400 IU/kg	PE: 12 h DVT: not approved
Tissue-type plasminogen activator (rt-PA)	2–6 min	None	50 mg	PE: 2 h DVT: not approved

DVT = deep venous thrombosis; h = hours; IU = international units; min = minute; PE = pulmonary embolism.

16. What are the long-term results for patients treated with thrombolytics?

Thrombolysis is advocated to reduce the acute morbidity and mortality from pulmonary embolism, reduce the recurrence rate of pulmonary emboli, preserve pulmonary microvasculature, and decrease the risk of chronic pulmonary hypertension from persistent pulmonary arterial clots. Over a decade it was shown that patients treated with thrombolytic therapy had better preservation of measurable lung diffusion (DLCO) than those treated with heparin. The investigators proposed that the pulmonary capillary blood volume (pulmonary microcirculation) is better preserved after thrombolytic therapy than after standard heparin anticoagulation. A preliminary report of follow-up hemodynamic evaluations of these patients 7 years later found that patients treated with thrombolytic agents had lower mean arterial pressures and pulmonary vascular resistance at rest and during exercise than patients who had been treated with heparin. However, the clinical and functional significance of these findings remains uncertain.

17. Is there a difference between local and systemic thrombolytic therapy for pulmonary embolism?

Thrombolytic therapy can be administered locally via a pulmonary arterial catheter directed either into or around an embolus. This procedure may lyse the clot with a lower dose of a thrombolytic agent in patients who are at risk for bleeding complications and have life-threatening pulmonary emboli. This procedure offers no advantage over systemic thrombolysis because local instillation often still results in a systemic lytic state.

18. What is the therapeutic role of an inferior vena cava filter in patients with pulmonary embolism?

The inferior vena cava (IVC) filter was introduced more than 25 years ago as a means of reducing the incidence of recurrent pulmonary emboli. These devices are placed in the inferior vena cava and trap thromboemboli from the lower extremity. The primary indication for placement of an IVC filter is the presence of deep venous thrombosis in a patient who cannot undergo systemic anticoagulation. A 20-year review of experience with the stainless steel Greenfield filter showed a 4% incidence of recurrence of pulmonary embolism in patients with contraindications to anticoagulation. In comparison, the incidence of recurrence of pulmonary embolism in anticoagulated patients is approximately 5.7% with heparin and 1.9% with coumadin.

Some physicians recommend the placement of a filter in patients with acute pulmonary embolism who have contraindications to thrombolytic therapy when recurrence of pulmonary embolism would be life-threatening. In trauma victims IVC filters may offer an important measure to prevent lethal pulmonary emboli. These patients have a high risk for the development of thromboembolic disease and often have contraindications to prophylactic anticoagulation. The clinical conditions associated with a particularly high risk are shown below. Prospective studies indicate that a prophylactic IVC filter may decrease the incidence of pulmonary embolism by 75% (1% to 0.25%) in these patients.

Trauma patients with the following conditions are at high risk for thromboembolism:
Spinal cord injury with paraplegia or quadriplegia (highest risk)
Severe head injury (Glascow coma scale < 8)
Age more than 55 years with isolated long bone fractures
Complex pelvic fractures involving posterior elements and associated long bone fracture

19. What is the relationship between pulmonary embolism and pregnancy?

Pulmonary embolism is five to six times more common in pregnant compared with non-pregnant women. Over a 5-year period of review in Australia, pulmonary embolism–associated mortality in pregnant women equalled the mortality caused by hypertensive complications of pregnancy. Pregnancy is associated with variations in the clotting cascade protein levels that may contribute to a relatively hypercoagulable state. Although the risk of pulmonary embolism is increased prenatally (particularly in the third trimester), the greatest risk occurs post partum, when the relative risk is approximately 20×. Other factors that contribute to the risk of pulmonary embolism during pregnancy are:
Previous pulmonary embolism (5–15% recurrence rate)
Immobilization
Age more than 40 years
Cesarean section
Gravida more than 4
African-American race
Hormonal therapy to promote fertility also increases the risk of thromboembolic disease.

20. Should pregnant patients with suspected pulmonary embolism undergo a conventional diagnostic evaluation?

Diagnosis of pulmonary embolism in pregnant women presents concerns about fetal radiation exposure. Undiagnosed and untreated pulmonary embolism represents a greater risk, however, to the well-being of the fetus. Current recommendations, therefore, encourage physicians to perform conventional diagnostic tests in pregnant patients with suspected pulmonary embolism. Some special precautions, however, should be initiated. Abdominal shields should be used during any radiographic procedure. Because the technetium used as the radiolabel in perfusion scans is excreted via the kidneys, we recommend hydration and placement of a Foley catheter to decrease the length of time that radionucleotide is in the bladder.

21. Can pregnant patients with pulmonary embolism be treated with systemic anticoagulation?

Coumadin is contraindicated in pregnant patients because of risk to the fetus. Heparin is the standard of care for use during the acute event and during long-term anticoagulation. Heparin therapy for longer than 5 months or at doses greater than 20,000 units a day, however, is associated with the development of osteoporosis.

BIBLIOGRAPHY

1. American College of Chest Physicians: Fourth Consensus Conference on Antibhrombotic Therapy. Chest 108(4 Suppl):225S–522S, 1995.
2. Becker DM, Philbrick JT, Walker FB IV: Axillary and subclavian venous thrombosis. Arch Intern Med 151:1934–1943, 1991.
3. Bell WR, Simon TL, DeMets DL: The clinical features of submassive and massive pulmonary emboli. Am J Med 62:355–360, 1977.
4. Braithwaite CEM, O'Malley KF, Ross SE, et al: Continuous pulse oximetry and the diagnosis of pulmonary embolism in critically ill trauma patients. J Trauma 33:528–531, 1992.
5. Dalen JE, Haffajec CI, Alpert JS, et al: Pulmonary embolism, pulmonary hemorrhage, pulmonary infarction. N Engl J Med 296:1431–1435, 1977.
6. Gefter WB, Hatabu H, Holland G, et al: Pulmonary thromboembolism: Recent developments in diagnosis using computed tomography and magnetic resonance imaging. Radiology 197(3):561–574, 1995.

7. Greenfield LJ, McCurdy JR, Brown PP, et al: A new intracaval filter permitting continued flow and resolution of emboli. Surgery 73:599–606, 1973.
8. Greenfield L, Proctor M: Twenty-year clinical experience with the Greenfield filter. Cardiovasc Surg 3:199–205, 1995.
9. Hull R, Delmore T, Carter C, et al: Adjusted subcutaneous heparin versus warfarin in the long-term treatment of venous thrombosis. N Engl J Med 306:189–194, 1982.
10. Jeffries WS, Bochner F: Thromboembolism and its management in pregnancy. Med J Aust 155:253–258, 1991.
11. Kelley MA, Carson JL, Palevsky HL, et al: Diagnosing pulmonary embolism: New facts and strategies. Ann Intern Med 114:300–306, 1991.
12. Morthy SS, Losasso AM, Gibbs PS: Acquired right-to-left intracardiac shunts and severe hypoxemia. Crit Care Med 6:28–31, 1978.
13. Overton DT, Bocks JJ: The alveolar-arterial oxygen gradient in patients with documented pulmonary embolism. Arch Intern Med 148:1610–1617, 1988.
14. Palevsky HL, Cone L, Alavi A: A case of "false-positive" high probability ventilation-perfusion lung scan due to tuberculous mediastinal adenopathy with a discussion of other causes of "false-positive: high probability ventilation-perfusion lung scans. J Nucl Med 32:512–517, 1991.
15. PIOPED Investigators: Value of the ventilation/perfusion scan in acute pulmonary embolism: Results of the Prospective Investigation of Pulmonary Diagnosis (PIOPED). JAMA 263:2753–2759, 1990.
16. Quinn DA, Thompson T, Terrin ML, et al: A prospective investigation of pulmonary embolism in women and men. JAMA 268:1689–1696, 1992.
17. Rogers FB, Schackford SR, Wilson J, et al: Prophylactic vena cava filter insertion in severely injured trauma patients: Indications and preliminary results. J Trauma 35:367–642, 1993.
18. Rutherford SE, Phelan JP: Deep venous thrombosis and pulmonary embolism in pregnancy. Obstet Gynecol Clin North Am 18:345–370, 1991.
19. Teigen CL, Maus TP, Sheedy PF, et al: Pulmonary embolism: Diagnosis with contrast-enhanced electron beam CT and comparison with pulmonary angiography. Radiology 194:313–319, 1995.

39. SPECIAL FORMS OF EMBOLIC DISEASE

Mark W. Geraci, M.D.

1. What is fat embolism syndrome?

Fat embolism syndrome (FES) is a clinical condition that can occur after fractures of long bones or other instances of marrow disruption. It is characterized by the appearance of free fat and fatty acids in the blood, lungs, brain, kidneys, and other organs. The classic triad of acute respiratory failure with diffuse pulmonary infiltrates, global neurologic dysfunction, and petechial rash occurs in only 0.5–2.0% of solitary long bone fractures; however, the incidence approaches 5–10% in multiple fractures with pelvic involvement. FES also has been associated with numerous nontraumatic clinical situations. The causes of FES are as follows:

Fractures (more than 90% of all cases)	Steroid therapy
Nontraumatic orthopedic procedures, mainly joint reconstruction	Alcoholic liver disease
	Parenteral infusion of lipids
Burns	Bone marrow harvesting and transplantation
Osteomyelitis	Liposuction
Diabetes mellitus	Decompression sickness
Pancreatitis	Cardiopulmonary bypass
Sickle cell disease	

2. What is the pathogenesis of FES?

The pathogenesis is controversial. Two major theories have been proposed. The mechanical theory postulates that bone marrow contents enter the venous system and lodge in the lungs as emboli. Smaller fat droplets (7–10 μ in diameter) may travel through the pulmonary capillaries into the systemic circulation and hence involve the brain and kidneys, as is commonly seen. Systemic embolization may also occur through a patent foramen ovale, a defect found in 20–34% of the population, but more likely occurs through intrapulmonary shunts. The biochemical theory suggests that circulating free fatty acids directly affect the pneumocytes, producing abnormalities in gas exchange. The most cogent therapy includes elements of both proposals. As the central inciting agent, embolic marrow fat is concentrated in the pulmonary bed and activates the clotting cascade, increases platelet function and fibrinolytic activity, and induces catecholamine-mediated mobilization of free fatty acids. These free fatty acids directly increase capillary permeability. Along with the release of inflammatory mediators, the final common pathway results in critical impairment of gas exchange and a form of ARDS.

3. How is the diagnosis of FES made?

The diagnosis is made on clinical grounds. The clinical presentation is usually marked by a latency period of 12–72 hours. Respiratory impairment leads to hypoxemia in up to 30% of patients. The chest radiograph often shows diffuse infiltrates. Cerebral symptoms may occur in 60% of patients and tend to follow the pulmonary symptoms. A petechial rash appears in 50% of patients and is usually found on the neck, axilla, trunk, or conjunctiva. The two most widely accepted clinical criteria for the diagnosis of FES are presented below.

Diagnosis of FES According to Gurd's (1970) Criteria

Major features	Minor features	Laboratory features
Respiratory insufficiency	Fever	Anemia
Cerebral involvement	Tachycardia	Thrombocytopenia
Petechial rash	Retinal changes	Elevated ESR
	Jaundice	Fat macroglobulinemia
	Renal changes	

A positive diagnosis requires the presence of one major feature plus four minor features and fat macroglobulinemia in the appropriate clinical setting.
From Gurd AR: Fat embolism: An aid to diagnosis. J Bone Joint Surg 52:732–737, 1970, with permission.

Diagnosis of FES According to Schonfeld's (1983) Criteria

SYMPTOM	SCORE
Petechiae	5
Diffuse alveolar infiltrates	4
Hypoxemia (Pao_2 = ≤ 70 torr)	3
Confusion	1
Fever (> 38° C)	1
Heart rate (≥ 120/min)	1
Respiratory rate (≥ 30/min)	1

FES is diagnosed when the cumulative score is 5 or more in the appropriate clinical setting.
From Schonfeld SA, Ploysongsang Y, DiLisio R, et al: Fat embolism prophylaxis with corticosteroids: A prospective study in high-risk patients. Ann Intern Med 99:438–443, 1983, with permission.

4. Are there specific tests to aid in the diagnosis of FES?

There is no single test to diagnose FES; rather, a pattern of biochemical abnormalities may be seen. Hematologic studies may reveal decreased hematocrit and platelets, whereas fibrin degradation products, prothrombin time, erythrocyte sedimentation rate, and C5a levels are often elevated. Biochemical abnormalities include lowered calcium level and the presence of fat microaggregates in samples of clotted blood. In a large series studied prospectively, the commonly held tenet of fat globules presenting in the urine was not found in any patient with FES. Similarly, after early reports of good predictive value, the presence of fat droplets in alveolar macrophages was shown not to be a reliable method for the diagnosis of FES.

5. How is FES treated?

A number of treatment modalities have been studied. The use of ethanol, heparin, low molecular weight dextran, and hypertonic glucose has shown inconsistent results, and these agents are not currently advocated. The first successful treatment of FES with corticosteroids was reported by Ashbaugh and Petty in 1966. In a well-designed, prospective, randomized, double-blind study of patients at high risk for FES, Schonfeld and colleagues showed that the prophylactic use of methylprednisolone (7.5 mg/kg IV every 6 hours for 12 doses) significantly reduced the incidence of FES. The use of steroids had no adverse effects on fracture healing. The mechanism of steroid effectiveness probably involves membrane stabilization, limitation in the rise of plasma free fatty acids, and inhibition of complement-mediated leukocyte aggregation. The effectiveness of steroids in situations other than prophylaxis remains to be tested. In summary, treatment includes aggressive supportive care, early ventilatory support, and early steroid use.

6. In what clinical settings has venous air embolism been described?

Air can enter the venous system when there is communication between gas (usually the atmosphere) and the open venous system and a pressure gradient favors the ingress of the gas. Gas may be forced into the venous system under high pressure, such as with laparoscopic procedures, pressurized infusion sets, or mechanical ventilation. Conversely, generating high negative intrathoracic pressures (as in hyperventilation, exacerbation of lung disease, hypovolemia, or upright positioning) may predispose patients to venous air embolism (VAE). With this pathogenic mechanism in mind, one can see VAE in surgical procedures (especially neurosurgery), central venous catheter placement, positive-pressure ventilation, trauma, laparoscopic procedures, contrast injections, and decompression sickness.

7. Describe the pathogenesis of VAE.

Once air enters the venous system, it migrates to the right heart and lungs. The major consequence to the circulatory system is obstruction to blood flow, causing both mechanical obstruction and profound vasospasm. Air may enter the arterial system from a right to left shunt, either from a cardiac defect or through microvascular intrapulmonary shunts. Moreover, a complex interaction occurs while air and blood mix in the right heart, causing a network of air bubbles, fibrin strands, platelet aggregates, erythrocytes, and fat globules. Factors other than simple mechanical obstruction may lead to pulmonary injury. The lungs can sequester neutrophils during VAE. Neutrophils gather around air bubbles, attach to the endothelium of the pulmonary arterioles, distort the microvascular architecture, and contribute to lung leak.

8. How much air is dangerous in VAE?

The factors that determine the severity of VAE were identified by Durant in 1947. The volume of air, the speed of entry, and the body position are all important factors; survival is greatest in animals recumbent on the left side. A volume of 3–8 ml air per kilogram body weight is necessary to produce death. Most VAE occurs in relation to central venous catheters (0–2% incidence). Mortality for VAE associated with central venous catheters has been reported to be as high as 32%. In humans, the lethal volume of air is estimated to be 300–500 ml. With a pressure gradient of only 5 cm water (as with normal tidal breathing) air can pass through a 14-g catheter at a rate of 100 ml per second.

9. What are the clinical manifestations of VAE? How can VAE be detected?

The clinical symptoms of VAE are often nonspecific. Patients may experience a gasping reflex, lightheadedness, dizziness, chest pain, or a sudden episode of dyspnea. If venous gas reaches the arterial circulation, evidence of myocardial or central nervous system injury may occur. Physical examination may reveal tachycardia, tachypnea, and signs of elevated right heart pressure. A mill-wheel murmur produced by movement of air bubbles in the right ventricle is considered the only specific sign, but it is a rare, transient, and late finding. Wheezing or rales may be present, possibly secondary to the vasospasm of the event. Detection of VAE may be difficult because the clinical signs and symptoms are often nonspecific. It is important to have a high index of suspicion in the correct clinical settings. Precoridal low frequency Doppler ultrasound is the most sensitive method for detection of venous air. During selected high-risk surgical procedures, continuous pulmonary artery pressure and end-tidal carbon dioxide monitoring (PET CO_2) are useful for early detection of VAE.

10. What is the treatment strategy for VAE?

Treatment of VAE is directed toward restoring flow within the cardiopulmonary circulation and promoting the reabsorption of intravascular air. If VAE is suspected, the patient should be placed left side down in a Trendelenberg position, allowing air to migrate toward the right apex of the heart, thus diminishing pulmonary outflow obstruction. Manual removal of air from an indwelling central line or pulmonary artery catheter may be attempted and is most effective at or above the right atrial junction, not in the right ventricle or pulmonary artery outflow tract. Closed-chest cardiac massage improves survival to the same extent as does proper positioning, presumably by mechanically forcing air out of the right ventricle and pulmonary outflow tract. Patients should be administered 100% FIO_2, and anesthetics containing nitrous oxide should be discontinued in an attempt to increase the rate of bubble absorption. For patients with persistent cardiopulmonary or cerebrovascular deficits despite these modalities, hyperbaric oxygen therapy should be initiated. If the patient needs to travel over a great distance, aircraft pressurized to 1.0 atmospheres should be used. High altitude (more than 300–500 feet) may increase bubble size.

11. What are the characteristics of amniotic fluid embolism?

Amniotic fluid embolism (AFE) is a rare but catastrophic syndrome occurring in 1 of 80,000 pregnancies. The cardinal signs of AFE are the sudden onset of respiratory distress, cyanosis, convulsions, and cardiovascular collapse during labor and delivery. Some 40% of patients also develop a major coagulopathy. AFE occurs during labor in 70% of cases, after vaginal delivery in 11%, and during cesarean section in 19%. Maternal mortality is 60–80%, and neurologically intact survival is seen in only 15% of women. Of fetuses in utero at the time of the event, only 40% survive.

12. Who is at risk for AFE?

AFE may occur during therapeutic abortion, abdominal trauma, amniocentesis, and labor and delivery. Although original reports stated that the incidence was greater with hypertonic labor, recently no correlation was found with the incidence of AFE and either prolonged labor or oxytocin use. Factors associated with increased risk for AFE include advanced maternal age, multiparity, premature placental separation, fetal death, fetal male sex, meconium staining, and a history of allergy or atopy in the mother.

13. How is AFE best treated?

Aggressive supportive care is imperative, as most maternal deaths occur within 1 hour of the onset of symptoms. New studies show that close hemodynamic monitoring with a pulmonary artery catheter often shows elevated wedge pressures and left ventricular dysfunction. Along with respiratory support that often includes mechanical ventilation, it is therefore recommended that close hemodynamic monitoring be instituted to optimize left ventricular function.

14. What is the pathogenesis of pulmonary tumor embolism?

Pulmonary tumor embolism occurs when solid tumors seed the systemic circulation with individual cells, clusters of cells, or large tumor fragments. These emboli travel to the pulmonary vasculature and are lodged largely in the microvasculature. Leukemic sequestration, seen most often in acute myelogenous leukemia (AML), is a similar clinical entity. Pulmonary tumor embolism has a different pathophysiologic mechanism than the more common mechanisms of tumor involvement of the lung, which include metastatic parenchymal disease, lymphangitic tumor spread, endovascular lymphomatosis, or large-vessel tumor occlusion. The pathologic spectrum of tumor embolism varies, ranging from large tumor masses that may mimic pulmonary embolism, to the more common microvessel embolism in small arterioles and capillaries that causes a subacute clinical syndrome. Most authorities believe that microvascular emboli are ultimately the source of lymphangitic carcinomatosis.

15. What tumors are associated with pulmonary tumor embolism?

Tumor embolism occurs in patients who are also at high risk for thromboembolic events, especially those with mucin-producing adenocarcinomas. It is therefore important to distinguish thromboembolic pulmonary disease from tumor embolism. The following tumors are associated with microvascular tumor emboli:

Hepatoma	Gynecologic	Gallbladder
Renal	Atrial myxoma	Thyroid
Stomach	Pancreas	Parotid
Prostate	Bladder	Lung
Choriocarcinoma	Breast	Skin
Colon	Esophagus	

16. How is the diagnosis of tumor embolism made? What treatment can be offered?

Most cases of pulmonary tumor embolism occur in patients with known malignant disease. The clinical course is usually subacute, with dyspnea developing over the course of weeks. Patients often show signs of pulmonary hypertension, including elevated venous pressures, a loud P2, and sometimes a right-sided gallop. The chest radiograph is often normal but may show evidence of focal metastatic disease. Ventilation-perfusion (V/Q) scans do not suggest thromboembolic disease; rather, the scans demonstrate peripheral subsegmental perfusion defects with a mottled appearance. The ventilation scan is usually normal. In this regard, the V/Q scan is similar to that seen with primary pulmonary hypertension or fat embolism yet is distinct from the focal abnormalities seen in pulmonary thromboembolic disease. Appropriate therapy for microvessel tumor embolism is poorly understood, because diagnosis is rarely made before death. Controlling the source of the primary tumor with surgical resection affords some benefit. Rarely, embolectomy has been performed; chemotherapy usually has no role in this disorder.

17. Describe the presentation of septic pulmonary emboli.

Septic pulmonary emboli result from the embolization of a distant endovascular infection. This is most often seen in right-sided endocarditis in intravenous drug abusers but may also be catheter-related or the result of septic pelvic thrombophlebitis. The clinical manifestations include fever, chills, rigor, dyspnea, pleuritic pain, cough, and hemoptysis. Physical examination reveals a cardiac murmur in only 20% of cases. The chest radiograph may be characteristic, showing multiple small, patchy peripherally located densities that can change rapidly on serial examinations. Complications include pulmonary gangrenous infarction, abscess formation, empyema, and pneumonia. Pulmonary vein septic thrombophlebitis can develop, and these infected emboli can serve as a source of systemic embolization.

18. What is the treatment for septic pulmonary emboli?

The mainstay of treatment is prolonged administration of high-dose antibiotics. Right-sided endocarditis is the most common cause of this syndrome. Four weeks of antibiotic therapy is generally indicated for endocarditis, but new regimens with a more aggressive initial course have been used in cases of sensitive strains of viridans streptococci and *Staphylococcus aureus*. Surgical resection of the tricuspid valve is recommended for organisms that do not respond to initial antibiotic therapy, fungal endocarditis, or coexistent infection with *S. aureus* and *Pseudomonas aeruginosa*. The prognosis for right-sided endocarditis in generally favorable when compared with that of left-sided disease.

BIBLIOGRAPHY

1. Ashbaugh DG, Petty TL: The use of corticosteroids in the treatment of respiratory failure associated with massive fat embolism. Surg Gynecol Obstet 123:493–500, 1966.
2. Bricker MB, Morris WP, Allen SJ, et al: Venous air embolism in patients with pulmonary barotrauma. Crit Care Med 22:1692–1698, 1994.
3. Chan C, Hutcheon M, Hyland R, et al: Pulmonary tumor embolism: A critical review of clinical, imaging, and hemodynamic features. J Thorac Imaging 2:4–14, 1987.
4. Clark SL, Hankins GDV, Dudley DA, et al: Amniotic fluid embolism: Analysis of the national registry. Am J Obstet Gynecol 172:1158–1169, 1995.
5. Dudney TM, Elliott CG: Pulmonary embolism from amniotic fluid, fat and air. Prog Cardiovasc Dis 36:447–474, 1994.
6. Durant TM, Long J, Oppenheier MJ: Pulmonary (venous) air embolism. Am Heart J 33:269–281, 1947.
7. Fabian TC: Unraveling the fat embolism syndrome. N Engl J Med 329:961–963, 1993.
8. Gurd AR: Fat embolism: An aid to diagnosis. J Bone Joint Surg 52:732–737, 1970.
9. Hanna PG, Gravenstein N, Pashayan AG: In vitro comparison of central venous catheters for aspiration of venous air embolism: Effect of catheter type, catheter tip position, and cardiac inclination. J Clin Anesth 3:290–294, 1991.
10. King MB, Harmon KR: Unusual forms of pulmonary embolism. Clin Chest Med 15:561–580, 1994.
11. Lantz PE, Smith JD: Fatal carbon dioxide embolism complicating attempted laparoscopic cholecystectomy—case report and literature review. J Forensic Sci 39:1468–1480, 1994.
12. Ordway CB: Air embolus via CVP catheter without positive pressure. Ann Surg 179:479–481, 1974.
13. Pell ACH, Hughes D, Keating J, et al: Fulminating fat embolism syndrome caused by paradoxical embolism through a patent foramen ovale. N Engl J Med 329:926–929, 1993.
14. Rementz MS, Quagliarello V: Endovascular infections arising from right-sided heart structures. Cardiol Clin 10:137–149, 1992.
15. Schonfeld SA, Ploysongsang Y, DiLisio R, et al: Fat embolism prophylaxis with corticosteroids: A prospective study in high-risk patients. Ann Intern Med 99:438–443, 1983.
16. Seidelin PH, Thompson AM: Central venous catheterization and fatal air embolism. Br J Hosp Med 25:438–439, 1987.
17. Vedrinne JM, Guillame C, Gagnieu MC, et al: Bronchoalveolar lavage in trauma patients for diagnosis of fat embolism syndrome. Chest 102:1323–1327, 1992.

40. PULMONARY HYPERTENSION

Lewis J. Rubin, M.D.

1. What is required to establish a diagnosis of primary pulmonary hypertension?

The criteria developed by the NIH Registry on primary pulmonary hypertension (PPH) required the demonstration of a mean pulmonary artery pressure at rest of more than 25 mmHg in the absence of a demonstrable cause, including left ventricular, valvular, or congenital heart disease; significant parenchymal lung disease; systemic connective tissue disease; or chronic thromboembolic disease. However, mild abnormalities in pulmonary function that are out of proportion to the hemodynamic abnormalities are common in PPH. Similarly, isolated Raynaud's phenomenon and connective tissue blood tests that are positive in low titers may also be seen in PPH.

2. Is a lung biopsy necessary to establish a diagnosis of PPH?

In most cases, a diagnosis of PPH can be made on clinical grounds by excluding other demonstrable causes. In rare cases, it may be necessary to obtain a biopsy specimen of lung tissue to exclude vasculitis or active interstitial lung disease when the clinical data are conflicting or inconclusive. Transbronchial biopsies should not be performed in this setting because the limited pathologic material is rarely diagnostic, and the hemodynamic derangements increase the risk of substantial and uncontrollable hemorrhage. Thoracoscopic biopsy is the preferred route.

3. Should every patient with unexplained pulmonary hypertension undergo polysomnography?

Sleep disordered breathing can produce a chronic pulmonary hypertensive state, although it is usually not as severe or progressive as PPH. Routine polysomnography in unexplained pulmonary hypertension is not recommended. Polysomnography should be performed when clinical suspicion of sleep apnea exists, based on a history of nocturnal snoring or apnea, daytime somnolence, or chronic hypercapnia.

4. Should every patient with unexplained pulmonary hypertension undergo pulmonary arteriography?

It is important to consider chronic thromboembolic disease in the differential diagnosis of every patient with unexplained pulmonary hypertension, since patients with this condition may be candidates for pulmonary thromboendarterectomy. A ventilation-perfusion (V/Q) lung scan should be performed on all patients. Most patients with chronic thromboembolic disease have multiple mismatched perfusion defects, whereas a normal scan is more consistent with PPH. Patients with an abnormal lung scan should undergo angiography in order to determine whether thromboembolic disease is present and potentially amenable to surgery.

5. When should pulmonary veno-occlusive disease be suspected?

Pulmonary veno-occlusive disease (PVOD) should be suspected when pulmonary hypertension is present and the chest radiograph shows pulmonary venous engorgement, often with Kerley's B lines. The pulmonary capillary wedge pressure in PVOD is usually normal, because the disease affects small and medium-sized veins in a patchy manner, thereby allowing transmission of postcapillary pressure through the larger veins. A clinical diagnosis of PVOD can be confirmed by the development of acute, reversible pulmonary edema with acutely infused prostacyclin, caused by an increased pulmonary blood flow in the presence of downstream vascular obstruction. The definitive diagnosis of PVOD requires histologic examination; however, this is rarely necessary. Patients with PVOD are unlikely to respond to medical therapy and should be referred for transplantation as soon as possible.

6. Which patients with pulmonary hypertension should be treated with anticoagulants?

Patients with chronic thromboembolic pulmonary hypertension and PPH should be treated with anticoagulants. The preferred approach is use of warfarin, adjusting the dose to achieve an international normalized ratio (INR) of 2.0–2.5. Adjusted dose subcutaneous heparin is a suitable alternative for patients who cannot tolerate warfarin. In addition to the risks of chronic anticoagulation, which exist for all patients, those with pulmonary hypertension are also at risk for pulmonary hemorrhage resulting from rupture of hypertensive pulmonary vessels. No data exist regarding the use of anticoagulants in other forms of pulmonary hypertension, such as connective tissue diseases and severe respiratory disease (cor pulmonale). Patients with severe pulmonary hypertension may benefit from anticoagulation as long as they have a low risk of complications.

7. Should all patients with pulmonary hypertension be started on calcium channel blocker therapy?

No. Treatment of pulmonary hypertension should be directed at the underlying mechanism. Patients with parenchymal lung disease should be treated with modalities that improve gas exchange and lung function, and supplemental oxygen therapy should be used to correct chronic hypoxemia. There are no data showing that long-term therapy with vasodilator drugs produces significant clinical improvement or prolonged survival in cor pulmonale. Additionally, these drugs can worsen gas exchange by increasing perfusion to poorly ventilated lung units. Patients with PPH or pulmonary hypertension caused by connective tissue disease should be treated with vasodilators only if acute pharmacologic testing shows evidence of pulmonary vasoreactivity.

8. What agents are available to test for acute vasoreactivity? What is the definition of a "beneficial response"?

The safest agents to use for acute testing are potent, titratable, short-acting, and fairly selective for the pulmonary vascular bed. Nitric oxide (NO), the endothelium-derived relaxing factor, is a selective pulmonary vasodilator when administered by inhalation, but it is investigational and cumbersome to administer. Prostacyclin (epoprostenol, Flolan), administered intravenously in incremental doses from 2–12 ng per kg per minute, is useful in predicting responsiveness to orally active drugs and is commercially available. Adenosine may be a suitable alternative to prostacyclin.

The ideal response to acute vasodilator testing is a reduction in pulmonary artery pressure and vascular resistance (preferably more than 20%) that is accompanied by unchanged or increased cardiac output and stable systemic blood pressure and arterial oxygen saturation. Patients who experience this pattern of response can be treated with oral calcium channel blockers and may show substantial and sustained clinical and hemodynamic improvement. In contrast, nonresponders should not be treated with oral vasodilators because they are unlikely to improve and the initiation of alternative approaches, which may be of greater benefit, will be delayed.

9. Is there a calcium channel blocker of choice? What dose should be used?

The two most widely used drugs are nifedipine and diltiazem, and neither appears to have a clear advantage over the other. Verapamil should not be used because it has less potent pulmonary vasodilator properties and has more negative inotropic effects than the others. Experience with the new calcium blockers is insufficient to recommend their use.

Therapy should be titrated based on tolerance, aiming for the maximally tolerated dose. Systemic blood pressure, heart rate, oxygen saturation, and physical examination should be monitored as the dose is titrated. Commonly achieved doses are 120–240 mg and 600–900 mg for nifedipine and diltiazem, respectively, using long-acting preparations.

10. What are the treatment alternatives for patients who do not respond to calcium blocker therapy?

Approximately 25–30% of patients with PPH can be treated with calcium blockers; the proportion of patients with connective tissue disease who respond is probably less. The two treatment alternatives for unresponsive patients are continuous IV prostacyclin infusion and transplantation.

Continuous prostacyclin therapy is approved by the U.S. Food and Drug Administration for the treatment of severe (New York Heart Association classes III and IV) PPH refractory to conventional therapy. Prostacyclin has been shown to improve hemodynamics, exercise tolerance, and survival, but it must be infused continuously using a portable infusion pump. Side effects include catheter-related infections and infusion interruptions. Prostacyclin therapy can be used as a bridge to transplantation or as a primary mode of therapy, depending on the clinical response.

11. Should prostacyclin therapy be reserved only for patients who respond acutely?

No. The long-term effects of continuous prostacyclin appear to be caused by other actions, in addition to its vasodilator properties, such as a beneficial effect on remodeling. The absence of an acute vasodilator response to prostacyclin does not preclude a beneficial effect of long-term therapy.

12. When should a patient with pulmonary hypertension be referred for transplantation?

Transplantation should be considered as an option for all patients with severe pulmonary hypertension. Patients who remain in functional classes III and IV despite aggressive therapy should be referred for listing. It is important to refer these patients as soon as it is evident that their condition is not improving, because the average waiting time for a lung transplant exceeds 1 year in most areas of the United States. Our approach with such patients is to initiate continuous prostacyclin and list for transplant concurrently. Repeat hemodynamic evaluation at 3- to 6-month intervals is useful in determining whether to use prostacyclin as a bridge to transplantation or to defer transplantation and continue prostacyclin indefinitely.

13. Are there any restrictions in lifestyle that should be discussed with patients who have pulmonary hypertension?

Yes. Pregnancy is poorly tolerated in patients with pulmonary hypertension because of dramatic hemodynamic stresses and hormonal changes that can affect the pulmonary circulation. Additionally, oral contraceptives can aggravate pulmonary hypertension. Accordingly, safe and effective alternative methods of birth control should be practiced. Extremes in altitude should be avoided, but air travel is generally safe. Commonly used over-the-counter decongestants should not be used because they frequently contain sympathomimetic drugs, which can produce tachycardia and vasoconstriction.

14. What do I tell may patients about survival?

Survival varies, but depends, in large part, on the severity of the hemodynamic abnormalities. Patients who respond to medical therapy with reduction in pulmonary artery pressure and preservation of right ventricular function may experience sustained improvement and prolonged survival, although the disease process may progress and be unresponsive to adjustments in medical therapy. The 3-year survival rate after lung transplantation is approximately 65–70%, with most deaths caused by chronic rejection or opportunistic infections. Despite these grim statistics, many patients have been maintained on long-term therapy for more than a decade, with sustained clinical stability.

BIBLIOGRAPHY

1. Bando K, Armitage JM, Paradis IL, et al: Indications for and results of single, bilateral, and heart-lung transplantation for pulmonary hypertension. J Thorac Cardiovasc Surg 108:1056–1065, 1994.
2. Barst RJ, Rubin LJ, Long WA, et al: A comparison of continuous intravenous epoprostenol (prostacyclin) with conventional therapy for primary pulmonary hypertension. N Engl J Med 334:296–301, 1996.
3. Barst RJ, Rubin LJ, McGoon MD, et al: Survival in primary pulmonary hypertension with long-term continuous intravenous prostacyclin. Ann Intern Med 121:409–415, 1994.
4. D'Alonzo GE, Barst RJ, Ayers SM, et al: Survival in patients with primary pulmonary hypertension: Results form a national prospective registry. Ann Intern Med 115:343–349, 1991.
5. Fuster V, Steele PM, Edwards WD, et al: Primary pulmonary hypertension: Natural history and the importance of thrombosis. Circulation 70:580–587, 1984.
6. Pasque MK, Trulock EP, Kaiser LR, et al: Single-lung transplantation for pulmonary hypertension: Three month hemodynamic follow-up. Circulation 84:2275–2279, 1991.
7. Rich S, Dantzker DR, Ayres SM, et al: Primary pulmonary hypertension: A national prospective study. Ann Intern Med 107:216–23, 1987.
8. Rich S, Kaufmann E, Levy PS: The effect of high doses of calcium-channel blockers on survival in primary pulmonary hypertension. N Engl J Med 327:76–81, 1992.
9. Rubin LJ: Primary pulmonary hypertension: An ACCP Consensus Paper. Chest 104:236–250, 1993.

IX. Interstitial Lung Diseases

41. GENERAL APPROACHES TO INTERSTITIAL LUNG DISEASE

Talmadge E. King, Jr., M.D.

1. What are the causes of interstitial lung disease (ILD)?

The most common causes of ILD are related to occupational and environmental exposures, especially to inorganic or organic dusts. Sarcoidosis, idiopathic pulmonary fibrosis (IPF), and pulmonary fibrosis associated with connective tissue diseases are the most common ILDs of unknown etiology.

Etiologic Classification of Interstitial Lung Disease

Occupational and environmental exposures
  Inorganic dust
    Silica, asbestos, hard metal dusts (i.e, cadmium, titanium oxide), beryllium
  Organic dusts (hypersensitivity pneumonitis or extrinsic allergic alveolitis)
    Thermophilic bacteria (i.e., *Macropolyspora faeni, Thermoactinomyces vulgaris, T. sacchari*)
    Other bacteria (i.e., *Bacillus subtilis, B. cereus*)
    True fungi (i.e., *Aspergillus, Cryptostroma corticale, Aureobasidium pullulans, Penicillin* spp.)
    Animal proteins (e.g., bird fancier's disease)
    Bacterial products (byssinosis)
  Chemical sources, gases, fumes, vapors, aerosols, paraquat, radiation

Drugs and poisons
  Chemotherapeutic agents (busulfan, bleomycin, methotrexate)
  Antibiotics (nitrofurantoin, sulfasalazine)
  Drug-induced lupus (diphenylhydantoin, procainamide)
  Gold salts
  Amiodarone
  Radiation

Connective tissue disease (CTD)
  Systemic lupus erythematosus (SLE)
  Rheumatoid arthritis
  Progressive systemic sclerosis
  Sjögren's syndrome
  Polymyositis and dermatomyositis
  Mixed connective tissue disease
  Ankylosing spondylitis

Other systemic diseases
  Sarcoidosis
  Vasculitides (Wegener's granulomatosis, Churg-Strauss syndrome)
  Hemorrhagic syndromes (Goodpasture's syndrome, idiopathic pulmonary hemosiderosis)
  Pulmonary histiocytosis X (eosinophilic granuloma of the lung)
  Chronic gastric aspiration
  Lymphangitic carcinomatosis
  Chronic pulmonary edema
  Chronic uremia
  Alveolar proteinosis

Idiopathic pulmonary fibrosis

Infections (residue of active infection of any type)

2. Describe the modes of clinical presentation of patients with ILD.

Patients with ILD commonly come to clinical attention in one of the following ways:

1. Onset of progressive breathlessness with exertion (dyspnea) and/or persistent nonproductive cough. Other important symptoms and signs include hemoptysis, wheezing, and chest pain.

2. Identification of interstitial opacities on chest x-ray.

3. Pulmonary symptoms associated with another disease, such as a CTD. Importantly, clinical findings suggestive of a CTD (musculoskeletal pain, weakness, fatigue, fever, joint pains or swelling, photosensitivity, Raynaud's phenomenon, pleuritis, dry eyes, dry mouth) should be carefully elicited. The CTD may be difficult to rule out since the pulmonary manifestations occasionally precede the more typical systemic manifestations by months or years (particularly in rheumatoid arthritis, SLE, and polymyositis-dermatomyositis).

4. Following the identification of lung function abnormalities on simple office spirometry, particularly a restrictive ventilatory pattern.

3. What are the presenting clinical manifestations of ILD?

Dyspnea. Shortness of breath is a common complaint of patients with cardiac or pulmonary disease. In most instances, the patient has attributed the insidious onset of breathlessness with exertion to aging, deconditioning, obesity, or a recent upper respiratory tract illness, and some patients deny the presence of dyspnea even when questioned. However, patients with sarcoidosis, silicosis, or pulmonary histiocytosis X may have extensive parenchymal lung disease without significant dyspnea, especially early in the course of their disease. Sudden worsening of dyspnea, especially if associated with pleural pain, may indicate a spontaneous pneumothorax.

Cough. A dry cough may be particularly disturbing for patients with processes that involve the airways, such as sarcoidosis, bronchiolitis obliterans with organizing pneumonia (BOOP), respiratory bronchiolitis, pulmonary histiocytosis X, hypersensitivity pneumonitis, lipoid pneumonia, or lymphangitic carcinomatosis. Although a productive cough is unusual for most ILDs, a mucoid salty-tasting sputum is sometimes reported with diffuse alveolar cell carcinoma.

Hemoptysis. Grossly bloody or blood-streaked sputum occurs in the diffuse alveolar hemorrhage syndromes, lymphangioleiomyomatosis, tuberous sclerosis, pulmonary veno-occlusive disease, long-standing mitral valve disease, and granulomatous vasculitides. Occasionally, diffuse alveolar bleeding may be present without hemoptysis; the clinical manifestations of dyspnea and an iron-deficiency anemia may be present. New onset of hemoptysis in a patient with known ILD should raise the possibility of a complicating malignancy.

Wheezing. Wheezing is an uncommon manifestation of ILD. It has been described in cases of lymphangitic carcinomatosis, chronic eosinophilic pneumonia, Churg-Strauss syndrome, and respiratory bronchiolitis.

Inspiratory squeaks. Scattered late inspiratory high-pitched rhonchi are frequently heard on chest examination in patients with bronchiolitis.

Chest pain. Clinically significant chest pain is uncommon in most ILDs, but pleuritic chest pain may occur in ILD associated with rheumatoid arthritis, SLE, mixed CTD, and some drug-induced disorders. Substernal chest pain or discomfort is common in sarcoidosis.

4. How long are clinical manifestations of ILD evident prior to presentation?

In the vast majority of ILDs, the symptoms and signs are chronic, i.e., months to years, as in idiopathic pulmonary fibrosis, sarcoidosis, and pulmonary histiocytosis X. In some, however, symptoms may be acute (days to weeks) or subacute (weeks to months). These latter processes are often confused with atypical pneumonias since many have diffuse radiographic opacities, fever, or relapses of disease activity; examples include acute idiopathic interstitial pneumonia, acute eosinophilic pneumonia, hypersensitivity pneumonitis, BOOP, some drug-induced ILDs, alveolar hemorrhage syndromes, and acute immunologic pneumonia that complicates either SLE or polymyositis.

5. Describe an initial evaluation of a patient suspected of having ILD.

The initial evaluation should include a complete **history** and **physical examination**. The initial laboratory evaluation should include biochemical tests to evaluate **liver** and **renal function** and **hematologic tests** to check for anemia, polycythemia, or leukocytosis. **Serologic studies** should be obtained if clinically indicated by features suggestive of a CTD or vasculitis: sedimentation rate, antinuclear antibodies, rheumatoid factor, hypersensitivity panel, anti-neutrophil cytoplasmic antibodies, anti-basement membrane antibody. A recent **chest x-ray** should be obtained, and it also is important to review all old chest x-rays to assess the rate of change in disease activity. Complete **lung function testing** (spirometry, lung volumes, diffusing capacity) and resting room air **arterial blood gases** should be obtained. Common diseases, such as COPD, anemia, heart failure, and mycobacterial or fungal disease, can mimic ILD, so they must be ruled out. Most causes of ILD will be identified by this process.

6. Why is the medical history so important in evaluating a patient with ILD?

Because the cause of the current illness is often recognized from the patient's history. Key areas of focus in the history include occupational and environmental exposures, smoking history, medication history, and family history.

Occupational history. A strict chronologic listing of the patient's lifelong employment must be sought, including specific duties and known exposures to dusts, gases, and chemicals. The degree of exposure, duration, latency of exposure, and use of protective devices should be elicited.

Environmental exposures. Review of the environment (home and work, including that of spouse and children) is valuable as well. It is especially important to determine if the patient has had exposures to pets (especially birds), air conditioners, humidifiers, hot tubs, evaporative cooling systems (e.g., swamp coolers), and water damage in the home or work environment. In hypersensitivity pneumonitis, respiratory symptoms, fever, chills, and an abnormal chest x-ray are often temporally related to the workplace (farmer's lung) or to a hobby (pigeon breeder's disease). Symptoms may diminish or disappear after the patient leaves the exposure for several days; similarly, symptoms reappear on returning to the exposure.

Smoking history. Some diseases occur largely among current or former smokers (pulmonary histiocytosis X, desquamative interstitial pneumonitis, idiopathic pulmonary fibrosis, and respiratory bronchiolitis) or among never or former smokers (sarcoidosis and hypersensitivity pneumonitis). Active smoking can lead to complications in some processes, such as Goodpasture's syndrome, in which pulmonary hemorrhage is far more frequent in current smokers.

Prior medication use. A detailed history of the medications taken by the patient, including over-the-counter medications, oily nose drops, and amino acid supplements, is needed to exclude the possibility of drug-induced disease. Lung diseases may occur weeks to years after the drug has been discontinued.

Family history. The family history is occasionally helpful since familial associations (with an autosomal dominant pattern) have been identified in cases of idiopathic pulmonary fibrosis, sarcoidosis, tuberous sclerosis, and neurofibromatosis. An autosomal recessive pattern of inheritance occurs in Niemann-Pick disease, Gaucher's disease, and Hermansky-Pudlak syndrome.

7. Is gender or age important in the evaluation of a patient with ILD?

Gender is important in lymphangioleiomyomatosis, which occurs almost exclusively in premenopausal women. Also, ILD in the CTDs is more common in women; the exception is ILD in rheumatoid arthritis, which is more common in men.

Age is helpful given that the majority of patients with sarcoidosis and CTD present between the ages 20–40 years. Conversely, most patients with idiopathic pulmonary fibrosis are over age 60 years.

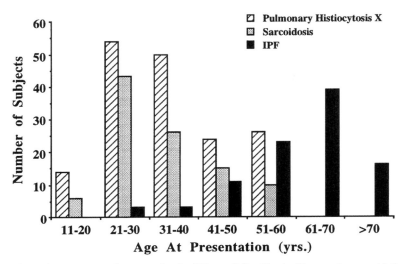

Comparison of age at onset of presentation in different ILDs. *Hatched bars,* pulmonary histiocytosis X (total subjects = 168); *shaded bars,* sarcoidosis (total subjects = 100); *solid bars,* IPF subjects (total subjects = 95).

8. How useful is the physical examination in the diagnosis of ILD?

The physical exam is commonly not specific but can be useful because it frequently reveals tachypnea, reduced chest expansion, and bibasilar end-expiratory dry crackles.

Crackles, or "Velcro rales," are common in most forms of ILD, although they are less common in the granulomatous lung diseases, especially sarcoidosis. Crackles may be present in the absence of radiographic abnormalities on the chest x-ray.

Cor pulmonale. The cardiac examination is usually normal except in the mid or late stages of the disease, when findings of pulmonary hypertension (i.e., augmented P_2, right-sided lift, and S_3 gallop) and cor pulmonale may become evident. Signs of pulmonary hypertension and cor pulmonale are generally secondary manifestations of advanced ILD, although they may be primary manifestations of a CTD (e.g., progressive systemic sclerosis).

Clubbing of the digits, i.e., the distal part of the finger is enlarged compared with the proximal part, is common in some patients (idiopathic pulmonary fibrosis, asbestosis) and rare in others (sarcoidosis, hypersensitivity pneumonitis, histiocytosis X). In most patients, clubbing is a late manifestation suggesting advanced derangement of the lung.

Cyanosis is uncommon and is usually a late manifestation indicative of advanced disease.

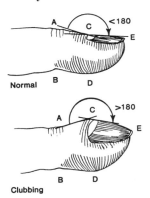

Clubbing of the fingers. In a normal finger, the length of a perpendicular dropped from point A to point B should be greater than a similar line from C to D. In clubbing, the relationships are reversed—that is, the distance C–D is greater than the distance A–B. The other important change is the angle described by A-C-E. In the normal finger this is usually < 180°, whereas in clubbing it is > 180°. (Reprinted with permission from DeRemee RA: Facets of the algorithmic synthesis. In DeRemee RA (ed): Clinical Profiles of Diffuse Interstitial Pulmonary Disease. Mount Kisco, NY, Futura Publishing Company, Inc., 1990, pp 9–44.)

9. What extrapulmonary physical findings may be helpful in arriving at a diagnosis of ILD?

Physical Findings	Associated Conditions
Systemic arterial hypertension	CTD, neurofibromatosis, some diffuse alveolar hemorrhage syndromes
Skin changes	
Erythema nodosum	Sarcoidosis, CTD, Behçet's syndrome, histoplasmosis, coccidioidomycosis
Maculopapular rash	Drug-induced, amyloidosis, lipoidosis, CTD, Gaucher's disease
Heliotrope rash	Dermatomyositis
Telangiectasia	Scleroderma
Raynaud's phenomena	Idiopathic pulmonary fibrosis, CTD (scleroderma)
Cutaneous vasculitis	Systemic vasculitides, CTD
Subcutaneous nodules	Von Reckinghausen's disease, rheumatoid arthritis
Calcinosis	Dermatomyositis, scleroderma
Eye changes	
Uveitis	Sarcoidosis, Behçet's syndrome, ankylosing spondylitis
Scleritis	Systemic vasculitis, SLE, scleroderma, sarcoidosis
Keratoconjunctivitis sicca	Lymphocytic interstitial pneumonia (LIP)
Salivary gland enlargement	Sarcoidosis, LIP
Peripheral lymphadenopathy	Sarcoidosis, lymphangitic carcinomatosis, LIP, lymphoma
Hepatosplenomegaly	Sarcoidosis, pulmonary histiocytosis X, CTD, amyloidosis, LIP
Pericarditis	Radiation pneumonitis, CTD
Myositis	CTD, drugs (L-tryptophan)
Muscle weakness	CTD

Adapted from Schwarz MI, King TE Jr, Cherniack RM: General principles and diagnostic approach to the interstitial lung diseases. In Murray JF, Nadel JA (eds): Textbook of Respiratory Medicine, 2nd ed. Philadelphia, W.B. Saunders, 1994, pp 1803–1826.

10. What is the role of the routine laboratory evaluation in a patient suspected of having ILD?

The routine laboratory evaluation is often not helpful because the findings are nonspecific. An elevated erythrocyte sedimentation rate and hypergammaglobulinemia are commonly observed but are nondiagnostic. Antinuclear antibodies, anti-immunoglobulin antibodies (rheumatoid factors), and circulating immune complexes are identified in many of these patients, even in the absence of a defined CTD. Elevation of lactate dehydrogenase may be noted but is a nonspecific finding common to many pulmonary disorders. An increase in the angiotensin-converting enzyme (ACE) level may be observed in sarcoidosis but is nonspecific, as elevated ACE levels have been noted in several interstitial diseases including hypersensitivity pneumonitis. Antibodies to organic antigens may be helpful in confirming exposure when hypersensitivity pneumonitis is suspected, although they too are nondiagnostic. The ECG is usually normal in the absence of pulmonary hypertension or concurrent cardiac disease.

11. What is the role of the routine chest x-ray in a patient suspected of ILD?

The diagnosis of ILD is often suspected initially on the basis of an abnormal chest roentgenogram. Unfortunately, the chest x-ray may be normal in as many as 10% of patients with some forms of ILD, particularly hypersensitivity pneumonitis. The physician should not ignore or incompletely evaluate a symptomatic patient with a normal chest x-ray or an asymptomatic patient with radiographic evidence of ILD. Failure to completely evaluate such patients often leads to progressive disease, which may be irreversible by the time the patient seeks additional medical attention.

12. Describe the common chest radiographic patterns seen in a patient with ILD.

The most common radiographic abnormality is a **reticular** or **reticulonodular** pattern; however, mixed patterns of alveolar filling and increased interstitial markings are not unusual. Most ILDs have predilection for the lower lung zones. As the disease progresses there is widespread infiltration associated with reductions in lung volume and the appearance of pulmonary hypertension. A subgroup of ILDs have predilection for the upper lung zones and often produce nodular infiltrates that result in upward contraction of the pulmonary hilus. With progression of the disease, small cystic structures appear, representing fibrous replacement of the normal alveolar architecture and radiographic **honeycombing**.

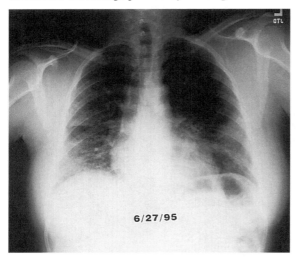

Idiopathic pulmonary fibrosis. The chest roentgenogram shows diffuse, reticular and hazy opacities in the lower lung zones.

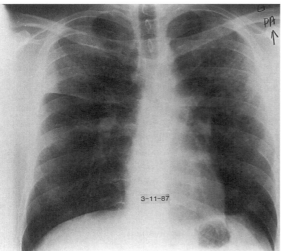

Sarcoidosis. This chest roentgenogram from a patient with sarcoidosis shows predominantly nodular and hazy opacities in the upper lung zones. The chest x-ray normalized following treatment with corticosteroids.

13. How useful is the routine chest roentgenogram in staging and follow-up of a patient with ILD?

The correlation between the x-ray pattern and the stage of disease (clinical or histopathologic) is generally poor. Only the radiographic finding of **honeycombing** (small cystic spaces) correlates with pathologic findings; it portends a poor prognosis.

14. What is the role of CT scanning of the chest in the evaluation of ILD?

High-resolution CT (HRCT) is well suited for evaluation of diffuse pulmonary parenchymal disease. Pattern recognition in diffuse lung disease is enhanced because HRCT avoids the problem of superimposition of structures and is exposure-independent. While still in the midst of research, HRCT offers:

    1. More accuracy than conventional chest x-ray in distinguishing air space from interstitial lung disease.

    2. Earlier detection and confirmation of suspected diffuse lung disease, especially in the investigation of a symptomatic patient with a normal chest radiograph.

    3. Better assessment of the extent and distribution of disease

    4. Ability to disclose coexisting disease, e.g., discern occult mediastinal adenopathy, carcinoma, or emphysema

    5. Utility in more specifically selecting appropriate type and site for biopsy

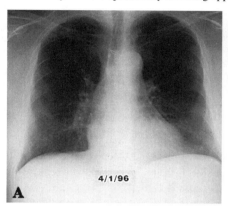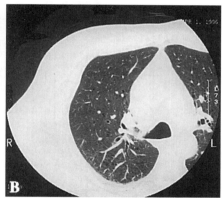

Hypersensitivity pneumonitis (bird fancier's disease). *A*, Chest roentgenogram is normal. *B*, HRCT scan of right lung reveals diffuse hazy or ground-glass increase in lung density (i.e., an increase in CT lung density that does not obscure the underlying lung parenchyma). Lung biopsy confirmed the presence of a granulomatous pneumonitis.

15. How is gallium-67 lung scanning of the chest used in the evaluation of a patient with ILD?

Gallium-67 lung scanning is of limited value. Ga-67 lung scanning has been tried as a means of evaluating the inflammatory component of ILD, since gallium is not taken up by normal lung parenchyma. Uptake may be diffuse or patchy and is believed to reflect an increased accumulation of inflammatory cells in the lung. To date, gallium scans have not been proven very useful in diagnosis, staging, or follow-up of ILD.

16. What is the role of pulmonary function testing (PFT) in the evaluation of a patient with ILD?

Measurement of lung volumes and spirometry function testing are important tests in assessing the severity of lung involvement. Also, the finding of an obstructive or restrictive pattern is useful in narrowing the possible diagnoses.

17. What is the most common pattern of lung function abnormality in patients with ILD?

Most of the interstitial disorders have a **restrictive defect** with reduced total lung capacity, functional residual capacity, and residual volume. Flow rates are decreased (FEV_1 and FVC), but this is related to the decreased lung volumes. The FEV_1/FVC ratio is usually normal or increased. Smoking history must be assessed.

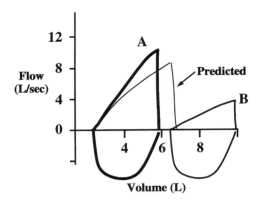

Maximal expiratory flow volume (MEFV curve) in idiopathic pulmonary fibrosis. *A*, MEFV curves at presentation in a 42-year-old nonsmoking man with a normal chest x-ray and lung biopsy-proven idiopathic pulmonary fibrosis. The FEV_1 and FVC values are low relative to the predicted values, but the FEV_1/FVC ratio is increased. However, at any given lung volume, the flow rates are higher than expected because of elevated driving pressure due to an increased elastic recoil. *B*, MEFV curve for a patient with COPD. FEV_1 and FVC are low relative to the predicted values, and the lung volumes are increased.

18. Does the presence of airflow obstruction on PFT rule out ILD as a major cause of the patient's illness?

A few disorders produce interstitial opacities on chest x-ray and obstructive airflow limitation on PFT, e.g., sarcoidosis, lymphangioleiomyomatosis, hypersensitivity pneumonitis, tuberous sclerosis, and COPD with superimposed ILD.

19. Is there a role for measurement of lung elastic recoil?

Yes, in symptomatic patients with a normal chest radiograph and minimal or no restrictive disease, measurement of elastic recoil (pressure-volume curve) may be helpful by identifying lung stiffness. Pressure-volume studies often yield a curve that is shifted downward and to the right, consistent with a stiff noncompliant lung. In general, as the disease progresses, lung compliance decreases and lung volumes fall.

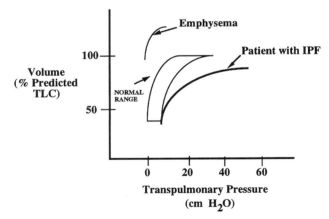

Relationship of the static deflation volume and pressure in a patient with idiopathic pulmonary fibrosis. The percent predicted total lung capacity (TLC) is plotted against the static transpulmonary pressure (cm H_2O) for a patient with ILD. In general, the compliance, maximum static transpulmonary pressure, and the coefficient of retraction (maximum transpulmonary pressure to TLC) tend to correlate with the extent of parenchymal lung involvement observed on lung biopsy.

20. Are there changes in the carbon monoxide diffusing capacity (DLCO) in ILD?

Yes, a reduction in the DLCO is commonly found, but it is not specific for a particular type of ILD. The decrease in DLCO is due in part to effacement of the alveolar capillary units but, more importantly, to the extent of ventilation-perfusion mismatching of the alveoli. Lung regions with reduced compliance due either to fibrosis or excessive cellularity may be poorly ventilated but still be well-perfused.

21. Do changes in DLCO correlate with disease stage in ILD?

No, the severity of the DLCO reduction does not correlate well with disease stage. In some ILDs, there can be considerable reduction in lung volumes and/or severe hypoxemia but normal or only slightly reduced DLCO, especially in sarcoidosis. The presence of moderate to severe reductions of DLCO in the presence of normal lung volumes should suggest ILD with associated emphysema, pulmonary vascular disease, pulmonary histiocytosis X, or lymphangioleiomyomatosis.

22. Are there changes in the arterial blood gases (ABGs) in ILD?

Yes, the resting ABGs may be normal or reveal hypoxemia (secondary to a ventilation-perfusion mismatching) and respiratory alkalosis. Carbon dioxide retention is rare and usually a manifestation of far-advanced end-stage disease.

23. Does a normal resting ABG rule out the need for measurement of gas exchange with exercise?

A normal resting PaO_2 (or O_2 saturation by oximetry) does *not* rule out significant hypoxemia during exercise or sleep. Further, although hypoxemia with exercise and sleep is very common, secondary erythrocytosis is rarely observed in uncomplicated ILD.

24. Why is the exercise gas exchange important in the evaluation of patients with ILD?

Because resting hypoxemia is not always evident and because severe exercise-induced hypoxemia may go undetected, it is important to perform exercise testing with serial measurement of ABGs. Arterial oxygen desaturation, a failure to decrease deadspace appropriately with exercise (i.e., a high V_D/V_T ratio), and an excessive increase in respiratory rate with a lower than expected recruitment of tidal volume provide useful information about physiologic abnormalities and extent of disease. There is increasing evidence that serial assessments of resting and exercise gas exchange are the best methods to identify disease activity and responsiveness to treatment.

CONTROVERSIES

25. What are the indications for referral and specialized testing?

Indications for specialized testing and referral to a pulmonologist include:
1. No specific cause of dyspnea or cough found
2. Symptoms exceed the physiologic or radiographic abnormalities identified
3. Empirical management (bronchodilators, diuretics, smoking cessation, etc.) resulted in atypical or unsatisfactory clinical outcome
4. Patient needs impairment or disability evaluation for worker's compensation or other reason
5. "Specialized" cardiopulmonary testing needed, such as:
    Fiberoptic bronchoscopy and bronchoalveolar lavage
    Lung biopsy required to confirm diagnosis
    Exercise testing with ABGs to determine if physiologic limitation exists and whether its cause is cardiac or pulmonary
    Determination of the pressure-volume relationship in a patient with relatively normal chest x-ray or minimal restriction on PFT
    Radionuclide scans (e.g., gallium)
    Right heart catheterization
    Pulmonary angiography
    Studies of respiratory drive
6. Therapeutic immunosuppressive or cytotoxic drug trial contemplated

26. Is bronchoalveolar lavage (BAL) analysis useful in the assessment of ILD?

In selected cases, BAL cellular analysis may be useful to (a) narrow the differential diagnostic possibilities between various types of ILD; (b) define the stage of disease; and (c) assess the progression of disease or response to therapy. However, the utility of BAL in the clinical assessment and management of ILD patients remains to be fully established.

Condition	Lavage Finding
Lymphangitic carcinomatosis, alveolar cell carcinoma, pulmonary lymphoma	Malignant cells
Diffuse alveolar bleeding	Hemosiderin-laden macrophages, RBCs
Alveolar proteinosis	Lipoproteinaceous intra-alveolar material (periodic acid–Schiff stain)
Lipoid pneumonia	Fat globules in macrophages
Pulmonary histiocytosis X	Monoclonal antibody (T6)-positive histiocytes Electron microscopy demonstrating Birbeck granule in lavaged macrophage
Asbestos-related pulmonary disease	Ferruginous bodies
Lipoidosis	Accumulation of specific lipopigment in alveolar macrophages
Berylliosis	+ Lymphoblast transformation test
Silicosis	Dust particles by polarized light microscopy
Wegener's	? Positive anti-neutrophil cytoplasmic antibodies

Adapted from Schwarz MI: Approach to the patient with interstitial lung disease. In Kelley W (ed): Essentials of Internal Medicine. Philadelphia, J.B. Lippincott, 1994, pp 1893–1897.

27. Should a lung biopsy be performed in all patients with suspected ILD?

No. However, following the initial evaluation, it is important to confirm the diagnosis and establish the stage of disease. In many instances, lung biopsy is indicated because:

1. It often provides a specific diagnosis, especially in alveolar proteinosis, sarcoidosis, pulmonary histiocytosis X, respiratory bronchiolitis, lymphangioleiomyomatosis, BOOP, veno-occlusive disease, vasculitis limited to the lung.

2. It excludes neoplastic and infectious processes that occasionally mimic chronic, progressive interstitial disease.

3. It occasionally identifies a more treatable process than originally suspected (e.g., hypersensitivity pneumonitis, BOOP, respiratory bronchiolitis-associated ILD, or sarcoidosis).

4. It provides the best assessment of disease activity.

5. Having a definite diagnosis makes the physician and patient more comfortable proceeding with therapies that may have serious side effects. Also, a definitive diagnosis avoids confusion (and anxiety) later if the patient is "failing" therapy or suffering serious side effects of therapy.

28. When should fiberoptic bronchoscopy with transbronchial lung biopsy be performed?

This is often the initial procedure of choice, especially when sarcoidosis, lymphangitic carcinomatosis, eosinophilic pneumonia, Goodpasture's syndrome, or infection is suspected. If a specific diagnosis is not made by transbronchial biopsy, then an open lung biopsy is indicated.

29. When should surgical lung biopsy be performed?

Open lung biopsy is the most definitive method to diagnose and stage the disease so that appropriate prognostic and therapeutic decisions can be made. Failure to secure a definitive diagnosis or determine the stage of disease prior to the initiation of treatment can result in unnecessary anguish for the physician caring for the patient with ILD and may result in potentially avoidable morbidity for the patient. Open lung biopsy via thoracotomy or video thoracoscopy is a relatively safe procedure with little morbidity and < 1% mortality. Currently, video-assisted thoracoscopic lung biopsy is the preferred method for obtaining multiple lung tissue samples for analysis.

30. When should a lung biopsy *not* be performed?

Relative contraindications to lung biopsy include serious cardiovascular disease, roentgeno-graphic evidence of diffuse end-stage disease (i.e., honeycombing), severe pulmonary dysfunction, or other major operative risks (especially in the elderly).

31. Describe the two major histopathologic patterns found in patients with ILD.

1. A **granulomatous** process characterized by an accumulation of T lymphocytes, macrophages, and epithelioid cells organized into discrete structures (granulomas) that result in derangement of normal tissue architecture.

2. **Usual interstitial pneumonitis** (UIP), a chronic inflammatory process characterized by a sequence of biological processes that result in pulmonary fibrosis. An alveolitis, composed of alveolar macrophages, with fewer numbers of lymphocytes, neutrophils, eosinophils, and mast cells, herald the onset of this process. This is followed by injury to the alveolar walls with changes in the epithelium and thickening of the alveolar walls with fibrosis, alveolar collapse, and finally marked derangement of the alveolar structures with loss of functioning alveolar-capillary units.

Patients with a granulomatous lung disease can progress to clinically significant pulmonary fibrosis. However, many of these patients remain free of severe impairment of lung function or even improve after immunosuppressive treatment (e.g., sarcoidosis or hypersensitivity pneumonitis). Conversely, patients with the UIP lesion often have a more devastating illness characterized by unrelenting progression to end-stage fibrosis and death, especially patients with IPF.

32. Which patients require treatment and when should it begin?

Management of most ILDs is difficult, and different approaches are taken depending on the specific entity. Regardless of etiology, end-stage fibrosis is irreversible and untreatable. An extensive and aggressive diagnostic evaluation early on, even in patients with relatively few symptoms, is recommended. Patients with evidence of lung function impairment, signs of progression, or evidence of active disease should be treated if no contraindications to therapy exist.

Pursuing a diagnosis and instituting appropriate therapy early in the disease course, prior to extensive fibrosis, is likely to improve responsiveness to therapy and hopefully delay or prevent the functional limitation and disability that commonly occur in these patients.

The major therapies for ILD involve corticosteroids with or without a cytotoxic agent (cyclophosphamide or azathioprine). Because many patients with ILD are elderly, the decision to treat elderly patients with immunosuppressive drugs should not be taken lightly, as the toxicity and side effects of these medications can be substantial.

33. Which patients require oxygen treatment and when should it be started?

Patients with ILD, especially idiopathic pulmonary fibrosis, typically are sufficiently dyspneic with exertion that they have stopped regular exercise. These patients need encouragement to develop a routine conditioning program to improve muscle strength and cardiovascular efficiency. Daily walks and stationary bicycling can help in weight control and improve the patient's sense of well-being. Supplemental oxygen is often required during exercise. Severe hypoxemia (PaO_2 < 55 mmHg) at rest or during exercise should be managed with supplemental oxygen.

Education in energy management techniques may provide the patient with the means to do more of their daily activities and hence improve quality of life. For example, using labor-saving devices to simplify work, planning daily priorities, pacing physical activity, and improving breathing and body mechanics can significantly contribute to energy conservation.

BIBLIOGRAPHY

1. Baughman RP, Lower EE, Lynch JP III: Treatment modalities for sarcoidosis. Clin Pulm Med 1:223–231, 1994.
2. Bitterman PB, Rennard SI, Keogh BA, et al: Familial idiopathic pulmonary fibrosis: Evidence of lung inflammation in unaffected family members. N Engl J Med 314:1343–1347, 1986.
3. Crausman RS, King TE Jr: Primary pulmonary histiocytosis X in the adult: Clinical features, diagnosis, and treatment. In Weinberger S (ed): UpToDate in Medicine [CD ROM Program]. Wellesley, MA, BDR, 1996.
4. DeRemee RA: Facets of the algorithmic synthesis. In DeRemee RA (ed): Clinical Profiles of Diffuse Interstitial Pulmonary Disease. Mount Kisco, NY, Futura, 1990.
5. Flint A: Pathologic features of interstitial lung disease. In Schwarz MI, King TE Jr (eds): Interstitial Lung Disease. Toronto, B.C. Decker, 1988, pp 45–62.
6. Hogg JC: Chronic interstitial lung disease of unknown cause: A new classification based on pathogenesis. AJR 156:225–233, 1991.
7. Hunninghake GW, Kalica AR: Approaches to the treatment of pulmonary fibrosis. Am J Respir Crit Care Med 151:915–918, 1995.
8. King TE Jr: Bronchoscopy in interstitial lung disease. In Feinsilver SH, Fein AM (eds): Textbook of Bronchoscopy. Baltimore, Williams & Wilkins, 1995, pp 185–220.
9. King TE Jr: Approach to the patient with interstitial lung disease. In Kelley W (ed): Textbook of Internal Medicine, 3rd ed. Philadelphia, J.B. Lippincott, 1996.
10. Mornex JF, Leroux C, Greenland T, Ecochard D: From granuloma to fibrosis in interstitial lung diseases: Molecular and cellular interactions. Eur Resp J 7:779–785, 1994.
11. Neville E, Walker AN, James DG: Prognostic factors predicting outcome of sarcoidosis: Analysis of 818 patients. Q J Med 52:525–533, 1983.
12. Panos RJ, Mortenson R, Niccoli SA, King TE Jr: Clinical deterioration in patients with idiopathic pulmonary fibrosis: Causes and assessment. Am J Med 88:396–404, 1990.
13. Rose C, King TE Jr: Controversies in hypersensitivity pneumonitis. Am Rev Respir Dis 145:1–2, 1992.
14. Rosenow EC III, Martin WJ II: Drug-induced interstitial lung disease. In Schwarz MI, King TE Jr (eds): Interstitial Lung Disease, 2nd ed. St. Louis, Mosby, 1993, pp 255–270.
15. Schwarz MI, King TE Jr (eds): Interstitial Lung Disease, 2nd ed. St. Louis, Mosby, 1993.
16. Schwarz MI, King TE Jr, Cherniack RM: General principles and diagnostic approach to the interstitial lung diseases. In Murray JF, Nadel JA (eds): Textbook of Respiratory Medicine, 2nd ed. Philadelphia, W.B. Saunders, 1994, pp 1803–1826.
17. Thurlbeck WM, Miller RR, Muller NL, Rosenow EC III: Diffuse Diseases of the Lung: A Team Approach. Philadelphia, B.C. Decker, 1991.
18. Wade JF III, King TE Jr: Infiltrative and interstitial lung disease in the elderly. Clin Chest Med 14:501–521, 1993.
19. Watters LC: Genetic aspects of idiopathic pulmonary fibrosis and hypersensitivity pneumonitis. Semin Respir Med 7:317–325, 1986.
20. Winterbauer RH: The treatment of idiopathic pulmonary fibrosis. Chest 100:233–235, 1991.

42. SARCOIDOSIS

Kevin G. Connelly, M.D.

1. What is the typical pathologic lesion of sarcoidosis?

Sarcoidosis is a multisystem granulomatous disease of unknown cause. Accordingly, the classic pathologic lesion is the granuloma. Sarcoidal granulomas are usually well formed and noncaseating. Although the granuloma is typical of sarcoid, granulomas are also seen in other diseases, such as tuberculosis (which is characterized by caseating granulomata) and other mycobacterial infections, fungal infections, hypersensitivity pneumonitis, and berylliosis. The latter syndrome represents a hypersensitivity reaction to beryllium and may be clinically indistinguishable from sarcoidosis. Because sarcoid is similar to infection pathologically, mycobacterial and fungal cultures should be obtained from biopsy specimens.

2. What type of inflammatory cells are thought to be involved in sarcoidosis?

Although the cause of sarcoidosis remains obscure, much is known regarding the immunology of the disease. The bronchoalveolar lavage fluid of patients with sarcoid shows increased numbers of lymphocytes and activated alveolar macrophages. The proportion of CD4-positive lymphocytes (T-helper cells) is increased, and the ratio of CD4-positive lymphocytes to CD8-positive lymphocytes is increased. Conversely, the ratio of CD4-positive cells to CD8-positive cells is reversed in peripheral blood from sarcoid patients. This finding has led to the concept of "compartmentalization" of immune cells at the site of inflammation in sarcoid.

3. Who is most likely to be affected by sarcoidosis?

Sarcoidosis most commonly occurs between the ages of 20 and 40 years and there is a slight female predominance. Sarcoid occurs worldwide, but certain groups are believed to have increased rates of disease. In the United States, African-Americans are affected more commonly than whites, but this is not seen in Europe. Northern Europeans, especially Scandinavians and Irish, also have higher rates.

4. How is the respiratory system involved in sarcoidosis?

The respiratory system is the organ system most frequently involved (90%) in sarcoidosis. Both the lungs and the intrathoracic lymph nodes are commonly involved. Pulmonary sarcoid may present asymptomatically with bilateral hilar and mediastinal adenopathy on chest radiograph. Sarcoid may also present with cough, dyspnea on exertion, or wheezing. The latter occurs when airway involvement by sarcoid granulomata leads to airflow obstruction. The following classification has been developed based on chest radiograph findings:

Stage 0	The absence of radiographic abnormalities
Stage I	Bilateral hilar and mediastinal lymphadenopathy without parenchymal pulmonary abnormalities
Stage II	Hilar and mediastinal adenopathy with parenchymal pulmonary abnormalities (generally a diffuse interstitial pattern)
Stage III	Diffuse pulmonary parenchymal disease without nodal enlargement
Stage IV	Pulmonary fibrosis with evidence of honeycombing (end-stage lung disease)

Although interstitial disease is more common, the airways (including the larynx, trachea, and bronchi) also may be involved. Sarcoidosis is almost always bilateral (95% or more of cases). Unilateral disease should encourage consideration of alternative diagnoses.

5. How does sarcoidosis affect pulmonary function testing?

The most common abnormalities seen on pulmonary function testing are reduction in the diffusion capacity for carbon monoxide (D_{LCO}) and reduction in lung volumes and vital capacity. Obstructive defects may also be seen and are generally believed to represent endobronchial involvement or airway distortion caused by parenchymal disease. Patients with such obstructive defects generally show little or no reversibility after inhalation of bronchodilators. Chest radiograph abnormalities do not necessarily correlate with abnormalities in pulmonary function testing.

6. Which extrapulmonary organ systems may be involved in sarcoidosis?

Sarcoidosis may affect essentially any organ system. The most common or importantly involved systems include the nervous system, skin, heart, eyes, and endocrine system.

7. What are the typical cutaneous manifestations of sarcoidosis?

Cutaneous involvement is common in sarcoidosis, and several findings are possible. The most classic findings are erythema nodosum and lupus pernio. The former is a painful, nodular panniculitis affecting the anterior aspects of the legs, which may be seen in the acute presentation of sarcoidosis. The latter is a bluish-purple raised lesion with a predilection for the eyes, lips, and nose, although it also occurs elsewhere, such as the extremities.

8. What are the cardiac manifestations of sarcoidosis?

Granulomatous involvement of the heart is found in 25% of patients at autopsy, but clinical evidence of cardiac disease occurs in only 5% of cases. The most common findings are heart block (which may be complete) and ventricular dysrhythmias (ranging from premature ventricular contractions to ventricular fibrillation). Although clinical cardiac involvement is uncommon, cardiac sudden death from conduction blocks or fatal ventricular dysrhythmias accounts for a significant number of deaths in patients who die from sarcoidosis. Cardiomyopathy also may occur but is rare.

9. What are the neurologic effects of sarcoidosis?

Clinical neurologic involvement occurs in 5–10% of cases. Neurosarcoidosis may be the presenting manifestation of sarcoidosis, and evidence of systemic involvement may be subtle. The neurologic manifestations of sarcoidosis are protean. Cranial nerve palsy (especially the facial nerve) is the most commonly reported finding. Basilar meningitis, peripheral neuropathy, and pituitary or hypothalamic involvement (or a combination of the two) are also seen. Neurosarcoidosis may be difficult to treat, and the mortality for patients with neurosarcoidosis is two to three fold higher than that in sarcoidosis patients without neurologic involvement.

10. How is the endocrine system involved in sarcoidosis?

The most important endocrine abnormality in sarcoidosis is disordered calcium metabolism. Excess production of 1,25 dihydroxy vitamin D by granulomas may lead to hypercalciuria and hypercalcemia, which may result in significant renal dysfunction and nephrocalcinosis. The syndrome of inappropriate secretion of antidiuretic hormone (SIADH) or diabetes insipidus may occur secondary to pituitary or hypothalamic involvement.

11. How may the eyes be involved in sarcoidosis?

Ocular involvement is an important and relatively common complication of sarcoidosis. Both anterior and posterior uveitis may occur. Lacrimal gland involvement may lead to sicca syndrome and retinal involvement may occur but is rare.

12. What is Heerfordt's syndrome?

Heerfordt's (Heerfordt-Waldenstrom) syndrome, also known as *uveoparotid fever*, is the constellation of fever, parotitis, facial nerve palsy, and anterior uveitis caused by sarcoidosis.

13. What is Lofgren's syndrome?

Lofgren's syndrome is the eponym given to the acute presentation of sarcoidosis characterized by the triad of bilateral hilar adenopathy, erythema nodosum, and arthralgias. Fever frequently accompanies this syndrome, which is more common in whites and Northern Europeans. The prognosis for this presentation of sarcoid is favorable, and disease resolves spontaneously in most patients.

14. How is sarcoidosis diagnosed?

The diagnosis of sarcoidosis generally requires a compatible clinical presentation and biopsy evidence of granulomatous inflammation of an involved organ. The majority of patients with sarcoidosis have pulmonary involvement; therefore, diagnostic measures are centered on the chest. In the appropriate clinical situation, the presentation of bilateral hilar adenopathy in an asymptomatic patient may be adequate to make a presumptive diagnosis of sarcoid. The major differential diagnosis in such patients with isolated intrathoracic adenopathy is lymphoma. However, patients with lymphoma generally have associated constitutional symptoms.

Currently, the most common method of confirming a diagnosis of sarcoidosis is fiberoptic bronchoscopy with transbronchial biopsies. In 60% of patients with stage I disease (i.e, without pulmonary parenchymal abnormalities on chest radiograph), noncaseating granulomas are found. The yield is more than 80% in patients with stage II or stage III disease. Endobronchial biopsies and transbronchoscopic needle biopsies also may be used. Mediastinoscopy and thoracoscopic or open lung biopsies have a near 100% sensitivity but are generally reserved for patients in whom fiberoptic bronchoscopy fails to ascertain the diagnosis. Biopsy of other organs such as the conjuntiva or skin is occasionally useful.

An elevated serum angiotensin-converting enzyme (ACE) level, the presence of anergy, and an abnormal gallium scan of the lungs are supportive but not diagnostic of sarcoidosis.

15. What is the Kveim reaction?

The Kveim reaction (also known as the Kveim-Siltzbach reaction or Kveim test) has been used in the diagnosis of sarcoidosis. Lymphoid tissue (lymph nodes, spleen) from patients with sarcoidosis is prepared in suspension and injected intradermally. A cutaneous reaction characterized by granuloma formation develops in 4–6 weeks and is not readily classifiable into classic type I–IV immunologic reactions. The exact antigen responsible for the reaction is not known. The sensitivity for this reaction may be as high as 90% in patients with stage I disease, but it may be less than 50% in stage III disease. The Kveim reaction is not currently utilized clinically in the United States.

16. What is the role of serum ACE levels in sarcoidosis?

Although elevated ACE levels have been noted in patients with sarcoidosis, the ACE level is neither sensitive nor specific enough to be relied upon as a definitive diagnostic tool for for sarcoidosis. Similarly, ACE levels on presentation may not accurately portend the clinical course of the disease. It is generally accepted that serial ACE levels may be of value in following the clinical course of disease. Therefore, ACE levels may be used as an adjunct measure for following disease activity. At present, the major measures for following disease activity are still clinical symptoms, pulmonary function testing, chest radiography, and other parameters of known extrapulmonary disease.

17. What is the prognosis for patients with sarcoidosis?

The prognosis for patients with sarcoidosis is generally good. The majority of patients with pulmonary sarcoidosis undergo spontaneous resolution or stabilization of their disease within 2–5 years of diagnosis. Patients with stage I disease have a higher rate of resolution (approximately 80%) than do patients with stage II (approximately 60%), who in turn fare better than patients with stage III (approximately 30%). A small number of patients may progress to end-stage lung disease. Patients with acute presentations of sarcoid (e.g., stage I disease with erythema nodosum, Lofgren's syndrome) have a particularly good prognosis. In general, older patients and those with extrapulmonary disease (except erythema nodosum) have a worse prognosis.

18. How and when should sarcoidosis be treated?

Sarcoidosis is often a self-limited syndrome and frequently does not require treatment. When treatment is required, corticosteroids are the agents of choice. Corticosteroids have been shown to improve symptoms and laboratory abnormalities (e.g, pulmonary function test abnormalities) in patients with sarcoidosis, but there is little evidence that corticosteroids alter the course of the disease.

The following situations require therapy:
- Hypercalcemia or hypercalciuria
- Central nervous system involvement (high-dose steroids used; response may vary)
- Ocular involvement (isolated anterior uveitis may be treated with topical corticosteroids, but posterior uveitis requires systemic therapy)
- Myocardial involvement (response is variable)
- Severe cutaneous, muscular, or other end organ involvement
- Respiratory symptoms (dyspnea, cough) or evidence of deranged pulmonary physiology as measured by pulmonary function testing (reduced diffusion capacity, reduced vital capacity). Patients who are asymptomatic and have only mild abnormalities in pulmonary physiology may be followed closely without treatment. If such patients show evidence of deterioration, therapy should be instituted promptly.

Therapeutic agents other than corticosteroids that have been used in small numbers of patients include hydroxychloroquine (primarily used for cutaneous disease), methotrexate, azathioprine, cyclosporin A, and cyclophosphamide. Whole brain irradiation has been used in a few cases of refractory neurosarcoidosis.

The acute presentation of sarcoidosis, Lofgren's syndrome, does not require corticosteroid therapy. Symptomatic treatment with nonsteriodal antiinflammatory agents generally is sufficient.

19. Are inhaled corticosteroids beneficial in pulmonary sarcoidosis?

Several small studies have been conducted; conclusions of some support whereas those of others refute a beneficial role for inhaled steroids in pulmonary sarcoidosis. At this point, systemic corticosteroids are the mainstay of therapy.

20. What should the preliminary work-up include in a patient with newly diagnosed sarcoidosis?

The major focus in evaluating a patient with sarcoidosis should be to identify problems that require treatment. Thus, the work-up includes:

A thorough history and physical examination

Pulmonary function testing and chest radiography

Blood studies including assessment of renal function and electrolytes, especially serum calcium level

A thorough ophthalmologic evaluation for evidence of eye involvement

Other evaluation is obtained as dictated by the particular findings of the individual patient.

BIBLIOGRAPHY

1. Consensus conference: Activity of sarcoidosis. Eur Respir J 7:624–627, 1994.
2. Fanburg BL, Lazarus DS: Sarcoidosis. In Murray JF, Nadel JA (eds): Textbook of Respiratory Medicine. Philadelphia, W.B. Saunders, 1994, pp 1873–1888.
3. Hunninghake GW, Gilbert S, Pueringer R, et al: Outcome of the treatment of sarcoidosis. Am J Respir Crit Care Med 149:893–898, 1994.
4. James GD: Clinical picture of sarcoidosis. In Schwarz MI, King TE (eds): Interstitial Lung Disease. St. Louis, Mosby Yearbook, 1994, pp 159–178.
5. Semenzato G, Agostini C: Immunology of sarcoidosis. In Schwarz MI, King TE (eds): Interstitial Lung Disease. St. Louis, Mosby Yearbook, 1994, pp 127–158.
6. Sharma OP: Extrapulmonary sarcoidosis: Part one. Semin Respir Med 13:1992.
7. Sharma OP: Extrapulmonary sarcoidosis: Part two. Semin Respir Med 13:1992.
8. Sharma OP, Maheshwari A, Thaker K: Myocardial sarcoidosis. Chest 103:253–258, 1993.
9. Stern BJ, Krumholz A, Johns C, et al: Sarcoidosis and its neurological manifestations. Arch Neurol 42:909–917, 1985.
10. Weissler JC: Southwestern Internal Medicine Conference: Sarcoidosis: Immunology and clinical management. Am J Med Sci 307:233–245, 1994.

43. IDIOPATHIC PULMONARY FIBROSIS

John E. Heffner, M.D.

1. What is idiopathic pulmonary fibrosis?

Also called cryptogenic fibrosing alveolitis, idiopathic pulmonary fibrosis (IPF) is the most common cause of ILD of unknown etiology. It has been estimated that 3 to 5 people per 100,000 population are affected by the disease. IPF is presumed to be an immunologic disease because many patients have circulating immune complexes, autoantibodies, and cryoglobulins. Moreover, IPF can occur in association with other conditions known to have an autoimmune basis of disease. These conditions include Hashimoto's thyroiditis, inflammatory bowel disease, chronic active hepatitis, and primary biliary cirrhosis. Lung inflammation develops during the early course of the disease apparently from the deposition of immune complexes that trigger the release of various cytokines, histamine, interleukins, proteases, and oxidants. Alveolar macrophages are initially activated and later participate in the recruitment of neutrophils, lymphocytes, and fibroblasts to the lung. Interstitial inflammation causes aveolar collapse and inactivation of surfactant. Unremitting inflammation results in the proliferation of fibroblasts causing the deposition of type I and type II collagen. Histopathologically, patients pass through the stages of cellular interstitial pneumonitis, desquamative interstitial pneumonitis, and usual interstitial pneumonitis. Unremitting disease terminates in severely deranged pulmonary function characterized by the radiographic and histologic appearance of honeycomb lung.

2. What anatomic region of the lung is affected by IPF?

IPF primarily affects the gas exchanging regions of the pulmonary parenchyma. This "interstitial" compartment of the lung is composed of parenchyma extending from the alveolar epithelial lining cells to the capillary endothelium. Normal constituents within the lung interstitium include matrix tissue containing collagen, elastin, glycoproteins, proteoglycans, fibronectin, and laminin in addition to occasional cellular elements including fibroblasts, myofibroblasts, and macrophages. Anatomic components of the interstitial space include the alveolar space, small conducting airways, arterioles, venules, and lymphatics. The normal architecture of the interstitial compartment is altered in IPF by an influx of inflammatory cells, proliferating fibroblasts, and the deposition of excess collagen.

3. What are the histologic features of IPF?

The histologic features of IPF depend on the stage of the disease in which patients present. Patients with early IPF may have cellular interstitial pneumonia (CIP–interstitial inflammatory cells) or desquamative interstitial pneumonia (DIP–alveolar macrophages). As lung inflammation progresses, patients then develop usual interstitial pneumonia (UIP), which is characterized by interstitial fibroblasts and excess collagen deposition. The terminal phases of the disease are associated with honeycomb lung, which is defined by the presence of endstage parenchymal changes with fibrotic cystic spaces. These histologic features are not diagnostic of IPF and occur in other conditions associated with ILD. Finding any of these patterns on a transbronchial lung biopsy specimen, therefore, warrants consideration of proceeding to a thorascopic or open lung biopsy to exclude a sampling error and an alternative diagnosis.

4. How do patients with IPF present?

Most patients are between 40 and 70 years of age and experience an insidious onset of dyspnea with exertion and a nonproductive cough. Crackles are audible at the lung bases and digital clubbing occurs in 40–70% of patients. Pulmonary hypertension may be apparent during the middle or late stages of the disease. The chest radiograph may have a diffuse ground-glass appearance at the onset of symptoms. As many as 15% of patients at initial presentation may have a normal chest radiograph. With progression of the disease, reduction in lung volume becomes apparent associated with a reticular or reticulonodular interstitial infiltrate primarily at the lung bases. Most patients do not have pleural or mediastinal lymph node abnormalities. High-resolution chest tomography (HRCT) demonstrates subpleural distribution of interstitial densities in a patchy pattern interspersed with normal appearing lung. HRCT may demonstrate significant abnormalities even in patients with normal chest radiographs. Although rare, patients with IPF on lung biopsy with normal HRCT results have been reported. Traction bronchiectasis creates multiple cystic lesions 2–4 mm in diameter. Early disease in the "alveolitis" phase may appear as a ground-glass pattern or as scattered areas of lung consolidation. Patients may have hypergammaglobulinemia, a positive antinuclear antibody test, rheumatoid factor, and circulating immune complexes.

5. What are the typical pulmonary abnormalities noted on pulmonary function testing?

Patients with ILD demonstrate a restrictive pattern on physiologic testing with decreased vital capacity, residual volume, total lung capacity, and thoracic gas volume. Compared to patients with other causes of ILD, such as sarcoidosis, they are more likely to have a low diffusing capacity for carbon dioxide. Flow rates are preserved in most patients.

Some patients with early IPF may have normal physiologic test results at rest. The presence of unexplained dyspnea in a patient with normal resting pulmonary function studies represents a need for exercise testing. Patients with IPF have "stiff lung" and ventilation-perfusion mismatching that cause rapid shallow breathing and hypoxia during exercise.

6. How should patients with IPF be diagnosed?

When the initial evaluation suggests the presence of IPF, thoracoscopic or open lung biopsy is required to establish the diagnosis. The lung biopsy is required to confirm the diagnosis, exclude alternative diagnoses, and establish the stage of the disease.

7. Is there any value to performing bronchoalveolar lavage (BAL)?

Bronchoalveolar lavage through a fiberoptic bronchoscope with analysis of cellular and noncellular components of the lavagate has improved our understanding of the pathophysiology of a number of conditions associated with ILD. The performance of these studies, however, has little value in making a specific diagnosis of IPF. BAL can suggest the probable prognosis in patients with established IPF. The presence of high numbers of lymphocytes in lavagates suggests that patients will have a good response to therapy. The presence of high numbers of neutrophils and eosinophils indicates that a response to therapy is unlikely to occur.

8. What are the therapeutic options available to patients with IPF?

Patients with IPF have a progressive disease with a median survival of less than 5 years without therapy. The presence of smoking is a major contributor to a poor clinical outcome. Spontaneous remissions rarely occur. Patients who present during the early inflammatory stages of the disease before the deposition of extensive collagen networks or the development of honeycomb lung have a better response to therapy. Available drug therapy is anti-inflammatory in nature. Corticosteroids have been reported to provide an improved clinical course in 25–35% of patients. Unfortunately, commonly used dosing regimens of 1.5 mg/kg/day of prednisone are associated with serious complications of therapy. Cytotoxic agents (cyclophosphamide and azathioprine) have been used as second-line therapy in patients who have failed corticosteroids. More recently, some investigators have reported a better initial response to cytotoxic agents than corticosteroids with fewer drug-related adverse reactions. Limited experience with chlorambucil has suggested that this may be a better tolerated drug and less expensive compared to other cytotoxic agents. Results of large scale randomized controlled trials comparing agents with each other or placebo are as of yet unavailable. Colchicine and penicillamine have been used in clinical trials but their efficacy remains unestablished.

Drug regimens should be continued for 3–6 months to determine response to therapy. Responsive patients generally require prolonged treatment with anti-inflammatory agents with close monitoring.

9. How can physicians know if a patient with IPF is responding to therapy?

As many as 70% of patients with IPF treated with corticosteroids will experience subjective improvement, whereas only 20–30% will have objective physiologic or radiographic evidence of a positive drug effect. It is important, therefore, to employ multiple markers to gauge a response to therapy. Responsive patients report a decrease in symptoms and demonstrate some evidence of radiographic or physiologic improvement or stabilization. Even the use of repeated pulmonary function or exercise testing, however, may often leave the clinician uncertain as to the benefits of ongoing therapy.

10. What can be done for patients who progress despite aggressive therapy?

Otherwise healthy patients younger than 55 years of age can be considered for lung transplantation. It is important to enroll patients early on a transplantation list before their disease progresses to the degree that they will not survive the wait for a donor organ. Ideal timing of transplantation has not been established.

BIBLIOGRAPHY

1. Homma Y, Ohtsuka Y, Tanimura K, et al: Can interstitial pneumonia as the sole presentation of collagen vascular diseases be differentiated from idiopathic interstitial pneumonia? Respiration 62:248–251, 1995.
2. Keogh BA, Crystal RG: Pulmonary function testing in interstitial pulmonary disease. What does it tell us? Chest 78:856–865, 1980.
3. Muller NL, Miller RR: Ground-glass attenuation, nodules, alveolitis, and sarcoid granulomas. Radiology 189:31–32, 1993.
4. Proceedings of the Fourth Annual Disease Lung Conference. Chest 100:230–254, 1991.
5. Raghu G: Idiopathic pulmonary fibrosis: A rational clinical approach. Chest 92:148–154, 1987.
6. Raghu G: Interstitial lung disease: A diagnostic approach. Are CT and lung biopsy indicated in every patient? Am J Respir Crit Care Med 151:909–914, 1995.
7. Raghu G, Depaso WJ, Cain K, et al: Azathioprine combined with prednisone in the treatment of idiopathic pulmonary fibrosis: A prospective, double-blind, randomized, placebo-controlled clinical trial. Am Rev Respir Dis 144:291–296, 1991.
8. Schwarz MI, King TE Jr (eds): Interstitial Lung Diseases, 2nd ed. Philadelphia, Mosby, 1993.
9. Watters LC, King TE, Schwarz MI, et al: A clinical, radiographic, and physiologic scoring system for the longitudinal assessment of patients with idiopathic pulmonary fibrosis. Am Rev Respir Dis 133:97–103, 1986.

44. COLLAGEN VASCULAR DISEASE

Marvin I. Schwarz, M.D.

1. Which components of the respiratory system are affected by the collagen vascular diseases?

Essentially, all components of the respiratory system can be primarily involved by collagen vascular disease, including the lung parenchyma (interstitium and pulmonary vessels), airways, pleura, and respiratory muscles. The respiratory system can also be affected secondarily in that drugs used to treat this group of diseases (especially methotrexate for rheumatoid arthritis and polymyositis-dermatomyositis and gold for rheumatoid arthritis) can induce an interstitial lung disease (ILD) that is difficult to distinguish from the ILD caused by the primary disorders.

2. Can any of the collagen vascular diseases initially present with pulmonary manifestations?

Although infrequent, ILD complicating rheumatoid arthritis and polymyositis-dermato-myosis and to a lesser extent scleroderma may precede the more typical manifestations of these disorders by months to several years. The onset of lupus erythematosus is occasionally heralded by an acute immunologic pneumonia, known as *acute lupus pneumonitis*. Pleuritis with or without pleural effusion can be the initiating event in rheumatoid arthritis, lupus erythematosus, and mixed connective tissue disease.

3. Are they any unique characteristics of the pleural effusions associated with the collagen vascular diseases?

In lupus erythematosus, pleurisy and pleural effusion, which occur in up to 60% of patients, represent the most frequent noninfectious pulmonary complication of this condition. Lupus-related effusions are exudates that contain both acute and chronic inflammatory cells. These effusions are characterized by high titers of antinuclear factor and low pleural fluid complement levels. Pleural effusions are also the most common noninfectious pulmonary complication of rheumatoid arthritis. Rheumatoid effusions are exudates with mixed inflammatory cell populations and occasionally low pleural fluid complement levels. Typically, a low pleural fluid glucose concentration (less than 30 mg/dl) with rheumatoid factor titers exceeding 1:320 is present in rheumatoid effusions.

4. What is the fate of a pleural effusion in either lupus erythematosus or rheumatoid arthritis?

The majority of these effusions are self-limiting and require no more than treatment of symptoms. In some instances, however, persistent pain or increasing pleural effusions may require corticosteroid therapy, which is usually effective. In both disorders, pleural effusions tend to recur, and occasional patients may experience extensive pleural inflammation that leads to fibrosis and pleural scarring. This, in turn, may lead to a "trapped lung" in which a fibrotic pleural peel prevents adequate lung expansion. Pleural infection leading to empyema is another complication of effusions related to collagen vascular disease.

5. In which collagen vascular disease is primary pleural involvement never a concern?

In the collagen vascular diseases, pleuritis and effusions occur most commonly in lupus erythematosus, mixed connective tissue disease, and rheumatoid arthritis. Pleural disorders occasionally develop in patients with systemic sclerosis (scleroderma) and Sjögren's syndrome. In systemic sclerosis, clinically apparent pleural disease occurs in only a few patients, but pleural fibrosis is common at postmortem examination. Primary pleural involvement does not occur in patients with polymyositis-dermatomyositis.

6. Which pulmonary problem is most common in patients with the collagen vascular diseases?

Community-acquired pneumonia—either from bacterial, viral, or mycoplasmal pathogens—or opportunistic pneumonia resulting from the immunosuppressive therapy used to treat the underlying disease are the most commonly experienced pulmonary problems. In immunosuppressed patients, *Pneumocystis carinii*, cytomegalovirus, *Nocardia*, and *Aspergillus* pneumonias must be considered when new infiltrates develop with fever. Additionally, patients with scleroderma or polymyositis-dermatomyositis frequently develop recurrent aspiration pneumonia. Aspiration occurs in patients with scleroderma because of esophageal dysmotility and dilatation with resultant gastroesophageal reflux. In polymyositis, inflammation of the upper esophageal and pharyngeal musculature leads to degeneration of the muscle bundles and resultant dysphagia and aspiration.

7. What causes pulmonary hypertension in patients with collagen vascular diseases?

Patients with collagen vascular disease may develop a primary form of pulmonary hypertension that is not associated with any other abnormalities of the lungs. The vessels undergo plexogenic changes characterized by intimal proliferation, medial thickening, luminal obliteration, and eventually recanalization. Primary pulmonary hypertension most commonly occurs in patients with scleroderma and develops to a lesser extent in those with systemic lupus erythematosus, rheumatoid arthritis, and mixed connective tissue disease. A secondary form of pulmonary hypertension occurs in any of the collagen vascular diseases if interstitial lung disease progresses to cause hypoxemia and resultant hypoxic vasoconstriction.

8. Which of the collagen vascular diseases is most likely to be complicated by pulmonary thromboembolism and why?

Patients with lupus erythematosus have a higher risk for pulmonary embolism compared with those who have other collagen vascular diseases. Patients with lupus often have a circulatory anticoagulant with procoagulant activity that predisposes them to deep venous thrombosis and subsequent pulmonary emboli. The circulating anticoagulant is an antiphospholipid antibody.

9. Can interstitial lung disease be present in a patient with collagen vascular disease who has a normal chest radiograph?

Symptomatic interstitial lung disease with a normal chest radiograph can occasionally occur in patients with any of the collagen vascular diseases. In this setting, pulmonary vascular disease (primary pulmonary hypertension or pulmonary emboli) is the first diagnostic consideration. After vascular disease is excluded, evaluation of these patients with a high-resolution CT scan usually shows parenchymal abnormalities even if the standard chest radiograph is normal. Physiologic testing, particularly rest and exercise arterial blood gas levels with measurement of alveolar-arterial gradients and dead space ventilation, demonstrate abnormalities before radiographic findings occur.

10. What is a necrobiotic nodule?

Necrobiotic nodules occur in patients with rheumatoid arthritis, appearing on standard chest radiographs as either multiple bilateral or solitary rounded lesions of varying sizes. They are histologically identical to subcutaneous rheumatoid nodules but can undergo cavitation when they occur in the lung. Necrobiotic nodules are more likely to occur in patients with high titers of rheumatoid factor and often appear during an active articular phase of the disease. They must be differentiated from other causes of lung nodules, such as tuberculosis and peripheral bronchogenic carcinomas.

11. What is Caplan's syndrome?

Caplan's syndrome was first reported in coal miners who developed rheumatoid arthritis and rapidly appearing lung nodules. The nodules are often confined to the upper lobes and may undergo cavitation. Patients with rheumatoid arthritis who inhale other inorganic dusts, such as silica and asbestos, may also develop this syndrome. The nodules themselves have been termed *pneumoconiotic nodules*.

12. What types of interstitial lung disease complicate the collagen vascular diseases?

Several histologic patterns of interstitial lung disease occur in patients with underlying collagen vascular disease. Usual interstitial pneumonia (UIP), characterized by an inflammatory-fibrotic process of the alveolar walls, is the most common pattern. It is the most difficult of the interstitial pneumonitides to treat and often results in end-stage honeycomb lung. Other histologic appearances include:

Bronchiolitis obliterans organizing pneumonia (BOOP)
Lymphocytic interstitial pneumonitis (LIP)
Diffuse alveolar hemorrhage (DAD)
Cellular interstitial pneumonitis (CIP)
Diffuse alveolar hemorrhage (DAH) caused by either bland hemorrhage or pulmonary
   capillaritis

The interstitial lung diseases listed above are much more responsive to antiinflammatory (corticosteroid preparation) and cytotoxic therapy (cyclophosphamide, azathioprine, and methotrexate) than is UIP.

13. What is the relative frequency of the various types of interstitial lung disorders that occur in patients with collagen vascular disease?

Systemic sclerosis has the highest incidence of ILD, which has been reported to be 100% in some patient series. The most common interstitial lesion in systemic sclerosis is UIP, which usually leads to end-stage honeycomb lung in these patients. UIP also appears in patients with rheumatoid arthritis and patients with polymyositis-dermatomyositis. LIP is the most common histologic pattern in patients with Sjögren's syndrome and rheumatoid arthritis. DAD occurs as an acute immunologic pneumonia in lupus erythematosus (termed *acute lupus pneumonitis*) and in patients with mixed connective tissue disease or polymyositis-dermatomyositis. DAH, with or without pulmonary capillaritis, is usually seen in patients with established lupus erythematosus and to a much lesser extent in the other collagen vascular disorders.

14. Most interstitial lung diseases and pleural diseases cause a restrictive defect as measured by pulmonary function testing. In which collagen vascular disease can an obstructive lung disease appear and why?

In rheumatoid arthritis, bronchiolitis obliterans (BO) can lead to a progressive, severe obstructive lung disease similar to the airway obstruction that develops secondary to smoking. Histologically, BO is an inflammatory process of the terminal and respiratory bronchioles that leads to a concentric fibrotic obliteration of the bronchiolar lumen. It was once thought that penicillamine was responsible for BO because many of the affected patients were treated with this agent. However, many cases of BO have been reported to occur in rheumatoid arthritis in the absence of penicillamine therapy. This condition rarely occurs with the other collagen vascular diseases.

15. What is a possible explanation for respiratory failure in a polymyositis-dermatomyositis patient who has no lung involvement?

Polymyositis-dermatomyositis is an inflammatory myopathy that leads to generalized muscle weakness. If the respiratory muscles are extensively involved, respiratory failure causing hypoventilation and hypoxemia will ensure. Respiratory failure occurs in up to 10% of patients and often requires mechanical ventilation. Subclinical involvement of the respiratory muscles does not cause overt respiratory failure but can cause tachypnea, dyspnea on exertion, and interference with cough generation leading to development of hypostatic pneumonia.

16. Which laboratory test helps predict the development of interstitial lung disease in patients with polymyositis-dermatomyositis?

Interstitial lung disease is more likely to occur in those patients who have positive titers to anti-Jo-1, an antibody to an acidic nuclear antigen. More than 60% of patients with polymyositis-dermatomyositis and interstitial lung disease have this antibody in their serum.

BIBLIOGRAPHY

1. Agarwal R, Sharma SK, Malaviya AN: Gold induced hypersensitivity pneumonitis in a patient with rheumatoid arthritis. Clin Exp Rheumatol 7:89–90, 1989.
2. Caplan A: Certain unusual radiographic appearances in the chest of coal miners suffering from rheumatoid arthritis. Thorax 8:29–37, 1953.
3. Geddes DM, Corrin B, Brewerton DA, et al: Progressive airway obliteration in adults and its association with rheumatoid disease. Q J Med 46:427–44, 1977.
4. Hochberg MC, Feldman D, Stevens MB, et al: Antibody to Jo-1 in polymyositis/dermatomyositis: Association with interstitial pulmonary disease. J Rheumatol 11:663–665, 1984.
5. Johnson DA, Drane WE, Currar J, et al: Pulmonary disease in progressive systemic sclerosis: A complication of gastroesophageal reflux and occult aspiration. Arch Intern Med 149:589–593, 1989.

6. Martin L, Chalmers IM, Dhingra S, et al: Measurements of maximum respiratory pressures in poly-myositis and dermatomyositis. J Rheumatol 12:104–107, 1985.
7. Matthay RA, Schwarz MI, Petty JL, et al: Pulmonary manifestations of systemic lupus erythematosus: Review of 12 cases of acute lupus pneumonitis. Medicine (Baltimore) 54:397–409, 1975.
8. Myers JL, Katzenstein AL: Microangitis in lupus-induced pulmonary hemorrhage. Am J Clin Pathol 85:552–56, 1986.
9. Petri M, Rheinschmidt M, Whiting-O'Keefe Q, et al: The frequency of lupus anticoagulant in systemic lupus erythematosus: A study of sixty connective tissue disease patients by activated partial thromboplastin time, Russel Viper venom time, and anticardiolipin antibody. Ann Intern Med 106:524–531, 1987.
10. Sahn SA, Kaplan RL, Maulitz RM, et al: Rheumatoid pleurisy: Observations on the development of low pleural fluid pH and glucose. Arch Intern Med 140:1237–1238, 1980.
11. Schuurawitzki H, Stiglbaver R, Graninger W, et al: Interstitial lung disease in progressive systemic scle-rosis: High resolution CT versus radiography. Radiology 176:755–759, 1990.
12. Tazelaar HD, Viggiano RW, Pickersgill J, et al: Interstitial lung disease in polymyositis and dermato-myositis: Clinical features and prognosis as correlated with histopathologic findings. Am Rev Respir Dis 144:727–733, 1990.

45. BRONCHIOLITIS AND SMALL AIRWAY DISEASE

Richard A. Helmers, M.D.

1. What is the clinical classification of the various forms of bronchiolitis (diseases affecting primarily the bronchioles)?

There are several ways to classify this fascinating group of disorders: bronchiolitis of known etiology versus idiopathic forms; clinical syndromes associated with constrictive bronchiolitis versus clinical syndromes associated with organizing pneumonia (descriptive pathologic terms discussed later); or bronchiolar disorders with airflow obstruction versus interstitial bronchiolar disorders. The last classification has the advantage of being based on clinical and pulmonary function information that is of most use to the respiratory practitioner and is most helpful in developing a differential diagnosis and a diagnostic and therapeutic plan.

2. What are the key bronchiolar disorders associated with airflow obstruction that are usually characterized by constrictive bronchiolitis on pathologic examination?

Bronchiolitis obliterans (also called *constrictive bronchiolitis*)
 Idiopathic
 Postinfectious
 Fume-related
 Associated with
  Connective-tissue diseases
  A drug reaction
  Posttransplant (bone marrow, heart-lung, or lung transplant recipients)
 Smoker's respiratory bronchiolitis
 Mineral dust bronchiolitis
 Diffuse panbronchiolitis

3. What are the key bronchiolar disorders associated with interstitial lung disease that are usually characterized by organizing pneumonia on pathologic examination?

These conditions include respiratory bronchiolitis-interstitial lung disease and bronchiolitis obliterans organizing pneumonia (BOOP). BOOP is often idiopathic, in which case it is also termed *cryptogenic organizing pneumonia* (COP). BOOP may also be seen with connective-tissue disorders, postinfection, and as a drug-related reaction.

4. What are the pathologic manifestations of constrictive bronchiolitis?

Constrictive bronchiolitis is characterized by alterations in the walls of membranous and respiratory bronchioles, often without extensive changes in the alveolar walls and ducts. The spectrum of changes ranges from bronchiolar inflammation to peribronchiolar fibrosis and ultimately concentric narrowing and obliteration of the bronchiolar lumen. The histologic findings are patchy, even in severely affected patients. Initially, intraluminal, mucosal, submucosal, and peribronchiolar inflammation occurs centered on membranous and respiratory bronchioles; the inflammatory infiltrate includes variable numbers of polymorphonuclear neutrophils, lymphocytes, and plasma cells. This early inflammatory stage is followed by peribronchiolar fibrosis that encroaches on the bronchiole lumen concentrically, eventually obliterating it.

5. What are the pathologic manifestations of BOOP?

The histologic hallmark is the presence of an organizing intraluminal exudate that results in patchy intraluminal fibrosis, consisting of polypoid plugs of immature fibroblastic tissue resembling granulation tissue. The characteristic intraluminal fibrotic buds are seen in respiratory bronchioles, alveolar ducts, and alveoli. Chronic inflammatory cells can be seen within the granulation tissue plugs. An acute and chronic bronchiolitis usually is noted away from the areas of intraluminal fibrosis and consists of a peribronchiolar infiltrate of acute and chronic inflammatory cells. Most patients also have an alveolar septal infiltrate of mononuclear inflammatory cells in the areas of intraluminal fibrosis. The fibroblastic plugs are eventually incorporated back into the interstitium and broken down by unclear mechanisms.

6. Describe the important features of toxic fume–related bronchiolitis.

Inhalation of toxic fumes is an uncommon cause of bronchiolitis. The nitrogen oxides are the most common cause. The gases are poorly soluble in water and are able to reach the smaller airways before they become hydrolyzed. Fume-related bronchiolitis may be associated either with classic bronchiolitis obliterans that has intraluminal polyps or with constrictive bronchiolitis. Nitrogen dioxide exposure is a significant industrial and environmental hazard in many settings, for example, agriculture; chemical, munitions, and missile industries; and arc welding. The clinical manifestations depend on the concentration of nitrogen dioxide inhaled and the duration of exposure. Acutely high concentrations can lead to ARDS and death. In those who recover or in those with only a mild illness after exposure, symptoms may recur a few weeks later. Cough and dyspnea are the major symptoms and generalized fine crackles are present on auscultation of the lungs. Pulmonary function tests (PFTs) may show either restriction and or obstruction, or both. Radiographic findings also vary. Usually there is a miliary or discretely nodular pattern scattered uniformly throughout both lungs. Pulmonary hyperinflation accompanied by an irreversible obstructive defect on PFTs occasionally may be seen. Corticosteroid therapy has been shown to be useful in the management of both acute-phase illness and late-phase illness. Once exposure has occurred, prevention of bronchiolitis obliterans may be possible by the administration of a short course of corticosteroids.

Sulfur dioxide, chlorine gas, ammonia, phosgene, smoke inhalation, and hydrogen chloride all can produce a disease with clinical, physiologic, and radiographic manifestations similar to those of disease caused by nitrogen dioxide.

7. Describe the important clinical characteristics of postinfection bronchiolitis.

The lung may develop bronchiolitis after either bacterial or viral infection. Respiratory tract infection in childhood may have long-term sequelae that include bronchiolitis or an increased risk of developing COPD in adulthood, or both. Respiratory tract infections acquired in adulthood occasionally have similar results. Compared with the pediatric population, however, relatively little information exists about the infectious agents of acute bronchiolitis in adults. Constrictive bronchiolitis (from fibrous obliteration of the small airways caused by healing of infection) may result from those infectious agents, which show a propensity to infect and injure epithelial cells of the respiratory tract with resultant bronchiolar inflammation and necrosis.

Clinically evident postinfectious bronchiolitis is uncommon in the adult general population, but pathologic evidence may be much more common. Smoking may potentiate bronchiolar injury associated with an infectious agent and predispose the individual to bronchiolitis. Only a limited number of agents have been reported to be causes of constrictive bronchiolitis; it is most commonly seen with adenovirus or influenza infection in children and in adults infected with *Mycoplasma pneumoniae*. Sporadic cases in adults have been associated with *Nocardia* spp., cytomegalovirus, and *Serratia, Legionella, Cryptococcus, Hemophilus,* and *Klebsiella* spp.

Adults present with nonproductive cough and dyspnea lasting for days to weeks. On examination, inspiratory crackles are a prominent finding, and wheezing is less common. Chest radiographs show hyperinflation and may show concomitant bronchiectasis. CT scans show marked heterogeneity of lung density and also may demonstrate bronchiectasis.

8. Can smoking cause bronchiolitis?

Cigarette smoking is a common cause of bronchiolitis today. Several studies have shown inflammation and fibrosis in membranous and respiratory bronchioles associated with cigarette smoking. The term *small airway disease* has also been used in several different ways to refer to chronic inflammation of distal bronchioles with physiologic evidence of airflow limitation, usually in cigarette smokers. This bronchiolar lesion may be important in the subsequent pathogenesis of centrilobular emphysema. The physiologic abnormalities in the small airways, however, do not predict the 15–20% of smokers who progress to chronic airflow limitation. Some radiologic studies have also suggested a relationship between duration and degree of cigarette smoking and the presence of small irregular opacities (so-called "dirty lungs") on chest radiographs. Because smoking appears to cause bronchiolitis, smoking cessation is important in these patients.

9. What is respiratory bronchiolitis-associated interstitial lung disease?

Respiratory bronchiolitis-associated interstitial lung disease (RB-ILD) is a relatively recently described syndrome with features consistent with interstitial lung disease among current or former smokers. It may be confused with other diffuse parenchymal lung diseases, especially idiopathic pulmonary fibrosis. Patients with RB-ILD probably represent a subset with a more severe stage on the spectrum of respiratory bronchiolitis–small airway disease of cigarette smokers. Lung biopsy is required for diagnosis because it is difficult to distinguish these patients from those with other causes of chronic interstitial lung disease.

Patients present with cough and dyspnea, diffuse fine reticulonodular interstitial infiltrates on chest radiograph, and a restrictive or mixed restrictive-obstructive pattern on PFTs. Coarse crackles are often heard throughout inspiration and sometimes continue into expiration. Finger clubbing has not been reported. CT scans show diffuse or patchy ground-glass density or fine nodules. Histopathologically, respiratory bronchiolitis is characterized by an inflammatory process involving the membranous and respiratory bronchioles. The clinical course and prognosis of RB-ILD is not known because there has not been a longitudinal study of a large group of patients. Smoking cessation appears quite important in the resolution of these lesions; patients may improve with smoking cessation only. A favorable response to corticosteroids, both functionally and radiographically, also has been reported. Overall, the prognosis is favorable.

10. What is COP?

COP or idiopathic BOOP is a distinct clinicopathologic syndrome consisting of an idiopathic illness that is responsive to corticosteroid therapy and has distinctive histopathologic findings. The disease occurs usually in the fifth and sixth decades and affects men and women equally. A persistent nonproductive cough is the most common presenting symptoms. Patients often have dyspnea on exertion and may note the onset of the disorder as a flu-like illness with cough, malaise, fatigue, fever, and weight loss. Less common symptoms are chest pain, hemoptysis, bronchorrhea, and night sweats. Most patients have had symptoms for less than 2–3 months. Cigarette smoking is not a precipitating factor. The symptoms often date to an acute upper respiratory tract infection of presumed viral etiology. Physical examination reveals bilateral crackles and, much less commonly, wheezes. In contrast to patients who have idiopathic pulmonary fibrosis (IPF), clubbing is not found. However, in one series, 25% of patients had no pulmonary physical findings. There are no other extrathoracic clinical physical findings.

A mild to moderate restrictive defect is the most common PFT finding. The diffusing capacity is reduced in the majority of patients. Resting and exercise arterial hypoxemia is common. An increased erythrocyte sedimentation rate is frequently found, often more than 100 mm per hour. C-reactive protein level is increased. A moderate leukocytosis with at most only a minor rise in eosinophils is seen. Autoantibodies are negative or slightly positive. Bronchoalveolar lavage reveals increased numbers of lymphocytes, neutrophils, and eosinophils.

11. Describe the radiographic features of COP.

The characteristic radiographic finding is bilateral, symmetric, patchy air space opacity (or opacities) ranging from 3–5 cm to the size of an entire lobe, often peripheral and pleural based, most profuse in the lower lobes. The opacities may migrate spontaneously. Small pleural effusions are common. The lung volumes may be normal or decreased. Interstitial opacities and irregular linear or nodular interstitial infiltrates, however, may be the dominant or only abnormality in a substantial minority of cases. These features may be difficult to distinguish from those of IPF. Rarely is the radiograph normal. The severity of radiographic abnormalities correlates with the extent of histologic involvement of the respiratory bronchioles and alveolar ducts.

CT scanning may reveal much more extensive disease than is expected by the plain chest radiograph. CT scans usually show a combination of consolidation and ground-glass density. Bronchial wall thickening and dilation are often seen as well. Moderate mediastinal adenopathy may occur. Round nodules up to 1 cm are found that correspond to involved bronchioles surrounded by a localized zone of organizing pneumonia.

12. How is COP diagnosed and treated?

The diagnosis of COP depends on both the clinical setting and the presence of characteristic pathology of the disease. An open lung biopsy is recommended to confirm the diagnosis. Ample lung tissue must be obtained and reviewed to rule out diseases such as IPF, hypersensitivity pneumonitis, or chronic eosinophilic pneumonia. Transbronchial lung biopsies generally do not provide an adequate sample to confirm COP and should be considered acceptable of diagnosis only in a patient with classic clinical-radiologic features.

The clinicopathologic syndrome of COP is a diagnosis of exclusion because a wide variety of clinical disorders are associated with the histologic finding of proliferative bronchiolitis in addition to COP. A thorough search must be performed to rule out these other possibilities, which include hypersensitivity pneumonitis, chronic eosinophilic pneumonia, connective tissue diseases, ARDS, vasculitides (especially Wegener's granulomatosis), ulcerative colitis, and drug-induced reactions. A variant of COP that has a rapidly progressive, fulminating, and life-threatening course has recently been reported.

Corticosteroid therapy is the most common treatment. It results in clinical recovery, usually with complete clinical and physiologic improvement and normalization of the chest radiograph in 66% of patients. Clinical improvement usually occurs within days to weeks. Treatment is usually continued for months. Often, patients relapse when corticosteroids are tapered but improve when treatment with corticosteroids is resumed. Patients with air space opacities on radiograph have a better outcome than those with interstitial opacities. The overall prognosis is much better than that of other interstitial lung diseases such as IPF.

13. What is cryptogenic bronchiolitis? Is it a separate disorder from COP?

Cryptogenic bronchiolitis (CB) is distinctly separate from COP. It is an idiopathic syndrome of chronic airflow obstruction in patients without evidence of underlying emphysema, chronic bronchitis, asthma, or bronchiectasis. Often these patients are misdiagnosed as having one of these processes, especially asthma. CB is often rapidly progressive. Some use the term *small airway disease* to describe CB, which has been estimated to cause approximately 4% of all obstructive lung diseases, although its true incidence may be higher. The disease usually occurs in middle age, and the most common symptoms are exertional dyspnea, nonproductive cough, and other nonspecific chest complaints, usually of 6 to 24 months' duration. Fever and chest pain usually do not occur. Wheezing and crackles may be present but are uncommon; the physical findings are generally unremarkable. The most important clinical feature is that most chronic obstructive lung disorders develop over many years, whereas CB develops much more rapidly. Half of patients are current or prior smokers. Chest radiographs may be normal but typically demonstrate hyperinflation. Varying degrees of interstitial infiltrates may also be present and, when seen in the presence of hyperinflation, are highly suggestive of CB. Pleural involvement is rare.

14. How is the diagnosis of CB made?

Although the radiographic features of CB are often nonspecific, the CT findings may be nearly diagnostic. Marked heterogeneity of lung density is seen with lobules of increased and decreased lung density that create a "mosaic" appearance. This heterogeneity of lung density is exaggerated on expiration. The areas of decreased density are thought to be caused by air trapping with associated reflex pulmonary oligemia; the increased density may the result of relative overperfusion of the more normal areas. Occasionally, patients with CB will have a near normal or normal CT.

PFTs generally reveal airflow obstruction, which is often severe. The diffusing capacity may be normal or decreased. Bronchoalveolar lavage reveals a marked increase in the number of neutrophils.

The cornerstone to the diagnosis of CB is a high index of clinical suspicion. Transbronchial biopsy is inadequate for diagnosis, and an open lung biopsy is often required for a definitive diagnosis. Because treatment generally requires prolonged, high-dose corticosteroid therapy, open lung biopsy should always be considered, especially if the diagnosis is in question or the risks of steroid therapy are substantial. Cyclophosphamide has also been used in those who fail to respond to corticosteroid therapy. In contrast to COP, the course of CB can, in some cases, be rapidly progressive and severe. Most patients have some response to corticosteroids but may remain dependent on steroids for prolonged periods.

15. Is bronchiolitis associated with connective tissue disease?

Pulmonary involvement in the connective diseases has been recognized for many years. Patients with connective tissue disease can have narrowing of the small airways as a result of either of two distinct clinicopathologic syndromes, i.e., bronchiolitis obliterans (constrictive bronchiolitis) or BOOP.

16. Describe the bronchiolopathy most commonly related to connective tissue disease.

The obstructive bronchiolitis seen in rheumatoid arthritis is the most common bronchiolopathy related to connective tissue disease. It is an increasingly recognized complication of rheumatoid arthritis and may be the most common form of lung involvement in this disorder. The majority of patients are middle-aged women with moderate to severe classic rheumatoid arthritis, high titers of rheumatoid factor, and at least 10 years of disease before the onset of symptoms. Many also have evidence of advanced autoimmune exocrinopathy (Sjögren's syndrome). A high clinical index of suspicion is necessary because the condition may be advanced by the time symptoms are noticeable. Symptoms usually consist of either the abrupt or insidious onset of dyspnea and dry cough. On examination one often hears early or mid-inspiratory crackles and "squeaks," believed to arise from opening and oscillation of narrowed bronchioles.

The chest radiograph shows normal or hyperinflated lungs; PFTs reveal obstructive physiology with a normal diffusing capacity. The CT scan reveals widespread patchy increases in attenuation that are accentuated by expiration ("mosaic" pattern). CT may have an increasing role in establishing a diagnosis if an open lung biopsy is contraindicated.

The prognosis in this disorder is often poor; the disease is invariably progressive and patients have a more rapid decline than those with smoking-related COPD. Some patients have a more chronic course of slow deterioration. There may be an association with penicillamine, but this is controversial.

Treatment with antibiotics and bronchodilators is ineffective. Corticosteroid therapy appears to be effective in some patients; the use of either cyclophosphamide or azathioprine also has been suggested.

Airflow or airway obstruction associated with bronchiolitis obliterans is a significant complication in both bone marrow transplant and lung transplant recipients. In these instances, the pathogenesis appears to be immune mediated; there is an association with graft-versus-host-disease (GVHD) in bone marrow recipients and transplant rejection in lung transplant recipients.

17. What is diffuse panbronchiolitis?

Diffuse panbronchiolitis (DP) is a disease of chronic inflammation confined mainly to the respiratory bronchioles. DP presents almost exclusively in subjects of Japanese descent. Almost all patients have a history of chronic paranasal sinusitis and develop chronic cough with copious sputum at the onset of this disease, which usually occurs in the second to fifth decades. One-third of patients have a smoking history; there is no gender predominance. Wheezing and crackles are noted on physical examination; clubbing is sometimes noted. Results of PFTs show marked obstruction and hypoxemia. Persistent marked elevation of cold agglutinins also occurs.

In DP, the chest radiograph reveals diffusely disseminated small nodular shadows up to 2 mm in diameter, most prominent in the lung bases, sometimes accompanied by lung hyperinflation caused by air trapping. CT scanning shows diffuse, small, rounded and linear opacities with dilatation of small bronchi and bronchioles and bronchial wall thickening. The nodules noted on chest radiograph and CT represent secretion-filled bronchioles.

Diagnosis of DP requires the constellation of findings described above. The presence of HLA-Bw54 is helpful; it is found in 66% of patients with DP and in approximately 11% of the Japanese population as a whole.

The natural history of DP is progressive respiratory dysfunction with episodic bacterial superinfection, often with *Pseudomonas* spp. Pseudomonal colonization appears to "accelerate" a destructive phase of the disease, leading to the development of diffuse bronchiectasis and cystic changes in the lung. The 10-year survival rate is as low as 25% for untreated disease. Long-term, low-dose (600 mg/day) erythromycin has been shown to be efficacious; some positive experience has also been reported with the quinolones. The mechanism of benefit is unclear.

18. Can exposure to mineral dust result in bronchiolitis?

Airflow obstruction is being increasingly recognized in individuals who have been exposed to inorganic mineral dust. Epidemiologic studies reveal that exposure to asbestos and other mineral dusts may cause obstructive pulmonary function in nonsmokers; animal exposure to asbestos or silica also produces airflow obstruction. A synergistic role with smoking appears probable.

Pathologic studies show fibrosis of the walls of respiratory and membranous bronchioles with minimal chronic inflammatory response. This lesion is morphologically recognizable and specific for dust exposure.

Terms used to describe this entity include *mineral dust–induced bronchiolitis* or *mineral dust-induced small airways disease* (MDAD). This condition has been observed after exposure to asbestos, silica, iron oxide, aluminum oxide, talc, silicates, and coal. The pathogenesis is unclear but probably involves the inflammatory response that follows the deposition of mineral particles or fibers in small airway walls.

BIBLIOGRAPHY

1. Davison AG, Heard BE, McAllister WAC, et al: Cryptogenic organizing pneumonitis. Q J Med 52:382–394, 1983.
2. Eber CD, Stark P, Bertozzi P: Bronchiolitis obliterans on high-resolution CT: A pattern of mosaic oligemia. J Comput Assist Tomogr 17:853–856, 1993.
3. Epler GR (ed): Diseases of the Bronchioles. New York, Raven Press, 1994.
4. Epler GR, Colby TV, McLoud TC, et al: Bronchiolitis obliterans organizing pneumonia. N Engl J Med 312:152–158, 1985.

5. Ichikawa Y, Hottam, Sumita S, et al: Reversible airway lesions in diffuse panbronchiolitis: Detection by high-resolution computed tomography. Chest 107:120–125, 1995.
6. Kindt GC, Weiland JE, Davis WB, et al: Bronchiolitis in adults: A reversible cause of airway obstruction associated with airway neutrophils and neutrophil products. Am Rev Respir Dis 140:483–492, 1989.
7. King TE: Bronchiolitis. In Schwarz MI, King TE (eds): Interstitial Lung Disease. St. Louis, Mosby-Year Book, 1993.
8. King TE (ed): Bronchiolitis. Clin Chest Med 14:4, 1993.
9. Myers JL, Veal CF, Shin MS, et al: Respiratory bronchiolitis causing interstitial lung disease: A clinico-pathologic study of six cases. Am Rev Respir Dis 135:880–884, 1987.
10. Niewoehner DE, Kleinerman J, Rice DB: Pathologic changes in the peripheral airways of young ciga-rette smokers. N Engl J Med 291:755–758, 1974.
11. Nizami IY, Kissner DG, Visscher DW, et al: Idiopathic bronchiolitis obliterans with organizing pneumo-nia: An acute and life-threatening syndrome. Chest 108:271–277, 1995.
12. Turton CW, Williams G, Green M: Cryptogenic obliterative bronchiolitis in adults. Thorax 35:805–810, 1981.
13. Yousem SA, Colby TV, Gaensler EA: Respiratory bronchiolitis-associated interstitial lung disease and its relationship to desquamative interstitial pneumonia. Mayo Clin Proc 64:1373–1380, 1989.

46. LYMPHANGIOLEIOMYOMATOSIS, EOSINOPHILIC GRANULOMA, AND NEUROFIBROMATOSIS

Kathleen Sutherland, M.D., and Robert B. Dreisin, M.D.

1. What do lymphangioleiomyomatosis, eosinophilic granuloma, and neurofibromatosis have in common?

All of these entities can cause interstitial lung disease characterized by diffuse reticulonodu-lar infiltrates on chest radiographs. All three may also be associated with airflow obstruction su-perimposed on the characteristic restrictive pattern seen in most interstitial lung diseases.

2. Describe the clinical profile of a patient with lymphangioleiomyomatosis.

Lymphangioleiomyomatosis (LAM) always occurs in females, usually in their reproductive years. As in other forms of interstitial lung disease, patients generally present with progressive dyspnea. The chest radiograph initially shows a fine, bilateral reticulonodular pattern, which may have a basilar predominance. One of the radiographic clues to the diagnosis of LAM is that the lungs actually appear normal or enlarged in size, as opposed to the reduced lung volumes common to most other interstitial lung diseases. High-resolution CT (HRCT) characteristically demonstrates several thin-walled cysts of varying sizes that are uniformly distributed throughout the central and peripheral lung fields. Despite evidence of interstitial lung disease on the chest ra-diograph, spirometry often shows an obstructive defect caused by the proliferation of immature smooth muscle cells in the small airways.

3. What causes LAM?

The cause of LAM is not known. However, the proliferation of smooth muscle cells is thought to be related to hormonal secretion because the disease occurs primarily in women in their reproductive years. Exacerbations have been documented during pregnancy, during menses, with the use of birth control pills, and after exogenous estrogen administration.

4. How does smooth muscle cell proliferation lead to the complications of LAM?

The common complications of LAM include pneumothorax, chylous effusions, and hemop-tysis. The peribronchial proliferation of smooth muscle cells leads to the obstruction of small airways and subsequent cyst formation. Rupture of these cysts results in pneumothorax in up to 40% of patients. Obstruction of lymphatic channels can lead to chylothorax. Similarly, the invasion of small veins and venules by smooth muscle cells may result in hemoptysis.

5. What is the best treatment for LAM?

The treatment of LAM is controversial. All forms of therapy are aimed at reducing circulating estrogen levels. Oophorectomy, antiestrogens, androgens, and progesterone have been tried. Because the disease is rare, there are few controlled treatment trials, and the evaluation of the various therapies is difficult. However, the best experience appears to be with progesterone. There are now several well-documented cases in the literature of improvement with progesterone and subsequent deterioration after the dose was tapered. No approach is curative, however; even with treatment, most women die within 10 years of the onset of symptoms. Lung transplantation has been successfully performed in a few patients with LAM, and this is a promising approach to the disease in its terminal stages.

6. What are the common pulmonary manifestations of neurofibromatosis?

Interstitial lung disease occurs in up to 25% of patients with neurofibromatosis. Dyspnea on exertion is the most common presenting symptom and appears between the third and sixth decades. The chest radiograph shows lower lobe infiltrates in the early stages of the disease. Eventually, bullous changes develop in the upper lung zones.

7. Describe the different tumors that can be found in the lungs of patients with neurofibromatosis.

Neurofibromatosis is a disorder of neural crest cells that results in the development of various neurogenic tumors including neurofibromas, schwannomas, and soft tissue sarcomas. All of these tumors can be found in the lung. In addition, schwannomas and sarcomas originating at peripheral sites can become malignant and metastasize to the lung.

8. What pulmonary function abnormalities are seen in neurofibromatosis?

Initially patients present with a restrictive defect and decreased $D_{L_{CO}}$, characteristic of interstitial lung disease. However, as the lung progresses to involve the small airways and as bullae are formed in the upper lung zones, spirometry may demonstrate a superimposed obstructive pattern.

9. How are eosinophilic granuloma, Hand-Schüller-Christian disease, and Letterer-Siwe disease related?

These three diseases are members of the histiocytosis X family and are characterized by proliferation of Langerhans' histiocytes. The growth of Langerhans cells in different parts of the body leads to distinct clinical syndromes. Eosinophilic granuloma is characterized by lytic bone lesions in the long bones, spine, skull, or jaw. Eosinophilic granuloma of the lung, also known as *pulmonary histiocytosis*, is a localized variant of eosinophilic granuloma, and results in interstitial lung disease. Patients with Hand-Schüller-Christian disease have membranous bone defects, exophthalmos, and diabetes insipidus. Letterer-Siwe disease, seen primarily in children, is a fulminant visceral form of this disorder that can mimic a malignant lymphoma.

10. What causes the pulmonary destruction seen in eosinophilic granuloma?

The proliferation and activation of the Langerhans cell, a histiocyte normally found in the skin and bronchiolar epithelium, leads to an uncontrolled inflammatory reaction in the lung. Initially Langerhans cells multiply in the tissue surrounding the respiratory and terminal bronchioles, causing bronchiolitis. As the granulomatous reaction progresses, alveolar structures are involved, resulting in progressive inflammation and fibrosis. Honeycombing is seen in the most severe forms of the disease.

11. Describe the pulmonary symptoms seen in eosinophilic granuloma.

Some patients with eosinophilic granuloma of the lung are asymptomatic, and the disease is discovered when a routine chest radiograph is taken for another reason. Most patients, however, present with the gradual onset of a dry, nonproductive cough and exertional dyspnea. These symptoms are nonspecific and may be present for months to even years before the diagnosis is made. Patients may also present with pleuritic chest pain or spontaneous pneumothorax.

12. What are the characteristic lung biopsy findings in eosinophilic granuloma of the lung?
Stellate-shaped lesions are scattered throughout the lung and consist of granulomas filled with atypical histiocytes (Langerhans cells), eosinophils, and lymphocytes. Outside the granulomas, normal alveolar structure is initially maintained, but as the disease progresses extensive fibrosis and prominent cyst formation develop. A positive immunohistochemical stain for S-100 protein can definitively identify the atypical histiocytes as Langerhans cells.

13. Why does the Langerhans cell proliferate in eosinophilic granuloma?
The cause of the proliferation is unknown. Eosinophilic granuloma is not associated with peripheral eosinophilia or any other evidence of atopy. Since the majority of patients with eosinophilic granuloma are smokers, it is postulated that cigarette smoke may stimulate the Langerhans cells.

14. How is eosinophilic granuloma treated? What is the prognosis of the disease?
Because the majority of patients who develop eosinophilic granuloma are smokers, the first line of treatment is smoking cessation. Steroids are sometimes prescribed in the most severe cases, but their benefit is unpredictable. The course of eosinophilic granuloma varies, but in most patients the disease is self-limited. Spontaneous remission after several months is common. Patients may be left with some dyspnea on exertion and a purely restrictive or combined restrictive-obstructive ventilatory defect.

15. How does bronchoalveolar lavage help in the diagnosis of eosinophilic granuloma?
Bronchoalveolar lavage (BAL) can be used to diagnose eosinophilic granuloma. A high percentage of alveolar macrophages and a slight increase in neutrophils and eosinophils are seen on differential cell count. Langerhans cells can be identified by the use of a monoclonal antibody, CDI (also known as OKT6). The Langerhans cell is also easily identified on electron microscopy by the characteristic appearance of cytoplasmic organelles, known as *Langerhans* or *Birbeck granules*. Because a few Langerhans cells may be seen in the BAL of patients with other interstitial diseases and even in asymptomatic cigarette smokers, at least 5% of total lavaged cells should be Langerhans cells to make the diagnosis. Conversely, eosinophilic granuloma often has a patchy distribution and BAL may be falsely negative. Therefore, if clinical suspicion of eosinophilic granuloma is high, an open or thoracoscopic lung biopsy should be pursued, even when no Langerhans cells are in the lavage.

16. What are the CT findings in eosinophilic granuloma and LAM?

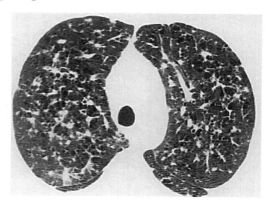

HRCT in a 50-year-old, asymptomatic male smoker shows irregular thick- and thin-walled cysts and scattered ill-defined nodules, predominantly in the upper lobes. These findings are typical of eosinophilic granuloma.

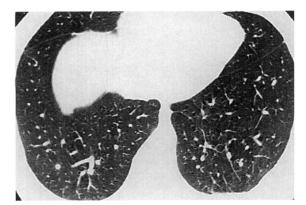

HRCT cuts through the lower lobes on the same patient show relative sparing of the lung bases.

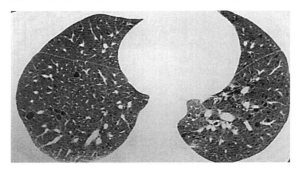

HRCT of a 43-year-old woman who presented with a spontaneous pneumothorax. Severe cystic obstruction of the lung parenchyma characteristic of LAM is seen.

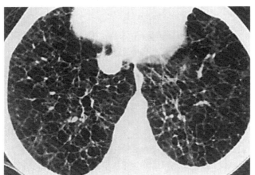

This 28-year-old woman presented during pregnancy with a spontaneous pneumothorax. She had a persistent air leak. Her HRCT revealed multiple thin-walled cysts consistent with LAM.

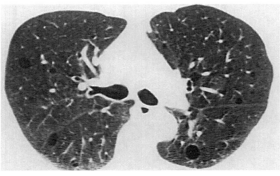

HRCT of a 66-year-old woman with dyspnea who was on estrogen replacement therapy. Scattered thin-walled cysts are shown. Biopsy confirmed LAM. There are now several case reports of LAM in postmenopausal women on estrogen replacement therapy. (The authors thank Chris Salmon of the Department of Radiology at Oregon Health Sciences University for all radiographic reproductions.)

BIBLIOGRAPHY

1. Baldi S, Papotti M, Valente ML, et al: Pulmonary lymphangioleiomyomatosis in postmenopausal women: Report of two cases and review of the literature. Eur Respir J 7:1013–1016, 1994.
2. Buckley KM, Deluca SA: Pulmonary lymphangiomyomatosis. Am Fam Phys 831–833, 1995.
3. Chollet S, Soler P, Duornovo P, et al: Diagnosis of pulmonary histiocytosis X by immunodetection of Langerhans cells in bronchoalveolar lavage fluid. Am J Pathol 115:225–232, 1984.
4. Danel C, Israel-Biet D, Costabel U, et al: The clinical role of BAL in pulmonary histiocytosis X. Eur Respir J 3:949–950, 1990.
5. Delgrange E, Delgrange B, Walton J, et al: Diagnostic approach to pulmonary lymphangioleiomyomatosis. J Intern Med 36:461–464, 1994 (Case report).
6. Eliasson AH, Pips Y, TeTolder M: Treatment of lymphangioleiomyomatosis: A meta-analysis. Chest 196:1352–1355, 1989.
7. Friedman PJ, Liebow A, Sokolof J: Eosinophilic granuloma of lung: Clinical aspects of primary pulmonary histiocytosis in the adult. Medicine 60:385–396, 1981.
8. George RB, Light RW, Matthay MA, et al: Chest Medicine: Essentials of Pulmonary and Critical Care Medicine. Baltimore, Williams & Wilkins, 1990.
9. Gillissen A, Kotterba S, Rasche K, et al: A rare manifestation of von Recklinghausen neurofibromatosis: Advanced neurofibromatous infiltration in lung of an HIV-positive patient. Respiration 61:292– 294, 1994 (Case report).
10. Guinee DG, Feuerstein I, Koss MN, et al: Pulmonary lymphangioleiomyomatosis: Diagnosis based on results of transbronchial biopsy and immunohistochemical studies and correlation with high-resolution computed tomography findings. Arch Pathol Lab Med 118:846–849, 1994.
11. Kitaichi M, Nishimura K, Itoh H, et al: Pulmonary lymphangioleiomyomatosis: A report of 46 patients including a clinicopathologic study of prognostic factors. Am J Respir Crit Care Med 151:57–33, 1995.
12. Massaro D, Katz S: Fibrosing alveolitis: Its occurrence, roentgenographic, and pathologic features in von Recklinghausen's neurofibromatosis. Am Rev Respir Dis 93:934–942, 1966.
13. Murray JL, Nadel JA (eds): Textbook of Respiratory Medicine, 2nd ed. Philadelphia, W.B. Saunders, 1994.
14. Patchefsky A, Atkinson WG, Hock WS, et al: Interstitial pulmonary fibrosis and von Recklinghausen's disease. An ultrastructural and immunofluorescent study. Chest 64:459–464, 1973.
15. Scully RE, Mark EJ, McNeely WF, et al: Case records of the Massachusetts General Hospital. Weekly clinicopathological exercises. Case 1-1992. N Engl J Med 326:454, 1992.
16. Scully RE, Mark EJ, McNeely WF, et al: Case records of the Massachusetts General Hospital. Weekly clinicopathological exercises. Case 18-1994. N Engl J Med 330:1300–1306, 1994.
17. Sleiman C, Mal H, Jebrak G, et al: Pulmonary lymphangiomyomatosis treated by single lung transplantation. Am Rev Respir Dis 14:964–966, 1992.
18. Taylor JR, Ryu J, Colby TV, et al: Lymphangioleiomyomatosis: Clinical course in 32 patients. N Engl J Med 323:1255–1260, 1990.
19. Unger PD, Geller SA, Anderson PJ: Pulmonary lesions in a patient with neurofibromatosis. Arch Pathol Lab Med 108:54–57, 1984.
20. Wahedna T, Cooper S, Williams J, et al: Relation of pulmonary lymphangioleiomyomatosis to use of the oral contraceptive pill and fertility in the UK: A national case control study. Thorax 49:910–914, 1994.

X. Vasculitis and Immunologic Disorders

47. WEGENER'S GRANULOMATOSIS AND CHURG-STRAUSS SYNDROME

Eugene J. Sullivan, M.D.

1. What is Wegener's granulomatosis?

Wegener's granulomatosis (WG) is a form of systemic vasculitis characterized by necrotizing granulomatous vasculitis of the upper and lower respiratory tract, glomerulonephritis, and variable degrees of small vessel vasculitis. According to the American College of Rheumatology, the following four criteria may be used to classify patients with vasculitis as having WG:

1. Nasal or oral inflammation
2. Abnormal chest radiograph (nodules, fixed infiltrates, or cavities)
3. Abnormal urinary sediment (hematuria or red cell casts)
4. Granulomatous inflammation on biopsy

In the presence of two or more of these criteria, WG can be classified appropriately with 88% sensitivity and 92% specificity.

2. What is limited Wegener's?

The term *limited Wegener's* refers to a form of the disease that does not involve the kidney. Although the term appears in the literature, its utility is unclear for two reasons. First, results of renal biopsies may be abnormal even in patients without clinical evidence of renal disease, thus blurring the distinction between limited and typical Wegener's. Second, with time, limited disease often progresses to involve the kidney.

3. How do patients with WG present?

Most patients present with complaints referable to the upper or lower respiratory tract. If the systemic illness is not apparent, these patients are often treated symptomatically for nasal or sinus complaints such as rhinitis, purulent or bloody nasal discharge, or nasal mucosal drying and crusting. Abnormalities are noted in chest radiographs of nearly 50% of patients at presentation. Pulmonary symptoms include cough, hemoptysis, and pleuritis. Approximately 20% of patients have evidence of glomerulonephritis on presentation, but it is usually asymptomatic. Eventually 75% of patients develop glomerulonephritis. Nonspecific musculoskeletal complaints such as myalgias and arthralgias are common.

4. What are the less common manifestations?

The majority of patients with WG eventually develop pulmonary; renal; and ear, nose, and throat (ENT) abnormalities of some sort. Less commonly, patients develop hearing loss, subglottic stenosis, ear pain, or oral lesions. Nonspecific ocular abnormalities such as conjunctivitis also may be seen. Proptosis is often painful and may be associated with diplopia and loss of vision. Fever and weight loss may be seen. Various skin lesions, though relatively uncommon at presentation, eventually develop in nearly 50% of patients. The central and peripheral nervous systems may also be involved.

5. What is the prognosis?

Historically WG was a uniformly fatal disease. Untreated, these patients died of disseminated vasculitis and renal failure after a mean of 5 months. The use of high-dose corticosteroids
improved the survival minimally. The addition of cyclophosphamide has greatly improved the
prognosis. With current treatment 90% of patients experience marked improvement and 75%
achieve complete remission. Relapses are experienced by 50% of those in remission, however. In
addition, significant morbidity is associated with both the disease and the treatment. Overall,
80% of patients now survive to 8 years.

6. How is WG treated?

The current standard therapy for WG was developed at the National Institutes of Health.
Treatment is initiated with both prednisone and cyclophosphamide. Unless patients are acutely
ill, these medications are given orally once daily. Cyclophosphamide is initiated at a dose of 2 mg
per kg and prednisone at 1 mg per kg. After 4 weeks the prednisone dose is tapered to 60 mg
every other day. This taper should occur over approximately 1–3 months. Subsequently the prednisone is slowly tapered off. The cyclophosphamide should be continued for at least 1 year after
clinical remission, at which time it is tapered off in 25 mg increments every 2–3 months.

Some suggest that methotrexate may be an effective alternative to cyclophosphamide, but the
data are limited. In addition, others report that trimethoprim-sulfamethoxazole may be effective,
especially in limited WG. There is, however, considerable controversy surrounding these reports.

7. What are antineutrophil cytoplasmic antibodies?

Antineutrophil cytoplasmic antibodies (ANCA) are a group of autoantibodies directed at
various constituents of neutrophils. ANCA are usually divided into two groups based upon the
staining pattern observed in ethanol-fixed neutrophils: p-ANCA results in a perinuclear staining
pattern and c-ANCA results in a cytoplasmic staining pattern. The specific antigens to which
these antibodies are directed continue to be identified. c-ANCA is usually directed against pro-
teinase 3 whereas the targets of p-ANCA seem to vary among patients and include myeloperoxi-
dase, elastase, lactoferrin, and other as yet unidentified leukocyte constituents.

8. What is the relevance of ANCA?

In the past several years a growing body of literature has developed regarding the use of ANCAs
as serologic markers for various diseases. Most of this work has related to vasculitic syndromes, but
more recently p-ANCA has been associated with such diverse diseases as inflammatory bowel disease, rheumatoid arthritis, and autoimmune liver disease. Because of its varied antigenic targets
and the diversity of associated diseases, p-ANCA is currently less helpful clinically than c-ANCA.

c-ANCA is somewhat more specific. It is most commonly seen in WG, although it has been
also noted in patients with microscopic polyangiitis and pauci-immune necrotizing glomerulonephritis. c-ANCA is present in more than 90% of patients with classic WG and approximately
70% of patients with limited WG. Overall, the sensitivity and specificity of c-ANCA for WG are
approximately 81% and 98%, respectively. As with any test, the actual positive predictive value
varies according to the pretest probability of the disease. Currently, ANCA represents a serologic
marker of disease. Whether these autoantibodies will be implicated in disease pathogenesis remains to be seen.

9. Can serial measurements of c-ANCA titers be used to follow disease activity and to justify altering immunosuppressive therapy?

Although the presence of c-ANCA is a sensitive and specific marker for WG, serial changes
in titers do not sufficiently correlate with changes in disease activity. Serial titers have been found
to temporally correlate with disease status in only 64% of patients. Clinical exacerbations are
preceded by increases in c-ANCA titers in only 24% of patients. Of patients in remission who
demonstrated a fourfold increase in c-ANCA titers, 44% did not have a relapse of the disease.
Thus, therapeutic decision making cannot be based upon changes in c-ANCA titers alone.

10. What is Churg-Strauss syndrome?

Churg-Strauss syndrome (CSS) is a form of systemic vasculitis that was first described in 1951 as a clinical syndrome characterized by asthma, eosinophilia, and systemic vasculitis. The three major pathologic findings are tissue infiltration by eosinophils, necrotizing vasculitis, and extravascular granulomas, although all three findings are not necessarily present. These pathologic findings are the reason why this disease is also referred to as *allergic granulomatosis and angiitis*.

Although a distinct clinical entity, CSS may be regarded as an overlap of Wegener's granulomatosis and polyarteritis nodosa. The American College of Rheumatology has developed criteria for classification of patients with vasculitis as having CSS. The presence of four or more of the following criteria allows appropriate classification with a sensitivity of 85% and a specificity of greater than 99%:

1. Asthma
2. Eosinophilia (more than 10%)
3. Neuropathy (mononeuritis of mononeuritis multiplex)
4. Pulmonary infiltrates (nonfixed)
5. Paranasal sinus abnormality
6. Extravascular eosinophils

11. How do patients with CSS present?

The course of CSS has several phases. Initially patients present with symptoms of allergic rhinitis. Asthma may develop concurrently or follow after several years. The second phase is characterized by peripheral blood eosinophilia and tissue infiltration with eosinophils. Patients at this stage may present with eosinophilic pneumonia or eosinophilic gastroenteritis. Finally, patients develop features of systemic vasculitis, which may include fever, weight loss, and general malaise. During this vasculitic phase involvement of other organ systems becomes apparent.

12. What is the treatment?

CSS is the most steroid responsive of the pulmonary vasculitides. Prednisone should be started at approximately 1 mg per kg per day and continued at this dose until a clinical response is achieved, whereupon the dose is tapered. After initiation of therapy the eosinophilia and allergic symptoms improve quickly, followed by the vasculitic features. Asthma symptoms frequently persist despite resolution of vasculitic illness. Steroid therapy is associated with a 62% 5-year survival. Cytotoxic agents such as cyclophosphamide may be added for patients who fail to respond to corticosteroids.

13. What are other manifestations?

Chest radiographic manifestations include pulmonary infiltrates that may be diffuse, patchy, or even nodular. These infiltrates are often migratory. Pleural effusions may also be seen. The eosinophilic infiltration and systemic vasculitis of CSS may involve any organ. If the gastrointestinal tract is involved, abdominal pain, mucosal ulceration, perforation, or obstruction may result. Skin involvement (such as palpable purpura, maculopapular rash, or subcutaneous nodules) is common and may be the site of a positive biopsy. Peripheral nervous system involvement (neuritis) is also common, and cranial nerve involvement such as optic neuritis may also be seen. Cardiac involvement is most commonly manifested by pericarditis and pericardial effusion, but coronary vasculitis also has been reported. Cardiac disease accounts for approximately 50% of deaths resulting from CSS. Musculoskeletal manifestations include arthralgia and myalgia. CSS may also involve the prostate and lower urinary tract leading to urinary retention or obstructive uropathy. Renal involvement in CSS is less common and less severe than in polyangiitis nodosa or WG.

14. When should the diagnosis of CSS be considered in patients who appear to have asthma?

Asthma is an extremely common disorder and CSS is uncommon; therefore, most patients with symptoms of asthma do not have CSS. CSS should be considered in patients with asthma if there is evidence of migratory pulmonary infiltrates or systemic vasculitis. Manifestations of systemic vasculitis may not be dramatic. CSS should should be considered in the asthmatic who has unexplained and seemingly unrelated complaints (such as recurrent unexplained abdominal pain) that might be a subtle manifestation of a systemic disorder. In addition, although patients with extrinsic asthma may have elevated eosinophil counts, they are seldom as high as those seen in CSS. Therefore, CSS should be considered in asthmatics whose peripheral blood eosinophil count exceeds 1.5×10^9 per liter.

15. Is the peripheral eosinophil count helpful in diagnosis? Can it be used for following treatment?

Peripheral eosinophilia is one of the diagnostic features of CSS and is present in almost all patients, although some patients may have normal eosinophil counts because of previous steroid therapy. In rare instances a patient may have an identical disease with tissue infiltration of eosinophils but without peripheral eosinophilia. The peripheral eosinophil count usually falls rapidly upon initiation of steroid therapy. Although the degree of eosinophilia may correlate with disease activity, other variables of disease activity should also be considered when therapeutic decisions are made. There is no consistent relationship between the severity of the asthma and the activity of the vasculitis.

CONTROVERSY

16. Is there a role for trimethoprim-sulfamethoxazole in the treatment of WG?

During the past decade there have been several reports of beneficial effects of trimethoprim-sulfamethoxazole (TMP/SMX) in patients with WG. These reports include patients who seemed to respond to TMP/SMX when used alone or in combination with corticosteroids or cyclophosphamide, or both. The dose of TMP/SMX is commonly one double strength tablet 2–3 times per day. Two mechanisms of action of TMP/SMX have been proposed: either TMP/SMX is effective against some unrecognized infectious etiology of WG or TMP/SMX may have some unknown immunosuppressive activity. Although some authors are quite convinced of its activity, others are more skeptical, citing the anecdotal nature of the published reports and the possibility that TMP/SMX may appear to be beneficial because of its effectiveness against bacterial superinfection. Although at some institutions TMP/SMX seems to be beneficial the National Institutes of Health experience with TMP/SMX is less promising. All agree that there is a need for prospective controlled trials of TMP/SMX in WG. Those who advocate its use recommend it only for patients with indolent courses who do not have clinical renal disease or active systemic vasculitis. Patients with more active disease should be treated with standard therapy.

BIBLIOGRAPHY

1. Chumbley LC, Harrison EG, DeRemee RA: Allergic granulomatosis and angiitis (Churg-Strauss syndrome): Report and analysis of 30 cases. May Clin Proc 52:477–484, 1977.
2. DeRemee RA: The treatment of Wegener's granulomatosis with trimethoprim/sulfamethoxazole: Illusion or vision? Arthritis Rheum 31:1068–1072, 1988.
3. Hoffman GS, Kerr GS, Leavitt RY, et al: Wegener's granulomatosis: An analysis of 158 patients. Ann Intern Med 116:488–498, 1992.
4. Kerr GS, Fleisher TA, Hallahan CW, et al: Limited prognostic value of changes in antineutrophil cytoplasmic antibody titre in patients with Wegener's granulomatosis. Arthritis Rheum 36:365–371, 1993.
5. Lanham JG, Elkon KB, Pusey CD, et al: Systemic vasculitis with asthma and eosinophilia: A clinical approach to the Churg-Strauss syndrome. Medicine (Baltimore) 63:65–81, 1984.
6. Leavitt RY, Fauci AS: Pulmonary vasculitis. Am Rev Respir Dis 134:149–166, 1986.
7. Leavitt RY, Fauci AS, Bloch DA, et al: The American College of Rheumatology 1990 criteria for the classification of Wegener's granulomatosis. Arthritis Rheum 33:1101–1107, 1990.
8. Leavitt RY, Hoffman GS, Fauci AS: Response: The role of trimethoprim/sulfamethoxazole in the treatment of Wegener's granulomatosis. Arthritis Rheum 31:1073–1074, 1988.
9. Masi AT, Hunder GG, Lie JT, et al: The American College of Rheumatology 1990 criteria for the classification of Churg-Strauss syndrome (allergic granulomatosis and angiitis). Arthritis Rheum 33:1094–1100, 1990.

48. DIFFUSE ALVEOLAR HEMORRHAGE SYNDROMES

Feroza Daroowalla, M.D., and Ganesh Raghu, M.D.

1. What are the diffuse alveolar hemorrhage syndromes?

Diffuse alveolar hemorrhage (DAH) syndromes are a group of disorders in which the small pulmonary vessels are the source of bleeding In many of the disorders that result in DAH, the alveolar capillary basement membrane is involved in an inflammatory process (pulmonary capillaritis). For example, DAH can occur as a complication of systemic vasculitis disorders, such as Wegener's granulomatosis and Goodpasture's syndromes. DAH can also be secondary to conditions in which the capillaries are not inflamed, such as mitral stenosis and coagulopathy. It is occasionally seen in patients exposed to drugs (e.g., D-penicillamine) and toxins (e.g,. trimellitic anhydride). Rarely, DAH occurs following bone marrow transplantation or as a manifestation of idiopathic pulmonary hemosiderosis/isolated pulmonary capillaritis.

Causes of Diffuse Alveolar Hemorrhage

WITH PULMONARY CAPILLARITIS*	WITHOUT PULMONARY CAPILLARITIS
Systemic lupus erythematosus	Systemic lupus erythematosus
Goodpasture's syndrome	Goodpasture's syndrome
Wegener's granulomatosis	Pulmonary veno-occlusive disease
Mixed cryoglobulinemia	Pulmonary capillary hemangiomatosis
Behçet's syndrome	Trimellitic anhydride
Henoch-Schönlein purpura	Mitral stenosis
Connective tissue disease	Coagulation disorders
Pauci-immune glomerulonephritis	D-Penicillamine
Immune complex glomerulonephritis	Idiopathic pulmonary hemosiderosis
Systemic necrotizing vasculitis	

* Can be present without systemic disease or vasculitis elsewhere.

2. How does DAH present?

Symptoms include cough, dyspnea, hemoptysis, and chest pain, which can persist for days to weeks and can be recurrent. Hemoptysis is not always present and may not occur despite extensive intra-alveolar bleeding. Iron-deficiency anemia can also occur. (It should be noted that DAH is not the most common cause of hemoptysis. Hemoptysis is most frequently associated with bronchitis, bronchiectasis, malignancy, pulmonary infarction, or necrotizing pneumonia.) Depending on the underlying cause of DAH, systemic signs and symptoms of vasculitis, sinusitis, ocular disease, arthritis, and glomerulonephritis may accompany the pulmonary symptoms.

The **chest radiograph** demonstrates diffuse or focal patchy alveolar infiltration with airspace filling. If the hemorrhages have been recurrent, interstitial infiltrates may be present. **CT scanning** demonstrates patchy alveolar filling with a homogeneous ground-glass appearance, but this finding is not specific for hemorrhage.

Among l**aboratory tests**, abnormal erythrocyte sedimentation rate (ESR), proteinuria, and elevated serum creatinine are present in systemic vasculitis or connective tissue disease.

3. What physiologic findings are associated with DAH?

Ventilation-perfusion abnormality results in hypoxemia in cases of extensive hemorrhage. Diffusing capacity for carbon monoxide (DLCO) is increased in patients with acute hemorrhage and, if measured, may show an increase as hemorrhage increases. In patients with associated interstitial fibrosis (that can result from chronic hemorrhage), DLCO may be reduced.

4. Discuss the association of systemic lupus erythematosus (SLE) with DAH.

DAH is seen rarely with SLE but can be catastrophic when it occurs. Mortality rates exceed 50%, and DAH can be recurrent in those who survive. It is usually seen in patients with active SLE with extrapulmonary disease and elevated titers of anti-DNA antibodies. Diffuse alveolar infiltrates, hypoxemia, dyspnea, and anemia are characteristic for this presentation. Pulmonary infiltrates are usually symmetric but can be asymmetric or unilateral. The differential diagnosis of the radiographic infiltrates includes congestive heart failure, pneumonia, uremia, pulmonary embolism (with infarct associated with lupus anticoagulant), and acute lupus pneumonitis.

5. Discuss the association of Goodpasture's syndrome and DAH.

Goodpasture's syndrome, also known as antiglomerular basement membrane (anti-GBM) antibody disease, is characterized by the binding of antibody to alveolar and glomerular basement membranes in a linear pattern. Men between the ages of 20–30 years are most commonly affected. Lung disease accompanies the renal disease in 60–80% of cases. DAH is more likely to occur in patients who smoke and is probably due to an increase in lung permeability. Exposure to volatile hydrocarbons has also been implicated in the development of DAH in these patients.

In the appropriate clinical setting, the diagnosis of DAH associated with Goodpasture's syndrome can often be made on clinical grounds if the patient has anti-GBM antibodies in serum and the typical renal abnormalities. In other patients, histologic confirmation with lung biopsy may be necessary. Of note, a high incidence of HLA-DRw2 and HLA-B7 is found in patients with Goodpasture's syndrome.

6. Are hemoptysis and DAH common in Wegener's granulomatosis? How are these patients diagnosed and treated?

DAH is rarely seen with Wegener's granulomatosis—only 50 cases of Wegener's and DAH with pulmonary capillaritis have been reported. However, hemoptysis due to capillaritis, *without* DAH, occurs in up to one-third of patients with Wegener's granulomatosis.

DAH can occur in an established case of Wegener's or can be the first manifestation of the disease. Clinical features of sinusitis, cavitary lesions, and nodular pulmonary infiltrates might be absent if the DAH is the initial manifestation. Histologic findings on lung biopsy may reveal pulmonary capillaritis in isolation or with granulomatous inflammation, vasculitis of medium-sized vessels, and parenchymal necrosis. Diagnostic tests include positive antineutrophil cytoplasmic autoantibodies in a cytoplasmic pattern (c-ANCA). ESR, c-ANCA levels, and DLCO are useful indicators of disease activity. Corticosteroids in combination with cyclophosphamide are the therapy of choice.

7. What is systemic necrotizing vasculitis?

Systemic necrotizing vasculitis disease involves small blood vessels (arterioles, capillaries, venules) and results in pulmonary capillaritis, DAH, and focal segmental necrotizing glomerulonephritis. The lungs are involved with capillaritis in 20–30% of cases. The lung disease tends to be severe and life-threatening. Cutaneous, gastrointestinal, neurologic, and sinus manifestations can also occur. The ESR and rheumatoid factor, antinuclear antibody, and circulating immune complexes are increased in the serum. Some patients may also exhibit cryoglobulinemia, elevated ANCA levels, or hepatitis B antigen. Treatment with a corticosteroid and cyclophosphamide or azathioprine has been successful.

8. Which cardiac disease should be considered in a patient with DAH?

DAH in a patient *without* renal or systemic vasculitic manifestations must raise the suspicion for **mitral stenosis**. This diagnosis should also be considered in any pregnant woman who presents with hemoptysis or DAH, because occult mitral stenosis, manifested as pulmonary hypertension, will become overt due to the increased pulmonary vascular volume associated with pregnancy. Mitral stenosis causes elevated pulmonary venous pressures and results in repeated intermittent hemoptysis with eventual organization of hemorrhage in the alveoli. Interstitial fibrosis can be a sequela of repeated hemorrhage into the pulmonary parenchyma. Massive hemoptysis can also occur in these patients with elevated left atrial pressure and resultant engorgement of bronchial varicosities.

9. Can occupational exposure be associated with the development of alveolar hemorrhage?

Workers exposed to **trimellitic anhydride** (TMA) can develop alveolar hemorrhage with associated dyspnea, hemoptysis, fever, pulmonary infiltrates, and anemia. TMA is used in the manufacture of plastics, paints, and epoxy resins, and workers inhale its fumes or the dry powder. The illness can occur 1–3 months after exposure.

On histologic exam of affected lung, no basement membrane changes or immune complex deposits are found. Serologic exam may reveal TMA antibodies, but these are found more commonly in patients with TMA-associated rhinitis or asthma. Therapy includes removal from exposure and supportive measures.

10. Which drug can result in diffuse alveolar hemorrhage?

D-Penicillamine, used to treat rheumatoid arthritis, progressive systemic sclerosis, Wilson's disease, or primary biliary cirrhosis, can produce DAH as well as an immune-complex-mediated glomerulonephritis. Histologic exam of glomerular capillaries reveals a granular immunofluorescent pattern for IgG and complement C3.

11. How is the diagnosis of idiopathic pulmonary hemosiderosis made?

This is a diagnosis of exclusion in patients with recurrent DAH in the absence of extrapulmonary disease, usually young adults and children. Patients may present with isolated hemoptysis or progressive dyspnea. The clinical course is variable, and the illness can follow a fulminant course leading to death or result in relapses over time leading to interstitial pulmonary fibrosis. Spontaneous remission with little residual effect can also occur.

Histologic examination reveals focal disruption of alveolar capillary basement membranes without vasculitis or immune complex deposition. Erythrocytes and hemosiderin-containing macrophages fill the alveolar space. Hemosiderin also collects in the interstitium. Although the pathogenesis remains unknown, there is an association with celiac sprue and elevation of serum IgA levels, which, in combination with responsiveness to immunosuppressive therapy, point to a possible immune mechanism.

12. What bronchoscopic findings are seen in a patient with DAH?

Bronchoscopy is indicated to localize an occult anatomic source of bleeding as an alternative explanation for pulmonary hemorrhage. The bronchoscopic exam in DAH may reveal diffuse bleeding from all or several bronchopulmonary segments. The bronchoalveolar lavage fluid may be mildly serous initially, but sequential aspirates of saline lavage may become grossly hemorrhagic. On microscopic exam, the lavage fluid reveals red blood cells and hemosiderin-laden alveolar macrophages. These findings are not diagnostic for DAH and merely reflect exposure of macrophages to blood in the alveoli.

13. What is the role of lung biopsy in the evaluation of DAH?

When the diagnosis cannot be made by clinical evaluation and bronchoscopy, a surgical lung biopsy (thoracoscopic-guided or open lung biopsy) can help clarify the diagnosis. The biopsy might reveal pulmonary capillaritis with inflammation of the capillaries in the alveolar walls. This is found in association with some systemic vasculitides but occasionally may be limited to the pulmonary vascular bed. Histologic examination reveals neutrophilic infiltration of the alveolar interstitium with resultant fibroid necrosis of the alveolar wall. Associated disruptions of the alveolar capillary membrane and leakage of red blood cells and neutrophils into the alveolar spaces may be present. Other features include collections of hemosiderin-containing macro-phages in the alveoli, hyperplasia of type II alveolar epithelial lining cells, and organization of intra-alveolar hemorrhage (organizing pneumonia). In recurrent DAH, varying degrees of pul-monary fibrosis may be seen.

In Goodpasture's syndrome, immunofluorescent staining reveals the characteristic pattern of linear attachment of anti-GBM antibody along the alveolar basement membrane. Transbronchial lung biopsy specimens may be sufficient to demonstrate this finding if adequate alveolar tissue is obtained.

14. How is DAH treated?

Treatment is directed toward the underlying cause of the hemorrhage. It also includes sup-portive measures for the hypoxemia and anemia associated with DAH. In severe cases, plasma-pharesis is indicated.

BIBLIOGRAPHY

1. Blanc PD, Golden JA: Unusual occupationally related disorders of the lung: Case reports and a literature review. Occup Med 7:403–422, 1992.
2. Leatherman JW, Davies SF, Hoidal JR: Alveolar hemorrhage syndromes: Diffuse microvascular lung he-morrhage in immune and idiopathic disorders. Medicine 63:343–361, 1984.
3. Orens JB, Martinez FJ, Lynch JP III: Pleuropulmonary manifestations of systemic lupus erythematosus. Rheum Dis Clin North Am 20:159–193, 1994.
4. Schwarz MI, Cherniak RM, King TE Jr: Diffuse alveolar hemorrhage and other rare infiltrative disorders. In Murray JF, Nadel JA (eds): Textbook of Respiratory Medicine, 2nd ed. Philadelphia, W.B. Saunders, 1994, pp 1889–1912.

XI. Ventilatory Disorders

49. SLEEP APNEA SYNDROMES

Lee K. Brown, M.D.

1. What is meant by a *sleep apnea syndrome*?

Sleep apnea is defined as the presence of an abnormal number of breathing cessations (apneas) or reductions in ventilation (hypopneas) during sleep. Although often used synonymously with sleep apnea, a *sleep apnea syndrome* is characterized more precisely as sleep apnea associated with nocturnal or daytime symptoms.

2. How many types of respiratory events have been described?

Three types of apneas or hypopneas are recognized:
- **Central**, typified by reduced or absent respiratory effort resulting in reduced or absent ventilation
- **Obstructive**, in which respiratory effort is maintained while ventilation decreases or disappears because of partial or total occlusion of the upper airway
- **Mixed**, which starts with one type of event (usually central) and concludes with the other. (Since it is believed that mixed and obstructive apneas are clinically the same disorder, they will not be discussed separately and both will be referred to as *obstructive sleep apnea.*)

3. How long must ventilation stop during sleep to be considered an apnea?

A widely accepted definition for apnea in adults requires ventilation to be absent for 10 seconds or longer. In children, many clinicians consider events as short as 3 seconds to be significant, especially in infants.

4. To what extent does ventilation have to be reduced to be considered hypopnea?

Hypopnea can be defined as a reduction in ventilation below a fixed percentage of baseline (70% of baseline is a common figure). However, many clinicians consider an event hypopneic only if the required reduction in ventilation is followed by significant oxyhemoglobin desaturation or evidence that the patient aroused out of sleep. This excludes events that seem to be of no pathologic consequence. In addition, a third type of obstructive phenomenon recently has been described in which ventilation does not decrease at all. The latter events, which are the hallmark of upper airway resistance syndrome, consist of repeated partial obstructions of the upper airway associated with sufficiently increased respiratory effort so that normal levels of ventilation are maintained. The increases in respiratory effort, however, are not without consequence: they can cause arousal out of sleep, resulting in many of the same symptoms that are associated with frank obstructive apneas and hypopneas.

5. How many apneas or hypopneas during sleep is considered abnormal?

There is currently no answer to this question, since only a few normative and longitudinal studies have been done. Severity of sleep disordered breathing is commonly assessed in terms of the apnea, hypopnea, and respiratory disturbance (or apnea-hypopnea) indices, calculated as the number of each event occurring per hour of actual sleep (not just time in bed). Based on currently available data, many clinicians consider a respiratory disturbance index (RDI) of more than 5 to be abnormal in adults. In children, an RDI as low as 1 may be abnormal, and several studies in the elderly have suggested that RDIs higher than 5 may occur commonly and are of uncertain significance in this age group.[8]

6. Where does the obstruction occur in obstructive sleep apnea?

The obstruction most commonly occurs in the oropharynx or hypopharynx, or both. In the oropharynx, the tongue and uvula prolapse posteriorly and invagination of lateral and posterior pharyngeal tissues occurs. Similarly in the hypopharynx, the root of the tongue and the epiglottis prolapse posteriorly. In certain rare neurologic disorders (e.g., Shy-Drager syndrome) obstruction can occur at the laryngeal level as the result of vocal cord paresis accentuated during sleep.

7. What causes the obstruction?

At least two contributing factors are thought to lead to the obstruction. First, many patients with obstructive apneas have some degree of narrowing of the upper airway from a variety of causes:

- **Obesity.** Significantly overweight individuals are more likely to have obstructive sleep apnea, and some workers have shown that collections of adipose tissue in the upper airway reduce its caliber.
- **Adenotonsillar hypertrophy.** More commonly a factor in children.
- **Macroglossia.** Most frequently attributed to hypothyroidism and myxedema.
- **Mandibular deficiency.** Micrognathia or retrognathia can result in posterior displacement of the tongue and compromise of the upper airway lumen. This may explain the tendency of obstructive sleep apnea to be inherited in some families because facial structure is largely an inherited trait. Abnormalities of the facial skeleton may also explain the high incidence of obstructive sleep apnea in acromegalics.
- **Upper airway tumors.** A rare cause of obstructive sleep apnea.

Second, the upper airway may collapse if excessive pressure is generated during inhalation; most often, this is attributed to the force necessary to overcome nasal obstruction (e.g., from allergic rhinitis or septal deviation).

Finally, an abnormality in the control of upper airway muscle tone is almost always implicated in the pathogenesis of obstruction during sleep. This situation stems from the number of roles that the upper airway must assume: it most frequently serves as a rigid conduit for airflow but at other times must become compliant to accommodate the passage of food to the esophagus or to phonate. Various muscles associated with the upper airway change its compliance depending on its function at the moment; obstructive apneas during sleep are accompanied by failure of these muscles to maintain the degree of tone necessary to keep the airway patent. It is not known why this occurs. Although obstructive sleep apnea can complicate several neurologic diseases associated with disordered ventilatory control or weakness of the upper airway dilator muscles, the majority of patients with obstructive sleep apnea have no demonstrable neurologic illness.

8. What are the symptoms of obstructive sleep apnea syndrome?

Obstructive apnea is an episode of asphyxia during sleep caused by upper airway occlusion. Progressive hypoxia, hypercapnia, and acidosis accompany each episode and progressively greater inspiratory effort must be made against an occluded upper airway, finally leading to arousal from sleep. Upper airway muscle tone is restored during the arousal, which allows effective ventilation to resume; this, in turn, allows a return to sleep. This sequence of events may occur repeatedly throughout the night, modulated to some extent by body position (events are usually worse in the supine position) and sleep state (worse during rapid eye movement [REM] sleep). The symptoms, many of which can be predicted based upon the known sequence of events, are conveniently divided into those occurring during sleep (nocturnal) and those during wakefulness (diurnal).

Nocturnal:

- **Snoring.** Almost always reported in obstructive sleep apnea. Snoring may be intermittent, occurring only in the interval between apneas (when large tidal volumes are drawn through an upper airway that is just beginning to achieve patency), or continuous if many events are hypopneas. It may also be described as resuscitative, a quality implying respiratory distress.

- **Abnormal motor activity.** The patient is essentially asphyxiating and may flail about, kick, or even sit up during respiratory events.
- **Nocturia.** Nocturnal diuresis and natriuresis are frequently associated with obstructive sleep apnea syndrome, at times leading to enuresis. The mechanism is not known but may involve atrial natriuretic factor.
- **Nocturnal acid brash.** The large negative intrapleural pressures generated during obstructed inspirations may promote gastroesophageal reflux.
- **Nocturnal awakenings.** Although each respiratory event typically is terminated by an arousal, the arousal is brief and usually the patient does not remember awakening. A few patients report awakenings, sometimes associated with air hunger or choking; rarely, obstructive sleep apnea syndrome results in insomnia.

Diurnal:

- **Excessive daytime sleepiness.** The recurrent arousals disrupt sleep architecture, with a resultant shift to lighter stages of sleep and less restorative sleep. Some studies have suggested that the severity of nocturnal hypoxemia may contribute to daytime sleepiness as well.
- **Cognitive impairment.** Difficulties with tasks involving memory or other cognitive functions may occur, and personality changes are sometimes reported. These may be largely related to the nocturnal hypoxemia.
- **Nocturnal or morning headache or nausea.** Recurrent hypercapnia from the nocturnal respiratory events may cause cerebrovascular dilatation and a "vascular" headache or related symptoms.

9. Are there physical findings typical of obstructive sleep apnea syndrome?

There are no physical findings specific to the disorder; that is, none can predict that any given patient will have the syndrome. However, the physical examination may reveal some of the following:

Obesity (common)

Enlarged uvula, which may be edematous or erythematous

"Crowded" oropharynx, which may be edematous or erythematous

Adenotonsillar enlargement (especially in children)

Retrognathia or micrognathia

Upper airway tumors (rare)

Systemic hypertension

Signs of pulmonary hypertension or cor pulmonale (usually confined to patients with daytime hypoxemia as well, i.e., those with obesity-hypoventilation (Pickwickian) syndrome or coexisting chronic obstructive lung disease.

Plethora (from secondary polycythemia)

Most obese or hypertensive patients do not have obstructive sleep apnea syndrome; further testing in these patients is warranted only if other clinical information supports the possibility of sleep apnea.

10. What laboratory studies should be performed when obstructive sleep apnea syndrome is suspected?

Arterial blood gas analysis is helpful if the question of obesity-hypoventilation (Pickwickian) syndrome is raised. A chest radiograph and an electrocardiogram should be obtained if pulmonary hypertension or cor pulmonale is suspected. A hematocrit aids in confirming a suspicion of secondary polycythemia. Although the association between hypothyroidism and obstructive sleep apnea is recognized, routine assay of thyroid-stimulating hormone has not been helpful if other clinical features of hypothyroidism are absent.

11. How is obstructive sleep apnea syndrome diagnosed?

The "reference standard" test for diagnosing obstructive sleep apnea syndrome is the overnight polysomnogram. This test is performed in a sleep laboratory with a technologist in attendance; the patient sleeps for at least 6–8 hours while the following signals are recorded on a standard or computerized polygraph:

- Electroencephalogram, submental electromyogram, electrooculogram. Sleep is divided into five different stages (I–IV and REM); these signals allow for the detection and staging of sleep.
- Respiratory effort (usually as a reflection of chest and abdominal movement) and ventilation (typically measured as airflow at the nose and mouth). These allow for the detection of apnea and hypopnea and their classification as obstructive or central. A microphone to detect snoring may also be included.
- Oxyhemoglobin saturation by pulse oximetry.
- Electrocardiogram (ECG); usually a single limb lead for assessment of cardiac rhythm.
- Body position (may be detected automatically or recorded manually by the technologist)

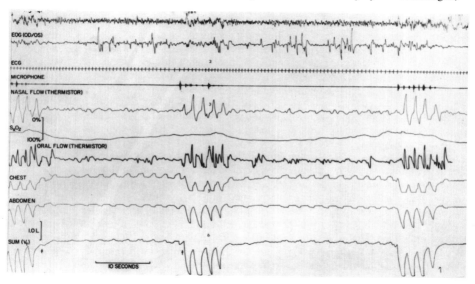

Polysomnogram showing obstructive sleep apneas. *Arrows* on the bottom tracing delineate one apnea. Note the marked reduction in nasal and oral flow (fifth and seventh tracings from the top) while respiratory effort continues (chest and abdomen recordings, second and third tracings from the bottom). Electroencephalogram (EEG) and electrooculogram (EOG) (first and second tracings) indicate REM sleep. EOG (OD/OS) = combined right and left eye oculogram; S_aO_2 = oxyhemoglobin saturation; V_t = tidal volume. (From Brown LK: Sleep apnea syndromes: Overview and diagnostic approach. Mt Sinai J Med 61:99–112, 1994; with permission.)

12. Can portable equipment record a polysomnogram in the patient's home?

Several devices are available that record some of the signals used in standard polysomnography while the patient sleeps in his or her own home. Although this technique has the advantages of reduced cost and increased comfort and convenience for the patient, it has drawbacks as well. The quality of the data recorded may be less than optimal because a technologist is not available to correct malfunctions; most systems record only a subset of the signals collected in the laboratory; therapeutic interventions cannot be made; and nocturnal events cannot be visualized directly by the technologist. Current standards of practice of the American Sleep Disorders Association limit portable recordings to the following situations:

• Patients with a high pretest probability of having obstructive sleep apnea syndrome based upon symptoms, who require an urgent diagnosis, but for whom standard polysomnography is not immediately available.
• Patients who cannot be studied in the laboratory.
• Follow-up of patients who have already been diagnosed and treated.

In addition, these standards require that the portable apparatus be capable of collecting multiple channels of cardiorespiratory information (e.g, chest or abdominal motion, airflow, pulse oximetry, heart rate). Systems that provide only pulse oximetry are specifically proscribed. Most studies have found oximetry to be relatively specific when the pretest probability of sleep apnea is high, but sensitivity varies widely depending upon what level of respiratory disturbance index is used to define the presence of the disorder. For instance, one group of investigators recorded a sensitivity for pulse oximetry alone of only 75%, when sleep apnea was defined as an RDI of more than 15, and only 60% using an RDI of more than 5.

13. What are the complications associated with obstructive sleep apnea syndrome?

Cardiac arrhythmias. Inspiratory effort against an occluded upper airway (the Müller maneuver) increases vagal tone, presumably through the mediation of baroreceptor reflexes. This results in a variety of bradyarrhythmias during the obstructive apnea itself, most commonly sinus bradycardia or sinus pauses. Various degrees of atrioventricular (AV) block also are commonly reported. Arousals from apnea are thought to be associated with sympathetic discharge and inhibition of parasympathetic tone, leading to sinus tachycardia. The combination of sinus bradycardia during apnea and sinus tachycardia in between apneas leads to cyclic variation in heart rate (CVHR); when detected serendipitously during 24-hour ambulatory ECG monitoring, this finding should prompt an inquiry into whether the patient has clinical evidence suggesting obstructive sleep apnea syndrome. However, the predictive value of CVHR is not high enough to warrant use of ambulatory ECG monitoring alone as a screening tool for apnea. The hypoxemia accompanying apneas, and possibly the sympathetic discharge at apnea termination, is thought to contribute to ventricular ectopy during sleep; ventricular arrhythmias are more common when oxyhemoglobin saturation falls below 60%. Hypoxemia may also lead to atrial tachyarrhythmias, such as atrial fibrillation or flutter or paroxysmal atrial tachycardia. The overall prevalence of cardiac arrhythmias in obstructive sleep apnea syndrome is a controversial topic. Earlier studies suggested that arrhythmias were quite common (approaching three out of four patients), whereas a recent study found no increased prevalence compared with a group without significant sleep-disordered breathing. Possibly, the earlier studies involved patients with more severe sleep apnea because patients with mild disease and fewer symptoms frequently went unrecognized at the time these studies were performed.

Systemic hypertension. Hypertension is often seen in patients with obstructive sleep apnea syndrome, but whether this is a confounding effect of the obesity and advanced age common to both groups or the result of a causal relationship has been controversial. A recent cross-sectional study made allowances for these confounding factors and still demonstrated a significant association, including a dose-response effect. Obstructive apneas are frequently associated with transient elevations of systemic blood pressure; among the mechanisms implicated are hypoxemia and increased sympathetic tone. The factors involved in converting this transient phenomenon in sleep to sustained diurnal hypertension are not known.

Myocardial infarction. Several studies have shown an association between myocardial infarction and obstructive sleep apnea, although causality has not necessarily been established. Sleep apnea may predispose the patient to myocardial infarction, or myocardial infarction may increase the likelihood of sleep-disordered breathing by leading to Cheyne-Stokes respiration. If obstructive sleep apnea does cause a predisposition to myocardial infarction, pathogenesis may involve the increased prevalence of hypertension in sleep apnea, recurrent hypoxemia during sleep, or other factors.

Stroke. Snoring and other clinical symptoms of obstructive sleep apnea have been associated with increased risk of stroke in several studies. This may also be an effect of systemic hypertension, although some investigators have demonstrated reduced cerebral blood flow during obstructive apneas.

Obesity-hypoventilation (pickwickian) syndrome. A small percentage of morbidly obese patients with obstructive sleep apnea syndrome hypoventilate during wakefulness; this disorder is obesity-hypoventilation, or Pickwickian syndrome. Although the pathogenesis of this syndrome is not known, intriguing evidence suggests that obstructive sleep apnea syndrome may be an important factor in some of these patients: in one study, eight patients with both disorders were identified, and awake hypoventilation resolved in four after effective therapy for sleep apnea was instituted.

Pulmonary hypertension and cor pulmonale. Pulmonary arterial pressure commonly is elevated transiently toward the end of an obstructive apnea and peaks shortly after the event terminates. This phenomenon is attributed largely to hypoxic pulmonary vasoconstriction and does not seem to lead to fixed, diurnal pulmonary hypertension or cor pulmonale unless awake hypoxia is also present. Thus, sleep apnea patients with pulmonary hypertension and right heart failure generally have coexistent COPD or obesity-hypoventilation syndrome.

Increased mortality. Given the known associations between obstructive sleep apnea syndrome and cardiovascular disease and stroke, it is not surprising that increased mortality has been demonstrated in this disorder. One study suggested that patients with an apnea index of more than 20 were at greater risk of death, and this value has been widely used as the criterion for mandatory treatment. Most studies have emphasized the predominantly cardiovascular origin of mortality, although increasing evidence suggests that vehicular accidents caused by hypersomnolence from the disorder may play an important role.

Some of the cardiac, vascular, and pulmonary complications thought to be associated with the obstructive sleep apnea syndrome and some presumed mechanisms are outlined in the figure on the following page.

14. When should a patient with obstructive sleep apnea syndrome be treated?

Both severity of disease (as assessed during polysomnography) and presence of daytime or nocturnal symptoms should be considered. Because mortality is increased in patients with an apnea index of more than 20, most clinicians treat patients in this group regardless of symptoms. In addition, because the difference between hypopnea and apnea may not be important in terms of physiologic effects, many clinicians extrapolate these mortality data to include any patient with a respiratory disturbance index of more than 20 in the "must treat" group. Patients with milder degrees of sleep-disordered breathing (respiratory disturbance index of 5–20) are generally treated if they have significant symptoms (e.g., daytime sleepiness, recurrent nocturnal awakenings).

15. What is the treatment of choice for obstructive sleep apnea syndrome?

Currently, nasal continuous positive airway pressure (C-PAP) represents the best treatment modality for most patients. It is applied via a nasal mask with a soft plastic cushion to provide an airtight seal and held in place by headgear that has velcro straps fastened around the back of the head. "Nasal pillows" may be used instead; these are soft plastic cushions inserted into the nares and also held in place by headgear with straps. A swivel connection and suitably long tubing connect the patient interface to a blower unit, so that the patient is free to move about in bed and change position at will. The blower unit incorporates either a pressure valve or other pressure regulatory apparatus so as to maintain a relatively constant system pressure regardless of the phase of respiration at any given time.

Several theories have been advanced and later discarded concerning the mechanism by which nasal C-PAP abolishes obstructive respiratory events. Current evidence supports the "pneumatic splint" theory, which holds that the positive pressure maintained in the upper airway by the C-PAP apparatus physically holds the airway open despite insufficient dilator muscle tone. Abundant evidence supports the efficacy of nasal C-PAP, including numerous studies showing resolution or improvement of daytime sleepiness, neuropsychologic deficits, cardiac arrhythmias during sleep, daytime hypoventilation in some patients, and cor pulmonale.

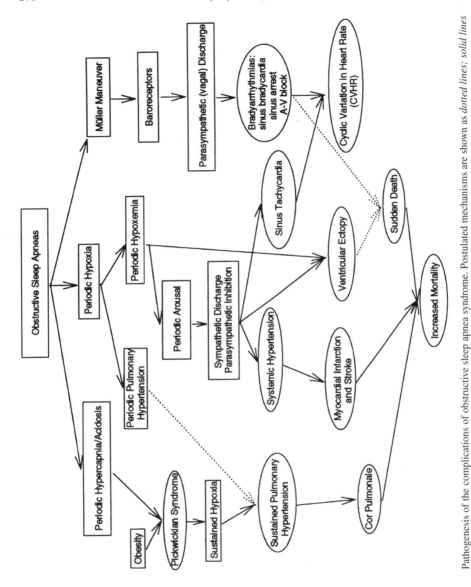

Pathogenesis of the complications of obstructive sleep apnea syndrome. Postulated mechanisms are shown as *dotted lines; solid lines* indicate mechanisms for which supporting data exist. A-V = atrioventricular

16. How is treatment with nasal C-PAP initiated?

Nasal C-PAP is initiated by a **titration** study, which has three purposes:

1. Determine the best interface (nasal mask, nasal pillows, need for chin strap or oronasal mask).

2. Determine the best C-PAP pressure (as evidenced by maximal elimination of apnea, hypopnea, snoring, and arousals) and verify efficacy during REM sleep and in the supine position.

3. Educate patient about the device.

Conventionally, C-PAP is titrated during a second night of polysomnography, after the first night has confirmed the diagnosis. Financial pressures from payors have largely driven the practice of "split-night" polysomnograms, in which an abbreviated diagnostic study during the first part of the night is followed by an abbreviated C-PAP titration, thus combining two assessments into one. One recent study suggested that adequate therapeutic data could be obtained from split-night studies when sleep apnea was moderate to severe (respiratory disturbance index more than 20), although this conclusion was at variance with results reported from earlier studies. Ample time is necessary to determine both the optimal C-PAP pressure and the most comfortable interface (type and size of mask or nasal pillows), and the split-night protocol may not always allow for this. In addition, the accuracy of the diagnostic phase may be questioned. It is likely that split-night protocols underestimate the severity of sleep apnea because the respiratory disturbance typically worsens during REM sleep, a stage that occurs more commonly toward the end of a night's sleep when the titration has already commenced.

17. Will patients really wear this apparatus and use it regularly?

Compliance with nasal C-PAP therapy varies depending upon how it is measured. Compliance can be evaluated by use of a patient questionnaire, by electrically timing how long the device is on each night, or by electronically recording how long the patient is actually breathing through it each night. Each method yields a progressively lower estimate of compliance. A recent, frequently quoted study indicated that patients reported an average of 6 hours of C-PAP use each night, and 60% said they used it every night. An electronic recorder indicated they actually used it an average of 5 hours each night. Usage patterns varied widely, with just under 50% of the patients using the device 4 or more hours a night for 70% or more of the nights. Usage did not decline significantly over the course of the 3-month study.

18. What factors affect nasal C-PAP compliance? What can be done about them?

C-PAP User Complaints*

COMPLAINT	SOLUTION
Claustrophobia	Try different interface (e.g., nasal pillows)
	Allow patient to become habituated to mask during the day
Discomfort from interface, including pain, air leaks, or contact allergy	Try different brands of mask, mask material, or different interface (e.g., nasal pillows)
	Change headgear or mask spacer size
	Custom-made mask
Nasal irritation; sneezing, rhinorrhea, epistaxis	Humidification
	Topical intranasal steroids
	Topical intranasal disodium cromoglycate
	Antihistamines (nonsedating types)
Nasal irritation: obstruction	See above; plus:
	Topical nasal decongestants
	Oral decongestants (e.g., pseudoephedrine)
	Antihistamines (nonsedating types)
Discomfort from air flow or pressure	Use ramp setting
	Convert to bilevel positive airway pressure
	Consider use of an "adaptive" C-PAP device[†]
Leakage from mouth	Chin strap
	Oronasal mask

* Various studies have reported the complaints listed, all of which presumably affect compliance.

† These devices are designed to adjust the C-PAP level periodically, maintaining just enough pressure to prevent respiratory events. They may result in lower average C-PAP levels and therefore may be better tolerated. Only limited data are available.

19. What role does surgery play in treatment of sleep apnea?

The most common surgical technique for treating sleep apnea is uvulopalatopharyngoplasty (UPPP), which involves resection of redundant lateral pharyngeal tissue, the margin of the soft palate, the palatine tonsils, and the uvula. This procedure increases the caliber of the oropharynx and may also reduce its compliance so that it is less likely to collapse. The success rate of UPPP depends upon how success is defined. Almost all patients report that snoring is reduced or eliminated and respiratory disturbance index declines. However, only 40–60% of patients have a reduction in respiratory disturbance index of 50% or more, and as few as 25% of patients record a fall in this index to below 20. UPPP failures are related to the persistence of obstruction in the hypopharynx, an area not treated by this procedure. Although numerous attempts have been made to identify a preoperative strategy capable of distinguishing hypopharyngeal from oropharyngeal obstruction, thus far no practical techniques are available. An additional hazard of treatment failure after UPPP relates to the fact that snoring may be alleviated while at the same time a serious degree of sleep apnea remains; thus, repeat polysomnography is mandatory following UPPP.

A few patients may develop velopharyngeal incompetence after UPPP, with symptoms of nasal reflux when swallowing liquids or change in voice quality (rhinolalia aperta). These complications often resolve spontaneously with the passage of time. The usual risks attendant to any surgery must also be considered (infection, bleeding) as must the particular risk of anesthesia and analgesia in the patient with sleep-disordered breathing. Careful monitoring is essential postoperatively, as some patients may develop worsening sleep apnea because of oropharyngeal edema; short-term use of nasal C-PAP is a consideration is such a patient.

For clinically important nasal obstruction refractory to medical treatment, consideration should also be given to nasal reconstructive surgery. This may be necessary in any case if C-PAP cannot be properly administered because of nasal obstruction.

More aggressive procedures are available if UPPP fails and the patient still cannot use nasal C-PAP. These are designed to address hypopharyngeal obstruction, and range from techniques that put anterior tension on the base of the tongue to prevent posterior displacement during sleep (anterior sagittal mandibular osteotomy with genioglossus-hyoid advancement) to procedures that also increase the size of the bony skeleton enclosing the tongue (maxillary and mandibular osteotomies with advancement). Midline glossectomy or lingualplasty have also been used in some centers, although the role of lingual surgery remains controversial.

20. What should I tell patients who ask about laser surgery for snoring and sleep apnea?

Laser surgery for sleep apnea usually consists of a staged uvulopalatoplasty, in which the carbon dioxide laser vaporizes the uvula and part of the soft palate over the course of several sessions. A single-session technique has also been described. Laser surgery usually relieves snoring by removing the vibrating tissues of the uvula and soft palate, but has not proved to be more effective for obstructive sleep apnea syndrome than conventional UPPP. In addition, laser surgery as usually described does not include the excision of lateral pharyngeal tissues (a component of conventional UPPP) and may therefore be less effective than the conventional technique. Laser surgery is said to be better tolerated by patients and more suitable for the outpatient setting. However, until more data are available, laser uvulopalatoplasty for treatment of sleep apnea is discouraged. If it is performed for sleep apnea, postoperative polysomnography is mandatory. Furthermore, patients who undergo laser surgery for snoring must be adequately screened preoperatively for the presence of sleep apnea.

21. What other treatments are available?

- **Weight loss.** Several studies have documented the salutary effect of weight loss in obese patients with sleep apnea. Adequate weight loss is often difficult to achieve and should not be the only modality employed, especially in severe disease. In patients with morbid obesity, bariatric surgery (e.g., gastric stapling) may be indicated.
- **Sleep position training.** Certain individuals have sleep-disordered breathing almost exclusively in the supine position. Such patients can sometimes be trained to remain in the lateral decubitus position by insertion of tennis balls into a pocket sewn into the top back of their nightwear.

- **Protriptyline or (possibly) fluoxetine.** Nonsedating antidepressant agents may be beneficial by suppressing REM sleep, the stage typically associated with the most severe apnea. Some data suggest that these agents also may increase upper airway muscle tone. Antidepressants should be considered for adjunctive use at best and reserved for only mild disease.
- **Oxygen.** Oxygen should usually be avoided as a single agent, because it frequently prolongs episodes of apnea by delaying hypoxemia-induced arousal. Oxygen may be used in combination with other modalities if hypoxemia remains despite suppression of discrete respiratory events.
- **Oral appliances.** Several devices are available that advance the mandible, hold the tongue anteriorally, or lift the palate. The mandibular advancement and tongue-retaining devices all have demonstrated efficacy, but the former are usually better tolerated. About 60% of patients achieve a respiratory disturbance index of less than 20 when wearing these appliances, which may represent a useful alternative for some patients.

22. How should I advise my patients with sleep apnea about driving and using heavy machinery?

Obstructive sleep apnea syndrome is a cause of hypersomnolence, and sleepy individuals who drive may be less vigilant or even fall asleep while driving. One recent study showed a sevenfold increase in the rate of automobile accidents with obstructive sleep apnea syndrome (respiratory disturbance index more than 5) compared with a normal control group. Laws concerning the reporting of impaired drivers to licensing authorities vary from state to state, and physicians who treat patients with sleep apnea should be familiar with local regulations and follow any reporting requirements. If no statutory duty exists, the physician is at the very least obligated in terms of good medical practice to warn such patients to refrain from driving or operating heavy machinery until their disorder is properly diagnosed and treated.

23. What causes central sleep apnea syndrome?

The term *central sleep apnea syndrome* is a misnomer because there is not one such disorder, but rather a group of disorders that all manifest as central apneas during sleep. The first major distinction involves separation of hypercapnic from eucapnic or hypocapnic central sleep apnea.

Hypercapnic central sleep apnea. Patients have alveolar hypoventilation caused by either defective central ventilatory control or respiratory muscle weakness. Disorders that affect brain stem respiratory centers include infarcts, encephalitis (including poliomyelitis), degenerative diseases, demyelinating diseases, congenital abnormalities, and iatrogenic injury (e.g, after cervical cordotomy). Many disorders can impair respiratory muscle strength, including primary muscle diseases (commonly, muscular dystrophies), diseases of the neuromuscular junction, neuropathies, motor neuron diseases, and spinal cord disorders.

Eucapnic or hypocapnic central sleep apnea. These syndromes are most often related to Cheyne-Stokes respiration, the waxing and waning respiratory pattern associated with congestive heart failure and stroke. Periodic breathing of high altitude is another Cheyne-Stokes ventilatory instability induced by hypoxemia. Central sleep apnea without the Cheyne-Stokes pattern may also occur in all of these disorders.

Additionally, central sleep apnea without the Cheyne-Stokes pattern may be seen in those with no known heart or central nervous system disease; an abnormality of medullary respiratory control is implicated, but the cause is not known. Some of these patients have upper airway obstruction coincident with the loss of respiratory effort, and reflex inhibition of ventilatory drive caused by the airway occlusion has been suggested as a possible mechanism. These patients often respond to nasal C-PAP treatment.

24. What are the symptoms and signs of the central sleep apnea syndromes?

The symptoms and signs depend on whether the syndrome is hypercapnic or eucapnic/ hypocapnic. Patients with hypercapnic central sleep apnea frequently snore and complain of daytime sleepiness, nocturnal or morning headache, and restless sleep. They are often hypoxemic during wakefulness and thus subject to developing pulmonary hypertension, cor pulmonale, and polycythemia. Eucapnic or hypocapnic central sleep apnea commonly results in complaints of insomnia and nocturnal choking or dyspnea; these patients may also experience daytime somnolence but rarely develop cor pulmonale.[1]

25. What treatments are available for the hypercapnic central sleep apnea syndromes?

In addition to effective treatment of the primary disease, hypercapnic central sleep apnea is most often managed with ventilatory support modalities. These are commonly noninvasive; i.e., they do not require tracheotomy or endotracheal intubation. Available techniques include positive pressure ventilation through a nasal or oronasal mask or negative-pressure ventilation administered through a cuirasse ("shell"), body wrap, or poncho. Nasal bilevel positive airway pressure is rapidly becoming the most common technique because of the availability of nasal masks (the same as used for C-PAP) and pressure-generating equipment. This equipment supplies higher pressure during inspiration than expiration; the expiratory pressure helps maintain upper airway patency, analogous to C-PAP, whereas the higher inspiratory pressure augments or generates tidal volume. In treatment of central sleep apnea, a timed mode is used that enables the apparatus to switch to its inspiratory pressure if no inspiratory effort is detected after a given length of time.

Other available treatments include diaphragmatic pacing and pharmacologic approaches. Commercially available systems for stimulating the phrenic nerves are available but have limited usefulness because they require intact phrenic nerve and neuromuscular junction and normal diaphragmatic function. Pharmacologic approaches include ventilatory stimulants such as progesterone or acetazolamide, REM-sleep suppressants such as the tricyclic antidepressants, or oxygen. Respiratory stimulants have limited utility in alveolar hypoventilation of central origin. Suppression of REM sleep may be of marginal benefit in patients whose sleep-disordered breathing occurs almost exclusively in REM. Oxygen must be used with care because it may potentiate hypercapnia.

26. Is the eucapnic /hypocapnic central sleep apnea syndrome treated differently?

Congestive heart failure, if present, should be treated aggressively since most central sleep apnea (especially of the Cheyne-Stokes type) is caused by this disorder. Nocturnal oxygen therapy has been useful, especially in congestive heart failure, but may also be tried when hemispheric stroke is implicated. Nasal C-PAP can be beneficial; mechanisms may include increasing P_{CO_2} or P_{O_2}, thus improving controller linearity, or relieving upper airway obstruction and thus any reflex inhibition of respiratory drive. Periodic breathing of high altitude usually resolves with time, or immediately upon returning to lower elevations; of course, supplemental oxygen can also be useful at high altitude.

BIBLIOGRAPHY

1. Bradley TD, McNichols WT, Rutherford R, et al: Clinical and physiologic heterogeneity of the central sleep apnea syndrome. Am Rev Respir Dis 134:217–221, 1986.
2. Bradley TD, Phillipson EA: Central sleep apnea. Clin Chest Med 13:493–505, 1992.
3. Brown LK: Sleep apnea syndromes: Overview and diagnostic approach. Mt Sinai J Med 61:99–112, 1994.
4. Brown LK: Sleep-disordered breathing in neurologic disease. Clin Pulm Med 3:22–35, 1996.
5. Cooper BG, Veale D, Griffiths CJ, et al: Value of nocturnal oxygen saturation as a screening test for sleep apnoea. Thorax 46:586–588, 1991.
6. Findley LJ, Unverzagt ME, Suratt PM: Automobile accidents involving patients with obstructive sleep apnea. Am Rev Respir Dis 138:337–340, 1988.
7. Flemons WW, Remmers JE, Gillis AM: Sleep apnea and cardiac arrhythmias. Is there a relationship? Am Rev Respir Dis 148:618–621, 1993.
8. Guilleminault C: Sleep and breathing. In Guilleminault C (ed): Sleeping and Waking Disorders: Indications and Techniques. Menlo Park, Addison-Wesley, 1982.
9. Guilleminault C, Stoohs R, Clerk A, et al: A cause of excessive daytime sleepiness. The upper airway resistance syndrome. Chest 104:781–787, 1993.
10. He J, Kryger MH, Zorick FJ, et al: Mortality and apnea index in obstructive sleep apnea. Experience in 385 male patients. Chest 94:9–14, 1988.

11. Hla KM, Young TB, Bidwell T, et al: Sleep apnea and hypertension. A population-based study. Ann Intern Med 120:382–388, 1994.
12. Jamieson AO: Split-night studies: A new standard? Forcing the examination of outcome. Sleep 14:381–382, 1991.
13. Keenan SA: Polysomnography: Technical aspects in adolescents and adults. J Clin Neurophysiol 9:21–31, 1992.
14. Klitzman D, Miller A: Obstructive sleep apnea syndrome: Complications and sequelae. Mt Sinai J Med 61:113–121, 1994.
15. Kribbs NB, Pack AI, Kline LR, et al: Objective measurement of patterns of nasal CPAP use by patients with obstructive sleep apnea. Am Rev Respir Dis 147:887–895, 1993.
16. Lin C-C, Tsan K-W, Chen P-J: The relationship between sleep apnea syndrome and hypothyroidism. Chest 102:1663–1667, 1992.
17. Maisel RH, Antonelli PJ, Iber C, et al: Uvulopalatopharyngoplasty for obstructive sleep apnea: A community's experience. Laryngoscope 102:604–607, 1992.
18. Rapoport DM: Treatment of sleep apnea syndromes. Mt Sinai J Med 61:123–130, 1994.
19. Rapoport DM, Garay SM, Epstein H, et al: Hypercapnia in the obstructive sleep apnea syndrome. A reevaluation of the "Pickwickian syndrome." Chest 89:627–635, 1986.
20. Schmidt-Nowara W, Lowe A, Wiegand L, et al: Oral appliances for the treatment of snoring and obstructive sleep apnea: A review. Sleep 18:501–510, 1995.
21. Shepard JW Jr, Garrison MW, Grither DA, et al: Relationship of ventricular ectopy to oxyhemoglobin desaturation in patients with obstructive sleep apnea. Chest 88:335–340, 1985.
22. Shephard JW Jr, Olsen KD: Uvulopalatopharyngoplasty for treatment of obstructive sleep apnea. Mayo Clin Proc 65:1260–1267, 1990.
23. Standards of Practice Committee of the American Sleep Disorders Association: Practice parameters for the use of laser-assisted uvulopalatoplasty. Sleep 17:744–748, 1994.
24. Standards of Practice Committee of the American Sleep Disorders Association: Practice parameters for the use of portable recording in the assessment of obstructive sleep apnea. Sleep 17:372–377, 1994.
25. Stoohs RA, Guilleminault C, Itoi A, et al: Traffic accidents in commercial long-haul truck drivers: The influence of sleep-disordered breathing and obesity. Sleep 17:619–623, 1994.
26. Strollo PJ Jr, Rogers RM: Obstructive sleep apnea. N Engl J Med 334:99–104 1996.
27. Yamashiro Y, Kryger MH: CPAP titration for sleep apnea using a split-night protocol. Chest 107:62–66, 1995.

50. ALVEOLAR HYPOVENTILATION

Thomas R. Vendegna, M.D., and Robert D. Ballard, M.D.

1. What is the definition of alveolar hypoventilation?

Alveolar hypoventilation is defined by an arterial Pco_2 greater than 45 mmHg and arises either when the respiratory system does not respond to the demand for ventilatory work or when the demand for ventilatory work exceeds respiratory capability. The former condition exists with decreased central ventilatory drive or respiratory muscle weakness, whereas the latter occurs with obstructive airway disease or parenchymal lung diseases. Therefore, hypoventilation can be subdivided into three broad categories: decreased central ventilatory drive, chest wall and neuromuscular disorders, and airway or parenchymal disease.

2. List the causes of alveolar hypoventilation.

Impaired Central Ventilatory Drive
Obesity-hypoventilation syndrome
Myxedema
Drugs
Structural (CVA, tumors, hemorrhage)
Idiopathic

Neuromuscular and Chest Wall Disorders
Central Nervous System
  Poliomyelitis
  Amyotrophic lateral sclerosis
  Syringomyelia
  Multiple sclerosis
  Cervical cord injury
Peripheral Nervous System
  Polyneuropathy (Guillain-Barré)
  Phrenic nerve injury
Motor-End Plate
  Myasthenia gravis
  Eaton-Lambert syndrome
  Botulism
Myopathy
  Muscular dystrophy
  Myopathy (inflammatory, metabolic, or hereditary)
Chest Wall Disorders
  Kyphoscoliosis
  Thoracoplasty
Airways/Parenchymal Disease
Upper Airway Obstruction
  Obstructive sleep apnea (not always a distinct entity, see obesity-hypoventilation)
  Tracheal stenosis
  Tonsillar hypertrophy
COPD
Cystic Fibrosis
Bronchietasis
Congestive Heart Failure
Interstitial Lung Disease

3. **How is the work-up of hypoventilation approached?**
Every good work-up begins with a **careful history** and **physical examination** focusing on the differential diagnosis. Because many forms of hypoventilation are initially asymptomatic and manifested only during sleep, detailed questioning of patients and family members about sleep patterns, snoring, daytime somnolence, fatigue, irritability, impotence, decreased mentation, and poor performance at work or school can be highly informative.

Laboratory tests include arterial blood gas analysis, hematocrit (looking for secondary erythrocytosis), and levels of electrolytes, magnesium, phosphate, and thyroid-stimulating hormone.

Pulmonary function tests can be helpful in diagnosing chest wall, neuromuscular disorders, and airway or parenchymal disease. In patients with obstructive lung disease, an FEV_1 of more than 1.0 liter suggests that a process other than the underlying airway disease is causing the hypercapnia. Likewise, in chest wall disorders kyphoscoliosis must be severe in association with a FVC of less than 1.0 liter to initiate hypercapnia. If the diagnosis remains unclear at this point, a nocturnal sleep study may be useful. Finally, voluntary hyperventilation with measurement of arterial Pco_2 may distinguish between those who cannot breathe and those who will not breathe.

Can't breathe	**Won't breathe**
Chest wall disorders	Impaired central ventilatory drive
Neuromuscular diseases	
Airways/parenchymal disease	

4. Why do we treat hypoventilation?

Hypoventilation and the associated hypoxia lead to progressive pulmonary hypertension. Pulmonary hypertension will lead to right heart strain and eventually failure. This will predispose the patient to edema and lethal arrhythmias. The hypoxia may also bring forth underlying atherosclerotic disease and increase the incidence of myocardial infarctions. Finally, hypoxia induces a secondary erythrocytosis that can create a hyperviscosity syndrome if the hematocrit exceeds 55%. Thus hypoventilation may lead to morbidity and mortality by many different avenues.

5. What defines the central respiratory control system?

In order to properly understand central hypoventilation, it is necessary to review the central respiratory control center. Breathing is regulated by three control systems within the central nervous system: behavioral, metabolic, and neural. The behavioral system originates in the forebrain and has motor outputs descending to the medullary pattern generator and through the corticospinal tracts to the respiratory lower motor neurons of the cervical cord. This system is under voluntary control and respiratory patterns are influenced by nonrespiratory variables such as emotion, phonation, and swallowing.

The metabolic system originates from the medullary pattern generator and output descends along the ventrolateral spinal tracts to the cervical cord. This system receives input from the peripheral and central chemoreceptors concerning arterial P_{O_2}, P_{CO_2}, and pH, and from the vagus nerves regarding mechanical events within the lungs.

Finally, breathing is influenced by a neural waking drive. The pathway of this system has yet to be fully described but probably involves the reticular activating system. Thus, during waking hours the respiratory system has a nonspecific excitation that enhances overall central output. During sleep, the waking drive is eliminated as is the behavioral system, leaving respiratory control critically dependent on the metabolic system.

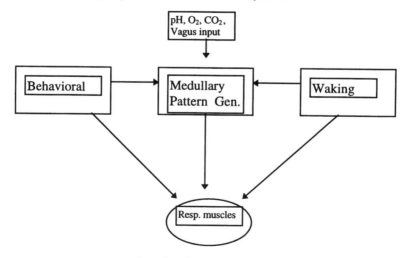

Central respiratory control systems.

6. In addition to sole dependence on the metabolic system, what other changes occur during sleep that alter respiration and predispose one to hypoventilation?

During sleep the reduced input from the waking and behavioral centers results in reduced tidal volume and increased upper airway resistance (secondary to decreased upper airway muscular activity). This results in a hypoventilatory state. Hypoventilation is allowed because the metabolic center during sleep shifts its ventilatory hypercapnic response curve to the right, resulting in a P_{CO_2} that is 2–4 mmHg higher than that in the awake state. These effects are most pronounced during rapid eye movement (REM) sleep when activity in both upper airway dilator muscles and chest wall respiratory muscles is eliminated and breathing becomes dependent on the diaphragm. Thus, during REM sleep individuals are predisposed to hypoventilation because upper airway tone is decreased, creating obstruction and increased ventilatory work. This occurs at a time when the respiratory system is dependent solely upon the diaphragm to meet these increased ventilatory demands.

7. How do central respiratory control and its alterations during sleep relate to disease states?

Autonomic dysfunction that occurs in diabetes mellitus or in Shy-Drager syndrome can lead to hypoventilation because the metabolic system utilizes autonomic neurons within its loop. These patients have normal behavioral and waking inputs but have difficulty during sleep when the system is metabolically dependent. Because patients are initially asymptomatic, disease is undetected unless an overnight sleep study reveals irregular breathing patterns and central sleep apnea.

Certain pharmacologic agents (e.g., opiates and sedatives or hypnotics) and disease states (e.g, encephalitis, meningitis, poliomyelitis, infarcts, and hemorrhages) can lead to central sleep apnea and hypoventilation secondary to alterations of input potentially from all three central respiratory systems. The incidence of poliomyelitis is currently low because of widespread vaccination. However, 25% of patients who once had polio can develop a postpolio syndrome 30–40 years later that involves peripheral nerves and results in muscle weakness, musculoskeletal pain, and dysphagia. Many such patients have been documented to have sleep apnea and hypoventilation that is most pronounced during sleep.

8. How does hypothyroidism cause hypoventilation?

Although the mechanism is not completely understood, hypothyroidism is a known cause of central hypoventilation. In 1961, Wilson and Bedell described the pulmonary function of patients with myxedema, noting that most subjects had hypercapnia and hypoxia that improved with thyroid supplementation therapy.[13] These authors also described a reduced hypercapnic ventilatory response, which also improved with therapy. Zwillich and colleagues subsequently reported a reduced hypoxic drive in patients with either myxedema or hypothyroidism, but only the patients with myxedema had a reduced hypercapnic drive as well.[14] After 3 weeks of thyroid supplementation therapy only the hypoxic drive was improved. Thus, it appears that hypothyroidism interferes with the central metabolic regulation of respiration. Hypothyroidism also can cause respiratory muscle weakness, as evidenced by reduced inspiratory and expiratory effort, which may also contribute to hypoventilation.

9. What is the pickwickian syndrome?

The pickwickian syndrome, or obesity hypoventilation syndrome, was first described by Burwell and associates in 1956 and named for a character in Charles Dickens' *Pickwick Papers*. As described by Burwell and colleagues, the syndrome is characterized by marked obesity, somnolence, cyanosis, periodic breathing, secondary erythrocytosis, and right ventricular heart failure.

Morbid obesity decreases total lung capacity, functional residual capacity, and tidal volume because of increased adipose tissue on the chest wall and elevation of the diaphragm caused by increased intraabdominal adipose tissue. The reduced lung volumes lead to atelectasis, which alters ventilation-perfusion matching and causes hypoxia. Most patients also have obstructive sleep apnea, which further increases ventilatory demand in a system predisposed to hypoventilation. Finally, hypoxic and hypercapnic metabolic central control centers are altered in most patients. Even though the mechanism is still unclear, it is easy to conceptualize that these patients with reduced lung volumes, atelectasis, hypoxia, upper airway obstruction, and altered metabolic central control can develop hypoventilation, especially during sleep.

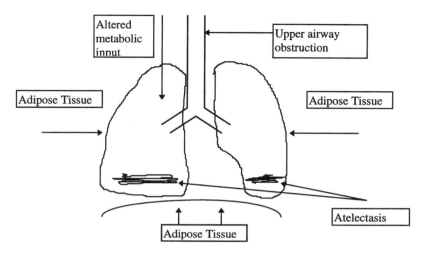

Pathologic factors involved in pickwickian syndrome.

10. How is central hypoventilation treated?

The first approach to treatment is the investigation of reversible underlying causes, such as space occupying lesions, central nervous system infections, thyroid disease, and the use of sedating agents. Once reversible causes are addressed, patients may be offered many noninvasive and, in more difficult cases, invasive methods of treatment. Obese patients should undergo aggressive weight reduction. Supplemental oxygen is effective in attenuating hypoxia induced by hypoventilation but may decrease hypoxic ventilatory drive and alter dead space within the lungs, further enhancing hypercapnia. Consequently, oxygen should be administered and titrated in a monitored setting both in the awake and sleep state.

Respiratory stimulants, such as theophylline and acetazolamide, augment ventilatory drive, but their effectiveness in long-term settings is poor. Medroxyprogesterone has been shown to increase central ventilatory drive, and some patients demonstrate prolonged benefits from this agent. Unfortunately it is difficult to predict who will respond, and many patients develop side effects, such as impotence.

An alternative mode of therapy is ventilatory assist devices. Negative-pressure assist ventilation, similar to the iron lung used to treat polio patients, has a predisposition to create or worsen upper airway obstruction secondary to the negative inspiratory pressure that is not typically coordinated with upper airway dilator activity. Positive-pressure ventilation (bilevel positive airway pressure) administered with a tight-fitting nasal mask during sleep can be effective in reversing both nocturnal and daytime hypercapnia as well as hypoxia. Unfortunately, compliance is a major issue in treatment success.

Other treatment options include diaphragmatic pacing and tracheostomy with a ventilatory assist device. Both of these strategies are invasive and are used only when noninvasive treatment fails. Diaphragmatic pacing is ineffective in many patients with neuromuscular and chest wall disorders. In addition, because it creates negative inspiratory pressure that is typically not coordinated with upper airway dilator activity, when used alone it may increase upper airway obstruction.

11. Why does chest wall disease sometimes lead to hypoventilation? Which patients are susceptible?

Chest wall diseases, such as kyphoscoliosis, distort the respiratory musculature. This is demonstrated by the lower inspiratory and expiratory pressures that these patients generate. The decreased muscular strength is also manifested by reduced lung volumes. When lung volumes decrease, atelectasis can occur, altering $\dot{V}/\dot{Q}$ matching and creating hypoxia. Thus, patients with chest wall disorders have reduced lung volumes and poor muscular function leading to poor ventilation. The chest wall disorder must be severe, with the angle of spinal deformity exceeding 100° and the vital capacity below 35% of predicted. In neuromuscular disorders, the muscular strength should be less than 30% of predicted and vital capacity below 55% predicted, or other disorders should be suspected as contributing to hypercapnia.

12. What is the treatment for hypoventilation in neuromuscular diseases and chest wall disorders?

Because these patients have more severe hypercapnia during sleep secondary to decreased behavioral and waking inputs, much of the focus has been on nocturnal therapy. Oxygen alone often results in unacceptably high levels of Pco_2, sometimes exceeding 95 mmHg. Although no randomized trial has confirmed that treatment prevents premature death, it is widely accepted that assisted ventilation decreases Pco_2, improves oxygen, and may prevent pulmonary hypertension. Negative-pressure ventilation may predispose patients to upper airway collapse. Thus, positive-pressure devices (bilevel positive airway pressure) are more widely accepted and may be more comfortable for the patient. In severe cases home ventilation through a tracheostomy can be instituted.

13. Why does nocturnal ventilation often improve daytime hypercapnia in chest wall disorders?

It has been speculated that nocturnal ventilation rests chronically fatigued respiratory muscles, thereby making them more effective during the day. Alternatively, improvement of nocturnal hypoxia may improve respiratory muscle endurance. Improvement of hypercapnia may lower the body's bicarbonate pool, which in turn may reset chemosensors and improve metabolic respiratory input. Thus, many theories exist but are not well supported by clinical trials.

14. How does obstructive sleep apnea cause hypercapnia?

Obstructive sleep apnea and its treatment are discussed at length in chapter 49, but approximately 5–10% of sleep apnea patients develop daytime hypercapnia. During sleep, in particularly REM sleep, postural respiratory muscle activity is reduced, making the respiratory system more dependent on the diaphragm. A decrease in upper airway muscle tone accompanies the loss of postural muscle groups. This loss in tone predisposes patients with enlarged soft tissues to upper airway collapse and obstruction. Such upper airway obstruction, at a time when the patient has little respiratory reserve (diaphragm only), potentiates a reduction in ventilation.

Patients may retain carbon dioxide, but in most this occurs only during sleep. However, in some patients the threshold for carbon dioxide response is raised and the patient's metabolic center allows hypercapnia. Although the mechanism for this is unclear, obesity and its subsequent effects may be necessary for hypercapnia to occur in the setting of obstructive sleep apnea. Thus, patients with obstructive apnea and daytime hypercapnia have obesity-hypoventilation syndrome.

15. Why do some patients with COPD develop hypercapnia?

Hypoxia and hypercapnia initially develop in patients with COPD during sleep and ultimately progress to become daytime alterations. During sleep, patients with COPD, as well as normal individuals, have a generalized decrease in respiratory input. The resultant decrease in accessory inspiratory muscle activity (observed most markedly during REM sleep), upon which many patients depend during wakefulness, leaves sleeping patients dependent solely upon the diaphragm, which may also be dysfunctional because of hyperinflation-induced distortion. Consequently, tidal volume is reduced and the amount of functional lung receiving adequate ventilation declines, creating dead space. Hypoventilation and increased dead space result in hypercapnia. As the disease progresses, dead space increases as a result of increasing tissue destruction. Despite accessory muscle use, the patient ultimately cannot meet ventilatory demands, and daytime hypercapnia ensues. Evidence exists that hereditary factors related to ventilatory control play a role in in determining who develops hypoventilation at a given level of disease, but these factors remain poorly understood.

16. Should a sleep study be done for all patients with COPD?

Connaughton and associates demonstrated that nocturnal measurements of hypercapnia and hypoxia were no more predictive of survival than awake measurements. Daytime hypoxia and hypercapnia have a poor prognosis and nocturnal measurements do not provide additional prognostic data unless obstructive sleep apnea is also suspected. However, when COPD patients require supplemental oxygen during wakefulness, many physicians advocate the increase of their nocturnal oxygen flow rate by approximately 1 liter per minute.

17. What therapies are available for patients with COPD and hypoventilation?

Long-term oxygen therapy is the only treatment demonstrated to improve survival in patients with COPD. Because supplemental oxygen may diminish hypoxic ventilatory drive, it is tempting to perform sleep studies on all patients to ensure that hypercapnia does not increase during sleep, although this is rarely done. The studies revealing that oxygen therapy improved survival in COPD patients had oxygen titration based on awake measurements, and whether patients should have nocturnal measurements remains unclear. Other therapies such as medroxyprogesterone, acetazolamide, theophylline, and negative-pressure ventilation have not been promising. Positive-pressure ventilation, such as bilevel positive airway pressure, may lower carbon dioxide acutely in patients with COPD, but no long-term studies of survival have been done.

BIBLIOGRAPHY

1. Bradley DT, Phillipson EA: Central sleep apnea. Clin Chest Med 13:493–505, 1992.
2. Connaughton JJ, Catteral JR, Elton RA: Do sleep studies contribute to the management of patients with chronic pulmonary disease? Am Rev Respir Dis 138:341–345, 1988.
3. Douglas NJ: Nocturnal hypoxia in patients with chronic obstructive pulmonary disease. Clin Chest Med 13:523–532, 1992.
4. Glauser FL, Fairman RP, Bechard D: The causes and evaluation of chronic hypercapnia. Chest 91:755–759, 1987.
5. Gold AR, Schwartz AR, Wise RA, et al: Pulmonary function and respiratory chemosensitivity in moderately obese patients with sleep apnea. Chest 103:1325–1329, 1993.
6. Goldstein RS: Hypoventilation: Neuromuscular and chest wall disorders. Clin Chest Med 13:507–521, 1992.
7. Hanly PJ: Mechanisms and management of central sleep apnea. Lung 1–18, 1992.
8. Hudgel DW: The role of upper airway anatomy and physiology in obstructive sleep apnea. Clin Chest Med 13:383–398, 1992.
9. Kopelman PG: Sleep apnea and hypoventilation in obesity. Int J Obes 16:S37–S42, 1992.
10. Kryger MH: Management of obstructive sleep apnea. Clin Chest Med 13:481–492, 1992.
11. McLear PW, Thawley SE: Airway management in obesity hypoventilation syndrome. Clin Chest Med 12:585–588, 1991.
12. Strumpf DA, Millman RP, Hill NS: The management of chronic hypoventilation. Chest 98:474–480, 1990.
13. Wilson WR, Bedell GN: The pulmonary abnormalities in myxedema. J Clin Invest 12:42–55, 1960.
14. Zwillich CW: Ventilatory control in myxedema and hypothyroidism. N Engl J Med 292:662–665, 1975.

XII. Occupational and Environmental Lung Diseases

51. SILICOSIS, COAL WORKERS' PNEUMOCONIOSIS, AND CHRONIC BERYLLIUM DISEASE

Lisa M. Maier, M.D., and Lee S. Newman, M.D., M.A.

1. What is silicosis?

Silicosis is probably the most prevalent chronic occupational disease in the world. Long-term exposure to free silica causes a nodular fibrotic lung disease in the interstitium. Disease presentation and severity depend on intensity and duration of exposure, nature of the silica inhaled, and poorly understood host susceptibility factors. Approximately 20% of the respirable silica particles inhaled are retained in the lung. Macrophages ingest the remaining silica particles, which leads to the release of oxidants, reactive oxygen species, and antiproteases that can cause lung injury. An inflammatory cascade is initiated, with interstitial accumulation and stimulation of numerous cell types and production of other inflammatory mediators. Subsequently, fibronectin may be released and fibroblast activation and collagen production ensue. The pathogenic mechanism remains obscure. The histologic hallmark of silicosis is the silicotic nodule composed of weakly birefrigent silica and a whorled hyalinzed central collection of collagen surrounded by dust-laden macrophages. These nodules coalesce to form larger masses, and more diffuse interstitial fibrosis can occur over time.

2. Who develops silicosis?

The element silicon is abundant and constitutes approximately 25% of the earth's crust. Exposure to silica occurs in numerous occupations. The prevalence of silicosis increased after the industrial revolution with the introduction of mechanized tools, such as the pneumatic drill, that amplified the amount of airborne silica dust in many industries. In this century the prevalence of silicosis has declined in the United States because of tighter regulation of silica dust levels. Although low dust levels are found in many industries, some industries fail to adhere to protective standards and silicosis still occurs in this country. Throughout the developing world, many workers are exposed to levels of silica high enough to cause silicosis.

Occupations and Industries in which Exposure to Silica Occurs

OCCUPATION/INDUSTRY	EXAMPLES OF SPECIFIC JOBS
Hard rock mining, excavating, tunneling	Miner, driller, blaster, crusher
Stonework	Sculptor, mason, monument carver
Stone quarrying	Crusher, trucker, laborer
Foundries	Casting, polishing, mold making
Construction	Sandblaster
Abrasives	Manufacturer of sandpaper, silica flour, sandblast grit
Tool grinding/sharpening	
Ceramics	Manufacturers of pottery, kilns, or refractory
Diatomaceous earth production	
Glass manufacture	

3. Does silicosis cause disease only after many years of exposure?

No. Silica exposure results in a spectrum of diseases ranging from acute to chronic. Chronic *simple silicosis* is the most common form, occurring slowly after 20–30 years of silica exposure. Silicosis is called *simple* when the chest radiograph shows discrete nodular shadows and *complicated* when these shadows coalesce to form larger conglomerate nodules or masses. Many individuals with chronic, simple silicosis are asymptomatic and have normal lung function, whereas others experience insidious onset of dyspnea, cough, sputum production, restrictive physiology, and derangement of gas exchange.

Acute silicoproteinosis develops within days to months after high level exposure, such as can occur with sandblasting. This disease is clinically and histologically indistinguishable from pulmonary alveolar proteinosis; its symptoms are dyspnea, radiographic findings of basilar alveolar infiltrates, and alveolar filling with protein-rich surfactant-like material. Individuals with this form of silicosis have a poor prognosis and may progress rapidly to respiratory insufficiency and death.

4. What are the radiographic manifestations of silicosis?

Silicosis can be diagnosed clinically in most individuals with a history of exposure and typical chest radiographic findings. Lung biopsy usually is not necessary for diagnosis of silicosis. The classic chest radiographic abnormalities consist of rounded opacities, 1–5 mm in size, predominantly in the upper lung zones, although sometimes throughout all lung fields. Egg-shell calcification of the hilar or mediastinal lymph nodes is almost pathognomonic of silicosis, although it is rarely seen. CT is more sensitive than plain radiography in detecting changes caused by silicosis.

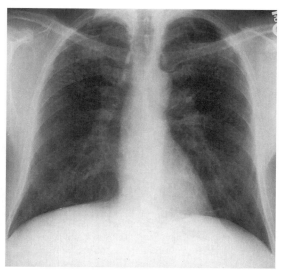

Chest radiograph shows typical findings of silicosis with upper lobe nodules predominant. Diffuse nodules are present and a conglomerate fibrotic mass consistent with progressive massive fibrosis is noted in the right upper lung.

5. What is progressive massive fibrosis?

Progressive massive fibrosis (PMF) is the coalescence of fibrotic upper lobe nodules into large conglomerate masses that cause restrictive pulmonary physiology and impaired gas exchange. PMF usually develops years after exposure ceases. It is associated with high cumulative levels of silica exposure. In addition to the professions listed in question 2, coal workers can develop PMF, especially if they mine coal from rock with a high quartz content.

6. Does silicotuberculosis still occur? How is it treated?

The association between silicosis and tuberculosis has been known since the nineteenth century. In the early part of this century silicotuberculosis was responsible for much morbidity and mortality and continues to plague developing countries. Any individual with silicosis or exposure to silica is at increased risk for tuberculosis. Screening silicotics, and possibly all workers exposed to silica, with a skin test for tuberculosis, has been recommended. Individuals with silicosis should be evaluated for tuberculosis if there are any signs, symptoms, or radiographic changes suggestive of the disease. Although the symptoms of tuberculosis and silicosis may be similar, typically they progress more quickly in silicotuberculosis than is expected in silicosis alone. Treatment of tuberculosis in silicotics consists of the conventional three- or four-drug therapy, if the organism is sensitive. Some have advocated a longer course of therapy (at least 12 months) because of higher relapse rates in some studies of silicotuberculosis.

7. Is there any therapy for silicosis?

There is no effective cure for silicosis. Individuals with silicosis are treated symptomatically in an attempt to prevent cor pulmonale. Supplemental oxygen should be given to individuals with hypoxemia. A high index of suspicion for tuberculosis should be maintained. Corticosteroids have been shown to produce short-term improvement in lung function, but long-term steroid therapy is not advocated because its long-term benefits are not known. Prevention of silicosis is far superior to treatment of the disease. Disease is prevented by reduction of the level of exposure to silica, although the level that is safe remains the subject of debate. For 100% respirable quartz, in an average 8-hour work day, the time weighted average of 0.1 mg per m^3 of air is the recommended upper limit of exposure. Even at this level, some individuals may develop silicosis. A clinician who diagnoses a case of silicosis should notify health authorities who can investigate whether the industry is in compliance with current exposure regulations.

8. What is black lung?

Black lung is a term usually applied to any respiratory disorder associated with work in the coal mines. Other terms have been applied to the lung diseases associated with coal dust, including *miner's asthma, anthracosis,* and *phthisis.* Coal workers' pneumoconiosis (CWP) is the fibrotic lung disease that results from inhalation and deposition of coal dust. The pathologic lesion observed in CWP consists of focal collections of macrophages laden with coal dust and is known as a *dust macule.* With more progressive disease these macules coalesce and form firm and palpable nodules. Chest radiographs may reveal small rounded opacities in the upper lung zones, not unlike those seen in silicosis. Many individuals with radiographic evidence of CWP may be asymptomatic. Those with advanced disease may report symptoms of dyspnea, cough, sputum production, or melanoptysis, the production of black-pigmented sputum. Symptoms and physiology generally correlate poorly with the severity of disease seen on radiographs in CWP.

9. Do nonsmokers exposed to coal dust develop airflow obstruction?

Exposure to coal dust causes emphysema, chronic bronchitis, and airflow obstruction. Focal emphysema is found commonly around coal macules and nodules. Emphysema is associated with the degree of fibrotic lung disease, the intensity of previous exposure, and the amount of retained coal dust. Pulmonary function tests may reveal reduced lung volumes, airway obstruction, or both. The pattern may be indistinguishable from that seen with tobacco abuse. This disease process occurs at a high rate in both smoking and nonsmoking individuals who are exposed to coal dust. Symptoms of chronic cough, sputum production, and wheezing are common. Emphysema, chronic bronchitis, and airflow limitation associated with coal dust are treated in the same way as these entities are when not associated with coal dust. Coal miners with emphysema, chronic bronchitis, or airflow obstruction should stop smoking, as should any emphysematous patient.

10. Are some miners more likely to develop CWP than others?

Not all coal miners are at equal risk for developing CWP. For example, miners working at the face of a mine, where higher exposure occurs, are more likely to develop CWP. Higher cumulative exposure levels are associated with higher rates of disease development. Anthracite coal found in the Eastern United States is more likely to cause disease than is bituminous coal found in the western part of the country. The prevalence of CWP has been decreasing over the past 20–30 years, probably because of reduced exposure levels and decreasing numbers of workers employed in the industry.

11. What is Caplan's syndrome (rheumatoid pneumoconiosis)? Who is at risk for this disease?

Anthony Caplan described the constellation of CWP, rheumatoid arthritis, and large nodular lesions, initially mistaken for PMF on chest radiograph. The nodules tend to be well defined, in contrast to those seen in PMF, and occur with little or no fibrotic lung disease. These necrobiotic nodules may cavitate or calcify and sometimes disappear. Caplan's syndrome also has been noted in individuals with silicosis. Some individuals with CWP or silicosis may have an elevated rheumatoid factor level or antinuclear antibody titer level without having rheumatoid arthritis.

12. Is berylliosis (chronic beryllium disease) extinct?

The metal beryllium became noted as a cause of lung disease in the 1940s when many workers in the fluorescent light industry became ill with a sarcoidosis-like disease or with acute pneumonitis. Today the acute form of disease is rare because levels of beryllium exposure in the workplace have decreased. However, chronic beryllium disease (CBD) continues to occur in many industries and among family members exposed to second-hand dust. CBD rates in industry range from 1–16% depending on the worker group studied. Although beryllium is no longer used in the manufacture of fluorescent lights, it is used in the aerospace, aircraft, nuclear weapons, electronics, ceramics, and automotive parts industries and in dental alloy manufacture.

13. Describe the symptoms of CBD.

The symptoms of CBD include slowly progressive dyspnea on exertion, dry cough, and chest pain. Constitutional symptoms of anorexia, fatigue, fevers, night sweats, and weight loss also may occur. Lung pathology includes noncaseating granulomas and diffuse mononuclear cell interstitial infiltrates. Skin involvement with granulomatous lesions may result from direct contact and inoculation with beryllium. Occasionally, a disseminated form of the disease may occur with granulomatous involvement of the liver, spleen, lymph nodes, bone, and kidneys.

14. How much beryllium exposure is too much?

Several studies and case reports indicate that chronic beryllium disease can occur at very low levels, probably below the existing federal standard. CBD has been observed in secretaries, office managers, and security guards; however, there is an exposure-response relationship. People who work in high-exposure jobs, such as machinists, are more likely to develop disease than are low-exposure workers. An allelic substitution in the HLA-DP locus appears to be a genetic marker of disease, suggesting that both exposure and host susceptibility contribute to the response to beryllium. Physicians should suspect CBD in any patient with granulomatous lung disease who has worked with metals, especially with beryllium, regardless of how low the reported exposure has been.

15. How is CBD distinguished from other granulomatous lung diseases such as sarcoidosis?

CBD is often misdiagnosed as sarcoidosis. A blood and bronchoalveolar lavage test called the *beryllium lymphocyte proliferation test* (BeLPT) helps in the differentiation of these diseases. Peripheral blood mononuclear cells or bronchoalveolar lavage cells from an individual with suspected CBD are exposed to beryllium salts in vitro. Because CBD results from an antigen-specific cell-mediated immune response to beryllium, cells from individuals with CBD proliferate, whereas those from patients with other granulomatous lung diseases do not. Most patients with CBD have an abnormal blood BeLPT. Some individuals become sensitized to beryllium, have an abnormal blood BeLPT, but have not yet developed granulomatous disease. Although 10–30% false-negative rates have been reported with the blood test, it is still more sensitive than chest radiograph or pulmonary function test in detecting disease. It also lends specificity to the diagnosis of granulomatous disease. In cases in which CBD is suspected but the blood BeLPT is normal, bronchoalveolar lavage BeLPT may improve the diagnostic yield. Most CBD patients have an abnormal bronchoalveolar lavage lymphocyte proliferation test, although tobacco smoke can interfere with the sensitivity of the bronchoalveolar lavage test.

BIBLIOGRAPHY

1. Caplan A: Certain unusual radiological appearances in the chest of coal-miners suffering from rheumatoid arthritis. Thorax 8:29–37, 1953.
2. Cowie RL: The epidemiology of tuberculosis in gold miners with silicosis. Am J Respir Crit Care Med 150:1460–1462, 1994.
3. Davis GS: Pathogenesis of silicosis: Current concepts and hypotheses. Lung 164:139–154, 1986.
4. Davis GS: Silicosis. In Harber P, Schenker MA, Balmes JR (eds): Occupational and Environmental Respiratory Disease. St. Louis, Mosby-Year Book, 1996, pp 379–399.
5. Graham WGB: Silicosis. Clin Chest Med 13:253–267, 1992.
6. Kreiss K, Mroz MM, Zhen B, et al: Epidemiology of beryllium sensitization and disease in nuclear workers. Am Rev Respir Dis 148:985–991, 1993.
7. Kreiss K, Wasserman S, Mroz MM, et al: Beryllium disease screening in the ceramics industry. J Occup Med 35:267–274, 1993.
8. Lapp NL, Parker JE: Coal workers' pneumoconiosis. Clin Chest Med 13:243–252, 1992.
9. Newman LS: Occupational illness. N Engl J Med 333:1128–1134, 1995.
10. Pairon JC, Brochard P, Juarand MC, et al: Silica and lung cancer: A controversial issue. Eur Respir J 4:730–744, 1991.
11. Rose CS, Newman LS: Hypersensitivity pneumonitis and chronic beryllium disease. In Schwartz MI, King TE (eds): Interstitial Lung Disease. St. Louis, Mosby-Year Book, 1993, pp 240–249.
12. Saltini C, Winestock K, Kirby M, et al: Maintenance of alveolitis in patients with chronic beryllium disease by beryllium-specific helper T cells. N Engl J Med 320:1103–1109, 1989.
13. Seixas NS, Robins TG, Attfield MD, et al: Exposure-response relationships for coal mine dust and obstructive lung disease following enactment of the Federal Coal Mine Health and Safety Act of 1969. Am J Ind Med 21:715–734, 1992.
14. Silicosis and Silicate Disease Committee: Disease associated with exposure to silica and nonfibrous silicate materials. Arch Pathol Lab Med 112:673–720, 1988.
15. Snider DE: The relationship between tuberculosis and silicosis. Am Rev Respir Dis 118:455–459, 1978.

52. ASBESTOS-RELATED LUNG DISEASE

E. Brigitte Gottschall, M.D., and Kevin P. Fennelly, M.D., M.P.H.

1. What is asbestos?

The word asbestos is derived from the Greek term for "inextinguishable." It refers to a family of six naturally occurring, flexible, fibrous hydrated silicate minerals that share the property of being relatively indestructible and heat resistant. Chrysotile, or white asbestos, is classified as a serpentine mineral because of its layered silicate structure. It constitutes 95% of the asbestos produced in the world. In the United States it is mined in California, Arizona, and Vermont. Crocidolite ("blue asbestos"), amosite, anthophyllite, tremolite, and actinolite are referred to as amphiboles because of their chained silicate structures. The toxicity of the various types of asbestos varies due in part to their morphology and physiochemical properties. The diameter and length of asbestos fibers are critically important in determining their potential pathogenicity. The amphiboles are more prone to be carcinogenic and to cause pleural fibrosis, but lung fibrosis seems to be equally associated with the amphiboles and chrysotile.

2. What are the pulmonary manifestations of asbestos exposure?

Asbestosis is fibrosis of the lung parenchyma. **Rounded atelectasis** is partial collapse of lung tissue caused by the retraction of adjacent fibrotic pleura and parenchyma. It is also called "pseudotumor" since on plain chest radiograph it appears as a pleural based mass. **Benign**

nodules may be seen in the lung parenchyma, and these may be due to localized areas of fibrosis and scarring, benign lymphoid nodules, or rounded atelectasis. There is also an increased incidence of **bronchogenic carcinoma** in asbestos-exposed workers.

3. What are the pleural manifestations of asbestos exposure?

Benign pleural effusion, also referred to as benign asbestos pleurisy, is a transient inflammation of the pleura associated with an exudative pleural effusion. **Pleural plaques** are discrete, well-circumscribed areas of fibrosis on the parietal pleura (on the inner surface of the rib cage or on the diaphragm) that are usually bilateral and often partially calcified. They are considered a "signature" of exposure to asbestos. **Diffuse pleural thickening** (also called pachypleuritis) refers to extensive fibrosis of both the parietal and visceral pleura, which is more likely to cause restrictive physiology on pulmonary function tests. **Malignant mesothelioma** is a malignant and invasive tumor of the pleura that is often fatal within 1–2 years of diagnosis.

4. How is the diagnosis of asbestosis established?

Asbestosis is an interstitial pulmonary fibrosis resulting from the inhalation of asbestos dust. The diagnosis of asbestosis is usually made on clinical grounds without histologic proof. A reliable and significant exposure history (there is a well-established dose-relationship for asbestosis), an appropriate time interval between exposure and detection of disease (10–40 years), radiographic evidence of diffuse lung fibrosis on chest radiograph or CT scan, pulmonary function tests with a restrictive pattern and decreased diffusing capacity, and a physical exam revealing fixed bilateral inspiratory crackles and clubbing will establish the diagnosis of asbestosis for medical and legal purposes. The first three criteria are mandatory, whereas the last three are considered confirmatory.

The assessment of the chest radiograph is based on the International Labor Organization (ILO) classification system for pneumoconiosis radiographs. This classification grades the classically reticulonodular pattern of pneumoconiosis radiographs based on profusion, size, shape, and extent. However, up to 10–20% of patients with asbestosis who are symptomatic and have physiologic abnormalities of gas exchange have a normal chest radiograph. High-resolution CT often shows early interstitial changes in these patients and has therefore become an important tool in the diagnosis of asbestosis.

5. What is the pathogenesis of asbestosis?

Following inhalation of asbestos for only one hour, animals develop evidence of lung injury within 48 hours. Increased numbers of alveolar macrophages gather at the alveolar duct bifurcations. These macrophages are activated by asbestos fibers, and there is a marked increase in the number of fibroblasts at these sites. The cytokines involved in this process include platelet-derived growth factor (PDGF), insulin-like growth factor (IGF-1), and fibroblast growth factor (FGF). A complex series of events results in fibroblast proliferation and the formation of scar tissue. Asbestos-activated macrophages also release cytotoxic oxygen-free radicals and plasminogen activator; the latter results in the formation of plasmin, a protease, which leads to further tissue destruction. Much of the toxicity of asbestos is due to the inability of macrophages to phagocytose the long fibers, which then move through the lung interstitium. There is coating of the fibers that leads to the formation of "asbestos bodies." Although this reduces the toxicity of the fiber, more than 85% of fibers in the lung remain uncoated. Some fibers tend to split longitudinally, which leads to persistence of the inflammatory process.

6. What occupations are associated with asbestos exposure?

The National Institute for Occupational Safety and Health (NIOSH) has estimated that up to 2.5 million workers in the U.S. are currently exposed to asbestos dust, but workers in the past have had much higher exposures. Asbestos was virtually ubiquitous in workplaces, so a listing of all occupations associated with exposure is not feasible. Some representative industries seen in our clinical practice and in the literature are listed below. In taking an occupational history, it is important to ask about job duties and whether the patient had ever worked with asbestos. A job title alone is often uninformative.

Asbestos miners	Maintenance/custodial workers
Automobile repair workers	Plumbers
Brake lining makers/repair workers	Pipe fitters
Boiler makers	Railroad workers
Construction workers	Roofers
Electricians	Sheet metal workers
Gasket makers	Shipyard workers
Insulation workers	Textile workers

7. Does everybody who is exposed to asbestos develop asbestosis?

With massive exposures to asbestos dust, all of the exposed workers developed disease. In more recent years with reduced exposure to the dust, it has become apparent that there is individual susceptibility to asbestosis. The capacity to clear asbestos from the lungs seems to be the most important risk factor for developing asbestosis. There is an exposure-response relationship, however, such that there is a higher incidence of asbestosis with increasing cumulative exposure. Recent studies have found no differences in the risks of asbestos-related diseases for women vs. men or for whites vs. blacks.

8. Is asbestosis treatable?

There is no specific treatment for asbestosis. Corticosteroid and immunosuppressive therapies are not indicated. Treatment is supportive and symptomatic. Intercurrent respiratory infections may occur commonly and should be treated aggressively. Oxygen therapy may be necessary to treat hypoxemia and right heart failure in the later stages of the disease. Influenza and pneumococcal vaccination are warranted. Cessation of exposure in an animal model has reduced the rate of progression. Patients should be counseled to abstain form smoking in order to decrease their risk for bronchogenic lung cancer, as well as to prevent other smoking-related diseases. The lack of viable treatment options emphasizes the critical need for primary prevention, i.e., reducing or eliminating asbestos dust exposure.

9. What is rounded atelectasis?

Rounded atelectasis is a form of partial lung collapse in the peripheral part of the lung. Synonyms include folded lung syndrome, Blesovskly's syndrome, shrinking pleuritis with atelectasis, atelactic pseudotumor, and pleuroma. The pathogenesis is controversial. The most accepted theory postulates that a pleural inflammatory reaction is followed by pleural shrinkage, causing atelectasis in the immediately adjacent lung parenchyma, which assumes a rounded configuration. The principal etiology is believed to be asbestos exposure; however, conditions such as parapneumonic effusions, CHF, Dressler's syndrome, pulmonary infarcts, chest trauma, and therapeutic pneumothoraces have been associated with rounded atelectasis. Its clinical significance lies in its presentation as a pulmonary mass that needs to be distinguished from a malignancy. It is often an incidental finding on chest x-ray, ranging from 2.5–7 cm in size. The angle between the pleura and the mass is usually sharp. Rounded atelectasis occurs predominantly in the lower lobes. The classic radiographic feature is a "comet tail" that extends from the hilum toward the base of the lung and then sweeps into the inferior pole of the lesion. No specific treatment is needed. In the past diagnosis often was made only at decortication, but now CT permits recognition of this benign condition noninvasively.

10. Are people still exposed to asbestos today?

Asbestos was used extensively in a large number of construction materials since early in the 20th century because of its heat resistance, flexibility, and tensile strength. The U.S. Environmental Protection Agency banned its use in many applications in 1973. Exposures to asbestos may occur today largely during the disruption of asbestos in building construction materials.

Such materials include acoustic ceiling tiles, vinyl floor tiles, insulation material on pipes, boilers, and structural beams, and within paints, walls, and plasters. The risk of disease is determined by exposures to airborne fibers, not simply the presence of asbestos-containing materials in buildings. Although the airborne concentrations in most buildings studied have been very low, there are rare buildings with higher levels. Some studies have found that about 11% of custodial and maintenance workers in buildings had radiographic evidence of asbestos-related diseases, but these studies were limited in several ways. These radiographs probably reflected significant past exposures. It is unlikely that there is a significant risk of asbestos-related diseases for such workers at current levels of exposure. If we assume a no threshold model of carcinogenesis, however, there may be a small risk of lung cancer and mesothelioma associated with similar low exposures.

11. What is "paraoccupational" exposure to asbestos?

"Paraoccupational" exposure refers to an exposure to a hazardous agent that is not directly associated with an individual's job or activity. Many workers who never used asbestos directly may have been significantly exposed to coworkers using asbestos in the vicinity. For example, electricians or maintenance workers might have been exposed when laborers were stripping off insulation materials containing asbestos. Inadvertent domestic exposures also occurred when asbestos workers carried large burdens of fibers into the home on clothing and in their hair. This led to an increased incidence of mesotheliomas in the families (including children) of asbestos workers.

12. What cancers are associated with asbestos exposure?

Bronchogenic carcinomas (lung cancers) in asbestos-exposed workers are similar to those seen in cigarette smokers, and the synergistic (multiplicative) effect of cigarette smoking and asbestos exposure is well documented. Cigarette smokers have a tenfold increased risk of lung cancer compared to nonsmokers; asbestos workers who are also smokers have a fiftyfold increased risk. These tumors usually occur at the bifurcations of large airways; thus, few of them are secondary to "scar" carcinoma.

Malignant mesothelioma is a relatively rare cancer in the general population, and it is clearly associated with asbestos exposure. Unlike bronchogenic carcinoma, cigarette smoking does not confer an increased risk of the disease. Exposure to crocidolite is associated with the highest rates of mesothelioma, but mesothelioma may occur after exposure to any type of asbestos. Dull, aching chest pain is a common presenting symptom. A biopsy obtained at open thoracotomy or by video-assisted thoracoscopy is usually needed to establish the diagnosis. New modalities of treatment have unfortunately extended survival for only a few months. Treatment is generally supportive, and death usually occurs within 2 years after the diagnosis. Malignant mesothelioma can rarely involve other mesothelial surfaces, including the pericardium, the peritoneum, and the tunica vaginalis testis.

A recently published study from Finland described an excess of **endometrial cancer** among female miners exposed to anthophyllite asbestos, and other studies have suggested an increased risk of female reproductive tissue cancers. These data are concerning but not yet conclusive.

Earlier studies had suggested that a wide range of malignancies were associated with exposure to asbestos, including cancers of the gastrointestinal tract, larynx and kidney, as well as lymphoma and leukemia. However, these studies were limited by potential confounding, and the data remain equivocal for the nonpleuropulmonary malignancies.

13. What hazards are associated with work in the asbestos removal industry?

Because of the known hazards of asbestos, regulatory agencies require extensive training and personal protective equipment for workers doing asbestos abatement. This involves using personal respirators and wearing impermeable protective clothing. Abatement sites may be hot. The use of water sprays to minimize airborne dust levels increases the humidity. These conditions can lead to significant heat stress as well as psychological stress. If the work area cannot be cooled to comfortable levels, a cool rest area should be provided, and it may be necessary to limit the working time between rest periods. Many respirators are made of rubber. Because of the increasing incidence of allergy to latex in some populations, it is prudent for clinicians to ask workers about skin or respiratory reactions to latex or rubber products.

BIBLIOGRAPHY

1. Adler BD, Kelsey PJ: Malignant mesothelioma of the tunica vaginalis testis. Australas Radiol 36:29–30, 1992.
2. Begin R, Samet JM, Shaikh RA: Asbestos. In Harber P, Schenker MB, Balmes JR (eds): Occupational and Environmental Respiratory Disease. St. Louis, Mosby, 1996, pp 293–329.
3. Brown DP, Dement JM, Okun A: Mortality patterns among female and male chrysotile asbestos textile workers. J Occup Med 36:882–888, 1994.
4. Browne K: Asbestos-related Disorders. In Parkes WR (ed): Occupational Lung Disorders. Oxford, England, Butterworth Heinemann, 1994, pp 411–504.
5. Magnani C, Terracini B, Ivalid C, et al: A cohort study on mortality among wives of workers in the asbestos cement industry in Casale Monferrato, Italy. Br J Ind Med 50:779–784, 1993.
6. Meurman LO, Pukkala E, Hakama M: Incidence of cancer among anthophyllite asbestos miners in Finland. Occup Environ Med 51:421–425, 1994.
7. McDiarmid MA, Weaver V: Fouling one's own nest revisited. Am J Ind Med 24:1–9, 1993.
8. Ohnaka T, Tochihara Y, Muramatsu T: Physiological strains in hot-humid conditions while wearing disposable protective clothing commonly used by the asbestos removal industry. Ergonomics 36:1241–1250, 1993.
9. Wagner GR: Mineral dusts. In Rosenstock L, Cullen MR (eds): Textbook of Clinical Occupational and Environmental Medicine. Philadelphia, W.B. Saunders, 1994, pp 825–837.

53. HYPERSENSITIVITY PNEUMONITIS AND OTHER DISORDERS CAUSED BY ORGANIC AGENTS

Cecile Rose, M.D., M.P.H.

1. What is meant by the term *organic agent*?

Substances of animal and vegetable origin are generally referred to as *organic agents*. Airborne organic agents are called *bioaerosols*, which are airborne particles, large molecules, or volatile compounds that are living or were released from a living organism. Sources of common bioaerosol components capable of causing human diseases include bacteria, fungi, protozoa, viruses, algae, green plants, arthropods, and mammals. For example, saliva bioaerosols from cats can cause asthma and rhinitis in cat-sensitive individuals. The necessary conditions and events required to produce aerosolization of an organism or its parts are the presence of a reservoir, amplification (increase in numbers or concentration), and dissemination (aerosolization). Human hosts are reservoirs for some organisms, for example, *Mycobacterium tuberculosis*. Others are found in environmental reservoirs that act as amplifiers or disseminators, such as *Legionella* bioaerosol dissemination from cooling towers.

2. Describe the spectrum of diseases caused by exposure to organic agents.

The wide spectrum of diseases associated with inhalation of organic agents includes:

Hypersensitivity pneumonitis

Rhinoconjunctivitis

Asthma

Inhalation fevers, such as grain fever, organic dust toxic syndrome (ODTS), and humidifier fever

Infections, such as legionella pneumonia or unusual infections from outbreaks in laboratory workers

Chronic airflow limitation and accelerated decline in lung function, such as the decline in FEV_1 often found in workers exposed to cotton dust, grain workers, and animal confinement workers

3. **What industries or occupational groups are most likely to be affected by exposure to organic agents?**

The most well-recognized occupational field associated with exposure to organic agents is the agricultural industry, in which the effects of exposure to grain dusts have been recognized since antiquity. The world produces more than 1.5 billion tons of grain annually, and the United States is a major producer and the greatest exporter of grain in the world.

Farmer's lung disease was the first form of hypersensitivity pneumonitis (HP) described. It is typically associated with inhalation of thermophylic bacteria and fungal contaminants in hay and grain. Mushroom workers, cheese workers, and wood workers are occupational groups in whom hypersensitivity lung diseases including both HP and asthma have been described. Proteins capable of causing hypersensitivity pneumonitis are also present in the serum and droppings of birds and can cause "bird breeder's" hypersensitivity pneumonitis.

Health care professionals are at risk of exposure to bioaerosols at work. The risk of occupational infectious illnesses such as tuberculosis has been widely reported, including multidrug-resistant tuberculosis. Laboratory animal workers are at risk for unusual infections such as Q fever (caused by *Coxiella burnetti*) and hypersensitivity lung diseases such as occupational asthma from exposure to aerosolized proteins present in the urine of laboratory animals.

More recently, bioaerosol exposures have been described in a wide variety of environmental settings. For example, organic agents in hot tub mists, contaminated humidifiers in office buildings, agents associated with decaying wood and damp walls in inner city dwellings have been associated with individual cases and outbreaks of hypersensitivity pneumonitis.

4. **What pathophysiologic mechanisms occur in the diseases caused by organic agents?**

Organic agents are capable of causing disease by both immune and nonimmune mechanisms. Hypersensitivity pneumonitis results from a cascade of inflammatory and immune mechanisms, the most important of which is T-lymphocyte activation. Bronchoalveolar lavage typically shows an increase in the total number of white blood cells, with a marked lymphocytosis. Rhinoconjunctivitis and allergic asthma from exposure to organic agents are associated with an IgE-mediated, immediate-type hypersensitivity reaction. The inhalation fevers associated with exposure to organic agents are noninfectious, nonallergic febrile responses to inhalation of high concentrations of grain dusts and some microbial bioaerosols. The chronic airflow limitation and chronic bronchitis associated with organic agents is also probably not an immune-mediated process, but rather a toxic effect from exposure to a variety of organic dust contaminants, probably including endotoxins from the cell walls of gram-negative bacteria.

5. **Describe the symptoms and signs of disease caused by exposure to organic agents.**

Hypersensitivity pneumonitis (allergic alveolitis) is characterized in its acute form by recurrent pneumonia with fever, chills, cough, chest tightness, shortness of breath, and myalgias. The subacute or chronic forms of HP are manifested by insidious and progressive dyspnea, fatigue, cough, weight loss, and decreased appetite.

Asthma is characterized by complaints of wheezing, chest tightness, cough, and shortness of breath. Symptoms may occur immediately after exposure or may be delayed 6–12 hours. Diagnosis usually relies on the patient's history, wheezing on examination, or reversible airflow limitation on pulmonary function testing, including methacholine challenge testing.

Allergic rhinitis is diagnosed by history, physical examination, the finding of eosinophils on nasal smear, elevated total or specific IgE antibody levels, and immediate skin prick testing to relevant aeroallergens.

Inhalation fevers are characterized by fevers, chills, malaise, and muscle aches but no prominent pulmonary symptoms or signs. Symptoms usually occur within 48 hours after exposure and subside within 24–48 hours, with no long-term effects.

6. **How is the diagnosis of HP established?**

Diagnosis is based on a careful clinical and exposure history followed by appropriate diagnostic testing. Results of pulmonary function testing may show restrictive, obstructive, or mixed abnormalities, sometimes with a decreased diffusion capacity for carbon monoxide. Gas exchange abnormalities are often present with exercise. The chest radiograph may be normal in early stages of disease but typically reveals small, discrete, scattered 1–3 mm nodules, often predominantly in the lower lobe. Diffuse, patchy infiltrates or a ground glass appearance may be present. Radiographic abnormalities in acute illness typically regress or resolve over 4–6 weeks if further exposure is avoided. In the subacute or chronic form of HP, linear interstitial markings become more distinct, often associated with progressive loss of lung volume. A high resolution CT (HRCT) scan also may be normal if disease is diagnosed early. In subacute or chronic HP, the predominant HRCT pattern is poorly defined centrilobular micronodules, often with ground glass attenuation. These findings probably reflect the histologic findings of cellular bronchiolitis, non-caseating granulomas, and active alveolitis.

7. Are precipitating antibodies useful in the diagnosis of HP?

The finding of specific precipitating antibodies in the serum of a patient with suspected HP indicates exposure sufficient to generate a humoral immunologic response; this may be a helpful diagnostic clue. Precipitins do not appear to have a role in disease pathogenesis but serve as markers of antigen exposure. Precipitins are often found in antigen-exposed individuals without clinically evident disease. Additionally, specific precipitating antibodies are frequently not demonstrable in patients with HP. Results may be negative because of poorly standardized commercial antigens or the wrong choice of antigen.

8. What information should be included in the occupational and environmental histories of patients with suspected exposure to organic agents?

The most important approach to diagnosis of diseases caused by organic agents is a high index of suspicion and careful occupational and environmental history-taking. The occupational history should contain a chronology of current and previous occupations, a description of job processes and specific work practices, and a list of specific exposures. Improvement in symptoms away from work or worsening of symptoms with specific workplace exposures can be a helpful diagnostic clue when present. Additionally, the presence of persistent respiratory or constitutional symptoms, or both, in exposed coworkers can be helpful in identifying exposure-related disease.

The environmental and home history should include:

A list of pets and other domestic animals

Hobbies and recreational activities that may involve exposures to organic dusts

Use of hot tubs, saunas, or indoor swimming pools

Presence of leaking or flooding in a basement or occupied space

Presence of humidifiers, dehumidifiers, swamp coolers, or cool mist vaporizers

Water damage to carpets and furnishings

Visible mold or mildew contamination in the occupied space

Use of feathers in pillows, comforters, or clothing

9. Is sick building syndrome caused by exposure to organic agents?

No. Sick building syndrome (SBS) is not included in the spectrum of diseases caused by exposure to organic agents. SBS is defined as an excess of nonspecific symptoms—including mucous membrane irritation, headache, and fatigue—associated with building occupancy. Specific causes of SBS are unknown and probably vary from building to building. Previous assumptions that SBS results from insufficient outdoor air are not well substantiated by existing epidemiologic studies. The possibility that SBS is associated with indoor exposure to bioaerosols has been raised. European studies suggest that SBS is associated with air conditioning systems with or without humidification. Additionally, occupant activities and furnishing can affect indoor air quality and complaint rates in buildings. Different buildings probably have different sources of poor indoor air quality; thus, SBS probably has several causes.

SBS is included along with building-related illnesses in the broad category of building-associated illnesses. Building-related illnesses (BRI) are distinct clinical entities such as asthma, hypersensitivity pneumonitis, allergic rhinitis, contact urticaria, infections, and toxic syndromes (for example, carbon monoxide poisoning) that result from building exposures. BRIs broadly overlap with the diseases that stem from exposure to organic agents.

10. How many people are affected by diseases resulting from exposure to organic agents?

The number is not known, but probably many more are affected than are clinically recognized. Our understanding of disease incidence and prevalence is hampered by the lack of a national database and reporting system, the nonspecificity of the symptoms associated with exposures to bioaerosols and other organic agents, and the fact that the symptoms mimic many other diseases such as viral illnesses and chronic bronchitis.

Most of the population-based studies of HP focus on the prevalence of illness among agricultural workers. In Scotland, the prevalence of farmer's lung in three agricultural areas ranged from 2.3–8.6%. A questionnaire survey of western Wyoming dairy and cattle ranchers elicited a history typical of acute farmer's lung disease in 3% of those surveyed. The prevalence of HP among bird hobbyists is estimated to range from 0.5–21%.

11. Describe the treatment options available for diseases caused by exposure to organic agents.

For the hypersensitivity diseases (rhinoconjunctivitis, asthma, and hypersensitivity pneumonitis), early recognition and removal from exposure to the antigen-containing environment is key in disease management. In some cases, removal will result in complete resolution of symptoms and physiologic and radiographic abnormalities. In patients with asthma or hypersensitivity pneumonitis who have severe abnormalities at presentation or persistent symptoms despite removal from exposure, short-term (2–3 months) treatment with oral corticosteroids may be helpful. No treatment for the inhalation fevers has been identified because these disorders are self-limited. Prevention of recurrent episodes is recommended because little information is available on the natural history of recurrent attacks.

12. How is antigen exposure eliminated in disease caused by bioaerosols?

Once a bioaerosol-related disease is diagnosed, eliminating antigen exposure is the most challenging part of the treatment. In some cases, an investigation aimed at assessing the bioaerosol status of the building or home can be undertaken. Although it is often difficult to prove the connection between specific exposures and disease, it may be possible to demonstrate bioaerosol reservoirs, amplifiers, and disseminators during an on-site inspection. The presence of potential bioaerosol sources may be sufficient to permit recommendations for remedial action without further investigation. If additional documentation of exposure is required, quantitative bioaerosol sampling can be considered. The primary objective of air sampling is to identify the source of bioaerosol components so that effective corrective action can be undertaken. Dose-response information is generally not available. Positive results may document the presence of a specific source; however, negative results are usually inconclusive with respect to confirming the presence or absence of sources. An exposure may be considered potentially significant when overall levels of the bioaerosol are at least an order of magnitude higher than those in outdoor air or when the types of bioaerosols differ between the control environment and the complaint environment. The mere presence of an unusual organism or antigen in an environment does not prove a causal relationship between the exposure and the illness.

13. Can diseases caused by organic agents be prevented?

There is little research on the prevention of these diseases. Appropriate design and maintenance of building heating, ventilation, and air conditioning systems is important in limiting microbial amplification and dissemination. Indoor microbial contamination is often related to problems with moisture control. Source control includes preventing leaking and flooding, removing stagnant water sources, eliminating aerosol humidifiers and vaporizers, and maintaining indoor relative humidity below 70%. Contaminants can be diluted by an increase in the amount of outdoor air in a building, and high efficiency filters can be added to the ventilation system to clean recirculated air. Complete elimination of indoor allergens is probably impossible, and it is often necessary to relocate immunologically sensitized individuals once hypersensitivity lung disease has occurred.

The efficacy of various types of respirators in preventing antigen sensitization and disease progression is unknown. Helmet-type powered air purifying respirators have been used to prevent episodic exposure in individuals with previous acute episodes of farmer's lung. Prolonged wearing of respiratory protection is limited by the fact that most respirators are hot and cumbersome; moreover, they may be expensive. Dust respirators offer incomplete protection against organic particulates and are not recommended once sensitization has occurred.

BIBLIOGRAPHY

1. Ando M, Konishi K, Yoneda R, et al: Difference in the phenotypes of bronchoalveolar lavage lymphocytes in patients with summer-type hypersensitivity pneumonitis, farmer's lung, ventilation pneumonitis and bird fancier's lung: Report of a nationwide epidemiologic study in Japan. J Allergy Clin Immunol 87:1002–1009, 1991.
2. Denis M, Bedard M, Laviolette M, et al: A study of monokine release and natural killer activity in the bronchoalveolar lavage of subjects with farmer's lung. Am Rev Respir Dis 147:934–939, 1993.
3. Enarson DS, Chan-Yeung M: Characterization of health effects of wood dust exposures. Am J Ind Med 17:33–38, 1990.
4. Kokkarinen JI, Tukiainen HO, Terho EO: Effect of corticosteroid treatment on the recovery of pulmonary function in farmer's lung. Am Rev Respir Dis 145:3–5, 1992.
5. Lynch DA, Rose CS, Way D, et al: Hypersensitivity pneumonitis: Sensitivity of high-resolution CT in a population-based study. AJR 159:469–472, 1992.
6. Remy-Jardin M, Remy J, Wallaert B, et al: Subacute and chronic bird breeder hypersensitivity pneumonitis: Sequential evaluation with CT and correlation with lung function tests and bronchoalveolar lavage. Radiology 189:111–118, 1993.
7. Rose C: Inhalation fevers. In Rom WN (ed): Environmental and Occupational Medicine, 2nd ed. Boston, Little, Brown, 1992, pp 373–380.
8. Rose C: Hypersensitivity pneumonitis. In Harber P, Schenker MB, Balms JR (eds): Occupational and Environmental Respiratory Disease. St. Louis, Mosby-Yearbook, 1996, pp 201–215.
9. Semenzato G, Zambello R, Trentin L, et al: Cellular immunity in sarcoidosis and hypersensitivity pneumonitis. Chest 193 (Suppl):139–143, 1993.
10. Shellito JE: Hypersensitivity and pneumonitis. Semin Respir Med 12:196–203, 1991.
11. Warren CPW: Health and safety in the grain industry. In Rom WN (ed): Environmental and Occupational Medicine, 2nd ed. Boston, Little, Brown, 1992, pp 381–390.

54. OCCUPATIONAL AIRWAYS DISEASE

Ronald Balkissoon, M.D.

1. What is the clinical significance of occupational asthma?

Deaths and morbidity due to asthma continue to be major health problems in the United States and other countries, and individuals with environmental allergies (atopy) are known to be at increased risk for developing asthma. A major source of varied and intense environmental exposures is the workplace. At the current time, over 250 different agents are recognized as potentially causing occupational asthma, and the list continues to grow. It is believed that approximately 10–15% of the cases of adult-onset asthma are work-related. In many industrialized countries, the annual number of reported cases of occupational asthma has surpassed that of dust-related lung diseases, such as silicosis and asbestosis.

2. Define the term occupational asthma.

Occupational asthma refers to disorders that are characterized by variable airflow limitation and/or airway hyper-responsiveness attributable to specific exposures found exclusively or predominantly in the workplace. Occupational asthma may be subclassified into two groups, occupational asthma with latency and occupational asthma without latency.

3. Define the term occupational asthma with latency.

Occupational asthma with latency generally implies an immune-mediated asthma caused by a workplace agent (sensitizer). After variable periods of exposure, susceptible individuals develop an immune response (sensitization) to a specific agent. Sensitization generally requires months to years of repeated exposure to the causative agent, although shorter latency periods are theoretically possible. Once an individual has become sensitized, he or she may report developing symptoms a few hours into the workshift, late in the workshift, after returning home, and even sometimes during sleeping hours. These latencies correspond to the well-recognized patterns of early, late, or dual asthmatic responses that were first described for inhalation challenge experiments with common environmental allergens (e.g., house dust or animal dander).

4. What is a sensitizer?

The term *sensitizer* has been used to refer to various agents that appear to cause asthma through immune-mediated mechanisms, i.e., they show characteristic patterns of early late or dual responses and/or demonstrate positive skin test, immunoglobulin response, radioallergosorbent test (RAST) response, or other evidence of immune system activation. Sensitizers have been somewhat arbitrarily divided into high-molecular and low-molecular weight compounds.

5. Give some examples of high-molecular-weight compounds that can induce asthma.

Products	Exposures
Animal products (proteins)	Lab workers, veterinarians
Bird proteins	Breeders, poultry workers
Insect proteins	Grain workers, researchers
Plant proteins	Bakers, food processors
Biologic enzymes	Detergents, pharmaceuticals
Vegetables (gums)	Printers, latex
Others	Crab, shrimp, oyster processing

Originally, it was believed that large-molecular-weight antigens found in flour, latex, or certain animal proteins caused typical IgE-mediated reactions, but now it is recognized that their mechanisms of immune activation leading to asthma may be more complex.

6. Give some examples of low-molecular-weight compounds.

Products	Exposures
Diisocyanates	Plastics, polyurethanes, auto paints
Anhydrides	Epoxy resins, plastics
Wood dust	Carpentry, saw mills, construction
Fluxes, colophony	Soldering, welders
Drugs	Pharmaceuticals (antibiotics, alpha-methyl dopa, albuterol, cimetidine, aminophylline, hydralazine), chemists, health care workers
Metal	Nickel, chromium, cobalt, zinc, vanadium, platinum, aluminum
Ethanolamines, ethylendiamines, aromatic amines, methacrylates	Cosmetics, manufacturing, rubber industry, fur industry
Glutaraldehyde	Hospital workers

It has been difficult to determine the mechanism of action for low-molecular-weight agents such as isocyanates, acid anhydrides, and plicatic acid (redwood cedar). It is thought that they typically require conjugation with a protein, such as albumen, to form an antigenic compound capable of stimulating an immune response. The pathophysiology is not completely understood and may differ for the various agents.

7. What is meant by the term occupational asthma without latency?

Occupational asthma without latency is considered to be nonimmunologically mediated. Common terms used to describe this phenomenon include irritant-induced asthma or reactive airways dysfunction syndrome (RADS). Individuals develop the clinical characteristics of asthma (i.e., variable airflow obstruction and airway hyper-responsiveness) immediately following high-level exposure to an agent that is recognized to have strong irritant properties. It is postulated that many of these compounds cause direct airway injury. Patients have been shown to have evidence of airway inflammation, but they do not seem to develop this inflammation through typical immune-mediated mechanisms. The pathophysiology thus remains unknown.

It remains controversial whether chronic occupational exposure to irritants such as acid mists or various types of dusts or smoke can lead to asthma or asthma-like conditions. Workers report the gradual onset of asthma-like symptoms following chronic exposure to irritants (i.e., latency period), but these disorders do not appear to be immune-mediated. The terms irritant-induced bronchitis or industrial bronchitis have been used to describe these patients.

Finally, irritant-induced asthma must be distinguished from preexisting asthma that may be aggravated by workplace irritants. The latter group of workers generally have underlying asthma that is suboptimally controlled, and workplace irritant exposures act like other nonspecific triggers, leading to increased symptoms.

8. What are some common irritants?

Agents that induce irritant-induced asthma are presumed to cause direct airway injury, although the precise mechanism remains unknown and likely varies with the agent in question. Numerous agents have been considered as potential causes for irritant-induced asthma or RADS. Some of these agents remain on this list only because an immunologic mechanism has not been identified as yet.

Fire smoke

Gases such as chlorine and ammonia

Atmospheric pollutants such as ozone and sulfur dioxide

Oil-based or certain acrylic-based paints

Formaldehyde used in hospitals, embalming, and rubber and plastic industries (may be immune-mediated)

Aluminum smelter emissions containing gaseous fluorides, hydrofluoric acid, sulfur dioxide, and cold tar volatiles (potroom asthma)

Machining lubricant and coolant fluids containing trace amounts of metals, additives, and bactericidal agents which are potential respiratory irritants

Machining fluids with inadequate bactericidal agents, allowing growth of bacteria and fungi

9. Is there a difference between occupational asthma and work-related asthma?

The term work-related asthma encompasses not only asthma caused by work (occupational asthma) but also preexisting asthma aggravated by workplace exposures. Excessively dusty environments or strong odors and vapors in the workplace can be irritating to asthmatics, causing increased symptoms but not necessarily increasing immune-mediated airway inflammation or bronchial hyperresponsiveness. Work-related asthma has a much broader definition than occupational asthma and is used for medicolegal and workers' compensation purposes. Some jurisdictions recognize workplace aggravation of underlying asthma as compensable, while many other jurisdictions do not.

10. Outline a practical working differential diagnosis in the initial evaluation of occupational asthma.

The initial differential should include underlying asthma or chronic bronchitis irritated by workplace exposures. Hypersensitivity pneumonitis, which is often work-related, should be considered because it can have an inflammatory airway component (i.e., reversible airflow obstruction and bronchial hyperresponsiveness). Less commonly, other respiratory diseases that may have airway involvement, such as sarcoid, may be aggravated by workplace exposures.

The remainder of the differential diagnosis is similar to that for nonoccupational asthma and includes such varied entities as gastroesophageal reflux disease, rhinosinusitis with postnasal drip, vocal cord/upper airway dysfunction, irritant tracheobronchitis, and psychogenic or factitious conditions (malingering).

11. What clinical criteria suggest reactive airways dysfunction syndrome (RADS)?

Stuart Brooks is credited for labeling this clinically defined entity, which is characterized by several criteria including:

1. No prior history of asthma-like respiratory disease.

2. Onset follows high-level exposures which typically occur with accidents or spills.

3. Toxicants are typically recognized irritant gases, vapors, fumes, aerosols, or dusts in very high concentrations.

4. Onset of symptoms is abrupt, occurring within minutes to hours but always within the first 72 hours (original definition was 24 hours) of exposure.

5. Symptoms are identical to those of asthma, i.e, chest tightness, wheezing, dyspnea, cough.

6. Spirometry may demonstrate reversible airflow obstruction (i.e., > 12% improvement in FEV_1 after administration of a bronchodilator).

7. Nonspecific bronchial provocation with methacholine or histamine reveals a positive response (i.e., $PC_{20} < 8$ mg/ml).

8. Other respiratory disorders that simulate asthma are ruled out.

12. Is the clinical course of RADS distinct in any ways from other asthmas?

RADS patients are distinguished from those with so-called irritant-induced asthma by the fact that symptoms in RADS patients occur abruptly following a single, memorable, high-level exposure due to an accident, spill, or inappropriate handling of an irritant material. It has been proposed that irritant-induced asthma may occur following chronic exposure to irritant.

The clinical course of RADS otherwise is very much like that of other asthma, having a variable response to steroids and a variable long-term prognosis. Some patients have complete recovery within days to weeks, and others never completely recover. Some studies suggest that early treatment with steroids (inhaled and oral) may improve prognosis.

13. What are the current methods used to evaluate patients for possible occupational asthma?

Current methods for the evaluation and diagnosis of occupational/environmental asthma remain suboptimal. In most centers, the available methods include obtaining a thorough medical and exposure history and documenting the temporal relationship between exposures and onset of symptoms. Next, one collects objective data, including physical signs and pulmonary function tests, which assess the presence of airway obstruction, reversibility, and hyper-responsiveness. Once the presence of asthma is confirmed, there are various ways in which doctors try to determine whether it is work or environmentally related.

The most common (and least satisfactory) method is to judge the plausibility of a causality based on the temporal relationship of the patient's occupational exposures and the onset of symptoms. Furthermore, obtaining a full environmental history (i.e., home, pets, hobbies, travel) is critical for ruling out other potential sources of significant exposures. Studies have shown that the occupational history may be reasonably sensitive but is not very specific.

Alternatively, patients may be followed for symptoms and objective measurements of breathing function over 2–4 weeks at work and 2–4 weeks away from work. Breathing function is evaluated using peak flow monitors, spirometry, and/or methacholine inhalation tests. One typically looks for significant changes in breathing test results between the time at work and the time away from work. Unfortunately, many individuals cannot afford to remain off work for 2–4 weeks.

14. How is the history useful in evaluating occupational asthma?

1. Positive answers to questions about whether symptoms are worse at work and/or better on weekends, holidays, and vacations are useful to raise the suspicion of possible work-related asthma, though they are not very specific.

2. Understanding the duration of exposure to a particular agent (including current and previous jobs) before the onset of symptoms will establish the latency period and whether it is more likely to be an immune versus irritant effect. Individuals may have first developed sensitization in a previous job without noting symptoms but report developing symptoms after a relatively short time at a new job.

3. Ask about the onset of symptoms during the workshift. Individuals who report symptoms developing right away (within minutes) after starting the workshift are more likely to have irritant effects rather than immune-mediated effects.

4. Individuals with chronic low level irritant exposures may report progressive symptoms during the day and/or week suggesting an immune-mediated mechanism.

15. What is the usefulness of peak flow measurements, spirometry, and methacholine inhalation tests in evaluating occupational asthma?

Serial **peak flow** measurements are highly operator-dependent, and recent studies have suggested that they are unreliable to diagnose occupational asthma. They may be used as an adjunct in patients thought to be reliable and compliant or in supervised situations.

Serial **spirometry** comparisons either cross-shift and/or are more difficult to obtain during periods at and away from work because of the requirements for a technician and more sophisticated equipment. Considering how highly variable spirometry can be, these factors limit the number of measurements obtained and therefore make it difficult to follow and interpret trends.

Serial **methacholine** challenge tests are fairly reliable measurements of nonspecific bronchial hyper-responsiveness and should show a significant improvement (i.e., a 2–3-fold increase in PC_{20}) during time away from exposure. Unfortunately, adequate time (often 4 or more weeks) has to transpire between the exposure and nonexposure measurements of bronchial hyper-responsiveness before a significant difference in PC_{20} may be detected.

16. Are tests of immunoreactivity useful in occupational asthma?

As a general rule, tests of immunoreactivity are supportive evidence but neither rule in or rule out the possibility of occupational asthma. Currently, they should not be considered as an essential part of the evaluation of occupational asthma.

17. Can skin testing be used to confirm sensitivity to a workplace irritant?

Skin tests are not very specific for asthma, because some individuals may have positive skin tests and no objective evidence for asthma. Nor are they sensitive, as individuals may have negative skin tests and positive inhalation challenges. This is not surprising since many occupational agents cause sensitization through mechanisms other than IgE. Further, it is not possible to perform skin prick testing for some agents. Epicutaneous skin prick testing is more reliable and specific than intradermal testing, which may produce erroneous artifactual positive reactions.

Patch testing is a test of classic type IV immunologic (T-cell-mediated) response and is typically used to assess occupational allergic contact dermatitis. A number of occupational exposures (e.g,. latex, formaldehyde, nickel, epoxy resins) can cause both skin and respiratory symptoms, suggesting that such agents work through more than one immune-mediated mechanism to cause symptoms. Patch tests are not sensitive or specific for occupational asthma and are not regarded as particularly useful tests in the evaluation of workers with predominantly respiratory symptoms.

18. What is the role of RAST, ELISA, and serum immunoglobulins in the evaluation?

Elevated specific immunoglobulin levels (IgE, IgG), positive radioallergosorbent tests (RAST), and enzyme-linked immunosorbent assays (ELISA) have been found to occur with a number of high-molecular-weight protein antigens (e.g., latex, flour, animal proteins) and also for some low-molecular-weight agents (e.g., isocyanates, platinum salts, acid anhydrides), but they are not particularly specific. Asymptomatic exposed workers with no objective evidence of asthma may also develop positive antibodies. Hence, these tests confirm exposure and immune sensitization but do not confirm a diagnosis of asthma. No prospective cohort studies have been performed to establish the proportion of individuals with positive immunoglobulin levels to a particular agent who go on to develop work-related asthma.

19. What are specific inhalation challenges?

These tests are considered the gold standard for establishing whether a particular agent is the cause of a person's asthma. Specific inhalation challenges involve testing individuals by direct exposure to the potential workplace agent in a controlled lab environment (i.e., a challenge chamber). This typically requires observing a person during control (sham) exposures and increasing doses of the putative causative agent over several days. After the final exposure for a given day, subjects need to be observed for up to 8 or more hours in a hospital to ensure that they do not have a significant late reaction. Because there are few reliable, specialized centers that perform these tests, the reliability and reproducibility of these methods have not been thoroughly documented.

20. What are appropriate clinical indications for specific inhalation challenges?

- Individuals who may have become sensitized to a specific agent and in whom confirming the diagnosis has significance for possible job modification or compensation purposes. Identifying a specific agent may allow job modifications, such as substitution of the causative agent or engineering controls (process isolation), or even worker relocation.
- Individuals having a prior history of asthma or other respiratory conditions in whom there is a question of whether a specific workplace agent is causing a true immune (sensitized) response. If the worker is truly sensitized, he or she may need to switch jobs; if it is only an irritant effect, then lowering exposure levels through relocation, substitution, engineering controls, or personal protective equipment may be sufficient.
- Individuals who report a compelling history for work-related symptoms when exposed to a specific agent that has not been previously recognized as causing occupational asthma.

21. Discuss the limitations of specific inhalation challenge tests.

A negative specific inhalation test does not rule out occupational asthma, as it is possible that exposure to the agent in the workplace may be different or another agent may be causing the asthma. In fact, there have been documented cases in which individuals have been found to be sensitized to agents in neighboring plants or facilities. Furthermore, if patients have been removed from work exposure for a prolonged period of time before being challenged in the laboratory, they may not demonstrate hyper-responsiveness. Hence, interpretation and reporting of these tests must be limited to identifying the presence or absence of sensitization to a particular agent. A negative test cannot always be used to definitively establish whether or not a person has occupational asthma.

22. How should occupational asthma be managed?

The primary management of **immune-mediated** occupational asthma should be avoidance of exposure (which usually requires a change of job), because this can result in a cure and continued exposure can lead to more severe asthma. Pharmacologic treatment is not unlike that for non-occupational asthma, involving the judicious use of systemic and inhaled steroids and bronchodilator medications. Prophylactic anti-inflammatory agents, such as cromolyn sodium, are not of any proven benefit in this group of patients. After a period of removal from the offending exposure, some individuals will be able to discontinue all asthma medication. Unfortunately, a significant proportion of individuals will have persistent symptoms and require long-term medication.

In contrast, patients with irritant-induced asthma or RADS may be able to remain in their job with certain process modifications, such as substance substitution, process isolation (i.e., enclosure), improved ventilation, and/or personal protective equipment (respirators). Pharmacologic treatment is the same as for immune-mediated occupational asthma.

23. What is the prognosis for individuals with occupational asthma?

The outcome for occupational asthma is quite varied and depends on a number of factors. Individuals who are identified early and managed appropriately generally have a better prognosis than those who are identified after prolonged periods of symptoms with ongoing exposure. Certain persons simply require removal from exposure, while others may require steroid and bronchodilator medication temporarily or permanently. Some unfortunate patients develop steroid-dependent asthma despite removal from exposure. To date, we do not know if there are significant differences in prognosis between immune-mediated, RADS, or irritant-induced occupational asthma.

24. How should impairment ratings be established?

Occupational asthma is one of the occupational respiratory disorders that requires special evaluation when assessing impairment and disability. Strict adherence to the American Medical Association's guidelines for the basic evaluation of the respiratory system is inadequate. The guidelines actually allude to this fact and place occupational asthma in a special category.

Evaluation of individuals with occupational asthma should incorporate the degree of symptoms and medication requirements during periods of clinical stability with measurements of spirometry and nonspecific bronchial hyperresponsiveness (methacholine challenge PC_{20}). Maximum medical improvement for individuals with occupational asthma should not be assessed until 2 years after the final exposure to the causative agent. Individuals requiring evaluation and impairment ratings of occupational asthma should generally be referred to pulmonary physicians with a particular interest and expertise in occupational asthma.

BIBLIOGRAPHY

1. American Thoracic Society: Guidelines for the evaluation of impairment/disability in patients with asthma. Am Rev Respir Dis 147:1056–1061, 1993.
2. Bardana EJ, Montanaro A, O'Hollaren MT (eds): Occupational Asthma. Philadelphia, Hanley & Belfus, 1992.
3. Bernstein IL, Chan-Yeung M, Malo JL, Bernstein DI (eds): Asthma in the Workplace. New York, Marcel-Dekker, 1993.
4. Brooks SM, Weiss MA, Bernstein IL: Reactive airways dysfunction syndrome (RADS): Persistent asthma syndrome after high level irritant exposures. Chest 88:376–384, 1989.
5. Chan-Yeung M, Lam S: Occupational asthma. Am Rev Respir Dis 133:686–703, 1986.
6. Chan-Yeung M, Enarson DA, Kennedy SM: The impact of grain dust on respiratory health. Am Rev Respir Dis 145:476–487, 1992.
7. Chan-Yeung M, Malo JL: Occupational asthma. Curr Concepts 333(2):107–111, 1995.
8. Clapp WD, Becker S, Quay J, et al: Grain dust-induced airflow obstruction and inflammation of the lower respiratory tract. Am J Respir Crit Care Med 150:611–617, 1994.
9. Kennedy SM: Acquired airway hyperresponsiveness from nonimmunogenic irritant exposure. Occup Med State Art Rev 7:287–300, 1992.

55. DRUG-INDUCED LUNG DISEASE

Andrew H. Limper, M.D., and Edward C. Rosenow, III, M.D.

1. How is the diagnosis of drug-induced lung disease made?

With rare exceptions, this is a diagnosis of exclusion. Other possible causes must be excluded because the findings of histology, radiology, history, and physical examination can represent a number of other disorders. Histologic studies are almost never characteristic, with the rare exceptions of drug-induced bronchiolitis obliterans with organizing pneumonitis (BOOP), mitomycin-induced hemolytic uremia syndrome, drug-induced eosinophilia (which more than 30 drugs are known to cause), oil granulomas, and dantrolene- and bromocriptine-induced pleural effusions with high lymphocytic differential in the effusion.

2. How can I be sure what drugs the patient is taking?

A physician can never be certain what drugs a patient takes unless the patient or the family brings in all medications from home, including all over-the-counter medications. It is not enough to ask patients which drugs they take because the answer is usually a list of the prescribed drugs used every day. For example, more than 50% of patients who take nitrofurantoin as needed for urinary tract symptoms will not list it as a regular medication because they take it at their discretion and not at a physician's discretion. Patients almost never list eye drops or oily eye solutions; these are not considered medications because they are not taken by mouth. Yet timolol (Timoptic) ophthalmic solution has caused many deaths in patients with COPD. Although patients never consider mineral oil a drug, it can cause pulmonary manifestations ranging from a solitary nodule all the way to diffuse respiratory disease and respiratory failure. There are more than 200 medications containing acetylsalicylic acid, which can be associated with a variety of pulmonary complications.

3. Why is it important to know all of the drugs that an asthmatic is taking?

In one series of asthmatic patients admitted to the ICU, unintentional salicylate ingestion was found to be the precipitating cause for the asthmatic exacerbation in up to 10% of the cases. As mentioned, more than 200 medications contain acetylsalicylic acid so a careful history is critical in these patients. In addition, β-blocker eye drops, such as timolol (Timoptic), can also precipitate an asthmatic exacerbation. A good philosophy regarding any unexplained medical problem is "look for the drug."

4. How do I find out if a drug I am not familiar with is known to cause drug-induced pulmonary disease?

The *Physician's Desk Reference* (PDR) lists almost every reaction known to the pharmaceutical firm and will mention the possibility of a bronchopulmonary reaction if it has been reported. The next step would be to call the "800" number listed in the pharmaceutical directory in front of the PDR and talk specifically about the drug to one of the medical directors, who may know of pulmonary complications that have not yet been published in the medical literature.

5. Does surgery pose an increased risk in a patient previously treated with bleomycin for a metastatic testicular tumor? Is this a unique situation?

Surgery itself does not pose an increased risk, but the administration of an excessive amount of oxygen to any patient who has previously received bleomycin brings with it the hazard of inducing acute bleomycin toxicity. It is imperative that the anesthesiologist be informed that the patient has previously received bleomycin. It is important to recognize that even if the patient received bleomycin in the distant past, toxicity may occur with oxygen exposure. The rule of thumb is to keep the FIO_2 below 25% whenever possible and monitor the patient during the first 4 hours after surgery for signs and symptoms of early ARDS. The development of toxicity after the administration of oxygen is not unique to bleomycin; evidence now exists that a high F_{IO_2} can precipitate ARDS in patients receiving amiodarone. So far this has occurred only during the immediate postoperative period.

6. What are the pulmonary complications associated with mitomycin C?

Mitomycin C can produce a hemolytic uremia syndrome; half of the patients who have it develop acute pulmonary edema resembling ARDS. There is no way to predict which patients will develop these complications. Renal and pulmonary biopsies show characteristic intravascular thrombi. The condition is serious and has a mortality rate of more than 50%.

7. A 26-year-old man with cerebral palsy has developed a left pleural effusion. He is afebrile and has no history of aspiration. The only medication he regularly takes is dantrolene to help control muscle spasms. The pleural fluid obtained by thoracentesis is an exudate with marked lymphocytosis. What other diagnostic studies are needed?

Nothing more needs to be done. Dantrolene and bromocriptine, which is used in Parkinson's disease, are both known to produce exudative pleural effusions with high lymphocyte counts. The pleural effusion resolves if the drug is stopped.

8. A 62-year-old female smoker with hypertension presents with acute pulmonary edema. Past medical history includes several admissions for the same problem. A recent work-up for cardiovascular disease had negative findings, including a normal coronary angiogram. The patient has hypertension, diabetes, peptic ulcer disease, and mild chronic lung disease. Her medications include glyburide, ranitidine, a long-acting theophylline preparation, atenolol, and hydrochlorothiazide. She takes the hydrochlorothiazide only occasionally, when her ankles swell. What is her diagnosis?

There are enough case reports of hydrochlorothiazide-induced noncardiac pulmonary edema to make this drug the likely culprit. Each time this patient was admitted to the hospital, all medications were stopped and her symptoms resolved. After discharge, however, she resumed taking the same medications. She might not have mentioned the hydrochlorothiazide as a regular medication because she is taking it at her discretion. The mechanism of this noncardiac pulmonary edema is unknown.

9. What drugs may produce acute respiratory insufficiency?

Bleomycin/oxygen
Mitomycin
Bleomycin (with eosinophilia hypersensitivity)
Procarbazine (with eosinophilia hypersensitivity)
Methotrexate (with eosinophilia hypersensitivity)
Amphotericin B
Nitrofurantoin (acute)
Acetylsalicylic acid
Interleukin-2
Heroin
Epinephrine
Fibrinolytic agents
Protamine
Blood products
Hydrochlorothiazide
Tocolytic agents
Tricyclic antidepressants
Complement-mediated leukostasis
Dextran-70 (Hyskon)
Tumor necrosing factor
Intrathecal methotrexate

10. You are asked to see a 22-year-old multiparous woman in labor who has acute pulmonary edema. The patient was admitted in premature labor, which was treated with a tocolytic agent that failed to stop the uterine contractions. The tocolytic agent was stopped and she was given intramuscular hydrocortisone to accelerate fetal lung maturation. There is no evidence that she aspirated during this hospitalization. Physical examination reveals no evidence of cardiac disease or deep venous thrombosis. What is the likely cause of her pulmonary edema?

Tocolytic agent–induced noncardiac pulmonary edema is well recognized. The tocolytic agent causes a peripheral vasodilation, which usually is well tolerated by the mother, but when the agent is stopped, the blood vessel tone returns to normal and squeezes intravascular fluid into tissues, including the lungs. In patients receiving tocolytic agents a drop in the hematocrit and blood pressure may be an indicator of hemodilution and may signal the healthcare provider to decrease the rate of administration of the tocolytic to prevent development of pulmonary edema. The mineralocorticoid effect of the hydrocortisone administered to the patient also causes fluid retention, further aggravating the situation. The presentation of tocolytic–induced pulmonary edema mimics that of a number of disorders, including aspiration, myocarditis with failure, amniotic fluid embolism, and even pulmonary embolism (a diffuse edematous picture is uncommon in the latter but must be considered). The treatment is supportive care.

11. A 30-year-old patient presents with diffuse patchy pulmonary infiltrates and peripheral eosinophilia. Could this be drug related?

The many drugs known to produce pulmonary infiltrates with eosinophilia include:

Acetylsalicylic acid	Imipramine	Procarbazine
Ampicillin	Mephenesin	Propranolol
Bleomycin	Naproxen	Sulfasalazine
Carbamazepine	Nitrofurantoin	Tetracycline
Chlorpropamide		

12. A patient presents with classic chest radiographic, high-resolution CT, and histologic findings for idiopathic pulmonary fibrosis. Are there any medications that could cause this?

The main drug to consider in this setting is nitrofurantoin, which is often taken by women on a long-term basis for recurring urinary tract infections. The histologic findings and radiographic images seen are classic for idiopathic pulmonary fibrosis, but the prognosis is better for nitrofurantoin-induced lung disease. In fact, about half of these cases will reverse spontaneously when the drug is withdrawn; however, the other half may require corticosteroids for 3–6 months in moderate doses such as 60 mg every other day. In our experience these patients frequently do not volunteer that they are on nitrofurantoin because they take it at their discretion.

13. A patient with seropositive rheumatoid arthritis has been receiving low-dose methotrexate once a week and now has a pulmonary infiltrate of insidious onset. Can a drug-induced infiltrate be separated from rheumatoid lung without separating the patient from her life savings?

Sometimes the distinction can be difficult without more elaborate testing, but if doubt exists, discontinuation of the methotrexate should reverse the process, especially if corticosteroids are added or increased. Approximately 50% of these patients have peripheral blood eosinophilia, which would not occur in rheumatoid lung. Granulomatous changes usually are seen on biopsy samples if the infiltrate is drug-induced. Their presence would again rule out a rheumatoid lung. Several cases of opportunistic infections, especially *Pneumocystis carinii* pneumonia, have been reported in patients taking low-dose methotrexate.

14. A 29-year-old patient who is a known drug addict was seen in the emergency department for diffuse pulmonary infiltrates and hemoptysis. Is this related to the drugs he has been taking?

Almost certainly, and the one to consider here is crack cocaine. The inhalation of crack cocaine can produce diffuse alveolar hemorrhage in some individuals. Fewer than 50% of the patients who present with noncardiogenic pulmonary edema complain of hemoptysis, which makes the diagnosis difficult. These patients are also at risk for cocaine-induced cardiac dysfunction, which also needs to be considered in the differential diagnosis.

15. How is amiodarone pneumonitis diagnosed?

Amiodarone may be associated with the following presentations: interstitial pneumonitis, ARDS (? oxygen precipitated), mass lesion (can cavitate), BOOP, eosinophilic pneumonitis, and asthma aggravation. Patients may present with either acute or insidious onset of symptoms, including shortness of breath and a nonproductive cough. The differential diagnosis includes subacute pneumonitis, congestive heart failure (which is seen commonly in this situation because all patients have cardiac disease), and pulmonary emboli. Usually the patient has been on amiodarone, 400 mg or more per day, for more than 2 months. The pattern seen on chest radiograph varies and can be quite asymmetric. Most patients with amiodarone lung have an erythrocyte sedimentation rate of more than 50 mm per hour. Bronchoalveolar lavage may be helpful in the diagnosis. Although even those patients on amiodarone who do not have pulmonary disease may have phospholipid-filled alveolar macrophages, their absence would exclude the possibility of amiodarone pneumonitis. Most patients respond to corticosteroids, but as many as 10–20% of patients can die from their respiratory complications.

16. Anigotensin-converting enzyme (ACE) inhibitor–induced cough can be a problem if the patient needs this drug. Is there anything that can be done?

As many as 15% of patients taking ACE inhibitors complain of cough. Some physicians have used nebulized cromolyn sodium or oral indomethacin to counter this cough when the cardiologist says it is essential for the patient to continue on the ACE inhibitor. Another alternative is to try the new drug, losartan, which is an angiotensin II inhibitor that does not affect bradykinin and is not associated with cough. It is worth noting that an under-recognized complication of the ACE inhibitors is angioedema of the face and upper airway.

17. I saw a 42-year-old patient on bleomycin with nodules in the lung that were presumed to be metastases. However, biopsy results showed they were consistent with BOOP. What caused this?

Bleomycin. Although there are many drugs known to be associated with BOOP, as shown below, bleomycin is the only one that we know of that produces nodules mimicking metastasis. The BOOP induced by other drugs appears as more of a patchy or semidiffuse pneumonitis.

Amiodarone	Gold	Penicillamine
Bleomycin	Methotrexate	Radiation
Cocaine	Mitomycin C	Sulfasalazine
Cyclophosphamide		

BIBLIOGRAPHY

1. Hargreaves MR, Mowat AG, Benson MK: Acute pneumonitis associated with low dose methotrexate treatment for rheumatoid arthritis: Report of five cases and review of published reports. Thorax 47:628–633, 1992.
2. Kavaru MS, Ahmad M, Amirthalingam KN: Hydrochlorothiazide-induced acute pulmonary edema. Cleve Clin J Med 57:181–184, 1990.
3. Lunde H, Hedner T, Samuelsson O, et al: Dyspnoea, asthma, and bronchospasm in relation to treatment with angiotensin converting enzyme inhibitors. BMJ 308:18–21, 1994.
4. Martin WJ II, Rosenow EC III: Amiodarone pulmonary toxicity. Recognition and pathogenesis (Part I). Chest 93:1067–1075, 1988.
5. Meisels IS, Loke J: The pulmonary effects of free-base cocaine: A review. Cleve Clin J Med 60:325–329, 1993.
6. Myers JL: Diagnosis of drug reactions in the lung. Monogr Pathol 36:32–53, 1993.
7. O'Donnell AE, Selig J, Aravamuthan M, et al: Pulmonary complications associated with illicit drug use. An update. Chest 108:460–463, 1995.
8. Pisani RJ, Rosenow EC III: Pulmonary edema associated with tocolytic therapy. Ann Intern Med 110:714–718, 1989.
9. Reed CR, Glauser FL: Drug-induced noncardiogenic pulmonary edema. Chest 100:1120–1124, 1991.
10. Rosenow EC III: Drug-induced pulmonary disease. Dis Mon 40:253–310, 1994.
11. Rosenow EC III, Myers JL, Swenson SJ, et al: Drug-induced pulmonary disease. An update. Chest 102:239–250, 1992.
12. Sahn SA: The pleura. Am Rev Respir Dis 138:184–234, 1988.
13. Salerno SM, Strong JS, Roth BJ, et al: Eosinophilic pneumonia and respiratory failure associated with a trazodone overdose. Am J Respir Crit Care Med 152:2170–2172, 1995.
14. Zitnik RJ: Drug-induced lung disease: Cancer chemotherapy agents. J Respir Dis 10:855–865, 1995.

56. RADIATION PNEUMONITIS

Ann M. Wierman, M.D., and Marie E. Wood, M.D.

1. What is radiation pneumonitis?

Radiation pneumonitis is a form of acute lung injury that develops in response to any type of ionizing radiation and causes a spectrum of symptoms. The total dose of radiation and the daily amount of radiation (fractionation) received are the most important factors influencing the development of radiation pneumonitis. At fractionated doses of 180–200 cGy (1 cGy = 1 rad), radiation is generally well tolerated and pulmonary toxicity is mild. Fractionated doses of 250 cGy or more greatly increase the incidence of symptomatic radiation pneumonitis, which may occur in more than 20% of patients treated with this dose.

2. What are the clinical characteristics of the acute phase of radiation pneumonitis?

Acute radiation pneumonitis occurs in a small subset of patients receiving therapeutic radiotherapy. The major symptoms are dyspnea, minimally productive or nonproductive cough, and tachypnea. Other potential manifestations include a low-grade fever, night sweats, leukocytosis, dyspnea on exertion, cyanosis, and increased sputum production, with or without mild hemoptysis. Some degree of histologic lung damage develops in any patient who receives radiation to the thorax. These microscopic tissue changes may be detectable as early as 24 hours after the initial radiation exposure. Patients usually do not manifest symptoms, however, until 2–3 months after the completion of radiation therapy. Symptoms may last from a few days to as long as 6 months.

3. What are the signs and symptoms of the chronic phase of radiation pneumonitis (radiation fibrosis)?

The chronic phase of radiation pneumonitis (also termed *radiation fibrosis*) may evolve over 6–24 months but generally stabilizes within 2 years. In this condition, the ionizing radiation precipitates chronic remodeling of the lung resulting in pulmonary fibrosis. Progressive thickening and fibrotic scarring of both the vascular and interstitial compartments of the lung occur.

Clinical manifestations of this disorder result from fibrotic changes that occur in the pulmonary parenchyma. Patients may be asymptomatic or have only mild dyspnea. In other instances, respiratory failure or the gradual development of cor pulmonale may occur. Radiation fibrosis may develop without antecedent episodes of acute pneumonitis.

4. Does a grading system exist for radiation-induced pulmonary toxicity?

The Radiation Therapy Oncology Group (RTOG) and the European Organization for Research and Treatment of Cancer (EORTC) have established scales of 0 to 5 to grade the severity of the acute and late phases of radiation-induced pulmonary injury. These scales incorporate the degree of symptoms, the intensity of radiographic changes, the requirements for oxygen support, and the eventual clinical outcome in severe instances of each condition. The latter variable is used for epidemiologic studies of radiation pneumonitis.

Acute Phase Scale

Grade 0   No symptoms
Grade 1   Mild cough or dyspnea on exertion
Grade 2   Cough with minimal exertion or requiring medical treatment
Grade 3   Oxygen and/or steroids required for symptoms at rest
Grade 4   Continuous oxygen or mechanical ventilatory support required
Grade 5   Death related to progressive fibrosis and/or radiation-induced respiratory insufficiency

Chronic Phase Scale

Grade 0   No symptoms
Grade 1   Asymptomatic or mild cough, with slight radiographic changes
Grade 2   Moderate symptoms caused by acute pneumonitis or chronic fibrosis
Grade 3   Severe symptoms with dense radiographic changes
Grade 4   Continuous oxygen or mechanical ventilatory support required
Grade 5   Death related to progressive fibrosis and/or radiation-induced respiratory
           insufficiency

5. Are there any other types of radiation pneumonitis?

Yes. Some authors believe that a hypersensitivity pneumonitis can occur in patients exposed to ionizing radiation. This reaction can develop even outside of the boundaries of the radiation port (even in the contralateral lung) and may result from tissue factors released from radiation damaged cells. Because this entity can produce pulmonary infiltrates in regions of nonradiated lung it may create a confusing clinical picture by simulating other lung conditions that can occur in patients with lung cancer, such as pneumonia, pulmonary infarction, or other drug-induced reactions.

6. What percent of individuals receiving radiation to the chest develop radiation pneumonitis?

The incidence of mild to moderate radiation pneumonitis approximates 10%; severe pneumonitis occurs in 1–3% of treated patients.

7. What radiographic changes are seen in radiation pneumonitis?

Radiographic abnormalities may be seen in radiation pneumonitis as soon as the first 2 weeks after the initiation of therapy, which is much earlier than the onset of clinical symptoms. Classically, only the lung parenchyma directly within the radiation port shows radiographic abnormalities, which are usually not defined by lung segments or lobes. In the 1970s and 1980s, infiltrates often corresponded to the square radiation ports used at that time, which gave rise to their description as "square pneumonias." This radiographic pattern is now less commonly seen because of innovations in radiation oncology, such as the use of individualized protective lung shields and modifications in the size of radiation ports as tumors shrink during the course of therapy. The earliest radiographic manifestation may be hyperlucency within the field of radiation, which corresponds to regional oligemia. Next, ground glass infiltrates develop that may progress over the next 3–4 months. Infiltrates may coalesce and appear nodular. Over the next 12–18 months, a fibrotic pattern generally occurs. Eventually, all of these patients develop histologic evidence of chronic fibrosis.

8. How should a patient with symptoms of radiation pneumonitis be evaluated.?

A chest radiograph should be obtained to evaluate symptomatic patients for radiographic abnormalities consistent with radiation pneumonitis. Often the radiographic findings are more impressive than the severity of the patient's symptoms and physical examination abnormalities. A chest radiograph may also assist the evaluation by excluding other causes of the patient's symptoms, such as pleural effusions, rib fractures, spontaneous pneumothoraces, and pulmonary hypertension. A CT scan affords the best radiographic visualization of the lung and may localize infiltrates to the radiation port, thereby supporting the diagnosis. Chest CT, however, may also demonstrate subtle infiltrates outside of the region exposed to radiation that appear to result from hypersensitivity reactions. CT scans can visualize tapering of the pulmonary vasculature entering the region of the radiation field, which is a common finding in radiation pneumonitis. Finally, CT may suggest the presence of opportunistic infections or other intrathoracic abnormalities independent of radiation-induced changes, such as tumor progression or lymphangitic spread of the cancer. Pulmonary function studies with diffusing capacity and room air arterial blood gas levels or pulse oximetry determination of oxygen saturation assist in the evaluation of these patients.

9. Is MRI helpful in the assessment of radiation pneumonitis?

MRI is not helpful in distinguishing acute radiation pneumonitis from other causes of lung injury. It may, however, assist in differentiating radiation fibrosis from recurrent tumor because fibrosis has low signals on T1 and T2-weighted imaging, in contrast to tumor, which is enhanced on T2 images.

10. What changes in pulmonary function occur with radiation pneumonitis?

In general, patients develop a decreased diffusing capacity (DLCO), decreased PaO_2, and decreased lung compliance. The changes in pulmonary function observed after radiation therapy, however, depend on the nature and degree of lung function abnormalities that existed before the radiation exposure. If pretreatment pulmonary reserve is compromised by baseline COPD, a minimal decline in pulmonary function can be expected in most patients after radiation therapy. However, if the pretreatment compromise of lung function resulted from effects of the tumor (obstructive pneumonia or infiltrative disease), patients may actually experience improvement in their pulmonary function.

11. Describe the histopathologic changes seen in radiation pneumonitis.

Histopathologic changes begin as early as 24 hours after radiation exposure and progress in a stereotypical pattern. Initially, type II alveolar cells react with an immediate increase in surfactant production. Type I alveolar cells are somewhat more radioresistant and do not demonstrate this early reactivity. Eventually, sloughing of alveoli occurs with an intraalveolar accumulation of debris and elements of the inflammatory response. These events have been termed the *exudative* or *latent phase*. Interstitial foam cells, abnormal fibroblast proliferation, and bizarre type II alveolar cells are also evident in tissue sections.

In some patients the lung may ultimately undergo structural changes that result in fibrosis and loss of functional lung volume 3–6 months after completion of therapy. Intimal thickening and obliterative vasculitis with sclerosis and loss of air spaces are the hallmarks of this fibrotic stage. Pleural effusions and eventual pleural thickening also can occur. Parenchymal and pleural fibrosis may combine to cause severe restrictive changes and compromised lung function. Symptoms may be exacerbated if severe scarring contracts the lung toward the hilum and mediastinal structures. Pulmonary fibrosis may progress over 12–18 months until it stabilizes.

12. How do other factors influence the development of radiation pneumonitis?

The following factors are known to influence the development of pneumonitis:

- **Technique of dose delivery.** Although the dose and fractionation of radiation therapy are the most critical factors in predicting pulmonary toxicity, the technique of dose delivery is also important. Anterior and posterior versus medial and lateral beams, tangential beams, compensating filters, and the amount of lung shielding dramatically affect the risk of developing radiation pneumonitis.
- **Prior radiotherapy.** Prior radiation exposure—even if it occurred years earlier—may contribute to radiation pneumonitis with subsequent exposures.
- **Comorbid disease.** The volume of irradiated lung does not usually correlate with the risk of radiation pneumonitis. If baseline pulmonary function abnormalities or comorbid cardiopulmonary diseases are present, however, larger radiation ports may be associated with a greater likelihood of pulmonary toxicity.
- **Concomitant chemotherapy.** Combination therapy with chemotherapeutic agents and lung irradiation may promote the toxic pulmonary effects of the drugs, the radiotherapy, or both.

13. What are some of the interactions commonly observed between radiation therapy and chemotherapeutic agents?

Combining radiation and chemotherapy may increase the incidence of radiation pneumonitis to as high as 20–30%. Certain drugs (especially the "radiosensitizing" agents methotrexate and *cis*platinum) given in a neoadjuvant, concurrent, sequential, or consolidative fashion may exacerbate lung injury induced by radiation. When cyclophosphamide is combined with a radiation regimen, radiation pneumonitis may increase substantially, unless the total dose of radiation is decreased by 30% or more. Cyclophosphamide in combination with total body irradiation for bone marrow transplantation may produce the "white lung syndrome" unless adequate lung filters are used. Conversely, bleomycin lung toxicity may be promoted by lung irradiation. The use of doxorubicin and dactinomycin may initiate "radiation recall," a condition in which previously irradiated lung is injured with the subsequent administration of these agents.

14. What is the therapeutic approach to radiation pneumonitis?

Prednisone is the treatment of choice for symptomatic radiation pneumonitis. Steroids rapidly decrease dyspnea and improve exercise tolerance in acute radiation pneumonitis. The effects of steroid therapy may be seen within 24 hours of initiation of treatment. Patients usually require 4–6 months of therapy followed by a slow and well-monitored tapering of prednisone doses. Treatment also should include serial evaluation using weekly pulse oximetry and intermittent spirometric measurements to monitor lung function. Symptoms may be exacerbated to pretreatment levels in some patients after prednisone is withdrawn. The prompt initiation of steroids for symptoms of acute pneumonitis has no impact on preventing radiation fibrosis or attenuating its eventual severity. Prednisone may delay the onset of fibrotic changes for several months, however.

15. How can radiation pneumonitis be prevented?

Careful dosing of patients and consideration of underlying risk factors for lung injury are the most important steps in preventing radiation pneumonitis. In the future, other preventive measures may become available. Free radical scavengers have been evaluated but to date no effective agent has been identified for clinical use. Several inflammatory cytokines, such as interleukin-1a and tissue growth factor-β, have been implicated in the generation of radiation-induced lung injury. Blockade of these cytokines perhaps combined with the inhibition of transcription of genes known to induce fibrosis may be prophylactic options in the future.

BIBLIOGRAPHY

1. Anscher MS, Murase T, Prescott DM, et al: Changes in the plasma TGF beta levels during pulmonary radiotherapy as a predictor of the risk of developing radiation pneumonitis. Int J Radiat Oncol Biol Phys 30:671–675, 1994.
2. Bai YH, Wang DW, Wang LP, et al: The role of free radicals in the development of radiation interstitial pneumonitis. J Environ Pathol Toxicol Oncol 12:199–204, 1993.
3. Cox JD, Stetz J, Pajak TF: Toxicity criteria of the Radiation Therapy Oncology Group (RTOG) and the European Organization for the Research and Treatment of Cancer (EORTC). Int J Radiat Oncol Biol Phys 31:1341-1346, 1995.
4. Jakacki RI, Schramm CM, Donahue BR, et al: Restrictive lung disease following treatment for malignant brain tumors: A potential late effect of craniospinal irradiation. J Clin Oncol 13:1478–1485, 1995.
5. Kao GD, McKenna WG: Genetics of radiation resistance. Molecular Biology and Genetics. 1994, pp 446–452.
6. Kimsey FC, Mendenhall NP, Ewald LM, et al: Is radiation treatment volume a predictor for acute or late effect on pulmonary function? A prospective study of patients treated with breast-conserving surgery and postoperative radiation. Cancer 73:2549–2555, 1995.
7. Lin M: Radiation pneumonitis caused by yttrium-90 microspheres: Radiologic findings. Am J Roentgenol 162:1300–1302, 1994.
8. Mah K, Keane TJ, Van Dyk J, et al: Quantitative effect of combined chemotherapy and fractionated radiotherapy on the incidence of radiation-induced lung damage: A prospective clinical study. Int J Radiat Oncol Biol Phys 28:563–574, 1994.
9. McDonald S, Rubin P, Phillips TL, et al: Injury to the lung from cancer therapy: Clinical syndromes, measurable endpoints, and potential scoring systems. Int J Radiat Oncol Biol Phys 31:1187–1203, 1995.
10. Morgan GW, Breit SN: Radiation and the lung: A reevaluation of the mechanisms mediating pulmonary injury. Int J Radiat Oncol Biol Phys 31:361–369, 1995 (Review).
11. Rubin P, Johnston CJ, Williams JP, et al: A perpetual cascade of cytokines postradiation leads to pulmonary fibrosis. In J Radiat Oncol Biol Phys 33:99–109, 1995.

57. INHALATIONAL INJURIES

David A. Kaminsky, M.D.

1. Name some common toxic inhalational agents and their sources.

The most common sources of toxic inhalational agents are industry, the home, and fire. Various industries involve the production of substances such as hydrogen sulfide (mining, petroleum), hydrogen chloride (plastics), ammonia (agriculture, plastics), chlorine (paper and textiles) oxides of nitrogen (agriculture, mining, welding), phosgene (welding, paint stripping), and sulfur dioxide (smelting, coal and oil combustion). Exposures in the home include chlorine gas (cleaning products) and carbon monoxide (heaters, automobiles, fires). Fires, in general, cause exposure to at least 75 different substances, the most important of which are carbon monoxide, carbon dioxide, nitrogen dioxide, hydrogen cyanide, phosgene, and aromatic compounds and aldehydes. Less common sources of toxic inhalational agents include hobbies (volatile hydrocarbons, metal fumes) and chemical warfare (organophosphates, phosgene, chlorine).

2. Describe the factors involved in determining the toxicity of inhalational agents.

The physical properties of a substance determine its major site of deposition and mechanism of injury. In general, substances that cause primarily upper airway injury tend to be larger (more than 5 microns) and more water soluble. In contrast, smaller (less than 1 micron), less water soluble agents are more likely to cause lower airway and alveolar damage. Substances may also be categorized as primarily irritating or asphyxiating, depending on their chemical effects. The intensity and duration of exposure are also important in dictating the severity of symptoms, as are any underlying host factors (preexisting pulmonary disease or other chronic medical illness). Since water-soluble agents tend to be quite irritating, they cause immediate symptoms that give the victim early warning of exposure. Less irritating substances, unfortunately, often result in more prolonged and intense exposure because the victim has little if any immediate warning.

Chemical Effect	Mechanism	Example
Irritant	Alkaline burn	Ammonia
	Acid burn, free radicals	Chlorine
	Acid burn, oxidation	Nitrogen dioxide
Inert	Asphyxiation (displacement of alveolar oxygen)	Carbon dioxide, methane
Binds to heme-containing proteins or cellular enzymes	Inhibit oxygen binding or utilization	Carbon monoxide, cyanide

3. What are the short-term and long-term consequences of exposures to toxic inhalational agents?

Severe upper airway irritation occurs within minutes after exposure to irritating gases. Pulmonary edema and pneumonia also may result from acute exposure to substances such as ammonia, chlorine, oxides of nitrogen, phosgene, and sulfur dioxide. In addition, many substances have immediate systemic effects as a result of cellular asphyxia (e.g., hydrogen cyanide), central nervous system dysfunction, or bone marrow suppression (e.g., benzenes). Weeks later, some substances cause more chronic respiratory problems, such as bronchitis (e.g., ammonia), bronchiolitis obliterans (e.g., oxides of nitrogen, sulfur oxide) and airway hyperreactivity (e.g., sulfur dioxide).

4. Describe the effects of exposure to ammonia, an upper airway irritant.

Ammonia is a highly water soluble, colorless, strongly alkaline gas with a pungent, irritating odor. It is widely used as an industrial chemical in the production of fertilizers, nitric acid, dyes, plastics, and pharmaceuticals. When ammonia combines with water in the upper respiratory tract, ammonium hydroxide and heat are both liberated. Thus, ammonia causes severe chemical injury from alkali-induced liquefaction of the mucosa as well as direct thermal injury. Clinically, patients who experience mild exposures may present with lacrimation, cough, and headache; those with more severe exposures present with upper airway edema manifested as chest tightness, dyspnea, wheezing, and stridor. Frank pulmonary edema or pneumonia may ensue, and the case fatality rate after severe exposure is approximately 40%. Treatment is mainly supportive, although antibiotics may prevent bacterial superinfection in patients with severe mucosal injury.

5. How does injury after exposure to the poorly soluble gas phosgene present?
    Unlike ammonia, phosgene exposure gives few warning signs because of its poor water solubility and consequent lack of upper airway irritation. Most exposures occur in chemical plants, although firefighters, dry cleaners, and welders are also at risk. Phosgene slowly hydrolyzes in mucosal water to form hydrochloric acid and carbon dioxide, so many minutes to hours may pass before symptoms develop related to direct epithelial damage and necrosis of small airways and capillary membranes. The clinical result is dyspnea, chest tightness, cyanosis, and hemoptysis, with progression to ARDS. Treatment is supportive.

6. What is silo filler's disease?
    Silo filler's disease occurs when a farmer develops respiratory failure after exposure to toxic levels of nitrogen dioxide that form within the first few days after storage of grain. Nitrogen dioxide is a reddish-brown gas that is heavier than air and has a characteristic sweet odor. It is representative of the oxides of nitrogen that form from the fermentation of grain nitrates. Because these gases are heavier than air they tend to accumulate in silos just above the grain surface, and a worker entering the silo from the top may be at risk of exposure. The pulmonary toxicity that develops is caused by the formation of nitric acid when the oxides of nitrogen react with water in the lower respiratory tract. Potent oxidation products released from the nitric acid cause local tissue inflammation, impairment of lung surfactant, and collagen damage.

7. Describe the clinical phases of silo filler's disease.
    • **Phase 1 (immediate).** Bronchospasm, dyspnea, nausea and vomiting, headache, and chest pain. Pulmonary edema may develop within 4–24 hours and patients may die before they reach a medical facility. Methemoglobin formation has been found in some cases.
    • **Phase 2 (2–5 weeks after exposure).** Symptoms abate during this time, but cough, malaise, and dyspnea may persist. Chest radiograph usually clears.
    • **Phase 3 (up to 5 weeks after exposure).** Development of bronchiolitis obliterans with interstitial miliary nodular pattern on chest radiograph, accompanied by fever, chills, cough, and progressive shortness of breath. Corticosteroids have been used with some success in this phase, but some patients develop persistent airflow limitation, and a small number die of respiratory failure.

8. What gas is well known for causing both upper and lower respiratory tract injury?
    Chlorine. Chlorine gas is a dense, heavy, irritating gas with a distinctive pungent odor. Exposure may occur in a variety of settings, including industry, home, and school. Because of its moderate water solubility, chlorine may affect the entire respiratory tree, depending on the duration and concentration of exposure. Chlorine reacts with water to form hydrochloric acid and oxygen-free radicals; it is estimated to be 20 times more irritating than hydrochloric acid alone. Tissue damage is manifested by epithelial sloughing and ulceration, purulent exudation, and increased capillary permeability and pulmonary edema. Symptoms include upper airway irritation and lacrimation in addition to chest tightness, dyspnea, and cough. Both obstructive and restrictive physiology may be found on pulmonary function testing. Treatment is supportive, but corticosteroids appear to be useful after chlorine exposure in patients with severe airflow limitation. Prophylactic antibiotics are generally not recommended despite the presence of significant airway mucosal disruption.

9. List other directly irritating inhalational agents and some of their characteristics.

- **Acrolein.** Clear yellow liquid with pungent odor; found in manufacturing, sewage treatment, cigarette smoke, smog, products of combustion of wood, paper and cotton; upper airway irritant; causes mucosal irritation, lacrimation, pulmonary edema.
- **Formaldehyde.** Colorless gas with pungent odor; commercial, medical, industrial sources; combustion product of gas stoves, heaters, cigarettes; component of smog; chronic home exposure may produce recurrent respiratory and systemic symptoms; causes upper airway irritation; airway hyperreactivity.
- **Hydrogen chloride.** Highly water soluble acid; used in manufacturing; produced from thermal combustion of polyvinyl chloride; immediate upper airway irritation with cough, dyspnea, and wheezing; possibly noncardiogenic pulmonary edema.
- **Ozone.** Naturally occurring form of oxygen produced in the upper atmosphere; occupational risks include welding, waste treatment, cold storage, food preservation; component of smog; sweet-smelling gas with moderate water solubility; causes upper and lower respiratory tract inflammation and may result in new or worsened airway hyperresponsiveness; clinical symptoms include chest pain, cough, and dyspnea.
- **Sulfur dioxide.** Highly water soluble, clear, dense gas; by-product of industry, component of smog; upper airway irritant; damage via formation of sulfurous acid; may cause upper airway obstruction, cyanosis, and pulmonary edema.

10. In what way are carbon dioxide, nitrogen, methane, ethane, helium, and hydrogen similar?

These gases cause toxicity upon inhalation by simple asphyxiation, because oxygen is displaced or removed from the ambient air. Such biologically inert gases must be in high concentration (more than 85% of inspired air) to exert this effect. Coal mining is the most important occupational hazard in this regard because exposures to high levels of methane gas may occur.

11. A patient presents with headache, weakness, and confusion. She recently had a new gas furnace installed. Her arterial blood gas shows a P_{O_2} of 80 on room air, but her arterial saturation is 97% by pulse oximetry. What is the most likely diagnosis?

Carbon monoxide (CO) poisoning. CO is a colorless, odorless gas produced by incomplete combustion of carbon-containing compounds such as wood, coal, and gasoline. Asphyxiation from CO is responsible for approximately 3,500 deaths per year in the United States. CO does not directly injure the lung. Instead, it displaces oxygen from hemoglobin with a binding affinity for hemoglobin that is 250 times higher than that of oxygen. In addition, CO shifts the oxyhemoglobin curve to the left, thereby reducing oxygen release at the tissue level, and binds to myoglobin in cardiac muscle, resulting in decreased oxygen availability to the heart. Finally, CO also binds to cytochrome oxidase, thus directly interfering with cellular respiration. Although the serum level of carboxyhemoglobin may not accurately reflect tissue levels of CO, blood levels and clinical signs tend to be correlated.

Carboxyhemoglobin Level (% of Total Hemoglobin)	Symptoms
0–5	None (normal value)
15–20	Headache, tinnitus
20–40	Disorientation, fatigue, nausea, weakness
40–60	Confusion, coma, respiratory failure
> 60	Shock, death (mortality > 50%)

12. What are some clinical clues in the diagnosis of CO poisoning?

The diagnosis of CO poisoning may not always be straightforward, especially if the exposure took place in the home. This was well illustrated in a recently published case report in

320 Inhalational Injuries

which a husband and wife repeatedly presented to the emergency department with acute cardiac ischemia caused by occult exposure to CO at home. Thus, epidemiologic clues may be very valuable. A further clue to the diagnosis is the classic cherry-red color to the skin; however, this sign is found in less than 10% of cases and usually only at high carboxyhemoglobin concentrations.

One of the most valuable clues is the discrepancy in the measured Po_2 and the saturation by pulse oximetry. The discrepancy is useful for the following reason. Pulse oximeters use only two wavelengths of light to assess the ratio of oxyhemoglobin and deoxyhemoglobin: 660 nm, at which absorption of deoxyhemoglobin is high relative to oxyhemoglobin, and 940 nm, at which absorption of oxyhemoglobin is high relative to deoxyhemoglobin. At 940 nm, carboxyhemoglobin has minimal light absorption, but at 660 nm, its absorption coefficient is similar to that of oxyhemoglobin; therefore, the pulse oximeter interprets carboxyhemoglobin as oxyhemoglobin and consistently overestimates the oxygen saturation when carboxyhemoglobin is present. To overcome this problem, CO-oximetry should be used, because this device uses four or more wavelengths capable of differentiating among various hemoglobin species.

13. Which toxic inhalational agent has the characteristic odor of bitter almonds?

Hydrogen cyanide. Hydrogen cyanide is another example (in addition to CO) of a chemical asphyxiant. Hydrogen cyanide inhibits intracellular cytochrome oxidase activity and thus poisons cellular respiration. Hydrogen cyanide exposure may occur in electroplating, photographic development, and polishing of metals; it also results from the burning of polyurethane, cellulose, nylon, wool, silk, and asphalt. Symptoms of headache, palpitations, giddiness, and dyspnea appear within seconds and may quickly progress to seizures, coma, and death. Clues to diagnosis are severe hypoxic symptoms without cyanosis, similar arterial and venous oxygen saturations, and an anion gap lactic acidosis. The smell of bitter almonds, although pathognomonic, is detectable only by approximately 60% of individuals.

14. Why is it vitally important to diagnose cyanide toxicity?

Hydrogen cyanide toxicity must not be overlooked because, unlike most other causes of toxic inhalation, specific antidote therapy is available. The traditional regimen is detoxification with amyl nitrate, sodium nitrite, and sodium thiosulfate. The nitrates are thought to convert hemoglobin to methemoglobin, which then competes with cytochrome oxidase for the cyanide ion. Thiosulfate further converts cyanide to the less toxic thiocyanide, which is then excreted in the urine. Excessive production of methemoglobin is a danger with this regimen, so methemoglobin levels must be monitored carefully.

15. A rotten egg odor is characteristic of which toxic inhalational agent?

Hydrogen sulfide. Hydrogen sulfide is a dense gas with a rotten egg odor, but this odor rapidly becomes undetectable upon continued exposure because of "olfactory fatigue." Exposure may occur in the petroleum industry as well as with sewage treatment and in volcanic gases, coal mines, and natural hot springs. Hydrogen sulfide is an even more potent inhibitor of cytochrome oxidase than is cyanide, causing disruption of the electron transport chain and cellular respiration. Unlike cyanide, however, hydrogen sulfide also causes upper airway irritation. Symptoms include rhinitis, bronchitis, and pulmonary edema, as well as significant central nervous system dysfunction, including headache, seizures, and respiratory failure. In addition to supportive measures, treatment includes the use of nitrites as in hydrogen cyanide toxicity.

16. A teenager presents to the emergency department appearing drunk but smelling of airplane glue. What is the likely diagnosis?

Solvent abuse. Many different volatile hydrocarbons are used as solvents in adhesives, airplane glue, dry-cleaning fluids, typewriter correctional fluid, and other materials. These compounds are highly volatile and therefore readily absorbed by the lung; they also are lipophilic, promoting their high concentration in the central nervous system. Inhalation, which may be either accidental or intentional, causes central nervous system effects of inebriation and depression, similar to those of alcohol, as well as perceptual changes similar to those of marijuana or hallucinogens. Other organ systems also may be affected, including the liver, kidneys, and bone marrow. Unfortunately, sudden death also has been reported, presumably secondary to cardiac dysrhythmia from direct myocardial toxic effects.

17. The recent subway terrorist attack in Japan involved which class of toxic inhalational agents?

Organophosphates (nerve gases). The nerve gas sarin was involved in the Japanese attack. It is representative of the class of potent organophosphate compounds used as nerve agents since World War I. Exposure may occur in agriculture also because organophosphates are used as insecticides. These substances block the enzyme acetylcholinesterase at cholinergic receptor sites and therefore result in a cholinergic crisis caused by the accumulation of acetylcholine. Increased muscarinic activity causes excessive secretions, miosis, bronchospasm, bradycardia, and intestinal hypermotility. Increased nicotinic activity results in fasciculations, weakness, and paralysis. Death from respiratory failure may occur within minutes. Treatment consists of rapid, thorough skin decontamination and several doses of atropine and pralidoxime.

18. What is metal fume fever?

Metal fume fever is a systemic illness that follows inhalation of the metallic oxides most commonly of zinc, copper, and magnesium and less commonly of beryllium, cadmium, mercury, nickel, vanadium, chromium, and osmium. Exposure may occur in industry as well as among craftsmen and artists. Symptoms typically occur several hours after exposure and include throat irritation, cough, dyspnea, weakness, myalgias, fever, and rigors. An elevated white blood cell count also may be seen. The illness resolves after 24–48 hours and is thought to be immunologically mediated. A similar illness, termed *polymer fume fever*, may be seen after inhalation of fumes generated from heated polytetrafluoroethylene (Teflon).

19. Is it true or false that the leading cause of death in fires is smoke inhalation and not burns?

True. Smoke inhalation both injures the lung directly and has systemic effects. The heat from a fire usually causes thermal injury above the vocal cords only, because the upper airway is extremely efficient at dissipating heat. Thermal injury takes the form of burns to the face, oropharynx, and upper airway and may result in airway edema and obstruction. Lower airway injury is usually due to the chemical effects of smoke, which cause direct mucosal irritation and result in bronchorrhea, bronchoconstriction, and airway edema. The chemical components of smoke are determined by the types of material undergoing combustion. Many of these components are gases, but many of these chemical components are also adherent to smoke particulates that may persist in the airway and perpetuate ongoing local injury. Systemic effects of smoke inhalation are primarily the result of cellular hypoxia and acidosis induced by the asphyxiants CO and hydrogen cyanide.

20. Describe the three phases of injury after smoke inhalation.

Phase 1 (0–36 hours). During this phase there are two main concerns: hypoxia and airway injury. Hypoxic injury may result from low inspired oxygen concentrations occurring during a fire or from the asphyxiant properties of CO and hydrogen cyanide. Airway injury from thermal or chemical causes results in upper airway obstruction, bronchorrhea, and bronchoconstriction.

Phase 2 (2–5 days). This period has been described as "the calm before the storm." During this phase, airway injury is resolving but tracheobronchial sloughing continues. Lung function may improve initially then decline as sloughing becomes severe and bronchopneumonia or ARDS develops.

Phase 3 (5+ days). During this period nosocomial pneumonia, respiratory fatigue, and ARDS may develop. Continued respiratory support and aggressive attention to fluid management and infection are crucial during this period until the lungs and burn wounds heal.

CONTROVERSIES

21. What is the role of hyperbaric oxygenation therapy in the treatment of CO poisoning?
Treatment of CO poisoning centers on the administration of 100% oxygen. The half-life for CO at room air is 240 minutes, but it decreases to 90 minutes on 100% oxygen and to only 20 minutes with hyperbaric oxygen (HBO) therapy at 2 atmospheres. The use of HBO is controversial, however, and has been the subject of a recent National Heart, Lung, and Blood Institute Workshop and many editorials. The theoretical benefit of HBO is that it provides a high enough dissolved oxygen content in plasma to meet the body's metabolic demands, even without functional hemoglobin. It also enhances CO elimination. These biologic effects do not necessarily translate into clinical benefits, however. In addition, HBO is costly, not widely available, and associated with some risk, including the theoretical harm of oxygen toxicity and free radical production. Most clinical trials have been observational only and not well controlled. Most have used neuropsychologic sequela of CO poisoning as endpoints, but these sequelae have not been consistently defined or measured. The most recent trial (reported in April 1995) was a prospective, randomized trial of HBO in patients with mild to moderate CO poisoning who presented within 6 hours of exposure. The trial found that HBO decreased the incidence of delayed neurologic sequela; however, it was criticized on many procedural grounds. Nevertheless, it appears to be one of the best controlled trials so far and certainly supports the call for further research.

22. What are the best methods for determining whether inhalational injury has occurred in a burn patient?
One of the most immediate concerns after smoke inhalation is patency of the upper airway. Many methods have been advocated for detecting whether airway injury has occurred and whether intubation is indicated. History and clinical signs are important in this evaluation but do not reliably predict upper airway injury. Such factors include exposure in a closed space or to steam, neck or facial burns, singed nasal hairs, sooty sputum, bronchorrhea, hoarseness, and wheezing. Haponick and colleagues advocate serial physiologic testing with spirometry and flow-volume loops to detect the earliest signs of injury. Such injury would manifest as upper airway edema, which would cause reduction in inspiratory flow rates and truncation of the inspiratory limb of the flow-volume loop, suggestive of variable extrathoracic obstruction. When serial studies remain stable and normal, the likelihood of significant upper airway obstruction is minimal and the patient may be safely observed. When serial measurements show progressive upper airway dysfunction, however, the likelihood of progressive anatomic injury is increased and dictates continued close follow-up if not immediate or prophylactic intubation.

Upper airway endoscopy, either by laryngoscopy or bronchoscopy, is thought by others to identify any anatomic changes sooner than might be evident by physiologic testing, and bronchoscopy also allows inspection of the lower airway for signs of injury. When signs of upper airway edema are present, intubation is recommended. If only mucosal irritation is seen, endoscopy should be repeated in 24 hours to reevaluate for edema. Once the tube is placed, however, the findings on bronchoscopy do not appear to predict the duration of mechanical ventilation, the level of support, or survival. Although hazards of endoscopy (precipitating upper airway closure) and intubation and mechanical ventilation (loss of cough, poor secretion clearance, nosocomial pneumonia) are recognized, the rule of thumb is "when in doubt, intubate."

BIBLIOGRAPHY

1. Blanc PD, Schwartz DA: Acute pulmonary responses to toxic exposures. In Murray JJ, Nadel JA (eds): Textbook of Respiratory Medicine, 2nd ed. Philadelphia, W.B. Saunders, 1994, pp 2050–2061.
2. Bingham HG, Gallagher TJ, Powell MD: Early bronchoscopy as a predictor of ventilatory support for burned patients. J Trauma 27:1286–1288, 1987.
3. Demling RH: Smoke inhalational injury. In Ayres SM, Grenvik A, Holbrook PR, et al (eds): Textbook of Critical Care. Philadelphia, W.B. Saunders, 1995, pp 1506–1516.
4. Haponik EF: Clinical and functional assessment. In Haponik EF, Munster AM (eds): Respiratory Injury: Smoke Inhalation and Burns. New York, McGraw-Hill, 1990, pp 137–178.

5. Haponik EF, Meyers DA, Munster AM, et al: Acute upper airway injury in burn patients. Serial changes of flow-volume curves and nasopharyngoscopy. Am Rev Respir Dis 135:360–366, 1987.
6. Mevorach DR, Heyman SN: Pain in the marriage. N Engl J Med 332:48–50, 1995.
7. NHLBI Workshop Summary: Hyperbaric oxygenation therapy. Am Rev Respir Dis 1414–1421, 1991.
8. Olson KR, Seger D: Hyperbaric oxygen for carbon monoxide poisoning: Does it really work? Ann Emerg Med 25:535–537, 1995.
9. Rorison DG, McPherson SJ: Acute toxic inhalations. Emerg Med Clin North Am 10:409–435, 1992.
10. Seger D, Welch L: Carbon monoxide controversies: Neuropsychologic testing, mechanism of toxicity, and hyperbaric oxygen. Ann Emerg Med 24:242–248, 1994.
11. Thom SR, Taber RL, Mendiguren II, et al: Delayed neuropsychologic sequelae after carbon monoxide poisoning: Prevention by treatment with hyperbaric oxygen. Ann Emerg Med 25:474–480, 1995.
12. Venus B, Matsuda T, Copiozo JB, et al: Prophylactic intubation and continuous positive airway pressure in the management of inhalation injury in burn victims. Crit Care Med 9:519–524, 1981.
13. Waldron HA: Non-neoplastic disorders due to metallic, chemical and physical agents. In Parkes WR (ed): Occupational Lung Disorders, 3rd ed. Boston, Butterworth-Heinemann, 1994, pp 593–643.
14. Weiss SM, Lakshminarayan S: Acute inhalation injury. Clin Chest Med 15:103–116, 1994.

58. PULMONARY DISABILITY EVALUATION

Akshay Sood, M.B.B.S., and Carrie A. Redlich, M.D., M.P.H.

1. What guides exist for the evaluation of pulmonary disability?

There are several guides with slightly varying standards for evaluating pulmonary disability. Social Security, the Department of Veterans' Affairs, and State Workers' Compensation Boards use different criteria. The most commonly used documents are the American Medical Association (AMA) guide to the Evaluation of Permanent Impairment and the American Thoracic Society (ATS) official statement. Physicians are encouraged to read through these documents before evaluating patients under different specific disability systems. Many, but not all, states use the AMA guidelines for determining workers' compensation.

2. What is the difference between impairment and disability?

Impairment means loss of physical or physiologic function. *Disability* refers to the impact of the impairment on the person's life. Impairment may occur without disability. For example, a patients with moderate emphysema working on a word processor may have measurable impairment and little resultant disability. Conversely, disability may occur without impairment. For example, an auto body shop painter with isocyanate asthma may be disabled from work but may have no measurable impairment if removed from work when the disease process is in an early stage. Two people with the same impairment may have different resultant disabilities.

3. What are the differences between permanent and temporary disability and between partial and total disability?

A disability may be characterized as either permanent or temporary. A permanent disability is not expected to improve with time and treatment. Temporary disability is thought to have a high probability of being short term and the patient can be expected to improve to a higher level of function. In addition, a disability may be characterized as partial or total. Total disability usually implies that an individual is unable to do any work.

4. What is workers' compensation?

Workers' compensation is a "no-fault" system of insurance in which insurers or employers pay benefits to an employee if he or she has an injury or illness caused by a workplace exposure or accident. In return, the worker gives up his or her rights to sue the employer for the injury. Workers' compensation laws vary from state to state. It is important for physicians to note their role in workers' compensation. Physicians are obligated to diagnose and treat work-related ill-ness and when attributing illness to an occupational exposure, to inform the patient and assist with the documentation to file claims for benefits.

5. How certain do I need to be that the impairment is the result of an occupational expo-sure when dealing with workers' compensation cases?

The level of certainty required in determining causation for workers' compensation is differ-ent from the usual standard of 95% certainty used in medical research. The commonly accepted standard of certainty that the illness was caused by an occupational exposure is one of "more probable than not" or a level of certainty greater than 50%.

6. What are the impairment criteria used in evaluating disability under the AMA guidelines?

The impairment criteria are based on the history, physical examination, pulmonary function tests, and chest radiograph of the patient. The relevant history to elicit includes dyspnea, cough, sputum production, wheezing, environmental exposures, tobacco use, and occupational expo-sures. Physical examination should include a description of breathing pattern, cyanosis, clubbing, adventitious lung sounds, and evidence of cor pulmonale. The findings on chest radiographs and pulmonary function tests are also important. Cardiopulmonary exercise testing and blood gas de-termination are usually not necessary.

7. What is the role of pulmonary function tests in evaluating lung impairment?

The most commonly used tests of pulmonary function are spirometry and DLCO. In obstruc-tive airway disease, the spirometry should be done after the administration of inhaled bron-chodilators. The test results are expressed as percentage predicted of the reference values based on the individual's height, age, race, and sex.

The AMA classification of respiratory impairment is outlined below. At least one of these measures of ventilatory function should be abnormal to the degree described in that class if the impairment is to be rated in that class.

American Medical Association Classification of Respiratory Impairment

TEST PARAMETER AS % PREDICTED	CLASS 1: NO IMPAIRMENT	CLASS 2: MILD IMPAIRMENT	CLASS 3: MODERATE IMPAIRMENT	CLASS 4: SEVERE IMPAIRMENT
FVC	$\geq 80\%$	60–79%	51–59%	$\leq 50\%$
FEV$_1$	$\geq 80\%$	60–79%	41–59%	$\leq 40\%$
FEV$_1$/FVC	$\geq 70\%$	60–69%	41–59%	$\leq 40\%$
DLCO	$\geq 80\%$	60–79%	41–59%	$\leq 40\%$

8. Should arterial blood gas levels be measured routinely in evaluation of pulmonary impairment?

Determinations of blood gas levels are considered invasive. There is relatively poor correla-tion between resting arterial PaO_2 and exercise capacity. For most persons with obstructive lung diseases, the FEV$_1$ correlates better with exercise capacity than does PaO_2. If hypoxemia is sus-pected, blood gas determinations are recommended. According to the AMA guidelines, resting hypoxia is defined as PaO_2 of 50 mm of Hg on room air or a PaO_2 of less than 60 mm of Hg on room air in the presence of pulmonary hypertension, cor pulmonale, or erythrocytosis. Hypox-emia should be documented on two occasions at least 4 weeks apart; its presence indicates severe impairment.

9. When should a cardiopulmonary exercise test be ordered?

In patients in whom subjective dyspnea is disproportionate to the pulmonary function test result or when the latter is difficult to interpret because of submaximal performance, cardiopul-monary exercise tests may be considered. These tests are also useful in determining whether a patient can perform a job with a known energy requirement. Under the ATS guidelines, the estimation of impairment from $\dot{V}O_2max$ (maximal oxygen consumption in ml per minute) is based on the premise that a worker can comfortably perform at 40% of his or her $\dot{V}O_2max$ and that oxygen requirements can be assigned to specific occupations. Those subjects whose $\dot{V}O_2max$ is less than 15 ml per kg per minute would be uncomfortable performing most jobs.

10. List some of the disease processes in which the subjective symptoms may exceed the measured pulmonary impairment.
- Reversible and episodic disease such as asthma
- Nonpulmonary diseases such as myocardial ischemia and anemia
- Psychogenic causes such as panic attacks
- Multiple chemical sensitivity syndrome
- Malingering

11. Does any test identify malingering?
There is no perfect test to identify a malingerer; however, the following steps can be taken to evaluate a malingerer:
- Make sure the patient understands the purpose and the performance of the pulmonary function testing.
- Review test results to ensure that patient has given a good effort that is reproducible.
- Cardiopulmonary exercise testing may be helpful in select situations in which there is a disparity between subjective symptoms and objective findings.

Fortunately, frank malingering is uncommon.

12. Are there any pulmonary diseases that have their own specific criteria for impairment and disability?
Several pulmonary diseases such as asthma and certain forms of pneumoconiosis have their own criteria for impairment and disability. The prevention of coal workers' pneumoconiosis is the goal of the Mine Safety and Health Administration, and miners suffering from pulmonary disability from dust inhalation can apply for compensation under a specific federal legislation popularly known as the "Black Lung Act."

According to the AMA guidelines, lung cancers are a cause of severe impairment at the time of diagnosis. If at reevaluation 1 year later, no evidence of tumor is found, impairment is calculated on the basis of the degree of physiologic impairment present at that time.

Some individuals with sleep apnea may develop a functional impairment that affects work activity. For example, long distance truck driving, operation of dangerous machinery, and the like should be proscribed for these individuals.

13. Since airflow obstruction in asthmatics varies at different times, how is their impairment rated?
Under the ATS guidelines, an asthmatic's impairment is scored on three parameters:
- Postbronchodilator FEV_1
- Percentage of change in FEV_1 after bronchodilator or degree of airway hyperresponsiveness as defined by PC_{20} (the concentration of the test agent, commonly methacholine, that provokes a fall in FEV_1 of 20% from baseline)
- Need for bronchodilators and steroids to control symptoms.

The sum of the above scores is used to calculate the degree of impairment. Before an asthmatic is permitted to return to work, the workplace should be assessed to insure that no triggers for asthma are present.

14. How is the impairment or disability determined in the case of occupational asthma?
The ATS statement places patients with asthma induced by sensitizers such as isocyanates in a unique category. The proper treatment for this condition is to remove the worker from further

exposure. In many such individuals, in the absence of exposure to the specific agent, physiologic tests may be normal and symptoms may be absent. Such patients are considered 100% disabled (even though they may not have measurable impairment) for any job that exposes them to the causative agent. Relocation to a new job and vocational retraining should be considered. A respirator may not be able to protect such a patient from low levels of the sensitizing agent that might trigger an attack. Assessment for long-term disability should be carried out 2 years after the removal from exposure when improvement has been shown to plateau. The evaluation should be done using the scaling systems for nonoccupational asthma.

15. When more than one factor is responsible for causing disease, how does a physician apportion the lung disease caused by each factor?

Apportionment describes the relative contribution of multiple factors to the total lung impairment and disability. For example, cigarette smoking can be a contributory factor in certain occupational diseases such as lung cancer. Often it is difficult, if not impossible, to determine the relative roles of different factors in disease causation. In these conditions, physicians are asked to state their opinion, taking into consideration the body of available knowledge in that area. The usual standard for workers' compensation is whether the occupational exposure has been a "substantial contributing factor" in causing or increasing the impairment.

16. Are patients with respiratory impairment unfit for certain jobs?

Yes, if the job entails a risk of exposure that could cause respiratory injury to already functionally impaired lungs. Also, some patients may not be able to tolerate wearing of protective devices. For example, an asthmatic requiring frequent inhaler therapy may have difficulty using respirators.

BIBLIOGRAPHY

1. American Thoracic Society: Evaluation of impairment/disability secondary to respiratory disorders. Am Rev Respir Dis 133:1205–1209, 1986.
2. American Thoracic Society: Guidelines for the evaluation of impairment/disability in patients with asthma. Am Rev Respir Dis 147:1056–1061, 1993.
3. Chan-Yeung M: Evaluation of impairment/disability in patients with occupational asthma. Am Rev Respir Dis 135:950–951, 1987.
4. Engelberg AL: Guides to the evaluation of permanent impairment, 3rd ed. Chicago, American Medical Association, 1988.
5. Harber P, Schenker MB, Balmes JR: Occupational and Environmental Respiratory Disease. St. Louis, Mosby-Year Book, 1996.
6. Murray JF, Nadel JA: Textbook of Respiratory Medicine, 2nd ed. Philadelphia, W.B. Saunders, 1994.
7. Oren A, Sue DY, Hansen JE, et al: Role of exercise testing in impairment evaluation. Am Rev Resp Dis 135:230–235, 1987.
8. Richman SI: Compensating victims of occupational lung disease: The physician's role in the system. J Occup Med 31:335–338, 1989.
9. Sue DY: Exercise testing in the evaluation of impairment and disability. Clin Chest Med 15:369–387, 1994.
10. U.S. Department of Health and Human Services, Social Security Administration: Disability Evaluation under Social Security. HHS Publication No. (SSA) 64-039. Baltimore, 1992.

XIII. Lung Neoplasms

59. SOLITARY PULMONARY NODULE

Elizabeth L. Aronsen, M.D.

1. Define a solitary pulmonary nodule.

A solitary solitary pulmonary nodule (SPN) is an isolated opacity seen on plain chest radiograph. SPNs are located entirely within the lung parenchyma, not associated with atelectasis or hilar adenopathy, and generally less than 4.0 cm in diameter.

2. How are SPNs usually discovered?

SPNs are usually asymptomatic and found on routine chest radiographs obtained for other reasons such as preoperative evaluation. Less often, local (such as hemoptysis or cough) or systemic (such as fatigue or weight loss) symptoms may prompt the clinician to obtain the chest radiograph that detects the SPN.

3. List some of the most common causes of SPNs.

Benign. Seventy-five to 85% of pathologically diagnosed SPNs are benign; benign SPNs can be classified as follows:

- **Granuloma.** More than half of all benign SPNs (40% of the total) are granulomas, which are categorized as follows:

  Infectious
  Histoplasmosis
  Coccidioidomycosis
  Tuberculosis
  Noninfectious
  Sarcoidosis
  Rheumatoid arthritis
  Vasculitides, such as Wegener's granulomatosis

- **Hamartoma.** Hamartomas represent the next most common benign cause, although they constitute less than 10% of all SPNs.

- **Other.** More than 100 benign causes of SPNs have been reported, including:
  Bronchiolitis obliterans with organizing pneumonia (BOOP)
  Parasitic infections
  Arteriovenous malformations
  Bronchogenic cysts
  Pulmonary infarction
  Eosinophilic granuloma
  Nodular pulmonary amyloidosis
  Anthrasilicotic intrapulmonary lymph nodes
  "Round" pneumonia, which is a less common presentation of acute pulmonary infection in which the alveolar space-filling disease assumes a more rounded nodular appearance.
  Rhodococcus equi pneumonia may present as a cavitating SPN in an immunocompromised patient.

Malignant
- **Primary bronchogenic**
  Non–small cell lung cancer
  Small cell lung cancer
  Primary pulmonary lymphoma
- **Metastatic disease from nonpulmonary sources**
  Kaposi's sarcoma
  Adenocarcinoma from any source
  Angiosarcoma

4. **What patient characteristics make the diagnosis of malignant disease more likely?**

Age. In patients under the age of 35 years virtually all SPNs are benign. The risk of malignant disease increases with increasing age, until by age 65 more than two-thirds of SPNs are malignant.

History of prior malignancy. Although primary bronchogenic carcinoma is the most frequent cause of resected malignant SPNs, metastatic disease, often originating from extrapulmonary adenocarcinomas of the breast, prostate, or colon, represent 30% of malignant SPNs. In one series, 50% of the patients with an SPN had a prior history of malignancy.

Smoking history. There is a well known association between smoking and the development of primary bronchogenic carcinoma, although the effect of smoking on malignancy in the setting of SPNs has not been specifically determined. Ten to 15 years after smoking cessation, the risk returns to that of the general nonsmoking population, making smoking discontinuation a health-care maintenance priority for physicians.

5. **What imaging techniques can be used to evaluate an SPN?**

Chest radiography. Chest radiography is the imaging modality that most often results in the initial diagnosis of an SPN. It is rarely relied upon, however, as the sole imaging technique in patients who appear to have an SPN because it often fails to detect additional parenchymal nodules.

Chest CT. Chest CT with contrast enhancement is almost always part of the work-up of the SPN to guide the clinician in assessing the most likely diagnosis and determining the best approach for obtaining a tissue sample. CT guidance is also used to localize the lesion with methylene blue or hook wires before surgical resection.

Positron emission tomography (PET). In the future, PET imaging of fluorodeoxyglucose uptake into SPNs may complement current conventional techniques.

6. **What CT characteristics make a diagnosis of malignant disease more likely?**

Nodule size. Twenty percent or fewer of SPNs less than 2.0 cm in diameter are malignant. In contrast, more than 80% of the SPNs larger than 3.0 cm in diameter are malignant.

Presence and pattern of calcification. Central, laminated, or diffuse patterns of calcification suggest a benign diagnosis such as granulomatous disease or hamartoma. Malignant disease only rarely shows evidence of calcification; when there is calcification, it more frequently exhibits an eccentric pattern.

Nodular density and configuration. Chest CT, with thin sections through the nodule, is very sensitive in defining the density and configuration of an SPN. The finding of a fat density within the nodule strongly suggests the diagnosis of hamartoma. A ground-glass appearance of the SPN is consistent with the diagnosis of bronchoalveolar carcinoma. The "halo sign" or ground-glass attenuation surrounding the SPN is characteristic of hemorrhagic nodules as seen in infectious processes (caused by fungus or virus) and, less frequently, noninfectious processes (Wegener's granulomatosis, Kaposi's sarcoma, metastatic angiosarcoma). The configuration of the SPN is less helpful in predicting malignancy, because well-marginated spherical nodules can be either benign or malignant. Poorly marginated or spiculated nodules strongly suggest malignancy.

Adenopathy. Both benign and malignant diseases may be associated with ipsilateral mediastinal or hilar adenopathy (defined as lymph nodes more than 1.0 cm in diameter).

Adenopathy involving the contralateral hemithorax, however, is highly suggestive of non-resectable malignant disease.

Contrast enhancement. Complete contrast enhancement by dynamic CT suggests malignancy, whereas capsular, peripheral, or no enhancement of the SPN is more consistent with benign causes such as hamartoma or tuberculoma. Pathologically, enhancement is thought to be caused by the distribution of small vessels within the mass. Further study is needed to determine the characteristics of other benign SPNs and whether enhancement can be used to reduce the number of surgical procedures needed to obtain definitive diagnoses.

7. How should the work-up of the SPN begin?

Obtain an old chest radiograph. A nodule is very likely to be benign if previous radiographs confirm that it has been present and unchanged in size for at least 2 years. In this setting, no further work-up is necessary. Malignant lesions usually have a doubling time measured in weeks to months. In effect, a lesion that grows either very rapidly (days) or very slowly (years) is likely to be benign. In the event of rapid growth, the patient usually has additional symptoms suggesting a benign diagnosis, such as infection or infarction. An SPN increasing very slowly in size may warrant further observation only for an additional period of time.

Obtain a chest CT. Contrast-enhanced dynamic chest CT with thin sections through the nodule helps to characterize the nature of the SPN, confirm its solitary nature, and stage the disease should it prove to be malignant. Often CT demonstrates several pulmonary nodules, suggesting the diagnosis of either granulomatous disease or pulmonary metastases. Less than 1% of primary bronchogenic cancers present as multiple synchronous lesions.

8. What step(s) should be taken next in the work-up and diagnosis of the SPN?

Observation. This is appropriate in many patients, particularly those with a very low likelihood of malignancy based on clinical and radiologic features, but also in those for whom an invasive diagnostic procedure would carry an unacceptably high risk of morbidity and mortality. The course of the SPN can be monitored with serial chest radiographs usually every 3 months for the first year, every 6 months for the second year, and on a yearly basis thereafter.

Biopsy. The alternative to observation is to obtain tissue for a definitive diagnosis. Biopsy can be performed using either CT- or fluoroscopy-guided transthoracic fine-needle aspiration (TTFNA) or fiberoptic bronchoscopy with transbronchial biopsy (TBBx). TTFNA and TBBx are often considered complementary procedures. The latter is associated with a lower diagnostic yield, particularly for small (less than 2 cm) peripheral SPNs. TTFNA can be considered diagnostic for malignant or some benign lesions only when definitively positive, because, as most clinicians would agree, nonspecific inflammation should not be construed as evidence of a benign lesion. Characteristic morphology seen after Gomori methenamine silver stain of biopsy specimens includes extracytoplasmic spheroids and cytoplasmic inclusions in the case of histoplasmosis. If diagnosis is not definitive, more aggressive attempts to obtain tissue must be pursued in most clinical situations. Open lung biopsy (OLBx) or video-assisted thoracoscopy (VATS) is performed in cases of high clinical suspicion with a nondiagnostic TTFNA or TBBx.

Resection. Patients at high risk for malignant disease (e.g., an older patient with a large, noncalcified, enhancing SPN and a smoking history) without significant comorbid illnesses or contraindications for general anesthesia are frequently referred directly for surgical resection of the mass. Thoracotomy has the advantage of often being both a diagnostic and a therapeutic procedure. Unfortunately, however, it is also associated with higher morbidity. A peripheral SPN may be amenable to surgical resection by a VATS approach rather than by open thoracotomy, thus reducing operating room costs, duration of anesthesia, and number of days in hospital.

BIBLIOGRAPHY

1. Gasparini S, Ferretti M, Secchi EB, et al: Integration of transbronchial and percutaneous approach in the diagnosis of peripheral pulmonary nodules or masses. Experience with 1,027 consecutive cases. Chest 108:131–137, 1995.

2. Harvey JC, Beattie EJ: Surgical treatment of solitary multiple pulmonary nodules. Compr Ther 19:238–241, 1993.
3. Kazerooni EA, Bhalla M, Shepard JA, et al: Adenosquamous carcinoma of the lungs: Radiologic appearance. Am J Roentgenol 163:301–306, 1994.
4. Lillington GA, Caskey CI: Evaluation and management of solitary and multiple pulmonary nodules. Clin Chest Med 14:111–119, 1993.
5. Midthun DE, Swensen SJ, Jett JR: Clinical strategies for solitary pulmonary nodule. Annu Rev Med 43:195, 1992.
6. Midthun DE, Swensen SJ, Jett JR: Approach to the solitary pulmonary nodule. Mayo Clin Proc 68:378–385, 1993.
7. Milman N, Faurschou P, Grode G: Diagnostic yield of transthoracic needle aspiration biopsy following negative fiberoptic bronchoscopy in 103 patients with peripheral circumscribed pulmonary lesions. Respiration 62:1–3, 1995.
8. Primack SL, Hartman TE, Lee KS, et al: Pulmonary nodules and the CT halo sign. Radiology 190:513–515, 1994.
9. Pugatch RD: Radiographic evaluation in chest malignancies. A review of imaging modalities. Chest 107(Suppl 6):294S–297S, 1995.
10. Santambrogio L, Nosotti M, Bellaviti N, et al: Videothoracoscopy versus thoracotomy for the diagnosis of the indeterminate solitary pulmonary nodule. Ann Thorac Surg 59:868–870, 1995.
11. Swenson SJ, Brown LR, Colby TV, et al: Pulmonary nodules: CT evaluation of enhancement with iodinated contrast material. Radiology 194:393–398, 1995.
12. Webb WR: Radiologic evaluation of the solitary pulmonary nodule. Am J Roentgenol 154:701–708, 1990.
13. Yamashita K, Matsunobe S, Tsuda T, et al: Solitary pulmonary nodule: Preliminary study of evaluation with incremental dynamic CT. Radiology 194:399–405, 1995.

60. LUNG CANCER

Teofilo L. Lee-Chiong, Jr., M.D., and Richard A. Matthay, M.D.

1. Is lung cancer the most prevalent cancer in men and women in the United States?

In 1996, 177,000 cases of lung cancer will be discovered in the United States (98,000 in males and 78,100 in females) and 158,700 deaths will occur from this disease (94,400 in males and 64,300 in females). Although lung cancer is, by a substantial margin, the number one cancer killer in men and women in the United States, it is not the most prevalent cancer. In 1996, it is estimated that 31% of new cancers diagnosed in women will be breast cancer, followed by lung cancer (13%) and colon and rectal cancer (11%). However, the estimated cancer deaths in the United States for women during the same year are lung (25%), breast (17%), and colon and rectum (10%).

For men, prostate cancer (41%) is projected to be the leading cause of new cancer cases in 1996 followed by lung (13%) and colon and rectum (9%). In contrast, 32% of the cancer deaths among men in 1996 will be the result of lung cancer, followed by prostate (14%) and colon and rectum (9%).

2. Why was there a marked delay in the acceleration of death rates due to lung cancer among women in the United States?

In contrast to men, substantial numbers of women did not start smoking cigarettes until they entered the labor force in the United States during World War II. A 15- to 20-year latency period followed, then beginning in the mid-1960s, the death rate from lung cancer accelerated among women. In fact, it is anticipated that this steep upward trend will not plateau until the year 2010 because of the difficulty women have in stopping smoking and in not starting smoking. Because men have been more successful in stopping cigarette smoking and in not starting smoking, death rates from lung cancer began to decline in the early 1990s in men.

3. What factors have been associated with a decreased incidence of lung cancer among cigarette smokers?

Cigarette smoking is clearly the number one cause of lung cancer. In the United States, between 25 and 27% of both men and women still smoke cigarettes, a marked decline over the 30 years since the Surgeon General's 1964 report on the hazards of cigarette smoking.

A later age of smoking initiation, lower tar content, and the use of filters are among the factors that have been found to reduce lung cancer risk in those who smoke cigarettes. Smoking cessation reduces the risk of lung cancer, but there is a latency period of approximately 3 years between cessation of smoking and evidence of a decline in the incidence of lung cancer.

4. Among the many substances encountered in the workplace that have been identified as causes of human lung cancer, which is the most frequent?

Asbestos is the most frequent occupational cause of lung cancer. Other agents found in the workplace that are associated with an increased incidence of lung cancer include arsenic, bis(chloromethyl) ether and chloromethyl methyl ether, chromium and certain chromium compounds (hexavalent chromium), ionizing radiation, gamma radiation (x-rays), mustard gas, nickel, radon progeny (decay products), and vinyl chloride.

Smoking prevalence has been high in most of the cohorts heavily exposed to asbestos, and there is a well recognized, important interaction between smoking and asbestos. In fact, it is estimated that the incidence of lung cancer is 50 times higher in heavy smoking men exposed to asbestos than in nonsmoking men who were not exposed to asbestos.

5. Does daily vitamin A or daily vitamin E ingestion decrease the death rate from lung cancer?

Unfortunately, the trials conducted in Finland and most recently in the United States have shown no benefit from either antioxidant, vitamin A or E, in preventing lung cancer deaths. Accordingly, neither of these agents is currently recommended for chemoprevention in candidates at high risk for lung cancer (e.g., heavy cigarette smokers).

6. What is the most frequent lung cancer cell type?

Adenocarcinoma has replaced squamous cell carcinoma as the most frequent histologic lung cancer cell type for all sexes and races combined. Over the past 20 years, the age-adjusted rates of lung cancer in the United States have increased by 30%, with the gain markedly greater in women (70%) than in men (17%). The largest percentage increases in age-adjusted rates were observed for small cell carcinoma and adenocarcinoma (approximately 60% each), with a more modest gain for squamous cell carcinoma (14%). The following is the current order of frequency of the major lung cancer cell types: adenocarcinoma, squamous cell carcinoma, small cell carcinoma, large cell carcinoma.

7. Are there differences in the manner of spread of specific cancer cell types?

Squamous cell carcinomas characteristically develop in chronically damaged airway lining cells. Their tendency to extend centrally toward the mainstem bronchi is responsible for the frequent occurrence of atelectasis, hemoptysis, and postobstructive pneumonitis with this type of cancer. Adenocarcinomas tend to metastasize early to the central nervous system, liver, adrenal glands, and bone. The gastrointestinal tract is commonly involved in metastatic large cell carcinoma. Finally, small cell cancers are often highly aggressive. It is not unusual to encounter extensive spread of cancer cells at the time of diagnosis. Bone, bone marrow, liver, and brain are frequent sites of metastatic small cell carcinomas.

8. What does *tumor growth doubling time* refer to?

The rate of tumor growth may be expressed in terms of its doubling time, the duration in which the tumor doubles in volume. Using the mathematical formula for determining the volume of a sphere, a 1-cm nodule detected on a chest radiograph doubles in volume when its diameter increases by 3 mm. An increase of 5 mm constitutes a doubling in volume of a 2-cm nodule. Doubling times for most malignant nodules range from 21–400 days. Benign processes typically exhibit growth rates that are either faster or slower.

9. What is Pancoast's tumor?

The Pancoast superior sulcus tumor syndrome defines a constellation of clinical features resulting from involvement of the cervical and first thoracic nerves by squamous cell carcinomas and other apical tumors. The first and second ribs may be destroyed. Patients may complain of shoulder and arm pain along the distribution of the ulnar nerve. Physical examination may disclose ptosis, myosis, and ipsilateral anhidrosis (Horner's syndrome).

10. What are the various paraneoplastic syndromes?

Approximately 10% of patients with lung cancer exhibit paraneoplastic syndromes. These clinical features do not result from the physical effects of tumor themselves; rather these phenomena are believed to arise from the excessive release of cellular products by tumors, ectopic production of hormones and other polypeptides, or neurovascular reflexes. The spectrum of clinical conditions includes the following:

- **Systemic disorders** such as anorexia, fever, and malaise
- **Cutaneous disorders** including digital clubbing and hypertrophic pulmonary osteoarthropathy. The latter, mostly related to non–small cell carcinoma, is characterized by painful arthropathy, periosteal proliferation, and neurovascular involvement of the extremities
- **Rheumatologic disorders** exemplified by polymyositis-dermatomyositis and systemic lupus erythematosus
- **Renal disorders** such as membranous glomerulonephritis and nephrotic syndrome
- **Endocrine disorders** including Cushing' syndrome, hypercalcemia (most frequently associated with squamous cell carcinoma), and the syndrome of inappropriate antidiuretic hormone (seen most commonly with small cell lung cancer)
- **Hematologic disorders** such as anemia, leukocytosis, eosinophilia, thrombotic diseases, and hemorrhagic diathesis
- **Neurologic disorders** including Lambert-Eaton syndrome (encountered usually in small cell lung cancer), subacute peripheral neuropathy, limbic encephalitis, necrotizing myelopathy and binocular visual loss
- **Miscellaneous disorders** consisting of nonbacterial thrombotic endocarditis, hypouricemia, and lactic acidosis

Several conditions may masquerade as paraneoplastic syndromes. Infections, fluid and electrolyte abnormalities, vascular defects, tumor metastasis, and drug reactions must be excluded before initiation of therapeutic regimens for these various syndromes.

Management involves eradication of the underlying tumor by surgical resection, chemotherapy, or irradiation. Specific treatments include:

Ketoconazole, aminoglutethimide, metyrapone, octreotide, adrenal arterial embolization or adrenalectomy for Cushing's syndrome

Biphosphonates and gallium nitrate for hypercalcemia

Demeclocycline and lithium carbonate for the syndrome of inappropriate antidiuretic hormone

3,4-Diaminopyridine, plasmapheresis, anticholinesterases, and immunosuppressive agents for Lambert-Eaton syndrome

11. How reliable is sputum cytology in the pathologic diagnosis of lung cancer?

The diagnostic yield of sputum examination is highest for central, upper lobe, and large (T3) lesions. Sputum cytology is less reliable for small (T1) tumors situated in the lower lobes or peripherally. The diagnostic yield also varies among the different cancer cell types. Sensitivity is greater for squamous cell carcinomas, which commonly involve the central airways, than for adenocarcinomas, small cell carcinomas, and large cell carcinomas. The diagnostic yield may be improved by sputum induction with an ultrasonic nebulizer and by the use of monoclonal anti-bodies, DNA image cytometry, and quantitative cytology.

12. When should CT scanning or MR imaging be performed in the evaluation of lung cancer?

Lung tumors detected on chest radiographs may be further evaluated using CT scanning or MRI. CT scanning makes possible accurate characterization and localization of lesions. In addition, CT scanning is useful for evaluation of uninvolved pulmonary parenchyma, mediastinum, chest wall, liver, adrenal glands, and brain. It can be used to guide transcutaneous needle biopsies.

Using a reference phantom, CT scanning can help clarify the nature of solitary pulmonary nodules. Lesions that are more dense than the phantom or contain more than 10% calcium are more likely to be benign. On the other hand, nodules that contain less than 10% calcium require further investigation. Phantom scanning is not recommended in patients with genitourinary or gastrointestinal mucinous carcinomas and integumentary sarcomas that are associated with calcium-rich metastatic lesions.

In contrast, MRI is capable of multiplanar imaging of anatomic structures and pathologic changes in the chest and is flow sensitive. It is valuable in assessing superior sulcus tumors; detecting tumor invasion of the brachial plexus, chest wall, heart, and great vessels; delineating tumor masses from adjacent atelectasis or dense infiltrates; distinguishing benign scars from residual or new tumors; and defining metastatic involvement of the liver, adrenal glands, and brain. Patients in whom CT scanning is not feasible because of allergy to iodinated contrast dye may safely undergo MRI testing.

13. What are the indications for mediastinotomy or mediastinoscopy?

Preoperative evaluation of the mediastinum by either mediastinotomy or mediastinoscopy is advisable for patients with either mediastinal lymph nodes larger than 1 cm or several smaller nodes. Lymph nodes involving the anterior mediastinal region may be reached by anterior mediastinoscopy or mediastinotomy via a limited parasternal thoracotomy (Chamberlain procedure). A cervical approach can be used to obtain specimens from the superior mediastinum. The diagnostic yield from mediastinal sampling is greatest for small cell and large cell carcinomas.

14. Explain the TNM descriptors used in assigning lung cancer stage.

The **T factor** describes the tumor size, location, and extent of invasion. T1 describes a lesion less than or equal to 3 cm in greatest diameter and completely surrounded by lung parenchyma or visceral pleura with no evidence of invasion proximal to a lobar bronchus. The T2 classification identifies one or more of four elements of tumor progression: (1) tumor size larger than 3 cm, (2) invasion of the visceral pleura, (3) invasion of the main bronchus more than 2 cm distant from the carina, and (4) atelectasis or obstructive pneumonitis extending to the hilar region. The T3 and T4 descriptors classify two levels of extrapulmonary extension of the primary tumor. Limited, circumscribed involvement of the parietal pleura, chest wall, diaphragm, or the mediastinal pleura (fat and pericardium) is classified T3. More extensive tumor growth involving mediastinal structures such as the esophagus, trachea, carina, heart, or great vessels or invasion of the vertebral body is classified as T4. The presence of a tumor-containing pleural effusion portends a poor prognosis and indicates T4 disease.

The **N factor** classifies regional lymph node metastases. If no evidence exists of regional lymph node metastasis, the designation is N0. Metastases limited to intrapulmonary nodes, including the ipsilateral hilar lymph nodes, within the lung and visceral pleura is classified N1. Metastasis confined to the ipsilateral mediastinal lymph group including the ipsilateral paratracheal, tracheobronchial, aortic, paraesophageal, subcarinal, and pulmonary ligament nodes is designated N2. More extensive metastasis to the contralateral mediastinal, contralateral hilar, ipsilateral or contralateral scalene or supraclavicular lymph nodes is classified N3.

The **M factor** identifies the absence or presence of metastasis to distant organ sites. Thus, M0 represents the absence of this finding and M1 represents its presence. Distant metastasis is associated with a fatal outcome in most cases.

15. How are the specific TNM descriptors used for stage groupings?

The stage groupings are used for patients with non–small cell carcinomas of the lung. Patients with small cell carcinoma of the lung are divided into two stages, limited stage disease or extensive disease. In patients with limited stage disease, the tumor is confined to one hemithorax and its regional lymph nodes (including mediastinal, contralateral hilar, and ipsilateral supraclavicular lymph nodes), whereas extensive stage disease is defined as disease beyond the definition of limited disease (including lymph nodes, brain, liver, bone, bone marrow, intraabdominal, and soft tissue metastases).

Stage Groupings of TNM Subsets

Occult carcinoma	TX N0 M0		
Stage 0	TIS Carcinoma in situ		
Stage I	T1 N0 M0	T2 N0 M0	
Stage II	T1 N1 M0	T2 N1 M0	
Stage IIIa	T1 N2 M0	T2 N2 M0	T3 N2 M0
	T3 N0 M0	T3 N1 M0	
Stage IIIb	T4 N0 M0	T4 N1 M0	T4 N2 M0
	T1 N3 M0	T2 N3 M0	T3 N3 M0
	T4 N3 M0		
Stage IV	Any T	Any N	M1

From Mountain CF: Lung cancer staging classification. Clin Chest Med 14:43–53, 1993; with permission.

16. How are stage groupings of TNM subsets used to assign therapy in patients with non–small cell lung cancer?

Patients with either stage I or stage II non–small cell carcinoma are candidates for surgical resection if they do not have medical contraindications to surgery. In most patients with stage I disease, a lobectomy is satisfactory for resection, although in some cases a bilobectomy or pneumonectomy is required. Patients with stage II disease often require a pneumonectomy for complete resection of tumor. Martini and colleagues at Memorial Sloan Kettering Hospital in New York City recently reported 5- and 10-year survival rates after resection for surgical stage I non–small cell lung cancer of 75% and 67%, respectively. In patients with stage II disease at surgery, the 5-year survival is approximately 30%.

Selected patients with stage IIIa disease are candidates for surgical resection, particularly those with localized chest wall involvement and no lymph node metastasis (T3N0M0). Patients with this lesion have a 35–40% 5-year survival rate after surgical resection. Studies are underway to assess preoperative chemotherapy with or without radiation therapy in patients with stage IIIa disease. Patients with stage IIIb disease, similar to stage IV disease with distant metastasis, are not considered surgical candidates and the prognosis is poor, with survival approaching 0% at 5 years.

17. What procedures can be used to determine surgical risk and predict postoperative outcome?

Spirometry, arterial blood gas measurements, and exercise testing are routinely employed in the preoperative risk assessment of patients undergoing pulmonary resection. Individuals with hypoxemia (PaO_2 less than 50 mmHg), hypercapnia ($PaCO_2$ more than 45 mmHg), calculated postoperative $DLCO$ of less than 40%, exercise-induced arterial desaturation of more than 2%, projected postresection FEV_1 of less than 800 ml or 30% of predicted value, or maximal oxygen-consumption less than 10 ml per kg per minute are considered at increased risk for postoperative morbidity and mortality. Although these criteria are widely quoted in the medical literature, they are by no means definitive and should not be the sole determinants of operability. Instead, significant abnormalities of these parameters should prompt additional evaluation to further stratify surgical risk. Patients with borderline measurements should undergo intensive perioperative pulmonary therapy. Less extensive surgical procedures (including nonanatomic resections, segmental resections, and thoracoscopic techniques) are increasingly available for individuals with prohibitively high risk of surgical complications.

18. How is the predicted postoperative FEV_1 calculated?

Individuals with preoperative FEV_1 and forced vital capacity (FVC) of 80% or greater of predicted values generally tolerate pneumonectomy well. If the preoperative FEV_1 is less than 80% of the predicted value, surgical morbidity and mortality may be determined by estimating the projected postoperative FEV_1. The latter is calculated by multiplying the preoperative FEV_1 by the percentage of remaining lung using a quantitative ventilation-perfusion lung scan. A projected postoperative FEV_1 less than 30% of the predicted value is commonly associated with a poor surgical outcome, whereas an estimate exceeding 40% of the predicted value typically suggests a benign postoperative course.

19. What surgical techniques are available for the management of lung cancer?

Tumors confined to a single lobe without regional nodal involvement may be managed successfully with lobectomy. Less extensive procedures can be performed for small, peripheral tumors (T1N0M0); segmentectomy and wedge resection are particularly appealing in individuals with reduced lung function. Compared with lobectomy, these limited procedures have higher recurrence rates. Bilobectomy and pneumonectomy are associated with higher mortality and complication rates but may be unavoidable in patients with more extensive local disease. The in-hospital postoperative mortality rates for patients who undergo surgical resection in a community hospital are 3.7% for segmental resections, 4.2% for lobectomies, and 11.6% for pneumonectomies. The mortality rates are lower in academic institutions and referral centers.

20. What role does thoracic irradiation play in the treatment of lung cancer?

Radiation therapy may be considered for patients with localized non–small cell lung cancer in whom surgical resection carries a significant risk because of concurrent illnesses. It may also be offered to patients who are eligible for surgery but refuse it. Irradiation after complete resection of stage II and IIIa lung cancer may diminish the incidence of local recurrent disease. It is routinely used as an adjunct after incomplete resection of non–small lung cancer, especially when residual tumor cells are detected at the margins of resection.

Radiation when combined with chemotherapy may improve survival rates over combination chemotherapy alone in patients with limited small cell lung cancer. Although chest irradiation has not been conclusively shown to improve survival in patients with extensive small cell cancers, it has been used for palliation of cranial, osseous, or orbital metastasis.

21. Which of the various cancer cell types is the most radiosensitive?

Small cell carcinoma is the most radiosensitive cancer type followed by squamous cell carcinoma and adenocarcinoma. Large cell tumors are the least radiosensitive.

22. What role does prophylactic cranial irradiation have in the treatment of patients with non–small cell or small cell carcinoma of the lung?

Although adenocarcinoma of the lung has a propensity for metastasizing to the brain, studies have not established that survival in patients with this tumor is improved by administration of prophylactic cranial irradiation (PCI). Patients with small cell lung cancer have a 40–50% risk of developing central nervous system metastases after successful chemotherapy. PCI has been shown to reduce the risk of brain metastases from approximately 23% to 6%. However, this reduction in the incidence of brain metastases is not translated into a survival advantage because relapse in the brain is typically accompanied by systemic recurrence in the majority of patients.

23. What are the potential complications of thoracic irradiation?

Acute pneumonitis is the primary complication of radiotherapy. It commonly occurs 1–3 months after therapy. Dyspnea and a nonproductive cough can present insidiously but generally improve over several weeks. A chest radiograph may reveal a sharply delineated infiltrate that approximates the size of the radiation port. Additional adverse sequelae of thoracic irradiation include subacute radiation pulmonary fibrosis, esophagitis, cardiomyopathy, spinal cord injury, and central nervous system dysfunction with memory loss, optic atrophy, or dysphonia.

24. What is the appropriate primary therapy for small cell carcinoma of the lung?

Approximately 20% of the estimated 177,000 annual cases of lung cancer in the United States are caused by small cell carcinoma of the lung (SCLC). The central therapeutic emphasis in patients with SCLC remains the use of combination chemotherapy. The most commonly used combinations of chemotherapy include etoposide and cisplatin (EP) and cyclophosphamide, doxorubicin, and vincristine (CAV) regimens. Although most patients with SCLC have a partial or complete response to chemotherapy, approximately 95% eventually die from their SCLC. Thus, in spite of an impressive response to chemotherapy in most cases, patients with this tumor still have a poor prognosis. Chest radiotherapy, 40–50 Gy administered for 3 to 5 weeks, can be given simultaneously with chemotherapy (concurrent therapy), interspersed between multiple cycles of chemotherapy (alternating), or at the completion of chemotherapy or while the chemotherapy is interrupted (sequential). Metaanalysis of prospective randomized trials comparing chemotherapy with the same chemotherapy plus radiation for patients with limited stage SCLC have shown 5% more patients alive at 2 and 3 years in the chemotherapy plus radiotherapy group. The latter group, however, has increased hematologic, esophageal, and pulmonary toxicity as well as more deaths from the toxicity of therapy compared with patients treated with chemotherapy alone.

BIBLIOGRAPHY

1. The Alpha-Tocopherol, Beta Carotene Cancer Prevention Study Group: The effect of vitamin E and beta carotene on the incidence of lung cancer and other cancers in male smokers. N Engl J Med 330:1029–1035, 1994.
2. Beckett WS: Epidemiology and etiology of lung cancer. Clin Chest Med 14:1–15, 1993.
3. Johnson BE: Management of small-cell lung cancer. Clin Chest Med 14:173–187, 1993.
4. Karsell PR, McDougall JC: Diagnostic tests for lung cancer. Mayo Clin Proc 68:288–296, 1993.
5. Lee-Chiong TL, Matthay RA: Lung cancer. In Harber P, Schenker MB, Balmes JR (eds): Occupational and Environmental Respiratory Disease. St. Louis, Mosby, 1996, pp 259–275.
6. Martini N, Bains MS, Burt ME, et al: Incidence of local recurrence and second primary tumors in resected stage I lung cancer. J Thorac Cardiovasc Surg 109:120–129, 1995.
7. Midthun DE, Swensen SJ, Jett JR: Approach to the solitary pulmonary nodule. Mayo Clin Proc 68:378–385, 1993.
8. Mountain CF: A new international staging system for lung cancer. Chest 89:225S–233S, 1986.
9. Mountain CF: Lung cancer staging classification. Clin Chest Med 14:43–53, 1993.
10. Parker SL, Tong T, Bolden S, et al: Cancer statistics, 1996. CA Cancer J Clin 46:5–27, 1996.
11. Patel AM, Davila DG, Peters SG: Paraneoplastic syndromes associated with lung cancer. Mayo Clin Proc 68:278–287, 1993.
12. Reilly JJ, Mentzer SJ, Sugarbaker DJ: Preoperative assessment of patients undergoing pulmonary resection. Chest 103:342S–345S, 1993.
13. Shields TW: Surgery therapy for carcinoma of the lung. Clin Chest Med 14:121–147, 1993.
14. Travis WD, Travis LB, Devesa SS: Lung cancer. Cancer 75:191–202, 1995.

61. MALIGNANT PLEURAL EFFUSIONS

Steven A. Sahn, M.D.

1. How is a malignant pleural effusion diagnosed?

The diagnosis is established by demonstrating exfoliated malignant cells in pleural fluid or by finding malignant cells in pleural tissue obtained by percutaneous pleural biopsy, thoracoscopy, thoracotomy or at autopsy.

2. What is a paramalignant effusion?

A paramalignant effusion is an effusion associated with a known malignancy but malignant cells cannot be demonstrated in pleural fluid or pleural tissue. Paramalignant effusions are caused by local effects of the tumor (lymphatic obstruction), systemic effects of the tumor (hypoalbuminemia), and complications of therapy (radiation pleuritis).

3. What is the most common cause of a malignant pleural effusion?

Lung cancer is the most common malignancy to metastasize to the pleura because of its close proximity to the pleural surface and its tendency to invade the pulmonary vasculature and embolize to the visceral pleural surface. Breast cancer, gastric carcinoma, and ovarian carcinoma are the next most frequent carcinomas to metastasize to the pleura.

4. How often is the primary site unknown when a malignant pleural effusion is diagnosed?

In approximately 10% of cases, the primary site is unknown at the time of diagnosis of a malignant pleural effusion. Work-up for the primary site should include an evaluation of the breasts in women and the prostate in men. Further work-up should be dictated by the patient's clinical presentation, physical examination, and ancillary laboratory tests.

5. What is the mechanism of formation of a malignant pleural effusion?

A blockage in lymphatic drainage of the pleural space at any point from the stoma of the parietal pleura to the mediastinal lymph nodes is the most important mechanism in the formation of a malignant pleural effusion and is responsible for large or massive effusions. Increased pleural capillary permeability plays a minor role in pleural fluid formation.

6. What are the most common symptoms in patients with malignant pleural effusions?

Patients most commonly present with dyspnea on exertion and cough. The presence and degree of dyspnea depend on the volume of pleural fluid and the patient's underlying pulmonary function.

7. Are all patients with malignant pleural effusions symptomatic at the time of diagnosis?

No. In a large series of patients with metastatic carcinoma to the pleura, almost one in four patients was relatively asymptomatic at presentation. In contrast, patients with malignant mesothelioma are virtually always symptomatic at the time the diagnosis is established, with chest pain being the most common symptom.

8. List the radiologic features that suggest a pleural effusion is caused by malignancy.

Massive pleural effusion (opacification of the entire hemithorax)
Bilateral pleural effusions with a normal heart size
Interstitial lung disease, mediastinal adenopathy and effusion (lymphangitic carcinomatosis)
Absence of contralateral mediastinal shift with an apparent large effusion

9. **What diagnoses should be considered when there is no contralateral mediastinal shift with an apparent large effusion?**

Lung cancer of the ipsilateral mainstem bronchus causing atelectasis

A fixed mediastinum caused by malignant lymph nodes

Malignant mesothelioma (the radiodensity represents predominantly tumor with only a small effusion)

Extensive tumor infiltration of the ipsilateral lung radiographically mimicking a large effusion

10. **Excluding cytologic examination, is pleural fluid analysis diagnostic for malignant pleural effusion?**

No. Malignant pleural effusions may be serous, serosanguinous, or grossly bloody and are usually exudates. The nucleated cell count is modest (approximately 2500–4000 cells/µl). The cell population generally consists of lymphocytes, macrophages, and mesothelial cells; lymphocytes often predominate (50–70%) in malignant effusions. In lymphoma, the majority of the nucleated cells are lymphocytes.

11. **Is pleural fluid eosinophilia common in malignant pleural effusions?**

No. Pleural fluid eosinophilia is inexplicably uncommon (5%) in malignant pleural effusions.

12. **What is the significance of a low pleural fluid pH (less than 7.30) in malignant pleural effusions?**

Patients whose malignant pleural effusion has a low pH have a high yield (95% positivity) on initial cytologic examination, a poor survival (2 months) from the time of thoracentesis, and a poor response (25–60%) to chemical pleurodesis.

13. **Which is the more sensitive test for the diagnosis of malignant pleural effusion, pleural fluid cytology or percutaneous pleural biopsy?**

Cytology is a more sensitive test for diagnosis than percutaneous pleural biopsy because pleural metastases tend to be focal and the latter is a blind sampling procedure. Yield from percutaneous pleural biopsy averages 50%, whereas yield from exfoliated cytology may be as high as 95%.

14. **What are the options for the patient with suspected malignancy and negative pleural fluid cytology and pleural biopsy?**

The options include observation for a few weeks followed by repeat studies, thoracoscopy, or open pleural biopsy. If the patient is anxious about the diagnosis, thoracoscopy should be done because, in expert hands, it provides a yield of 80–95% in patients with malignant disease.

15. **What is the prognosis for the patient with a malignant pleural effusion?**

Lung, gastric, and ovarian cancers tend to have a survival time of only a few months from the time of diagnosis of a malignant effusion. Patients with breast cancer may survive for several months to years depending on the response to chemotherapy. Patients with lymphomatous pleural effusions tend to have survival times intermediate between those of breast cancer and other carcinomas.

16. **What are the usual clinical and physiologic responses to therapeutic thoracentesis?**

Therapeutic thoracentesis generally rapidly relieves dyspnea. However, the volume of pleural fluid removed at thoracentesis dose not correlate closely with the improvement in lung volumes; in addition, Pao_2 may fall in some patients despite relief of dyspnea.

17. **What causes dyspnea in patients with large pleural effusions?**

Dyspnea appears to be caused by several factors including decrease in the compliance of the chest wall, contralateral shift of the mediastinum, and decrease in the ipsilateral lung volume. Reflex stimulation from the lungs and chest wall is also important.

18. Which patients are candidates for chemical pleurodesis?

Patients who have recurrent, symptomatic pleural effusions, are not terminal, and have a pH of more than 7.30 should be considered for chest tube drainage and instillation of a chemical agent.

19. What are the success rates for the available chemical pleurodesis agents?

Complete success rates (no recurrence of any fluid) for the available agents vary from 93% for talc to 0% for etoposide. The tetracyclines (tetracycline, doxycycline, and minocycline) have complete success rates of 67%, 72%, and 86%, respectively. Bleomycin and *Corynebacterium parvum* have complete success rates of 54% and 76%, respectively.

20. How should talc be administered?

Talc given by poudrage through the thoracoscope or by talc slurry through a chest tube is equally effective in the control of malignant pleural effusions. Talc slurry is less expensive than poudrage because the latter requires thoracoscopy.

21. How much talc should be used?

Five grams of talc is probably the optimum dose because it results in a high success rate with minimal adverse effects. Patients who have been reported to have adverse effects such as ARDS, pneumonitis, and respiratory failure usually received higher doses (10 g).

22. When should the chemical agent be instilled in the pleural space for pleurodesis?

Instillation should take place when the lung has reexpanded and minimal or no pleural fluid is observed on chest radiograph.

23. Does the patient have to be rotated after instillation of the chemical agent?

No. It has been shown with radiolabeled tetracycline that distribution is rapid and complete within seconds of pleural space instillation.

24. When should the chest tube be removed during the pleurodesis procedure?

Success rates tend to be higher when 24-hour chest chest tube drainage is less than 150 ml.

25. What are the adverse effects of talc?

Fever and chest pain are the most common adverse effects of talc and most other chemical agents instilled into the pleural space. Other adverse effects that have been reported with talc include empyema, arrhythmias, and respiratory failure; the latter appears to be related to high doses.

26. Which patients should not be treated with chemical pleurodesis?

Patients whose disease appears to be terminal, those with a pleural fluid pH of less than 7.30, those with a trapped lung, and those with mainstem bronchial occlusion with tumor should not be treated with chemical pleurodesis.

BIBLIOGRAPHY

1. Chernow B, Sahn SA: Carcinomatous involvement of the pleura: An analysis of 96 patients. Am J Med 63:695–702, 1977.
2. Kennedy L, Sahn SA: Talc pleurodesis for the treatment of pneumothorax and pleural effusions. Chest 106:1215–1222, 1994.
3. Lorch DG, Gordon L, Wooten S, et al: The effect of patient positioning on the distribution of tetracycline in the pleural space during pleurodesis. Chest 93:527–529, 1988.
4. Myer PC: Metastatic carcinoma of the pleura. Thorax 21:437–443, 1966.
5. Sahn SA: Pleural effusion in lung cancer. Clin Chest Med 14:189–200, 1993.
6. Sahn SA: Malignant pleural effusions. In Fishman AP, Elias JA, Fishman JA, et al (eds): Pulmonary Diseases and Disorders, 3rd ed. New York, McGraw Hill, 1996.
7. Sahn SA, Good JT Jr: Pleural fluid pH in malignant effusions: Diagnostic, prognostic, and therapeutic implications. Ann Intern Med 108:345–349, 1988.
8. Walker-Renard PB, Vaughan LM, Sahn SA: Chemical pleurodesis for malignant pleural effusions. Ann Intern Med 120:56–64, 1994.

62. SYSTEMIC COMPLICATIONS OF LUNG CANCER

Alejandro C. Arroliga, M.D., and Richard A. Matthay, M.D.

1. What are the causes of paraneoplastic syndromes in bronchogenic carcinoma?

Patients with bronchogenic carcinoma may experience systemic manifestations involving the endocrine, connective tissue, osseous, vascular, hematologic, skin, and neuromuscular systems. The term *paraneoplastic syndrome* refers to systemic manifestations that result from hormone precursors, growth factors, or cytokines produced by the tumor or from host antibodies directed against tumor antigens that cross-react with normal structures. The antigen-antibody reactions commonly affect the nervous system, causing histopathologic and functional alterations. Paraneoplastic syndromes in patients with bronchogenic carcinoma are more often associated with small cell lung cancer than with non-small cell lung cancer.

2. Name the most common paraendocrine syndromes associated with bronchogenic carcinoma.

Paraendocrine syndromes are paraneoplastic syndromes caused by hormones or hormone precursors produced by the neoplasm. The most common paraendocrine syndromes are inappropriate antidiuresis (SIAD), ectopic secretion of proopiomelanocortin peptides (ectopic Cushing's syndrome), and the hypercalcemia of malignancy.

3. What are the clinical characteristics of the paraneoplastic syndrome of inappropriate antidiuresis?

The syndrome of inappropriate antidiuresis (SIAD) is characterized by hyponatremia (serum sodium concentration < 135 mmol/L), plasma hypo-osmolality (< 280 mOsm/kg), inability to maximally dilute the urine in the presence of hyponatremia (urine osmolality > 100 mOsm/kg) and absence of other conditions that cause hyponatremia (e.g., certain drugs, hypovolemia, hypotension, and abnormalities of cardiac, renal, thyroid, and adrenal function). SIAD affects up to 16% of patients with small cell lung cancer, more commonly in patients with extensive rather than limited disease.

4. What are the more important pathogenetic factors of paraneoplastic SIAD?

Pathogenesis of SIAD consists primarily of the ectopic production by the tumor of the peptide arginine vasopressin (AVP), then inappropriate thirst, and, least importantly, production of atrial natriuretic factor (ANF) by the tumor. Dilution and concentration of urine occur in the distal tubule under the influence of AVP, which is normally secreted by the neurohypophysis. The secretion of AVP is affected by plasma osmolality and intravascular volume. When plasma osmolality decreases, the AVP level normally decreases, allowing the excretion of free water in hypotonic urine. AVP secretion makes the epithelium of the collecting duct permeable to water, thereby allowing the fluid in the collecting tubules to equilibrate with the hypertonic medullary interstitial fluid and making the urine hypertonic. In patients with paraneoplastic SIAD, the tumor produces AVP which is not regulated by plasma osmolality. In vitro, the tumor cells behave as if they were hypothalamic cells under constant stimulation. The level of AVP remains relatively increased, and the urine is not maximally diluted in patients with SIAD.

In the presence of plasma hypo-osmolality, satiety usually occurs, but patients with SIAD have excessive fluid intake caused by inappropriate thirst, which is as important as the presence of elevated AVP. In vitro, small cell lung cancer cells produce ANF, a hormone with natriuretic properties that may contribute to the pathogenesis of SIAD.

5. How is SIAD managed in patients with bronchogenic carcinoma?

Paraneoplastic SIAD is managed by both treating the tumor and correcting the hyponatremia. In 88% of affected patients, the hyponatremia is corrected by chemotherapy for the tumor. Fluid restriction (< 800 ml/day) causes a modest rise in serum sodium. Lithium carbonate has been used to treat SIAD, but it is effective in only 20% of patients and has significant toxicity. Therapy with demeclocycline (a tetracycline derivative), 0.9–1.2 gm/day, and fludrocortisone (a synthetic mineralocorticoid), 0.1–0.3 mg twice a day, is useful. Therapy with hypertonic 3% saline is reserved for patients with neurologic symptoms.

6. What is the pathogenesis of paraneoplastic Cushing's syndrome?

Up to 50% of patients with small cell lung cancer have biochemical evidence of hypercortisolism and elevated plasma immunoreactive adrenocorticotropin (ACTH) and proopiomelanocortin (POMC), but only 5% of patients with small cell lung cancer develop clinical manifestations of Cushing's syndrome. POMC/ACTH, which is produced by the tumor independent of the hypothalamic-pituitary-adrenal axis, is not suppressed by corticosteroid therapy. The secretion of POMC/ACTH induces bilateral adrenal hyperplasia and hyperfunction of the adrenal cortex, resulting in high plasma cortisol levels.

7. Describe the clinical characteristics of paraneoplastic Cushing's syndrome.

Paraneoplastic Cushing's syndrome has a rapid onset of symptoms (< 6 months). Affected patients usually present with peripheral edema, systemic hypertension, proximal muscle weakness, pigmentation of the skin, and moon facies. Metabolic abnormalities, such as hypokalemic metabolic alkalosis and hyperglycemia, are common, and patients have increased susceptibility to infections.

8. How is paraneoplastic Cushing's syndrome diagnosed?

At the time of onset of the paraneoplastic Cushing's syndrome, the bronchogenic carcinoma is usually clinically evident. Patients with this syndrome have elevated plasma and urine free cortisol and elevated ACTH. Unlike patients with Cushing's disease, patients with paraneoplastic Cushing's syndrome do not have suppression of ACTH, urine 17-hydroxycorticoids, and urine free corticoids during the high-dose dexamethasone suppression test (2 mg every 6 hr for 8 doses). In selected cases, the finding of abnormal fragments from the POMC molecule (e.g., corticotropin-like intermediate lobe peptide, γ-melanocyte-stimulating hormone) and abnormal ratio of β-lipotropin to γ-lipotropin in plasma suggest the ectopic origin of ACTH.

9. How are these patients treated?

Paraneoplastic Cushing's syndrome is managed primarily by treating the tumor. Combination chemotherapy and radiation often completely suppress the ectopic production of POMC. Patients who respond partially usually need additional therapy to control the effects of hypercortisolism. Therapy for the peripheral edema, muscle weakness, hypertension, and metabolic abnormalities characteristic of Cushing's syndrome consists of adrenal enzyme inhibitors, such as ketoconazole, metyrapone, and aminoglutethimide, given alone or in combination. Therapy with ketoconazole (400–800 mg/day), which blocks the 14-demethylation of cholesterol, is effective in two-thirds of affected patients. Mifepristone, a peripheral glucocorticoid antagonist, and octreotide, a somatostatin analogue, may also be used alone or in combination with adrenal enzyme inhibitors.

10. What are the two mechanisms for the development of hypercalcemia in patients with bronchogenic carcinoma?

Hypercalcemia of malignancy affects 6–38% of patients with bronchogenic carcinoma, most commonly (72%) in squamous cell carcinoma. These patients have a large tumor mass, and their prognosis is poor, with the median survival after the onset of hypercalcemia of only

1.5 months. The two mechanisms for the development of hypercalcemia in patients with cancer are local osteolysis, which occurs in < 20% of cases, and humoral hypercalcemia of malignancy. **Local osteolysis** occurs in patients with widespread bony involvement and is caused by osteoclastic bone resorption in areas adjacent to the tumor. **Humoral hypercalcemia** of malignancy is the predominant mechanism in up to 80% of cases. These lung cancer cells produce parathyroid hormone-related peptide (PTHrP), a potent resorbing agent that increases osteoclastic activity and the renal tubular reabsorption of calcium and causes renal phosphate wasting. Patients with humoral hypercalcemia are usually hypovolemic, a condition that favors the reabsorption of calcium together with water and sodium from the proximal renal tubules.

11. How do you treat patients with symptomatic hypercalcemia of malignancy?

Because some treatments for humoral hypercalcemia have toxic effects, only patients with debilitating symptoms, such as polyuria, polydipsia, dehydration, or altered mental status, or with a serum calcium concentration > 14 mg/dl should be treated. The first step in therapy is to correct dehydration, restoring intravascular volume to increase calcium filtration at the level of the kidneys. Loop diuretic therapy prevents volume overload and aids calciuresis. However, the serum calcium rises after the saline infusion is stopped, and other therapy is usually necessary. Salmon calcitonin inhibits bone resorption and increases the renal excretion of calcium. Although a weak hypocalcemic agent, calcitonin has a fast onset of action. Plicamycin, another hypocalcemic agent, has toxic effects on the osteoclast and normalizes serum calcium concentration, usually after a single dose. Gallium nitrate and the bisphosphonates etidronate and pamidronate are the treatments of choice for patients with hypercalcemia of malignancy. Although they have a slow onset of action (2–3 days), they are effective in 60–100% of cases, and the effect may last for 1–3 weeks.

12. What are the most common paraneoplastic neurologic disorders associated with bronchogenic carcinoma?

Subacute sensory neuronopathy and the Lambert-Eaton myasthenic syndrome. They affect about 3% of patients with bronchogenic carcinoma, most commonly patients with small cell lung cancer. **Subacute sensory neuropathy** is characterized by sensory ataxia, absence of deep tendon reflexes, and normal motor function. Asymmetric abnormalities of the extremities, including pain, paresthesias, and numbness, are common. Most affected patients have a panneuronal IgG antibody in cerebrospinal fluid and serum.

The **Lambert-Eaton myasthenic syndrome** is caused by an immune response in which the tumor expresses an antigen and the host produces an IgG antibody against the antigen that cross-reacts with a subunit of the calcium channel complex in the presynaptic area. The antibody blocks the function and reduces the number of voltage-gated calcium channels, causing a deficit of acetylcholine release at the motor nerve terminals. The most common symptoms of the syndrome are fatigability and muscle weakness, mainly of the proximal muscles of the legs. Other symptoms include aching, stiffness, and symptoms of autonomic dysfunction (e.g,. dry mouth and impotence). Deep tendon reflexes are depressed.

13. What are the most common causes of the superior vena cava syndrome? What are its clinical features?

Up to 90% of cases of the superior vena cava syndrome are caused by malignancy, with bronchogenic carcinoma (70–80% of cases) being the most common causative malignancy and small cell lung cancer the most common histologic type. Other tumors that cause this syndrome include lymphoma, primary mediastinal tumor, and metastatic carcinoma. In the syndrome, blood flow to the superior vena cava is obstructed either by compression by the tumor or lymph nodes or by thrombosis of the vein.

The syndrome evolves over a few days to weeks and is characterized by edema of the upper extremities, face, and larynx. Cerebral edema may also occur. On physical examination, affected patients commonly have dilated veins in the upper part of the body, facial ruddiness, and proptosis. Conjunctival suffusion and edema of the nasal mucosa and tongue may occur. The pathologic diagnosis of the superior vena cava syndrome can be made by biopsy of the lung tumor or by mediastinoscopy or anterior mediastinotomy. Transthoracic needle aspiration biopsy of the tumor under ultrasound guidance has recently been shown to be useful (diagnostic yield of 83%).

Patients with the syndrome should avoid lying supine and diuretic therapy may be used carefully to decrease venous pressure. After the histologic diagnosis has been established, the underlying malignancy must be treated, but the prognosis of patients with the superior vena cava syndrome caused by bronchogenic carcinoma is poor.

14. What is the pathogenesis of the cancer anorexia-cachexia syndrome?

The anorexia-cachexia syndrome, which occurs in up to 80% of patients with advanced malignancy, is characterized by loss of appetite, weight loss, nausea, constipation, and muscle weakness. The syndrome is probably caused by the production of proinflammatory cytokines by tumor cells and reactive host cells. This release of cytokines leads to anorexia and lean tissue wasting. There is convincing evidence from animal models that interleukin-1, interleukin-6, tumor necrosis factor-α, and interferon-α are important factors in the pathogenesis of this syndrome.

15. How is the cancer anorexia-cachexia syndrome managed?

Metoclopramide, a prokinetic agent, 10 mg given orally before meals and bedtime, may improve appetite and relieve early satiety caused by dysmotility and gastroparesis.

Megestrol acetate, started at a dosage of 160 mg/day, improves appetite and reverses weight loss. The effects of the drug are dose-related, and its mechanism of action is unknown. Although the drug causes few side effects, the dosage should be kept in the lower range and the drug should not be given to patients with a history of deep vein thrombosis.

Other drugs that may be useful include dronabinol (a synthetic form of Δ9-tetrahydrocannabinol), pentoxifylline, and thalidomide. Nutritional supplementation, preferably by the enteral route, is advisable in patients with the cancer anorexia-cachexia syndrome. The role of total parenteral nutrition in this disorder is unclear.

16. Describe the clinical characteristics of hypertrophic osteoarthropathy.

Hypertrophic osteoarthropathy is a disorder of bones, joints, and soft tissues that is either idiopathic or associated with disease of the gastrointestinal tract, cardiovascular system, and, more commonly, the respiratory system. The disorder has been reported in up to 10% of patients with bronchogenic carcinoma and pleural tumors; it is more commonly associated with squamous cell carcinoma, although it can occur in patients with adenocarcinoma and large cell carcinoma. Hypertrophic osteoarthropathy is rarely associated with small cell lung cancer. Other associated respiratory disorders include infectious processes of the lung (e.g., abscesses, bronchiectasis, and empyema) and cystic fibrosis.

Hypertrophic osteoarthropathy is characterized by clubbing of the digits, bilateral symmetrical periosteal new bone formation affecting mainly the long bones of the distal extremities, noninflammatory arthritis, thickness of the subcutaneous soft tissue in the distal extremities and occasionally the face, and evidence of autonomic dysfunction (e.g., flushing, blanching, increased sweating of hands and feet).

17. What factors are involved in the pathogenesis of hypertrophic osteoarthropathy? How is it managed?

The pathogenesis of this disorder is not well understood. The condition of some patients with bronchogenic carcinoma and hypertrophic osteoarthropathy improves significantly after the vagus nerve on the side of the tumor is cut, suggesting a neurogenic cause. The production of a humoral substance, either by the tumor or the host, has also been suggested as a cause. The commonly mentioned humoral agents are growth hormone produced by the tumor and platelet-derived factors.

The management of hypertrophic osteoarthropathy includes treatment of the tumor and symptomatic therapy. Clubbing by itself is frequently asymptomatic. The symptoms related to periostitis and synovitis respond to therapy with nonsteroidal anti-inflammatory drugs. Corticosteroids and propantheline bromide may provide symptomatic relief.

BIBLIOGRAPHY

1. Altman RD: Hypertrophic osteoarthropathy. In McCarty DJ, Koopman WJ (eds): Arthritis and Allied Conditions. Philadelphia, Lea & Febiger, 1993, pp 1511–1517.
2. Arroliga AC, Matthay RA: Paraneoplastic syndromes in bronchogenic carcinoma. Clin Pulm Med 1:322–332, 1994.
3. Bigsby R, Greengrass R, Unrou H: Diagnostic algorithm for acute superior vena caval obstruction (SVCO). J Cardiovasc Surg 34:347–350, 1993.
4. Bilezikian JP: Management of acute hypercalcemia. N Engl J Med 326:1196–1203, 1992.
5. Burtis WJ, Brady TG, Orloff J, et al: Immunochemical characterization of circulating parathyroid hormone-related protein in patients with humoral hypercalcemia of cancer. N Engl J Med 322:1106–1112, 1990.
6. Dalmau J, Posner JB: Neurologic paraneoplastic antibodies (anti-Yo; anti-Hu; anti-Ri): The case for a nomenclature based on antibody and antigenic specificity. Neurology 44:2241–2246, 1994.
7. Dalmau J, Graus F, Rosenblum MK, et al: Anti-Hu-associated paraneoplastic encephalomyelitis-sensory neuronopathy. Medicine 71:59–72, 1992.
8. Elrington GM, Murray NMF, Spiro SG, et al: Neurological paraneoplastic syndrome in patients with small cell lung cancer: A prospective study of 150 patients. J Neurol Neurosurg Psychiatry 54:764–767, 1991.
9. Espat NJ, Moldawer LL, Copeland EM: Cytokine-mediated alterations in host metabolism prevent nutritional repletion in cachectic cancer patients. J Surg Oncol 58:77–82, 1995.
10. Gosney MA, Gosney JR, Lye M: Plasma growth hormone and digital clubbing in carcinoma of the bronchus. Thorax 45:545–547, 1990.
11. Gross AJ, Steinberg SM, Reilly JA, et al: Atrial natriuretic factor and arginine vasopressin production in tumor cell lines from patients with lung cancer and their relationship to serum sodium. Cancer Res 53:67–74, 1993.
12. Ko JC, Yang PC, Yuan A, et al: Superior vena cava syndrome: Rapid histologic diagnosis by ultrasound-guided transthoracic needle aspiration biopsy. Am J Respir Crit Care Med 149:783–787, 1994.
13. Kovacs L, Robertson GL: Syndrome of inappropriate antidiuresis. Endocrinol Metab Clin North Am 21:859–875, 1992.
14. Lennon VA, Kryzer TJ, Griesmann GE, et al: Calcium-channel antibodies in the Lambert-Eaton syndrome and other paraneoplastic syndromes. N Engl J Med 332:1467–1474, 1995.
15. List AF, Hainsworth JD, Davis BW, et al: The syndrome of inappropriate secretion of antidiuretic hormone (SIADH) in small-cell lung cancer. J Clin Oncol 4:1191–1198, 1986.
16. Moses AM, Scheinman SJ: Ectopic secretion of neurohypophyseal peptides in patients with malignancy. Endocrinol Metab Clin North Am 20:489–505, 1991.
17. Nelson KA, Walsh D, Sheehan FA: The cancer anorexia-cachexia syndrome. J Clin Oncol 12:213–225, 1994.
18. Odell WD: Ectopic ACTH secretion: A misnomer. Endocrinol Metab Clin North Am 20:371–379, 1991.
19. Ortho DN: Cushing's syndrome. N Engl J Med 332:791–803, 1995.
20. O'Neal JH, Murray NMF, Newsom-Davis J: The Lambert-Eaton myasthenic syndrome: A review of 50 cases. Brain 111:577–596, 1988.
21. Patel AM, Davila DG, Peters SA: Paraneoplastic syndromes associated with lung cancer. Mayo Clin Proc 68:278–287, 1993.
22. Schteingart DE: Ectopic secretion of peptides of the proopiomelanocortin family. Endocrinol Metab Clin North Am 20:453–471, 1991.
23. Shepherd FA, Laskey J, Evans WK, et al: Cushing's syndrome associated with ectopic corticotropin production and small-cell lung cancer. J Clin Oncol 10:21–27, 1992.
24. Stewart MF, Orosby SR, Gibson S, et al: Small cell lung cancer cell lines secrete predominantly ACTH precursor peptides not ACTH. Br J Cancer 60:20–24, 1989.

63. BENIGN NEOPLASMS OF THE LUNG

John P. Wilkins, M.D., and Melvin L. Morganroth, M.D.

1. What percentage of primary pulmonary neoplasms are benign?

Less than 10% of all primary pulmonary neoplasms are benign.

2. What is the most common benign pulmonary neoplasm?

The most common benign pulmonary neoplasm is a pulmonary hamartoma. Hamartomas are mesenchymal tumors that originate from undifferentiated multipotential cells in connective tissue of bronchial walls. Histologically, hamartomas consist of the same tissues seen normally in the lung such as collagen and smooth muscle; they occasionally contain fat or cartilage. Generally hamartomas occur as single tumors, although rarely they can present as multiple pulmonary nodules and their size can slowly increase over time. Hamartomas are seen in patients in their 60s and rarely in patients less than 30. They are three times more common in men than women.

3. Where in the lung do hamartomas usually occur?

Hamartomas usually occur in the lung peripherally; therefore, patients tend to be asymptomatic when the "mass" is found on routine chest roentgenograms. They are generally well circumscribed solitary pulmonary nodules that are less than 4 cm in diameter, although occasionally they can be enormous and can grow over time (sometimes filling a hemithorax). Approximately 10% of hamartomas grow endobronchially, producing symptoms of cough, fever, hemoptysis, or wheeze. Lesions that grow endobronchially are visible bronchoscopically and occasionally diagnosed during bronchoscopy.

4. Describe the radiographic appearance of a hamartoma.

A hamartoma appears as a homogeneous, lobulated peripheral mass between 1 and 8 cm, averaging about 4 cm in diameter. In rare instances they have visible "popcorn" calcifications. When these lesions are located endobronchially they show signs of atelectasis or pneumonia, or both. Rarely, hamartomas present as cystic structures or as multiple lesions. CT of the chest can be helpful in diagnosing hamartomas, particularly when the chest roentgenogram does not show any calcifications. High resolution CT scans are helpful in establishing the diagnosis in patients who have masses less than 3 cm in diameter that show fat with or without calcification.

5. How is a hamartoma diagnosed?

Because hamartomas are usually peripheral, sputum cytology and bronchoscopy are of little value in diagnosis. Pathologic diagnosis is obtained either by CT-guided biopsy or by surgery. CT-guided biopsies can establish the diagnosis in approximately 85% of cases with low overall morbidity and mortality. Although hamartomas are considered benign, some controversy exists as to whether they can undergo malignant transformation. For this reason, after diagnosis, patients should be followed with serial chest radiographs. In patients in whom CT-guided biopsy is not diagnostic or in whom the mass shows growth on serial roentgenograms, surgical intervention is indicated. The surgical options include video assisted thoracoscopic surgery or an open lung biopsy via an open thoracotomy.

6. What are bronchial carcinoids?

Bronchial carcinoids are the third largest group of lung tumors after bronchogenic carcinomas and hamartomas. They account for 4% of all primary lung neoplasms. Although they have been considered "adenomas" in the past, they may act like low-grade carcinomas and, therefore, should be considered potentially malignant. Carcinoids have neuroendocrine origins and a spectrum of malignant potential: small cell carcinoma is the most malignant, "atypical" carcinoids have an intermediate grade, and "typical" carcinoids have the most benign course.

7. Who gets bronchial carcinoids?

Bronchial carcinoids are generally seen in adults in their mid-40s and occur equally in men and women. Although there is no association with smoking in patients with typical carcinoids, there is a correlation with smoking in patients with atypical carcinoids and small cell carcinoma.

8. How do bronchial carcinoids present?

Clinical presentation depends on location. The majority of bronchial carcinoids (approximately 80%) occur centrally and endobronchially and therefore present with symptoms of obstruction: cough, wheeze, hemoptysis, chest pain, or fever. The remaining 20%, which are peripheral, are usually found accidentally on a routine roentgenogram in an asymptomatic patient. In such patients the diagnosis can be delayed for up to 3 years. Occasionally, patients may present with the carcinoid syndrome resulting from vasoactive material produced by the tumor (see question 11).

9. How are bronchial carcinoids diagnosed?

On chest roentgenogram carcinoids can result in atelectasis or obstructive pneumonitis because of an endobronchial location. Lymphangitic spread and pleural-based masses can also be seen in atypical carcinoids. In addition, atypical carcinoids can show evidence of peripheral cavitation in contrast to typical carcinoids, which are generally well demarcated and central.

Because of their endobronchial nature carcinoids are generally seen during bronchoscopy. They often appear reddish-brown, which gives them a hypervascular appearance. Bronchoscopists have been reluctant to biopsy these lesions because they were thought to be at increased risk of hemorrhage during the procedure. Recent studies, however, have shown that these lesions can be safely biopsied if care is taken.

10. List the differences between typical and atypical carcinoids.

Feature	Typical Carcinoid	Atypical Carcinoid
Sex difference	None	None
Age (years)	55	60
Smoking	No association	~60% occur in smokers
Frequency	~75% of carcinoids	~15% of carcinoids
Location in the lung	Usually central	Usually peripheral
Roentgenographic appearance	Well circumscribed; can be associated with obstructive pneumonia, atelectasis	Spiculated or smooth margins; may show evidence of necrosis, hilar adenopathy
Pathologic appearance	Rare mitotic figures, prominent mosaicism, argyrophilic	Increased mitotic figures, prominent mosaicism, argyrophilic
Lymph node involvement	Rarely, ~7%	45%
Metastasis	Essentially never	20%
Recurrence after resection (5-year disease-free interval)	95%	40%
Malignant potential	Low	High

11. What is carcinoid syndrome?

Carcinoid syndrome occurs in approximately 4% of patients with carcinoid tumors and always reflects metastasis of the tumor, usually to the liver. The syndrome is caused by the production of high levels of 5-hydroxytryptamine that enter the systemic circulation and cause severe flushing, hypotension, anxiety, nausea, and vomiting. Lesions isolated to the liver usually do not produce this syndrome because the 5-hydroxytryptamine is metabolized by the liver and inactivated later if it enters the systemic circulation. The difference between metastatic abdominal carcinoids and metastatic thoracic carcinoids is that the systemic symptoms of flushing, hypotension, anxiety, nausea, and vomiting are much more profound in thoracic tumors than in abdominal tumors. In addition, thoracic tumors can spread to the left atrium, whereas abdominal tumors spread to the right atrium.

12. Describe tracheobronchial papillary tumors.

Only a tough attending would ask this question on rounds! Tracheobronchial tumors most commonly occur in young children in the larynx and are generally squamous papillomas. Human papillomavirus has been implicated in their development. Tracheobronchial papillomas tend to cause "central" symptoms, e.g., cough, wheeze, stridor, or hemoptysis. These tumors are generally benign and tend to regress before adolescence without treatment. In adults, these tumors can undergo malignant transformation and generally are removed either endobronchially with a carbon dioxide laser or surgically.

13. Which benign tumors arise from mucous glands in the tracheobronchial tree? Describe them.

Adenoid cyst carcinomas grow from the minor and major salivary glands and the mucous glands of the upper respiratory tract. They occur in the lower respiratory tract 15% of the time, originating in the submucosa. Despite the fact that these are slow growing, they are true carcinomas and tend to recur locally. Adenoid cyst carcinomas infrequently metastasize. They usually present in patients in their 50s and, because of their site of origin, tend to cause airway symptoms, such as cough, choking, chest pain, hemoptysis, wheeze, or stridor. The chest roentgenogram shows a pattern of chronic pneumonia. During bronchoscopic examination of the airways, these tumors appear in a variety of patterns, from a single pedunculated mass to a diffusely infiltrative lesion.

14. What are teratomas?

Teratomas are included in the differential diagnosis of anterior mediastinal masses, in addition to thymomas, thyroid cancers, and lymphomas (usually the terrible ones). Remember the four T's and you'll impress everyone during rounds. Teratomas are very rarely seen within the pulmonary parenchyma. They contain every embryonic cell line—endoderm, mesoderm, and ectodermal layers—and arise from the third pharyngeal pouch. These tumors may have a malignant component. When the diagnosis of teratoma is considered the possibility of a metastatic lesion from the gonads should be ruled out. Teratomas are more commonly seen in younger patients, between the ages of 20 and 30 years, and occur equally in men and women. Patients commonly present with central symptoms including chest pain, hemoptysis, trichoptysis, pneumonia, or bronchiectasis. Radiographically, teratomas are seen in the anterior mediastinum or in an upper lobe; they appear irregular and lobulated and may have calcifications. Surgery is usually required to make the diagnosis.

15. Are there any other benign tumors that occur in the lung?

The two most common benign tumors of the lung, hamartomas and carcinoids, have already been discussed. For the rest, make "THE CALL:"

T Teratomas/tracheobronchial papillomas (central)
H Hemangiomas: usually subpleural (peripheral) benign tumors arising from blood vessels
E Endometriosis: think of this one in a young woman with recurrent right-sided pneumothoraces around her menstrual period; generally occur peripherally

C   Chondromas: rare; arise from bronchial cartilage (endobronchial)
A   Adenomas, adenoid cystic carcinoma: rare, seen endobronchially, and arise from the submucosa of the lower respiratory tract
L   Leiomyomas: 2% of benign tumors; about 33% occur peripherally in patients under the age of 20; 90% of patients are women; can mimic asthma if it occurs in the trachea
L   Lipoma (the shape changers): usually occur around the bronchus and can change in appearance roentgenographically depending on the patient's position

Endobronchial lesions present with central symptoms (e.g., cough, fever, wheeze, hemoptysis, or chest pain). Peripheral lesions are found by luck, usually, and rarely cause symptoms unless they involved the pleura, e.g., pain or pneumothorax.

BIBLIOGRAPHY

1. Bharani SN, Arbeit JM, Hyde JS, et al: Mucoepidermoid tumor of the trachea. Chest 70(6):782–784, 1976.
2. Dusmet M, Mckneally MF: Bronchial and thymic carcinoid tumors: A review. Digestion 55(Suppl 3): 70–76, 1994.
3. Fraser RG, Pare JAP, Pare PD, et al: Diagnosis of Diseases of the Chest, 3rd ed. Philadelphia, W.B. Saunders, 1989.
4. Freidman PJ: Classification of leiomyomatous lung lesions. Am J Roentgenol 142(4):851–852, 1984.
5. George R, Light R: Essentials of Pulmonary and Critical Care, 2nd ed. Philadelphia, W.B. Saunders, 1990.
6. Hasleton PS: Histopathology and prognostic factors in bronchial tumors. Thorax 49(Suppl):S56–S62, 1994.
7. Kvols LK: Metastatic carcinoid tumors and the malignant carcinoid syndrome. Ann N Y Acad Sci 733:464–470, 1994.
8. Murray JF, Nadel JA: Textbook of Respiratory Medicine, 2nd ed. Philadelphia, W.B. Saunders, 1994.
9. White SH, Ibrahim NB, Forrester-Wood CP, Jeyasingham K: Leiomyomas of the lower respiratory tract. Thorax 40:306–311, 1985.

64. PULMONARY METASTATIC DISEASE

R. Hal Hughes, M.D., and Stephanie M. Levine, M.D.

1. How common are pulmonary metastases?

At autopsy, evidence of lung metastases is seen either grossly or microscopically in 30–40% of patients with extrathoracic primary tumors. However, only 10–30% of these are recognized before death. Although many tumor types may metastasize to the lungs, the malignancies that are most consistently associated with pulmonary metastases are malignant melanomas, genitourinary carcinomas, soft-tissue and osteogenic sarcomas, and germ cell neoplasms.

2. Describe the usual radiographic patterns of pulmonary metastatic disease.

Solitary and **multiple** metastatic nodules tend to occur in the periphery of the lungs presumably because they spread hematogenously. The lower and middle lung fields tend to be involved more commonly because these are the zones of greatest blood flow. Often the multiple metastatic lesions are bilateral, well circumscribed, and occur in varying sizes. Chest CT is understandably superior in detecting small metastases involving the subpleural, apical, and costophrenic angle regions as well as in assessing mediastinal lymphadenopathy.

Lymphangitic carcinomatosis often simulates interstitial pulmonary edema, in that it has irregular coarse bronchovascular markings and prominent septal or Kerley B lines. However, the linear pattern may have a nodular component, thus creating a coarse reticulonodular pattern. High resolution CT in these patients may show an increased number of irregular thickened septal lines arranged in polyhedral patterns. The lines predominate in the central chest and may be termed *Kerley A lines*. Often knot-like thickening or beading occurs along the course of the lines, which is the most specific finding for lymphangitic carcinomatosis.

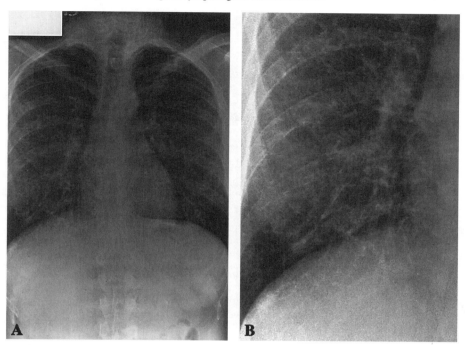

A, Posteroanterior chest radiograph from a 47-year-old man shows an interstitial pattern consistent with lymphangitic carcinomatosis. He was found to have adenocarcinoma by transbronchial biopsy. **B,** Enlargement of the periphery of the same radiograph shows Kerley B lines *(arrow)*.

3. What primary extrathoracic tumor can result in *solitary* pulmonary metastases?

It is estimated that 25% of all metastases to the lung are solitary. Moreover, 3–5% of all *solitary pulmonary nodules* are actually solitary metastases. The most common tumor types that result in solitary metastases are colon carcinomas (usually rectosigmoid), sarcomas (especially osteogenic), renal cell and breast carcinomas, testicular neoplasms, and melanomas. On rare occasions, bladder and hepatocellular carcinomas present as solitary pulmonary metastases.

4. What primary extrathoracic tumor types occur as *multiple* pulmonary metastases?

Although multiple metastases may present in numerous forms, the following radiographic patterns may suggest certain tumor types. **Cannonball** lesions are associated with colorectal and renal cell carcinomas, sarcomas, melanomas, and choriocarcinomas. **Miliary** patterns are noted with medullary thyroid carcinomas, melanomas, renal cell carcinomas, and ovarian carcinomas. **Cavitary** masses are most commonly seen with squamous cell carcinomas of any origin (usually head and neck tumors in males and genitalia-related tumors in females), colon carcinomas, osteogenic sarcomas, and rarely pancreas or bladder carcinomas. Osteogenic sarcomas are commonly associated with pneumothoraces, which may be the initial presentation of this disease. **Calcified** metastases are unique to osteogenic sarcomas, chondrosarcomas, and synovial cell sarcomas.

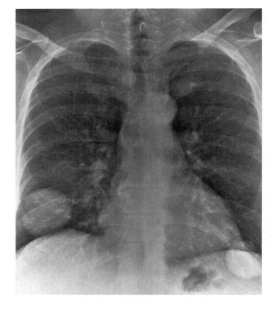

Posteroanterior chest radiograph from a 52-year-old man who had undergone a prior partial left humoral resection and reconstruction secondary to a soft tissue sarcoma. Metastatic cannonball lesions are seen.

5. Which primary extrathoracic malignancies are associated with lymphangitic pulmonary metastases?

The most common tumor types are breast, pancreatic, gastric, and colon carcinomas. Less commonly, germ cell tumors (especially testicular), prostate carcinomas, and cervical carcinomas metastasize in this fashion. Lung carcinomas and lymphomas are intrathoracic malignancies that can present with a lymphangitic pattern.

6. What are the common clinical manifestations of lymphangitic spread of carcinoma to the lungs?

Dyspnea often begins insidiously and characteristically progresses rapidly, during which time pulmonary function tests may reveal decreased diffusion capacity, reduced lung volumes and lung compliance, and hypoxemia. Cough is also a frequent complaint and is usually nonproductive.

7. Name the extrathoracic tumors that metastasize endobronchially.

Renal cell carcinoma, breast carcinoma, melanoma, and colorectal carcinoma all occur commonly. Occasionally other tumors such as cervical carcinomas, uterine carcinomas, Kaposi's sarcomas, and other sarcomas are found endobronchially.

8. Which extrathoracic tumor types are associated with pleural effusions?

The most common malignancies presenting with pleural effusions are breast, pancreas, gastric, ovarian, and renal cell carcinomas.

9. How is metastatic disease of the lung usually diagnosed?

Sputum cytology may be positive in up to 35% of patients; the yield is higher with larger masses and endobronchial disease. Fiberoptic bronchoscopy with transbronchial biopsy is especially useful if patients have hemoptysis, localized wheezing, or radiographs suggesting atelectasis or diffuse infiltrates. Bronchoalveolar lavage may be diagnostic of metastatic tumor, especially when lymphangitic spread has occurred. Transthoracic fine needle aspiration or biopsy is often diagnostic with peripheral lesions or lymphangitic spread. Aspiration of wedged capillary blood via pulmonary artery catheters has been reported to be diagnostic for lymphangitic carcinomatosis when cytologic examination of the buffy coat is performed. Newer techniques such as radiolabeled monoclonal antibodies directed toward specific primary tumor antigens may ultimately be useful.

10. Does a new solitary pulmonary nodule (SPN) discovered after a primary extrathoracic tumor has been found always represent metastatic disease?

The answer often depends on the primary tumor pathology. SPNs after resection of sarcomas or melanomas are ten times more likely to represent a metastasis than a second primary tumor. However, new SPNs after genitourinary or colorectal primaries have a 50% chance of being a metastasis. Those after head and neck tumors are twice as likely to be new primaries.

CONTROVERSIES

11. What are the criteria for surgical resection of pulmonary metastases?

Most authors agree on the following criteria: (1) the primary tumor must be controlled, (2) there is no other evidence of extrathoracic metastatic disease, (3) the metastatic lung disease must be amenable to complete resection, (4) the patient must be physiologically able to tolerate the proposed surgery, and (5) there is no other *effective* systemic therapy. More controversial issues regarding the potential success of metastasectomies include a smaller number of lung nodules, a longer disease-free interval before recurrence, and longer tumor doubling time.

12. What are the usual surgical approaches for metastasectomies?

The majority of cases require only a wedge resection or a limited segmentectomy. Lobectomies are required in approximately 25% of cases and pneumonectomies in only 8%. New techniques such as laser or needle-tipped electrocautery have been used successfully in some instances. Video-assisted thoracoscopic surgery (VATS) also holds promise but relies heavily on CT findings, which may limit its use to staging in this setting. For bilateral resections, either a median sternotomy or a "clam shell" thoracotomy (bilateral anterior thoracotomy with a transverse sternotomy) is used in selected patients. The reported surgical mortality of pulmonary metastasectomies is 1%.

13. How successful are surgical resections of pulmonary metastases?

The overall success of these surgeries is directly related to the type of tumor; in many cases, a smaller number of nodules, a slower growth rate, and a longer disease-free interval portend a better prognosis. For instance, patients with metastatic disease from soft tissue sarcomas undergoing metastasectomy, have an overall 5-year survival rate ranging between 21 and 38%, but most series show improved survival with less than five nodules, a disease-free interval of more than 1 year, and tumor doubling time of more than 40 days. Patients undergoing metastasectomy for colorectal carcinoma have an overall 5-year survival rate of 31–43%, with a trend toward longer survival in those with a solitary metastasis 3 cm or less in size. Melanomas tend to metastasize to extrathoracic locations, but when metastases are limited to the lungs, patients undergoing metastasectomies have a 5-year survival rate of 11–25% and a better prognosis with two or fewer nodules and a disease-free interval of more than 1 year. Rarely, metastatic tumors may regress spontaneously without any specific therapy, such as reported with renal cell carcinoma, trophoblastic carcinoma, and transitional cell carcinoma of the bladder.

BIBLIOGRAPHY

1. Chiles C, Ravin CE: Intrathoracic metastasis from an extrathoracic malignancy: A radiographic approach to patient evaluation. Radiol Clin North Am 23:427–438, 1985.
2. Filderman AE, Matthay RA: Metastatic malignant tumors. In Bone RC (ed): Pulmonary and Critical Care Medicine. St. Louis, Mosby, 1994.

3. Fraser RG, Paré JAP, Paré PD, et al: Diagnosis of Diseases of the Chest, 3rd ed. Philadelphia, W.B. Saunders, 1989.
4. Luce JA: Metastatic malignant tumors. In Murray JF, Nadel JA (eds): Textbook of Respiratory Medicine, 2nd ed. Philadelphia, W.B. Saunders, 1994.
5. Marincola FM, Mark J: Selection factors resulting in improved survival after surgical resection of tumors metastatic to the lungs. Arch Surg 125:1387–1393, 1990.
6. Masson RG, Krikorian J, Lukl P, et al: Pulmonary microvascular cytology in the diagnosis of lymphangitic carcinomatosis. N Engl J Med 321:71–76, 1989.
7. Mountain CF, McMurtrey MJ, Hermes KE: Surgery for pulmonary metastasis: A 20 year experience. Ann Thorac Surg 38:323–330, 1994.
8. Nadich D, Zerhouni EA, Siegelman SS: Computed Tomography of the Thorax. New York, Raven Press, 1985.
9. Ochs RH: Neoplasms of the lung other than bronchogenic carcinoma. In Fishman AP (ed): Pulmonary Diseases and Disorders, 2nd ed. New York, McGraw-Hill, 1988.
10. Pugatch RD: Radiologic evaluation in chest malignancies: A review of imaging modalities. Chest 107:294S–297S, 1995.
11. Rusch VW: Pulmonary metastasectomy: Current indications. Chest 107:322S–330S, 1995.
12. van Halteren HK, van Geel AN, Hart A, et al: Pulmonary resection for metastases of colorectal origin. Chest 107:1526–1531, 1995.

XIV. Respiratory Failure

---

65. ACUTE RESPIRATORY FAILURE

Hyun Joo Kim, M.D., and David H. Ingbar, M.D.

---

1. Define acute respiratory failure and list the causes.

Acute respiratory failure (ARF) is characterized by the inability to maintain adequate oxygenation or ventilation that develops over a short period of time. For practical purposes, the onset is usually over several hours or days. Subacute respiratory failure usually occurs over several weeks to 1–2 months. The oxygenation criteria defining ARF are PaO_2 of less than 50–55 mmHg or an arterial oxygen saturation by pulse oximetry of less than 85% on room air. Some authorities say patients with less severe, "relative hypoxemia" (compared with normal) have respiratory insufficiency, but this is not well defined. The ventilation criteria for acute respiratory failure are $PaCO_2$ of more than 50 mmHg or an increase of more than 10 mmHg over the baseline $PaCO_2$.

ARF has several causes, including infection (pneumonia), pulmonary edema, diffuse alveolar hemorrhage, lobar atelectasis, airway obstruction (mechanical or caused by asthma or COPD), neuromuscular or chest wall disease, drug overdose, sleep-disordered breathing, pleural effusion, pneumothorax, and ascites. Sometimes ARF is superimposed on chronic respiratory failure, as in exacerbations of COPD.

2. How can the causes of ARF be classified for practical clinical use?

ARF can be classified into hypercapnic respiratory failure (defined by a very high $PaCO_2$) or hypoxemic respiratory failure (very low PaO_2). Hypercapnic or ventilatory failure commonly occurs with problems in the function of the respiratory muscles ("pump failure"), such as drug overdose decreasing ventilatory drive or diaphragm paralysis. Oxygenation failure usually occurs because of problems with alveolar disease (pulmonary edema, acute lung injury), severe ventilation-perfusion mismatching (COPD, asthma) or loss of functional alveolar-capillary surface area (pulmonary emboli, vasculitis). Some diseases have abnormalities of both oxygenation and ventilation. For example, COPD can have both hypoxemia and hypercapnia. In most COPD patients, minute ventilation is actually increased above normal, so the inability to excrete carbon dioxide really is not caused by pump failure per se, but rather the inability to compensate for very inefficient alveolar ventilation.

The chest radiograph provides another way to classify ARF. The common causes of ARF can be divided into those with a normal or abnormal chest radiograph. ARF with normal lung parenchyma on chest radiograph often is the result of COPD, asthma, pulmonary embolism, or neuromuscular dysfunction. In contrast, infection, pulmonary edema, atelectasis, very large pleural effusions, and pneumothorax result in abnormalities on the radiograph.

3. What is the prognosis for a patient with ARF?

In a recent multicenter, international study, the overall in-hospital mortality rate for patients with ARF was 44.4%.[11] Obviously, the prognosis in a specific individual is a function of the cause, the severity of pulmonary dysfunction, other acute medical conditions, and concomitant underlying lung or systemic disease. Patients with ARF caused by sepsis had average survival rates (46%), whereas those with ARF caused by pneumonia or postshock lung injury had higher survival rates (63% and 67%, respectively). Factors associated with poor survival included greater severity of lung injury, FIO_2 requirement of 80% or more on the ventilator, peak inspiratory pressure on the ventilator of more than 50 cm H_2O, longer periods of mechanical ventilation, and concomitant multiorgan failure.

4. How can the clinician monitor a patient for development of ARF?

To monitor a patient, the clinician should follow vital signs, oxygenation via oxygen saturation or arterial blood gas (ABG), the chest radiograph, and the function of vital end organs (central nervous system and kidney function, especially). Clues to the development of ARF include complaints of dyspnea, cough, chest tightness, or chest pain. Physical examination may reveal tachycardia, tachypnea of more than 30 breaths per minute, and diffuse crackles in pulmonary edema or signs of lobar consolidation in pneumonia. Cyanosis is not a reliable physical examination finding because it is observer dependent and, in the best circumstances, requires more than 5 g/dl of desaturated hemoglobin. Because some patients with severe hypoxemia have no shortness of breath, only by measuring blood gas levels can respiratory failure be completely excluded. Laboratory assessment by ABG analysis, supplemented if appropriate by oximetry, is essential. In addition, the chest radiograph may demonstrate abnormalities such as diffuse alveolar infiltrates or effusions.

5. Calculate the normal PaO_2.

The normal PaO_2 is calculated based on the normal alveolar arterial oxygen gradient (A-a gradient) and a normal alveolar PO_2 (PAO_2). The alveolar gas equation is used to calculate the PAO_2, based on the principle that at sea level, the total alveolar gas pressure is equal to the pressures of all the gases in the alveoli.

$$760 \text{ mmHg} = PAO_2 + PACO_2 + PAN_2 + PAH_2O$$
$$PAO_2 = 760 - PAH_2O - PAN_2 - PACO_2 = 760 - 47 - 563 - 40 = 110 \text{ mmHg}$$

Normal PaO_2 is calculated by the A-a gradient:

A-a oxygen gradient $= PAO_2 - PaO_2$

$PAO_2 = FIO_2$(atmospheric pressure - water pressure) $- 1.25(PaCO_2)$

At sea level:

$PAO_2 = FIO_2(760 - 47) - 1.25(PaCO_2)$

For room air with an FIO_2 of 0.21:

$PAO_2 = (0.21 \times 713) - 1.25(PaCO_2) = 150 - 1.25 (PaCO_2)$

The A-a oxygen gradient normally is 8–15 mmHg and increases with age. Thus, the normal PaO_2 is 95–102 mmHg. The PaO_2 decreases with age as ventilation-perfusion mismatch increases.

6. Name the 5 mechanisms of hypoxemia.

Shunt occurs when areas of lung are perfused but not ventilated, leading to hypoxemia that does not correct with increasing FIO_2. Shunt can be anatomic, e.g., with an arteriovenous malformation, or physiologic, as with alveolar flooding and collapse in acute lung injury. Shunt does not correct with 100% FIO_2 because the alveoli do not participate in gas exchange. The opposite of shunt is dead space—alveoli that are ventilated but not perfused—which occurs in pulmonary emboli. Dead space does not cause hypoxemia, however, because the blood does not flow to these regions.

Ventilation/perfusion ($\dot{V}/\dot{Q}$) mismatch refers to ventilation and perfusion that are not matched normally. Two types of abnormalities coexist: alveoli that are normally ventilated but poorly perfused; and alveolar areas that are normally perfused but poorly ventilated. The extreme of the former is dead space, whereas the extreme of the latter is shunt. The latter contributes much more to hypoxemia. The hypoxemia usually improves relatively easily with supplemental oxygen because a small change in FIO_2 leads to a large increase in the PAO_2 in the poorly ventilated alveoli and significantly increases oxygenation of the red blood cells traveling past these alveoli.

Diffusion block is an uncommon cause of hypoxemia that results from marked thickening of the interstitial tissue between the alveolar space and the capillary. In the past, this mechanism was believed to operate in patients with interstitial lung disease. Recently, however, it has been appreciated that capillary destruction is probably more important as a cause of hypoxemia in these diseases. Diffusion block may cause hypoxemia when patients with interstitial disease exercise, and the time that red blood cells spend in the capillaries decreases to the point that equilibration with P_{AO_2} is incomplete. One pulmonary function test gives some insight into these problems. The diffusing capacity for carbon monoxide measures the overall functional alveolar capillary surface area and incorporates problems in diffusion, loss of capillaries, and incomplete equilibration.

Low F_{IO_2} causes hypoxemia based on the alveolar gas equation at high altitudes where F_{IO_2} is less than 21%.

Hypoventilation, or decrease in total and alveolar ventilation, increases the P_{ACO_2} while decreasing P_{AO_2}, as predicted by the alveolar gas equation. This occurs in persons with decreased respiratory drive, including neuromuscular disease, narcotic drug overdoses, or sleep apnea.

7. Can the A-a gradient help to determine the mechanism of hypoxemia?

Yes. ARF in the setting of a normal A-a gradient indicates hypoventilation, whereas an increased A-a gradient indicates shunt, $\dot{V}\dot{Q}$ mismatch, low F_{IO_2}, or decreased diffusing capacity as the mechanism. A-a gradient is particularly useful in patients with a drug overdose who hypoventilate but also may have components of chemical or bacterial aspiration pneumonia or atelectasis.

8. Describe the consequences of hypercapnia.

Hypercapnia may lead to:

Hypoxemia

Acidemia

Tachycardia

Decreased work of breathing as a consequence of hypoventilation

Decreased blood pressure, but the secondary release of systemic catecholamines counterbalances this tendency

Changes in cerebral vascular autoregulation so that cerebral vasodilation increases cerebral carbon dioxide washout, thus reducing the effect of hypercapnia on the brain by lowering cerebral P_{CO_2} and cerebral acidosis

9. What are the indications for endotracheal intubation?

Endotracheal intubation is beneficial in patients with inadequate oxygenation or ventilation during conventional therapy; it is also indicated in some patients for upper airway obstruction, airway protection, or secretion management. The difficult clinical decision is choosing the time when intubation is necessary. In some patients who are rapidly deteriorating or tiring and do not have prospects for a rapid reversal and improvement, intubation should be done semiurgently under controlled circumstances. Patients who are slowly deteriorating or who are likely to improve rapidly with the initiation of therapy (acute congestive heart failure, untreated asthma) sometimes may be carefully observed and repeatedly assessed before the decision to intubate is made. Most patients who cannot maintain oxygenation (P_{aO_2} less than 60 mmHg with F_{IO_2} 50% or more) or ventilation (rising P_{aCO_2} with worsening acidemia) should be considered seriously for intubation. Another situation in which intubation is needed is the patient who is tiring from the increased work of breathing, manifested by increased respiratory and heart rates and paradoxical or dyskinetic motion of the abdominal muscles. Airway protection may be needed for a patient who is somnolent or lethargic or at high risk of aspiration (e.g., patients with neurologic disorders or drug overdoses and some individuals undergoing upper gastrointestinal endoscopy or lavage with a large-bore gastric tube). Rarely, patients may need intubation for secretion management because they are unable to clear increased secretions resulting from an acute bronchitis or pneumonia superimposed on severe chronic lung disease or neuromuscular disease.

10. What is noninvasive ventilation? What are its advantages and disadvantages?

Noninvasive ventilation refers to positive-pressure mechanical ventilation using a facial or nasal mask, which may avoid or delay the need for endotracheal intubation. Several modalities can be used noninvasively: continuous positive airway pressure (CPAP), bilevel positive airway pressure (BiPAP), pressure support ventilation (PSV), and pressure control ventilation (PCV). CPAP provides positive pressure throughout the respiratory cycle and thus helps avoid atelectasis and maintain airway and alveolar recruitment. A tightly fitting facial or nasal mask is required to maintain positive end-expiratory pressure (PEEP). With BiPAP inspiratory and expiratory pressures can be set independently; BiPAP may be triggered to augment the patient's spontaneous inspiration, or it may work independently. PSV assists the patient's inspiratory efforts without necessarily imposing PEEP and is more comfortable for some patients. PCV is similar to PSV in supporting only inspiration, but it does not require patient triggering or effort.

- **Advantages**
  Avoidance of endotracheal intubation and its complications
  Patient comfort
  Preservation of speech and swallowing when nasal ventilation is used
- **Disadvantages**
  Difficulty (for some patients) in keeping on a tight-fitting device
  With a face mask, the inability to talk, eat, or swallow
  The risk of aspiration caused by vomiting with increased air in the stomach

11. Can noninvasive ventilation prevent endotracheal intubation?

Noninvasive ventilation devices can be used continuously in the tenuous patient or intermittently for short-term or long-term therapy. Recent studies have shown that noninvasive ventilation is effective in preventing intubation in patients with exacerbations of COPD and useful for patients with congestive heart failure who have pulmonary edema. In addition, it may shorten the length of hospital stay and the in-hospital mortality in patients with COPD. Noninvasive ventilation also has been used successfully to prevent intubation in patients with ARF of other causes (such as neuromuscular disease) or for patients who refuse intubation. Intermittent long-term use of these modes also provides respiratory muscle rest, which may avoid gradual deteriorations and worsening chronic respiratory failure in patients with neuromuscular diseases.

12. What other therapies exist for ARF?

Treatment of ARF is supportive care and therapy for the specific cause of the ARF. The clinician should use antibiotics for pneumonia; diuretics and vasodilators for pulmonary edema; and bronchodilators for obstructive lung disease. In addition, supplemental oxygen, support of blood pressure, correction of electrolyte abnormalities, adequate nutrition, and prophylaxis for deep venous thrombosis are encouraged.

It is important to have detailed information about a patient's prior pulmonary status. In particular, baseline ABG levels are helpful for predicting the best possible $Paco_2$ to expect when the patient's pulmonary function has completely improved. A common mistake in ventilated patients is overventilation so that the $Paco_2$ is "normal," but at a level significantly lower than the baseline hypercapnia. The kidneys then excrete bicarbonate; when weaning starts and the $Paco_2$ rises because of limited optimal lung function, respiratory acidosis occurs.

13. Why are perioperative patients at risk for ARF?

Patients in the perioperative period are susceptible to atelectasis, which can lead to ARF. Factors predisposing patients to the development of postoperative atelectasis include obesity, supine position, upper abdominal incision, ascites or peritonitis, airway secretions, fluid overload, and anesthesia. The chest radiograph helps in the decision of how aggressively to treat atelectases, i.e., whether bronchoscopy is necessary. If air bronchograms are present on the radiograph, bronchoscopy is not beneficial, and the patient can be managed with bronchodilators, chest physiotherapy, and frequent suctioning. In contrast, if no air bronchograms are seen, bronchoscopy is helpful in diagnosis and treatment of an obstructing plug or copious secretions in the airways.

14. What systemic complications may develop in patients with ARF?

Complications of ARF

Cardiopulmonary	Gastrointestinal
Deep venous thrombosis	Acute gastric ulceration or inflammation
Pulmonary emboli	with hemorrhage
Myocardial ischemia	Malnutrition
Cardiac arrhythmias	Complications of enteral and parenteral
Nosocomial pneumonia	nutrition
Neurologic	Acalculous cholecystitis
Delirium	Drug-associated hepatic dysfunction
Stupor and coma	**Renal**
"ICU psychosis"	Acute renal failure (caused by hypoperfusion, acute
Infectious	tubular necrosis, or nephrotoxic drugs)
Line sepsis	Hypomagnesemia
Abscesses	Hypophosphatemia
Nosocomial pneumonia	Electrolyte disorders
Decubitus ulceration	
Other infections	

In addition to systemic complications, many complications occur related to the presence of an endotracheal tube, such as barotrauma, endotracheal tube problems, tracheal stenosis or dilatation, nosocomial sinusitis or otitis, self-extubation, and laryngeal trauma.

15. What should be done routinely to prevent these complications?
It is important to carefully monitor the patient with ARF. Symptoms and physical examination should be assessed at least once daily. In patients who are sedated and paralyzed, paralytics should be stopped daily if possible to assess the patient's neurologic status, pain in different regions, and level of sedation. Blood pressure must be optimized to maintain adequate perfusion of end organs, and vasopressors should be used if blood pressure cannot be maintained with intravenous fluid administration alone. Urine output should be kept optimal with fluids or diuretics, or both. Because patients with ARF are at risk for cardiac complications, the cardiac rhythm should be monitored continuously. In addition, the following routine laboratory tests may be needed daily until the patient's condition is stabilized: electrolyte, blood urea nitrogen, and creatinine levels; liver function tests; hemoglobin; white cell count; and platelets, as heparin-associated thrombocytopenia is often seen even with the use of heparin flushes alone. Blood, sputum, urine, and any other drainage sites should be cultured if the patient develops a fever. A daily chest radiograph is useful while the patient's condition is critical, because it can indicate worsening pulmonary status.

Ventilated patients should have their secretions assessed daily and the airway peak and static pressures, the presence of auto-PEEP, the minute ventilation, and the actual respiratory rate and achieved tidal volume measured. In some institutions, more complete respiratory variables—including peak negative-inspiratory pressure and spontaneous respiratory rate, tidal volume, and vital capacity—are assessed daily in patients who are not paralyzed.

Some specific preventive measures include:
Routine use of prophylaxis for deep venous thrombosis and stress gastrointestinal bleeding
Daily measurement of endotracheal cuff pressure
Daily assessment of endotracheal tube position
Provision of adequate nutrition beginning early in the ICU stay
Adequate sedation or restraint, if necessary
Insuring adequate sleep in a day-night cycle

16. Describe the advanced modes of ventilation.

Recent advances in ventilator therapy have provided additional options in the management of critically ill patients with ARF who are difficult to ventilate or oxygenate. The most commonly used new mode is **PCV**. The clinician sets inspiratory pressure and inspiratory time or fraction, and this pressure is maintained without guaranteeing a delivered tidal volume. The actual tidal volume delivered is primarily a function of lung compliance and may change with altered patient status (mucus plug, pneumothorax, pulmonary edema). PCV may be set up to have a higher mean intrathoracic pressure, increasing the functional residual capacity and keeping more alveoli open. It also provides greater inspiratory flow early during inspiration, which may aid in opening more alveoli and allowing better distribution of the inspired gas. Consequently, it may help patients with inhomogeneous lung disease or acute lung injury. The major disadvantage of PCV is the lack of guaranteed tidal volume. New ventilators offer this back-up option and also have sensitive triggering of PCV breaths by patient inspiration.

Inverse ratio ventilation (IRV) refers to mechanical ventilation in which the ratio of inspiration to expiration is reversed to greater than 1. This allows longer time at higher pressure for alveoli to fill with oxygen and less time during expiration for alveoli to collapse. IRV may be beneficial in patients with acute lung injury who are difficult to oxygenate with conventional mechanical ventilation. It also may help patients with heterogenous lung disease. Possible consequences of IRV include hypotension from the increased mean intrathoracic pressure and increased auto-PEEP and hypercapnia from the decreased expiratory time. IRV is not a comfortable mode of ventilation and usually requires that the patient be paralyzed or heavily sedated.

Proportional assist ventilation (PAV) is a recent experimental mode that is used only in spontaneously breathing patients. PAV is designed to optimize the relationship between patient effort and ventilator response by adjusting inspiratory pressure to patient effort. This allows the patient to better control his or her breathing pattern and minute ventilation. PAV provides greater patient comfort, lower peak airway pressures, and improved control over respiratory pattern.

High frequency ventilation (HFV) uses very small tidal volumes with high respiratory rates; several variants are available with different frequencies and delivery mechanisms. Minute ventilation is maintained by using very high rates. Some patients may benefit from improved healing of bronchopleural fistulas or more uniform distribution of ventilation leading to improved gas exchange. However, in large randomized series of patients with ARF, HFV has not shown any benefit over other modes of ventilation, and barotrauma still occurs. The theoretical benefit of a lower risk of barotrauma with smaller tidal volumes has not been clinically substantiated, possibly because the alveolar pressures may be much higher than the measured proximal airway pressure.

Split lung ventilation refers to differential ventilation of the lungs accomplished by blocking one main bronchus while ventilating the other lung or using a double-lumen endotracheal tube to ventilate both lungs independently. Split lung ventilation allows each lung to be ventilated and inspected separately. This is useful in the setting of unilateral massive hemoptysis, a large bronchopleural fistula, or radically unequal degrees of lung injury.

CONTROVERSIES

17. When can oximetry be used instead of arterial blood gas monitoring? What are the limitations of oximetry?

Oximetry is a useful, quick, noninvasive indicator of arterial oxygenation. It is helpful when the oxygen saturation has to be determined but knowledge of arterial Pa_{CO_2} or pH is not required, e.g., it is an easy way to ensure adequate oxygenation as FI_{O_2} is reduced.

There are three limitations to the use of oximetry. First, the readings may be inaccurate or misleading in the presence of an abnormal hemoglobin (methemoglobin or carboxyhemoglobin) or increased tissue or intravascular pigment (bilirubin, methylene blue, and indocyanine green). In these cases, oximetry must be correlated with the oxygen saturation obtained by direct measurement of the ABG. Second, oximetry becomes relatively inaccurate with poor tissue perfusion and with low oxygen saturation (less than 70%). Third, and most important, oximetry may not be sufficient in patients with obstructive lung disease, metabolic abnormalities, shock, or hypoventilation because it does not measure $PaCO_2$ or arterial pH. The flat upper portion of the oxygen-hemoglobin saturation curve means that large changes in PaO_2 above 60 mmHg result in only small changes in oxygen saturation. A common error is that a patient with acute onset of shortness of breath is placed on supplemental oxygen, then undergoes oximetry, which shows adequate oxygen saturation but gives no indication of the patient's ventilatory status. Therefore, ABG measurements are required in the initial evaluation of a patient with shortness of breath or other signs of ARF because it is important to know the $PaCO_2$ and arterial pH and the response of the PaO_2 and $PaCO_2$ to supplemental oxygen. It also is necessary to obtain ABG levels in the initial period after extubation to follow the $PaCO_2$ as a sign of ventilatory insufficiency.

18. Are measurements of mixed venous oxygen saturation useful?

Mixed venous oxygen saturation ($S\overline{v}O_2$) is an indirect reflection of tissue oxygen delivery and consumption. When this value is very low, tissues are extracting almost all the oxygen that is delivered to them and they may be inadequately supplied with oxygen and other metabolic substances. Anaerobic metabolism with lactic acidosis is probably occurring or incipient. $S\overline{v}O_2$ typically is measured in blood drawn from the proximal pulmonary artery, because the blood has been mixed in the right ventricle, but can be measured continuously with an oximetric pulmonary artery catheter. Mixed venous blood gas is less useful than the $S\overline{v}O_2$ because the mixed venous blood oxygen partial pressure ($P\overline{v}O_2$) varies with hemoglobin's affinity for oxygen, even in the presence of stable oxygen content. $S\overline{v}O_2$ is dependent on cardiac output, hemoglobin concentration, arterial oxygen saturation, oxygen blood flow pattern, and oxygen consumption. A change in one variable can alter $S\overline{v}O_2$, especially if changes in the other variables do not compensate. Venous PO_2 should not be measured on blood specimens that have not had complete mixing of all the venous return, because there is wide range in normal venous PO_2 from different tissue beds and results are misleading.

When $S\overline{v}O_2$ is measured continuously, falling values may be an early indication of clinical deterioration in a patient in the ICU. An isolated reading also may confirm acute clinical deterioration. These measurements are particularly helpful in patients with isolated cardiac disease, because $S\overline{v}O_2$ varies with cardiac output. Decreasing $S\overline{v}O_2$ may signal occult bleeding, early cardiac failure, inadequate tissue oxygen delivery, or impending cardiac arrest; however, interpretation of $S\overline{v}O_2$ values is often not straightforward. First, the normal range varies significantly. Second, altered distribution of organ blood flow alone can affect $S\overline{v}O_2$. Third, rising $S\overline{v}O_2$ may indicate clinical deterioration, as in sepsis, in which blood is shunted away from mesenteric beds and through skin capillaries without much oxygen consumption. Finally, continuous $S\overline{v}O_2$ monitoring may be affected too much by variations in patients' oxygen consumption with exertion and anxiety, so that transient decreases in $S\overline{v}O_2$ lead to expensive evaluations without a clinical change. In summary, use of $S\overline{v}O_2$ along with clinical observations, ABG analysis, and measurement of cardiac output may offer early diagnostic information in the setting of sepsis, cardiac failure, blood loss, and other complications that can occur in a critically ill patient in the ICU; however, little data are available to suggest that using $S\overline{v}O_2$ continuously or intermittently improves outcome.

BIBLIOGRAPHY

1. Borg UR, Stoklosa JC, Siegel JH, et al: Prospective evaluation of combined high-frequency ventilation in post-traumatic patients with adult respiratory distress syndrome refractory to optimized conventional ventilatory management. Crit Care Med 17:1129–1141, 1989.
2. Brochard L, Mancebo J, Wysocki M, et al: Noninvasive ventilation for acute exacerbations of chronic obstructive pulmonary disease. N Engl J Med 333:817–822, 1995.
3. Chapman KR, D'Urzo A, Rebuck AS: The accuracy and response characteristics of a simplified ear oximeter. Chest 83:860–864, 1983.
4. Elliott MW, Aquilina R, Green M, et al: A comparison of different modes of noninvasive ventilatory support: Effects on ventilation and inspiratory muscle effort. Anaesthesia 49:279–283, 1994.

5. Hall JB, Schmidt GA, Wood LDH: Principles of critical care for the patient with respiratory failure. In Murray JF, Nadel JA (eds): Textbook of Respiratory Medicine, 2nd ed. Philadelphia, W.B. Saunders, 1994, pp 2545–2588.
6. Hill NS: Noninvasive ventilation: Does it work, for whom, and how? Am Rev Respir Dis 147:1050–1055, 1993.
7. Marcy TW, Marini JJ: Inverse ratio ventilation in ARDS: Rationale and implementation. Chest 100:494–504, 1991.
8. Marini JJ: Respiratory Medicine. Baltimore, William & Wilkins, 1987.
9. Marini JJ, Pierson DJ, Hudson LD: Acute lobar atelectasis: A prospective comparison of fiberoptic bronchoscopy and respiratory therapy. Am Rev Respir Dis 119:971–978, 1979.
10. Meduri GU, Fox RC, Abou-Shala N, et al: Noninvasive mechanical ventilation via face mask in patients with acute respiratory failure who refused endotracheal intubation. Crit Care Med 22:1584–1590, 1994.
11. Vasilyev S, Schaap RN, Mortensen JD: Hospital survival rates of patients with acute respiratory failure in modern respiratory intensive care units. Chest 107:1083–1088, 1995.

66. ACUTE RESPIRATORY DISTRESS SYNDROME

Marc Moss, M.D.

1. What is the acute respiratory distress syndrome (ARDS)?

ARDS is a unique form of acute lung injury that occurs in association with a variety of diagnoses and produces a clinical triad of severe hypoxemia, decreased static pulmonary compliance, and diffuse infiltrates on chest radiograph. Pathologically ARDS is characterized by the nonspecific pattern of diffuse alveolar damage in association with a proteinaceous alveolar edema. Because the left ventricular filling pressure is not elevated in ARDS patients, this syndrome is sometimes identified as a noncardiogenic form of pulmonary edema.

2. How is ARDS defined?

Until 1994, this was a difficult question to answer, as ARDS had been defined in a variety of ways. In 1994, the American-European Consensus Conference on ARDS established a uniform definition of ARDS based on four criteria:

1. Acute onset
2. $Pao_2:Fio_2$ ratio of 200 mmHg or less (regardless of PEEP level)
3. Bilateral infiltrates seen on frontal chest radiograph
4. Pulmonary artery wedge pressure of 18 mmHg or less when measured or no clinical evidence of left atrial hypertension

A mild form of ARDS, called *acute lung injury* (ALI), was also defined. The criteria for ALI are the same as for ARDS except the $Pao_2:Fio_2$ ratio is only 300 mmHg or less.

3. How common is ARDS?

In 1977, the incidence of ARDS was estimated to be 75 cases per 100,000 people. More recently, three studies have reported much lower incidence rates for ARDS, ranging from 1.5–7.1 cases per 100,000 people. One explanation for these different rates of incidence is the use of different definitions of ARDS.

4. Which patients are at risk for developing ARDS?

Although ARDS has been reported to occur in a variety of patients, the most common diagnoses associated with ARDS are:

Sepsis   Hypertransfusion of blood products
Trauma   Drug overdose
Aspiration of gastric contents Pancreatitis

The incidence of ARDS has been consistently the highest in patients with sepsis (40%), trauma (10–34%), and aspiration (10–36%).

5. Describe the postulated pathogenesis of ARDS.

Investigators have artificially divided the pathogenesis of ARDS into three phases: initiation, amplification, and injury. During initiation, the precipitating event, such as sepsis, triggers a general inflammatory response, involving endotoxin, tumor necrosis factor, interleukin-1, and other cytokines. Subsequently, during amplification, effector cells such as neutrophils are recruited, activated, and retained in the endothelial cell bed of the lung, from which they migrate into the pulmonary parenchyma. Finally, during injury, these effector cells release harmful substances, such as superoxide anion and hydrogen peroxide, that damage the surrounding lung tissue.

6. How quickly do patients develop ARDS?

Most patients develop ARDS within 5 days of their acute event. For patients with sepsis, the onset of ARDS is rapid: more than 50% develop ARDS within a 24-hour period. For trauma patients, ARDS develops slightly more slowly: less than 33% develop ARDS within 24 hours.

7. What is the mortality rate of patients with ARDS?

Historically, the mortality rate for patients with ARDS has been reported to be more than 50%. Over the past few years, the mortality rate has appeared to be declining, and one study has reported a mortality rate as low as 36%. The reason for improved survival is presently unknown.

8. What is the cause of death in patients with ARDS?

Classically, the cause of mortality in patients with ARDS has been divided into early causes (within 72 hours) and late causes (after 72 hours). The original presenting illness or injury causes the majority of early deaths. Late deaths were most commonly caused by sepsis syndrome (36%) and cardiac dysfunction (23%). Irreversible respiratory failure was responsible for only 16% of late deaths. However, more recent studies have reported that irreversible respiratory failure is becoming a more common cause of late mortality in patients with ARDS and can account for up to 40% of all deaths.

9. What is the outcome for the survivors of ARDS?

Respiratory symptoms are more commonly present in survivors of ARDS than was initially appreciated. The most common respiratory symptom is mild dyspnea on exertion, but occasionally the shortness of breath is severe enough to significantly limit normal activity. The most common pulmonary function abnormalities are decreased diffusing capacity and restrictive defects. The majority of improvements in pulmonary function tests (PFTs) and quality of health scores occur in the first 3 months after extubation. However, PFTs have been reported to be abnormal in 50% of ARDS patients at 6 months after extubation, and in 25% of ARDS patients at 1 year.

Patients with severe ARDS had significantly worse PFT results than did individuals with mild ARDS. The best predictors of persistently abnormal PFT results are increased FIO_2, higher levels of PEEP, and decreased static pulmonary compliance during the acute clinical course of ARDS.

10. Does the inflammatory cascade postulated to cause ARDS produce injury to other organs?

ARDS must be viewed as the pulmonary expression of a systemic disease. The inflammatory cascade and effector cells that are postulated to be involved in the pathogenesis of ARDS also affect other organ systems. Clinically, in acutely ill patients a pattern of progressive organ dysfunction has been described that is called the multiple organ dysfunction syndrome (MODS). The other organ systems commonly affected in MODS include renal, hepatic, cardiovascular, hematologic, and central nervous.

11. Is there any proven therapy for ARDS?

Although a variety of therapeutic modalities have been tested in patients at risk for ARDS and those with documented ARDS, there is presently no standard medical treatment for ARDS.

12. What is the role of inhaled nitric oxide in the treatment of ARDS?

Nitric oxide (NO) is a potent endogenous mediator that is released from the endothelium and produces vasodilatation. When inhaled, NO diffuses from the alveoli to the vascular smooth muscle and subsequently is tightly bound to hemoglobin. NO vasodilates the pulmonary blood vessels that are adjacent to well ventilated alveoli, thereby improving ventilation-perfusion mismatching. Because NO is inactivated when it is bound to hemoglobin, inhaled NO causes selective pulmonary vasodilatation without altering systemic vascular resistance. In a small study of patients with ARDS, inhaled NO reduced mean pulmonary artery pressures and intrapulmonary shunting and improved oxygenation without affecting systemic blood pressure or cardiac output. Although these initial results are exciting, NO has potential toxicities including the inactivation of heme-based enzymes required for electron transport. Further controlled trials are necessary before the role of inhaled NO in patients with ARDS can be determined.

13. Describe the CT scan appearance of the lungs in a patient with ARDS.

Despite diffuse infiltrates on plain chest radiographs, CT scanning reveals patchy areas of dense infiltrates and areas of normal appearing lung tissue. Posterior and gravitationally dependent areas of the lung are more infiltrated than nondependent areas. With the addition of positive end-expiratory pressure (PEEP), a portion of the consolidated lung parenchyma can be recruited for gas exchange.

14. What is the optimal mode of mechanical ventilation for patients with ARDS?

The primary goal of mechanical ventilation in patients with ARDS is to achieve ventilation and oxygenation that will adequately support all organ systems. Based on evidence that large tidal volumes and high airway pressures produce barotrauma to the lung both macroscopically (pneumothorax, pneumomediastinum, and subcutaneous emphysema) and microscopically (alveolar edema, hyaline membrane formation, and disruption of type I pneumocytes), strategies in mechanical ventilation have been redirected. Lower initial tidal volumes (6–10 ml per kg) that do not produce a transpulmonary pressure exceeding 30–35 cm H_2O are now recommended. If necessary, $Paco_2$ should be allowed to rise, in order to avoid high transpulmonary pressure, a strategy termed *permissive hypercapnia*. Additionally, the least amount of PEEP necessary (usually in the range of 5–12 cm H_2O) should be used to maintain an arterial oxygen saturation of more than 90% at an Fio_2 of less than 60%.

CONTROVERSIES

15. What is the role of steroids in the treatment of ARDS?

Due to their antiinflammatory effects, corticosteroids have been studied in patients at risk for ARDS and those with ARDS. Well designed, randomized, prospective multicenter trials have shown no benefit from steroid administration in early ARDS. In spite of these results, the utility of corticosteroids given later in the course of ARDS has been examined. Five to 10 days after the onset of ARDS, collagen deposition starts to occur in the lung, which can rapidly progress to fibrosis. This phenomenon has been termed the *fibroproliferative phase* of ARDS. Nonrandomized studies have reported that steroid administration during the fibroproliferative phase of ARDS may lead to significant improvement in oxygenation, radiologic abnormalities, and survival. Based on these studies, it has been recommended that a 7–14 day trial of 2–4 mg per kg of prednisone be administered 1–2 weeks after the onset of ARDS in patients with severe ARDS and no clinical signs of improvement. Before corticosteroids are prescribed, systemic infection should be either ruled out or appropriately treated. In contrast, other investigators argue that the role of steroids during the fibroproliferative phase of ARDS is not presently known, and has the potential to be harmful. These researchers believe that steroids should not be prescribed late in the course of ARDS until proper prospective and randomized studies have been performed.

16. What is the role of increased oxygen delivery in the treatment of ARDS?

Patients with ARDS who develop failure of other organ systems (MODS) often have worse clinical outcomes. The development of MODS may be in part the result of suboptimal tissue perfusion and cellular energy deficits caused by inadequate systemic oxygen delivery (DO_2). DO_2 is defined as the arterial oxygen content times the cardiac output. Increases in oxygen delivery with volume expansion or the infusion of inotropic agents such as dobutamine can improve tissue perfusion and potentially eliminate cellular energy deficits. Initial studies involving primarily surgical patients demonstrated an improvement in mortality when the systemic organ delivery was elevated to supranormal levels. However, more recent studies involving septic patients and critically ill individuals with a variety of diagnoses failed to detect a beneficial effect. Therefore, therapies aimed at maximizing DO_2 should not presently be used in patients with ARDS.

17. What is the proper fluid management in patients with ARDS?

The endothelial cell damage observed in patients with ARDS produces an increase in the microvascular permeability of the lung. Protein molecules traverse more easily from the vascular lumen into the pulmonary parenchyma, which reduces the osmotic gradient. Therefore, the fluid flux across the capillary membrane, as described by Starling's law of transcapillary exchange, becomes primarily related to the microvascular hydrostatic pressure. In light of the endothelial cell damage, elevation in the microvascular hydrostatic pressure leads to an exaggerated increase in extravascular lung water content, further pulmonary damage, and potentially the need for higher levels of inspired oxygen. Therefore, a reasonable overall strategy for patients with ARDS would be to reduce the pulmonary microvascular hydrostatic pressure in order to minimize the accumulation of extravascular lung water. However, this plan needs to be balanced with optimal systemic DO_2 and adequate nonpulmonary organ function.

Clinical assessment of the volume status in critically ill patients is notoriously inaccurate. Therefore, the placement of a pulmonary artery catheter that can measure pulmonary capillary wedge pressure (PCWP) is often necessary. Volume expansion is indicated for patients who are severely volume depleted (low PCWP) and whose cardiac output is insufficient for nonpulmonary organ perfusion. If the patient is anemic (hematocrit less than 30%), transfusion of packed red blood cells can be used for volume expansion. Otherwise, crystalloid should be used, because albumin or colloid substitutes are not indicated for patients with ARDS. Volume depletion by diuresis or hemofiltration is reasonable when PCWP is high and cardiac output and nonpulmonary organ perfusion are adequate.

18. Is there a role for prone position ventilation in patients with ARDS?

An improvement in oxygenation has been reported when patients with ARDS are turned from a supine to a prone position. In some studies, switching a patient to the prone position increased the mean PaO_2 by as much as 69 mmHg. This improvement in oxygenation may last for up to 3 days. Mechanisms for the improved prone PaO_2 have been postulated to be an increase in the functional residual capacity (FRC), a more efficient diaphragmatic motion, better postural drainage of secretions, and an improvement in $\dot{V}/\dot{Q}$ mismatching. Recently, animal studies have shown that the prone position leads to a more uniform gravitational distribution of pleural pressures and therefore improves $\dot{V}/\dot{Q}$ mismatching. Although these results appear promising, the use of prone ventilation should be restricted to ICUs that are experienced with this technique.

BIBLIOGRAPHY

1. Bernard GR, Artigas A, Brigham KL, et al: Report of the American-European Consensus Conference on Acute Respiratory Distress Syndrome: Definitions, mechanisms, relevant outcomes, and clinical trial coordination. Am J Respir Crit Care Med 151:818–824, 1994.
2. Bernard GR, Luce JM, Sprung CL, et al: High-dose corticosteroids in patients with the adult respiratory distress syndrome. N Engl J Med 317:1565–1570, 1987.
3. Gattinoni L, Brazzi L, Pelosi P, et al: A trial of goal-oriented hemodynamic therapy in critically ill patients. N Engl J Med 333:1025–1032, 1995.
4. Hudson LD: Epidemiology of the adult respiratory distress syndrome. Semin Respir Crit Care Med 15:254–259, 1994.
5. Hudson LD, Milberg JA, Anardi D, et al: Clinical risks for development of the adult respiratory distress syndrome. Am J Respir Crit Care Med 151:293–301, 1995.
6. Kollef MH, Schuster DR: The adult respiratory distress syndrome. N Engl J Med 332:27–37, 1995.
7. Lamb WJE, Graham MM, Albert RK: Mechanism by which the prone position improves oxygenation in acute lung injury. Am J Respir Crit Care Med 150:184–193, 1994.
8. Matthay MA, Broaddus VC: Fluid and hemodynamic management in acute lung injury. Semin Respir Crit Care Med 15:271–288, 1994.
9. McHugh LG, Milberg JA, Whitcomb ME, et al: Recovery of function in survivors of the adult respiratory distress syndrome. Am J Respir Crit Care Med 150:90–94, 1995.
10. Meduri GU, Belenchia JM, Estes RJ, et al: Fibroproliferative phase of ARDS: Clinical findings and effects of corticosteroids. Chest 100:943–952, 1991.
11. Milberg JA, Davis DR, Steinberg KP, et al: Improved survival of patients with acute respiratory distress syndrome (ARDS): 1983–1993. JAMA 273:306–309, 1995.
12. Montgomery AB, Stager MA, Carrico CJ, et al: Causes of mortality in patients with the adult respiratory distress syndrome. Am Rev Respir Dis 132:485–489, 1985.
13. Moss M, Parsons PE: Mechanical ventilation and the adult respiratory distress syndrome. Semin Respir Crit Care Med 15:289–299, 1994.
14. Rossaint R, Falke KJ, Lopez F, et al: Inhaled nitric oxide for the adult respiratory distress syndrome. N Engl J Med 318:1481–1486, 1993.
15. Suchyta MR, Clemmer TP, Elliot CG, et al: The adult respiratory distress syndrome: A report of survival and modifying factors. Chest 101:1074–1079, 1992.

67. AIRWAY MANAGEMENT

Stuart G. Rosenberg, M.D., and James Duke, M.D.

1. What is airway management? Why is it important?

To maintain homeostasis in humans, all tissues require oxygen delivery and carbon dioxide removal. Although tissues require a surprisingly small oxygen tension, it is essential that delivery to the lungs (and ultimately the tissue and cellular level) be reliable and constant. Hence, maintenance of a patent airway for oxygen delivery and carbon dioxide excretion is paramount. Airway management also encompasses protection of the airway from obstruction or other insults such as aspiration of gastric contents. It is important to distinguish tracheal intubation from mechanical ventilation of the lungs, as one does not necessarily imply the other. For example, a patient may require tracheal intubation for airway protection only and continue to breathe spontaneously without the need for mechanical ventilation. For the purposes of this chapter, airway management is defined as direct laryngoscopy with tracheal intubation. Mask ventilation and creation of an airway surgically also may be integral components of airway management.

2. List several indications for tracheal intubation.

Need for mechanical ventilation
Protection of the respiratory tract from pharyngeal secretions or gastric contents

Pulmonary toilet

Delivery of anesthetic agents or other therapeutic agents

Relief of or protection from upper airway obstruction

In cases of massive hemoptysis or lung abscess, a dual lumen endotracheal tube may be used to isolate the lungs from each other so that the healthy lung is protected from spillage from the diseased lung.

3. What is a "difficult airway"?

There is no standard definition of difficult airway. Most authors agree that there is a spectrum of difficulty in performing laryngoscopy and tracheal intubation ranging from easy to impossible. The diagram below illustrates the four grades of laryngoscopic view as described by Cormack and Lehane.

A severe grade III or grade IV view often results in an impossible intubation, although occasionally a "blind" attempt is successful. An impossible tracheal intubation implies the trachea cannot be intubated despite optimal positioning, several attempts with different operators and laryngoscope blades, manual posterior and cephalad displacement of the larynx, and muscle paralysis. The incidence of difficult airways varies depending on the patient population studied. In surgical patients, some difficulty can be encountered in up to 15% of patients. A definite grade III view occurs 1–4% of the time, and the incidence of failed intubations is approximately 0.05–0.35%. A recent study investigated 297 intubations in an ICU population and found 8% to be difficult. British anesthesia studies estimate that difficult airways with failed tracheal intubation cause approximately 600 deaths worldwide annually.

Grade I   Grade II   Grade III   Grade IV

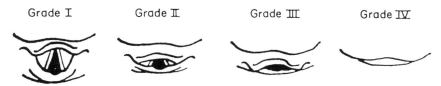

The four grades of laryngoscopic view. (From Benumof JL: Management of the difficult airway. Anesthesiology 75:1087–1110, 1991; with permission.)

4. How is the airway assessed for potential difficulty?

A patient's airway is assessed by historical review, physical examination, and occasionally through inspection of radiographs, pulmonary function tests, and direct fiberoptic examination. Review of previous anesthetic records may be invaluable if time permits. The urgency of the problem requiring airway management significantly affects the extent of evaluation allowable.

If possible, a **focused examination** of the airway should be undertaken. Examination of the oral cavity includes assessment of the extent of the opening (three fingerbreadths is optimal), the quality of the teeth (prominent teeth may interfere with direct laryngoscopy, whereas visualization of the larynx in an edentulous patient is less of a problem), size of the tongue, and shape of the palate (a high, arched palate may be associated with difficulty). If the patient can cooperate by opening his or her mouth and protruding the tongue, the inability to visualize posterior soft tissue structures (such as the uvula and tonsillar pillars) suggests that the larynx is difficult to visualize.

A mandibular body of less than three fingerbreadths (measured from the mental process to the thyroid notch) is indicative of a larynx that will be superior to the field of view. A short, large neck poses similar problems.

Any stigmata of airway pathology, such as healed burns, tracheostomy scars, or abnormal masses or swelling, should be viewed with the greatest of concern. If these conditions are not producing airway obstruction, they may do so once the patient is sedated or paralyzed.

Patients with a limited range of motion of the head and neck may prove problematic, because direct laryngoscopy requires some amount of extension of the upper cervical spine and flexion of the lower cervical spine. Pain, paresthesia, or weakness on neck motion should alert one to the possibility of cervical instability.

Dynamic sources of airway obstruction include mediastinal or extrathoracic tumor. Sedation, paralysis, or supine position may exacerbate the degree of obstruction. These dynamic obstructions may be characterized by pulmonary function testing (flow-volume loops). Imaging of the neck and chest also may suggest these diagnoses.

5. Describe the anatomy of the larynx.

The larynx is located at cervical spine levels 4–6 in adults. It protects the entrance to the respiratory tract and provides for phonation. The larynx is composed of three unpaired cartilages (thyroid, cricoid, and epiglottic) and three paired cartilages (arytenoid, corniculate, and cuneiform). The thyroid cartilage is the largest and most prominent (the "Adam's apple"), forming the anterior and lateral walls. The cricoid cartilage is shaped like a signet ring, faces posteriorly, and is the only complete cartilagenous ring of the laryngotracheal tree. The cricothyroid membrane connects these structures anteriorly and is important to identify for cricothyroidotomy if needed. The arytenoid cartilages articulate on the posterior aspect of the larynx and are the posterior attachments of the vocal cords. In the patient whose anterior larynx is difficult to view, the arytenoids may be the only visible structures; their identification allows for a successful intubation.

6. What reflexes are produced by laryngeal stimulation? How is the larynx anesthetized?

The larynx is richly innervated and stimulation produces intense autonomic and spinal reflexes. Stimulation of the larynx may produce a laryngosympathetic reflex (causing tachyarrhythmias, hypertension, and myocardial ischemia), a laryngovagal reflex (responsible for laryngospasm, apnea, bradycardia, and hypotension), or a laryngospinal reflex (causing coughing, bucking, and retching or vomiting). The larynx is innervated primarily by the vagus nerve via the superior and recurrent laryngeal nerve branches. The internal branch of the superior laryngeal nerve provides sensory innervation of the larynx above the vocal cords and may be anesthetized directly at the point where it perforates the thyrohyoid membrane just cephalad to the cornu of the thyroid cartilage. The ninth cranial nerve provides sensation to the vallecula epiglottica (the space anterior and superior to the epiglottis where the curved Macintosh blade makes contact) via the lingual nerve and can be anesthetized in the trough of the glossopalatal arch just to the side of the tongue.

7. What instruments and devices should be readily available for routine and difficult airway management?

Of paramount importance are devices that can supplement inspired oxygen concentration (FIO_2) and deliver oxygen by positive-pressure ventilation such as a bag and mask.

Devices that help maintain airway patency include **oral and nasal airways** (trumpets). The tongue is the most common cause of airway obstruction in obtunded patients and these devices elevate the tongue off of the posterior pharyngeal wall. In semiconscious patients, nasal trumpets are better tolerated. Care should be taken on insertion, as epistaxis can complicate airway management. These airway adjuncts are available in graduated sizes.

Laryngoscope handles and blades are available in several shapes and sizes. Slender handles are available for pediatric patients and short, stubby handles are available for patients with large chests. The most commonly employed blades are the curved Macintosh (sizes 3 and 4) and the straight Miller (sizes 2 and 3) blades.

Endotracheal tubes, commonly manufactured from polyvinyl chloride, have a radiopaque line from top to bottom, standard size connectors, high-volume low pressure cuff and pilot balloon, and a hole in the beveled, distal end (Murphy eye). The internal diameter ranges from 2.0–10.0 mm in 0.5-mm increments. Plastic-coated malleable metal stylets that may be inserted into the tube are useful in directing it during intubation.

Airway adjuncts that have been developed for difficult airway situations include esophageal obturators or combitubes, malleable stylets, light wands, retrograde intubation kits, fiberoptic endoscopes (flexible and rigid), and surgical airway devices for needle or open cricothyroidotomy.

8. Describe placement of a laryngoscope blade.

The curved blade is inserted into the mouth, sweeping the tongue to the left, and the tip of the blade is placed in the vallecula. With a gentle lift (not pry) of the handle the epiglottis should flip out of the visual axis revealing the glottic inlet. The straight blade can be placed in the vallecula or inserted past the epiglottis, lifting it directly. It is of the utmost importance to control the tongue, keeping it out of the field of view. If this is not done, further efforts at intubation may prove futile. Although clinicians tend to have a preferred blade, facility with the use of both is optimal. Many agree that in the difficult airway situation, when the larynx is situated anterior to the visual axis or the epiglottis is particularly long or floppy, the straight blade frequently affords improved visualization.

9. Once the need for tracheal intubation is established, what options are available to safely secure the airway?

The following important issues must be addressed first:

• How urgent is the situation?

Although a patient in or near cardiac arrest requires immediate airway intervention with little or no time for airway evaluation, there may be more latitude in patients experiencing gradually worsening respiratory failure or who need airway control for a diagnostic or therapeutic procedure.

• Is the patient awake or obtunded?

Awake patients will probably need some form of anesthesia (IV or topical sedation) and possibly neuromuscular blockade. Obtunded patients may need nothing further, although with stimulation they may become agitated and uncooperative requiring sedation or paralysis, or both.

• What is the risk of aspiration of gastric contents?

Few, if any patients in urgent circumstances are likely to have empty stomachs. The risk of aspiration is real and the sequelae may be significant. Maneuvers available to decrease the risk of significant aspiration include awake intubation, application of cricoid pressure (Sellick maneuver), "rapid sequence intubation" (RSI), and if time permits, pretreatment with an antacid or gastric motility agent.

• Is a difficult intubation anticipated?

Remember the adage, hypoventilation is better than no ventilation! If difficult ventilation or intubation is likely, an awake intubation in the spontaneously breathing patient would be wise. Options in the awake individual include a flexible fiberoptic technique, blind nasal approach, retrograde technique, or a surgical airway. Some practitioners perform laryngoscopy while the patient is awake (blocking the lingual nerve allows placement of the laryngoscope blade into the vallecula). If an adequate view is obtained, further sedation or paralysis is administered and intubation proceeds.

• Is an oral or nasal approach preferred?

A blind nasal approach may be useful in the spontaneously breathing patient. It obviates the need for deep sedation and neuromuscular blockade. If time permits, topical anesthesia and vasoconstrictors applied to the nasal mucosa improve working conditions as well as patient comfort and cooperation. Complications include epistaxis, submucosal tracking of the tube, sinusitis, and potential weaning difficulty resulting from the use of a smaller endotracheal tube.

• Is sedation or paralysis a viable option?

If the assessment suggests that ventilation and intubation are likely to be successful, the patient is probably a candidate for some degree of sedation and neuromuscular blockade. Use of any of these pharmacologic agents should never be taken lightly. Apnea and hypoxia may occur rapidly, and the patient loses protective airway reflexes.

10. Describe the techniques for awake intubation, application of cricoid pressure, and RSI.

Awake intubation is usually performed with some sedation, topical anesthesia of the airway, and possibly airway nerve blocks. Cricoid pressure may be used to occlude the esophagus against the cervical spine, preventing entry of regurgitated material into the respiratory tract. This maneuver also prevents passage of gas into the stomach during positive-pressure mask ventilation and may help to bring an "anterior" larynx into view. RSI, a technique developed in the operating suite to decrease the incidence of aspiration, is performed only if the airway appears readily manageable. The patient is preoxygenated, given an induction agent immediately followed by a neuromuscular blocker (without mask ventilation). Cricoid pressure is applied and intubation rapidly proceeds. Critically ill patients tend to desaturate rapidly after induction of anesthesia and paralysis and therefore need a modified RSI in which mask ventilation is performed with cricoid pressure applied.

11. What medications are used to facilitate intubation?

In the setting of impending respiratory failure or need for rapid airway protection, possibly the only neuromuscular blocking agent to be considered is succinylcholine (Sch). Its onset of action is rapid (about 45 seconds), and its duration of action is brief (about 5–10 minutes). If difficulties arise during airway management, spontaneous respirations will return sooner than with any other relaxant. Rocuronium, the only other relaxant with an onset nearly as fast as that of Sch, lasts 30–45 minutes or more. The most serious complication to occur with Sch (other than loss of the airway) is the hyperkalemic response seen in patients with burn, crush, or spinal cord injuries. This response has been reported in other critically ill populations also. Calcium is the immediate treatment.

Useful Medications for Awake Endotracheal Intubation

PURPOSE	MEDICATION	DOSE	ROUTE	COMMENTS
Antisialagogue	Glycopyrrolate	0.2–0.4 mg	IV or IM	Give 30 minutes before procedure
Sedation	Midazolam	1–2 mg*	IV	Amnestic
	Fentanyl	50–250 µg*	IV	Analgesic
	Propofol	10–20 mg aliquots	IV	Sedative-hypnotic in small doses
	Droperidol	1.25–2.5 mg*	IV	Neuroleptic
Topical anesthesia	1% Phenylephrine/ 4% lidocaine	1–2 cc 2–4 cc	Intranasal	Vasconstrictor and local anesthetic
	2% Viscous lidocaine	5–20 cc	Oral	"Swish and swallow"
	Cetacaine spray	2–4 sprays	Oral	Contains benzocaine; excessive use may produce methemo-globinemia
	1% Lidocaine	2–3 cc	Airway blocks	Aspirate before injection
	4% Lidocaine	2–3 cc	Transtracheal injection	Aspirate before injection

* All sedatives should be slowly titrated to effect. Excessive doses may worsen respiratory depression, hypoxemia, and carbon dioxide retention. These are only suggested doses and these medications should always be titrated slowly and carefully to effect, especially in elderly patients or those with compromised cardiovascular and respiratory function.

Medications Useful for Paralysis and Induction of Unconsciousness

PURPOSE	MEDICATION	DOSE	ROUTE	COMMENTS
Neuromuscular blockade	Succinylcholine	1–2 mg/kg	IV	Produces apnea! Onset 45 seconds Duration 5–10 minutes See text for side effects
Induction of unconsciousness	Etomidate	0.1–0.3 mg/kg	IV	Adrenal suppression Myoclonus Relatively cardiostable

12. Suggest a management strategy for a patient who cannot be intubated despite institution of sedation and neuromuscular blockade.

Never underestimate the utility of bag-mask ventilation with 100% oxygen. If the patient can be adequately oxygenated and ventilated by mask, the clinician has the luxury of time to reassess the situation and call for help. Prolonged attempts at intubation in a patient experiencing oxygen desaturation do not serve the patient well. Repeated attempts at intubation may lead to airway edema and bleeding, which may then progress to difficulty mask ventilating the patient. Inability to intubate and mask ventilate is a true emergency, usually requiring surgical creation of an airway.

Reassessment of the airway after failed intubation should include the following:

- Is the patient well positioned? The "sniff" position is optimal, i.e., the occiput resting on a folded towel or blanket, creating lower cervical spine flexion and upper cervical spine extension.
- Would a change of laryngoscope or laryngoscopist be of benefit? After two or three attempts, the procedure should be turned over to a more experienced person.
- Is the assistant applying proper cricoid pressure?

If intubation remains impossible there are several options:

- Allow the drugs to wear off while supporting with mask ventilation.
- Attempt flexible fiberoptic laryngoscopy and intubation.
- Try one of the other airway adjuncts mentioned above.
- Perform blind nasal intubation.
- If the ability to mask ventilate adequately also is lost, perform a needle cricothyroidotomy, which usually achieves adequate oxygenation, although hypercapnia may ultimately become a problem.
- Further attempts at intubation could then be tried in the oxygenated patient or a surgical airway (e.g., tracheostomy) established.

13. What is a dual-lumen endotracheal tube?

A dual, or double-lumen, endotracheal tube consists of an endobronchial lumen (left or right sided) that seats in a mainstem bronchus and a tracheal lumen that is in continuity with the other mainstem bronchus. Inflatable tracheal and bronchial cuffs allow for isolation of each lung.

14. What are the indications for its use?

Isolation of the lungs can be lifesaving in patients with massive hemoptysis or lung abscess by protecting the healthy lung from spillage. Isolation of the lungs also allows for "split-lung" ventilation, i.e., independent differential ventilation of each lung by two ventilators. Split-lung ventilation has been shown to improve oxygenation in patients with severe unilateral pneumonia, pulmonary edema, and lung contusion and has been used for whole lung lavage. It is also useful in the treatment of bronchopleural fistula.

15. What airway management problems may be encountered in an obese patient?

A large tongue, redundant oropharyngeal tissue, and short thick neck combine to make tracheal intubation difficult and also may make mask ventilation difficult, as may decreased chest wall compliance. Gastric volume and acidity predispose these patients to significant aspiration.

16. How does rheumatoid arthritis affect airway management?

- Abnormalities of the **cervical spine** are commonly seen. Cervical myelopathy may occur because of spinal cord compression. Neck manipulation during tracheal intubation should be minimized to prevent further spinal cord injury.
- **Temporal-mandibular joint** involvement may make adequate opening of the oral aperture difficult.
- **Cricoarytenoid arthritis** causes erythema and edema of the vocal cords and may decrease the glottic inlet size. A small endotracheal tube should be considered if the patient exhibits hoarseness, dysphagia, or stridor. The incidence of postextubation stridor may be increased.

17. Should difficult airway management be anticipated in acromegalic patients?

These patients have facial and mandibular abnormalities including macroglossia, redundant soft tissue folds in the oropharynx, an enlarged epiglottis, and often subglottic narrowing, all of which may make airway management difficult.

18. What is the proper airway management of a patient whose cervical spine is injured?

Proper airway management of the patient with a suspected or actual cervical spine injury or instability is controversial. Blind nasal intubation techniques have historically been recommended but may be technically difficult. More recently, direct oral intubation after sedation or paralysis (e.g., RSI) with in-line stabilization of the head and neck has been advocated. Cervical spine movement occurs with both techniques; however, the incidence of new neurologic deficits with either is rare. The technique preferred by the most skilled operator should be used. Optimally, a flexible fiberoptic technique with the head and neck in neutral position should be used. Other options include use of the "light wand" or Bullard laryngoscope. These devices decrease the amount of cervical motion required to visualize the larynx. Again, the most familiar technique should be chosen.

19. How should the airway be managed in a patient with intracranial hypertension?

Laryngoscopy, tracheal intubation, coughing, and bucking are powerful stimuli that elevate intracranial pressure (ICP). One should consider use of an anesthetic induction agent that lowers ICP (such as a barbiturate or etomidate) before airway management. Opiates and intravenous lidocaine also blunt airway reflexes. Pharmacologic paralysis should be considered to improve intubating conditions and prevent coughing and bucking. The effect of succinylcholine on ICP is controversial, although probably not clinically significant. The key to success is a rapid, smooth intubation procedure (followed by hyperventilation if warranted).

20. In what ways does pregnancy make airway management difficult?

Enlarged breasts and potential airway edema (in the preeclamptic patient) may make tracheal intubation difficult. In addition, pregnant patients are predisposed to aspiration of gastric contents, hypoxia, acidosis, and hypotension during intubation.

21. How is the airway managed when an obstruction is present?

Obstruction may be secondary to soft tissue infection, tumor, edema, or other causes. The approach to airway management depends on the urgency of the situation. Head tilt with jaw thrust or use of an oral or nasal airway device relieves soft tissue obstruction. Suspected tumor or infection may be evaluated, if time permits, by radiographic imaging, flow-volume loops, or direct laryngoscopy via a small flexible fiberoptic nasal laryngoscope. The airway may be secured using an awake, flexible fiberoptic approach or retrograde technique (a wire is passed through the cricothyroid membrane up and out the mouth or nose and an endotracheal tube is inserted over the wire). If a more urgent situation presents, awake laryngoscopy is the safest approach. If the patient cannot tolerate awake manipulation of the airway, consider airway management in the operating suite where inhalational anesthesia can be administered in the spontaneously breathing patient. Equipment for a surgical airway should always be readily available.

22. What are the airway implications of diabetes mellitus?

The "stiff joint syndrome" seen in diabetics may affect the jaw and neck, making tracheal intubation difficult.

23. Address the major concerns in the period immediately after intubation.

- Verification of proper placement of the endotracheal tube should be the first concern. Methods of verification include:

  Direct observation of the tube through the cords

  Bilateral chest movement during positive-pressure inspiration

  Water vapor in the tube on expiration

  Auscultation of bilateral, equal breath sounds

  Palpation of the cuff in the sternal notch

  "Feel" of the ambu-bag

  Qualitative or quantitative measurement of end-tidal carbon dioxide

  Use of an esophageal detector device

  Direct visualization via a flexible fiberoptic scope through the tube

  Do not rely on the pulse oximeter as an immediate indicator of proper intubation because desaturation may take several minutes after preoxygenation or mask ventilation with 100% oxygen.

  Always follow-up with a chest radiograph for proper tube placement as well.

- Deterioration of gas exchange may result from mainstem intubation; bronchospasm; aspiration; heart failure; tube obstruction from kinking, plugging, or biting; pneumothorax; cuff leak; worsened ventilation-perfusion matching; or severe coughing and bucking.
- Significant hemodynamic changes that may occur include: hypertension or hypotension, tachycardia or bradycardia, and the potential for cardiovascular collapse secondary to autoPEEP generated by vigorous bagging or bronchospasm.
- The endotracheal tube must be secured with proper taping and continuation of sedation or paralysis if needed.
- A nasogastric tube should be placed to decompress the stomach.

24. How is the patient extubated? What should you watch for in the newly extubated patient?

Extubation and weaning from mechanical ventilation are two different processes. Once it is demonstrated that the patient can breathe spontaneously on a reasonable F_{IO_2}, consideration is given to extubation. The next important issue is whether or not the patient can protect and maintain a patent airway. If airway obstruction (e.g., from edema or tumor) is a concern, deflate the endotracheal tube cuff and check for an air leak. The absence of an air leak indicates the potential for airway obstruction upon extubation. Once it is determined the patient is a candidate for extubation, a controversy exists as to the timing of extubation during the respiratory cycle. Historically, the tube has been removed during active expiration to ensure that secretions are expelled as opposed to aspirated. Some authors recommend that the tube be removed during inspiration when the vocal cords open, decreasing trauma and potentially laryngospasm. In either case, thorough suctioning should precede extubation. The patient should receive nothing by mouth before extubation in the event that reintubation is required. Patients should not receive anything by mouth for several hours after extubation to prevent aspiration from loss of the coordinated swallowing mechanism. Postextubation stridor is common because of airway edema and may be treated with racemic epinephrine and corticosteroids. Hoarseness results from vocal cord trauma, and airway obstruction may be caused by vocal cord dysfunction. Subglottic stenosis is a late complication that may require surgical therapy.

BIBLIOGRAPHY

1. American Society of Anesthesiologists' Task Force on Management of Difficult Airway: Practice guidelines for management of the difficult airway. Anesthesiology 78:597–602, 1993.
2. Baker GS, Duke J: Airway management. In Duke J, Rosenberg SG (eds): Anesthesia Secrets. Philadelphia, Hanley & Belfus, 1996, pp 41–50.

3. Benumof JL: Management of the difficult airway. Anesthesiology 75:1087–1110, 1991.
4. Bogdomoff DL, Stone DJ: Emergency management of the airway outside of the operating room. Can J Anaesth 39:1069–1089, 1992.
5. Cormack RS, Lehane J: Difficult tracheal intubation in obstetrics. Anesthesia 39:1105–1111, 1984.
6. Hastings RH, Kelley SD: Neurologic deterioration associated with airway management in a cervical spine-injured patient. Anesthesiology 78:580–583, 1993.
7. Marks JD, Bogetz MS: New concepts in the management of the difficult airway. Clin Anesth 5:1–11, 1994.
8. Schwartz DE, Matthay MA, Cohen NH: Death and other complications of emergency airway management in critically ill adults. Anesthesiology 82:367–376, 1995.
9. Wood PR, Lawler PGP: Managing the airway in cervical spine injury. Anesthesia 47:792–797, 1992.

68. NONINVASIVE VENTILATION

Sangeeta Mehta, M.D., and Nicholas S. Hill, M.D.

1. What is noninvasive ventilation?

Noninvasive ventilation (NIV) refers to the delivery of mechanical ventilation to the lungs without an invasive (endotracheal) airway.

2. Why should I use NIV?

The most compelling reason to use NIV is to avoid the adverse effects of intubation or tracheostomy, which may be divided into three groups: those occurring during the process of intubation and mechanical ventilation, those resulting from loss of airway defense mechanisms, and those that occur after removal of the endotracheal tube.

Aspiration of gastric contents and trauma to the teeth, hypopharynx, larynx, and trachea may occur during airway intubation, particularly with inexperienced intubators. The cardiovascular complications of intubation and mechanical ventilation include arrhythmias and hypotension. Sequelae of prolonged intubation attempts include cardiac arrest, generalized seizures, and gastric distention.

Chronic bacterial colonization and inflammation associated with intubation impair the function of airway cilia and incapacitate the natural pulmonary defense mechanisms, predisposing patients to the development of nosocomial pneumonia and sinusitis, both potentially life-threatening infections. An over-reliance on airway suctioning can further aggravate this problem by irritating airway mucosa, which increases airway inflammation, edema, and secretions.

After extubation, hoarseness, sore throat, cough, sputum production, hemoptysis, and tracheal stenosis may be significant. In addition, intubation may prolong ICU and hospital stays, and thus increase cost, because additional time may be necessary for weaning or for management of complications of intubation.

In contrast, NIV avoids many of the traumatic complications of intubation; preserves airway defense mechanisms; may reduce weaning time; and may be more comfortable for patients, allowing them to eat, drink, talk, and expectorate secretions. In addition, NIV is easily applied and portable; its use may avoid or reverse tracheostomy, thus simplifying patient care.

3. Name the different types of NIV.

The available noninvasive methods include "body" ventilators, positive-pressure ventilators (PPV), and continuous airway pressure (CPAP).

Body ventilators assist ventilation by applying pressure to the thorax or abdomen and by using the force of gravity. They can be categorized by the way in which they assist ventilation. The negative-pressure ventilators (i.e., the iron lung, pneumowrap, or chest cuirass) produce a vacuum around the thorax and abdomen, which results in chest expansion and air being drawn into the lungs through the mouth and nose. When the pressure around the chest wall returns to that of the surrounding air, expiration occurs passively as result of the elastic recoil of the lungs and chest wall. In contrast, the intermittent abdominal pressure ventilator (IAPV or pneumobelt) uses direct pressure on the abdomen (for expiration) and the force of gravity (for inspiration), and the rocking bed relies on positional shifts and the force of gravity to assist diaphragmatic movement.

PPVs actively assist inspiration by delivering either a preset positive airway pressure or tidal volume during inspiration. The technique can be used to control ventilation entirely or to assist spontaneous respiratory effort. Exhalation occurs by passive lung recoil to some preset positive end-expiratory pressure (PEEP) or to atmospheric pressure. Unlike invasive ventilation, noninvasive positive-pressure ventilation (NPPV) is delivered through a mask (or interface) that provides no direct access to the lower airways. Thus, it is by design "leaky," and successful ventilation relies on intact upper airway function and patient cooperation.

CPAP delivers a constant pressure during inspiration and expiration, so that airway pressure is held positive in relation to atmospheric pressure throughout the respiratory cycle. CPAP is not a true ventilatory mode in that inspiration is not actively assisted. However, it can reduce work of breathing in spontaneously breathing patients either by improving compliance or counterbalancing intrinsic PEEP. Pressures of 5–10 cm H_2O are most commonly used; pressures above 15 cm H_2O are rarely needed or tolerated.

4. Why aren't body ventilators used as often today?

Body ventilators are used less often because they all have disadvantages in comparison to NPPV, which is the noninvasive ventilatory mode of first choice for most applications. The rocking bed is bulky, and both the rocking bed and pneumobelt are relatively ineffective ventilators. In addition, the pneumobelt requires at least a semi-upright position, and is therefore useful primarily for daytime ventilatory support. The negative pressure devices, despite their efficacy, have several shortcomings, including bulk and lack of portability, time-consuming application, problems with correct fitting, and asynchronization with patient respiration. Patient discomfort, mainly musculoskeletal shoulder and back pain, is related to the necessity to sleep in the supine position during use of a negative pressure ventilator. In addition, and probably of greatest concern, is the potentiation of obstructive apneas and oxygen desaturations with negative pressure ventilators during sleep. Nonetheless, body ventilators are still used in selected patients with chronic respiratory failure who have failed or cannot tolerate NPPV. Some patients prefer body ventilators because they leave the face free or, as is the case with the rocking bed, are very simple to use.

5. Are there any indications for intermittent positive-pressure breathing?

Intermittent positive-pressure breathing (IPPB) was used widely to administer aerosolized medication to patients with acute exacerbations of COPD until the NIH-sponsored multicenter trial showed that it has no benefit over nebulizer therapy. Since then the use of IPPB, at least as traditionally administered (via a mouthpiece powered by simple pressure-limited ventilators at pressures of 15–20 cm H_2O for 10–20 minutes, three or four times daily), has waned. IPPB was also used to assist ventilation short term in hypoventilating patients but never gained wide acceptance for this application, possibly because the duration of use was too short to show significant benefit. NPPV has supplanted IPPB for this application; but in a sense, the difference between the two is largely semantic. NPPV is more often administered nasally or oronasally for sustained periods of time, but in reality, it works in a similar manner and can be administered by many of the same ventilators. Although supportive data are scant, the following would be acceptable current indications for IPPB according to American Association of Respiratory Care (AARC) guidelines:
- To improve lung expansion:
  In patients with clinically important atelectasis when other forms of therapy (incentive spirometry, chest physiotherapy, deep breathing) have been unsuccessful
  In patients unable to adequately clear secretions because of ineffective cough

• To deliver aerosolized medications:
  When metered dose inhaler or nebulizer has been unsuccessful in patients with acute severe bronchospasm
  To patients with respiratory muscle weakness or chronic conditions in which intermittent ventilatory support is indicated (e.g., patients on chronic home ventilatory support)

6. What types of interfaces (or masks) are used for NPPV?

Three types of interfaces are used to deliver NPPV: nasal masks, which cover only the nose; oronasal masks, which cover both the nose and mouth; and mouthpieces that may be standard plastic devices held in place using a lip seal or custom-fitted orthodontic device. Mouthpieces have been used to deliver noninvasive ventilation mainly to patients with chronic respiratory failure who require continuous ventilation, but any of the three interfaces can be employed, depending on patient preference.

Nasal and oronasal masks are commercially available in several sizes (pediatric; small, medium, large, adult; and so forth) and types. Recently, custom-molded, individualized masks constructed to conform to facial contours have been used for the delivery of NPPV. Both nasal and oronasal masks are applied to the face with straps that encircle the head; chin straps can be added if a significant amount of air leaks through the mouth.

7. What types of mask should be used to deliver NPPV to the patient with acute respiratory failure?

For acute respiratory failure, nasal or oronasal masks are used most often. Regardless of the type of mask used, studies have reported similar complication and success rates in acute respiratory failure, defined as the percentage of patients who tolerate the device, have improved gas exchange, and avoid endotracheal intubation. However, both masks have advantages and disadvantages. Nasal masks allow eating and conversation but permit more air leakage through the mouth, and thus may maintain delivered air pressure to the lungs less effectively. Oronasal masks, on the other hand, interfere with speech and swallowing and may be less well tolerated than nasal masks, particularly by claustrophobic patients. Theoretically, the risk of aspiration in the event of emesis is greater with oronasal masks, as is the risk of asphyxiation if the ventilator malfunctions or is disconnected and the patient is unable to remove the mask. The recent incorporation of antiasphyxia valves into some oronasal masks, however, reduces the latter risk.

8. What types of ventilators are used for NPPV?

Virtually any positive-pressure ventilator currently in use may be used noninvasively in a variety of modes (e.g., controlled mechanical ventilation, intermittent mechanical ventilation, or pressure support). However, the increasing use of long-term home ventilatory support has given rise to a variety of smaller, portable, inexpensive, easily applicable devices that are either volume or pressure limited and offer fewer features than critical care ventilators. Recently, the so-called bilevel positive airway pressure (BiPAP) devices have gained popularity. These are pressure-limited devices that cycle between adjustable (up to 20–30 cm H_2O) inspiratory (IPAP) and expiratory positive airway pressures (EPAP), using either patient flow-triggered (S) or time-triggered (T) modes. The S/T mode combines the two triggering modes and functions like the assist/control mode on a standard volume ventilator. Ventilatory augmentation with BiPAP is determined by the level of pressure support (i.e., the pressure difference between IPAP and EPAP). Some models have no disconnect alarm, making them inadvisable for use in patients requiring continuous ventilation, unless appropriate alarms are added.

In contrast to the pressure-limited ventilators, volume-limited ventilators deliver a preset tidal volume during inspiration. Although heavier and more expensive than the portable pressure-limited ventilators, volume-limited ventilators are capable of delivering higher airway pressures, have more sophisticated alarms, and have back-up batteries, and these are preferred in patients who require high inflation pressures or continuous ventilation.

9. What are the indications for NPPV in acute respiratory failure?

Patients should be at risk for requiring endotracheal intubation. In addition to clinical signs of acute respiratory distress (including severe dyspnea, tachypnea, tachycardia, and use of accessory muscles or paradoxical abdominal motion), patients should have physiologic evidence of acute respiratory failure or insufficiency (i.e., acute respiratory acidosis or acute hypoxemia). Patients should be cooperative but need not be alert, as some authors have used NPPV successfully with confused or obtunded patients. Patients should be able to protect their airway and have controllable secretions. NPPV should not used in any patient suffering a respiratory or cardiac arrest and probably should not be used in patients with hemodynamic instability, uncontrolled cardiac arrhythmias, myocardial ischemia, or other unstable medical conditions.

The underlying cause of respiratory failure and its reversibility are also important. NPPV is clearly successful in avoiding intubation in patients with acute respiratory failure caused by COPD. Anecdotal reports have also demonstrated success in patients with cardiogenic pulmonary edema, cystic fibrosis, obstructive sleep apnea, chest wall impairment, and respiratory failure after trauma. NPPV may be useful in patients who have refused or are not candidates for endotracheal intubation. Patients who are likely to require heavy sedation or paralysis for slowly reversible respiratory failure, such as that caused by severe ARDS or pneumonia, are poor candidates.

Selection Guidelines for NPPV Use in Acute Respiratory Failure

Physiologic signs of acute respiratory insufficiency	Appropriate patient
	Able to protect airway
Acute or acute-on-chronic hypercapnia	Cooperative
Hypoxemia without hypercapnia*	Minimal secretions
Clinical signs of respiratory distress	Hemodynamically stable
Tachypnea	Appropriate diagnostic category
Abdominal paradox	Obstructive lung disease (COPD, asthma,
Accessory muscle use	cystic fibrosis)
	Restrictive lung disease
	Acute pulmonary edema
	"Do not intubate"

* Data are insufficient on the use of noninvasive ventilation in such patients, with the exception of CPAP for acute pulmonary edema.

10. What are the initial settings for NPPV in acute respiratory failure?

Studies using volume ventilation have administered tidal volumes of 1.5–2.0 times those required during conventional intermittent positive-pressure ventilation (i.e., 10–15 ml per kg). This is partly to compensate for air leaking through the mouth or around the mask. Also, dead space may be greater with mask ventilation than with invasive ventilation because the entire upper respiratory tract is included in the ventilating volume. Most studies of pressure support ventilation have used inspiratory pressures of 8–20 cm H_2O and PEEP of 0–5 cm H_2O. When using BiPAP, we usually start with an IPAP of 8–11 cm H_2O and EPAP of 3–5 cm H_2O.

When the timed mode or a mode with a timed back-up is used, such as assist/control (or spontaneous/timed in BiPAP), ventilator rate must be selected. We usually select a rate lower than spontaneous (12–16 breaths per minute) to allow the patient to trigger. In fatigued patients or those with neuromuscular disease, however, rates of 18–22 breaths per minute may control breathing and allow for complete respiratory muscle rest. Oxygen is usually connected directly to the mask or in-flow tubing, with the flow rate titrated to maintain oxygen saturation at 90% or more.

11. How should patients with acute respiratory failure using NPPV be monitored and how should settings be adjusted?

Once the mask is applied and delivery of assisted ventilation begins, patients require coaching and encouragement to leave the mask in place, relax as much as possible, and let the ventilator "breathe for them." Patients may request more or less inspiratory assistance, and their preferences for particular settings should be respected as much as possible. Tired or breathless patients often allow the ventilator to control their breathing as soon as they feel they are receiving sufficient volume. Within 60 minutes after NPPV is started, successful patients usually appear much more comfortable, with an obvious reduction in accessory muscle activity. Respiratory and heart rates decrease rapidly, and the relief of dyspnea may induce sleep almost immediately.

Patients with acute respiratory failure receiving NPPV should be monitored as closely as any intubated patient until their condition stabilizes. These patients are at risk for abrupt oxygen desaturations related to events such as mucus plugging or mask removal and should be admitted to an ICU or respiratory step-down unit. Pulse oximetry, vital signs, and cardiac rhythm should be monitored, and arterial blood gas measurements should be obtained within the first hour and periodically thereafter as indicated clinically, for accurate assessments of carbon dioxide tension. Further ventilator adjustments should be made based on arterial blood gas results and patient tolerance. If hypercapnia does not improve, the level of pressure support or tidal volume should be increased, within the limits of patient tolerance. Persistent hypoxemia can be treated by an increase in either the supplemental oxygen flow or the EPAP. The former is preferable, at least initially, as the disadvantage of increasing the EPAP is a decrement in the absolute level of pressure support, and thus less ventilatory assistance, resulting in smaller tidal and minute volumes and possibly an elevation in $Paco_2$.

12. When should a nasogastric tube be inserted in patients with acute respiratory failure receiving NPPV?

Some investigators use nasogastric tubes routinely when delivering NPPV to patients with acute respiratory failure via an oronasal mask. The concern is that vomiting into the mask will lead to aspiration. In our experience, this approach is unnecessary unless the patient has other indications for nasogastric drainage, such as a recent history of nausea and vomiting, abdominal distention, or excessive gastric insufflation. If selection guidelines for administration of NPPV are observed carefully, patients who are unable to protect their airway will not receive NPPV. Exceptions may occur among patients who have "do not intubate" orders. When these patients are obtunded or are unable to adequately protect the airway, nasogastric drainage is a consideration. However, no controlled studies relating to this question are available, so clinical judgment must be exercised.

Nasogastric tubes for enteral feeding are usually unnecessary because patients are able to eat when using NPPV. Nasogastric tubes may interfere with mask sealing and increase air leaking. However, if mask tension and ventilator tidal volume are adjusted to compensate for the leak, ventilatory assistance is usually not compromised.

13. How should NPPV for acute respiratory failure be discontinued?

As patients stabilize, NPPV can be interrupted for short periods to allow eating, drinking, and conversation. Patients often resume NPPV without prompting when they feel dyspneic or fatigued. Complete discontinuation of NPPV should await clinical improvement as manifested by a reduction in respiratory rate to less than 24 breaths per minute and an improvement in gas exchange. $Paco_2$ should be stable or slightly improved and oxygen saturation should be adequate (more than 90%) on low oxygen flow rates. Patients often communicate to their caretakers that they no longer require assisted ventilation. Ventilation can be either discontinued abruptly, followed by close monitoring of vital signs, oximetry, and blood gases, or reduced gradually, as is done with pressure support weaning. Once NPPV is discontinued, patients should be closely monitored so that it can be reinstituted if they deteriorate.

14. What are the indications for NPPV in chronic respiratory failure?

NPPV is indicated when symptoms of hypoventilation and daytime hypercapnia develop in a wide variety of slowly progressive neuromuscular disorders such as limb girdle muscular dystrophy, the postpolio syndrome, and multiple sclerosis. Some patients with nocturnal hypoventilation and no daytime carbon dioxide retention may be candidates, particularly if they have symptoms, but firm guidelines have not been established. Other appropriate candidates are those with hypoventilation associated with severe kyphoscoliosis or central disorders. Obstructive sleep apnea or obesity-hypoventilation syndrome with persistent hypoventilation despite nasal CPAP are also appropriate indications, although the very obese may be difficult to ventilate.

Use of long-term NPPV in patients with COPD is controversial (see question 21), but it has been used successfully in cystic fibrosis patients with hypercapnic respiratory failure as a bridge to potential lung transplantation. Patients who would be at higher risk using noninvasive instead of invasive techniques should be excluded. Thus, noninvasive ventilation should be used with caution, if at all, when upper airway function is compromised, which often occurs in rapidly progressive neuromuscular syndromes such as amyotrophic lateral sclerosis or Guillain-Barré syndrome.

Selection Guidelines for NPPV Use in Chronic Respiratory Failure

Chronic stable or slowly progressive respiratory failure
    Significant carbon dioxide retention (Pa_{CO_2} > 50 mmHg)
    Mild carbon dioxide retention with symptoms
        Morning headache
        Daytime hypersomnolence
    Nocturnal hypoventilation or severe oxygen desaturation*

Appropriate condition
    Slowly progressive neuromuscular disorder
    Chest wall deformities
    Obstructive sleep apnea unresponsive to CPAP
    Obesity-hypoventilation
    Idiopathic hypoventilation
    Cystic fibrosis
    Chronic obstructive pulmonary disease*

Inappropriate candidates excluded
    Upper airway function adequate
    Ability to clear secretions
    Reversible underlying disorders (hypothyroidism, congestive
        heart failure, and so forth) adequately treated
    Cooperative, motivated patient

---

* Tentative indications.

15. How do you initiate and help patients adapt to long-term NPPV?

Initiation for patients with chronic respiratory failure is similar to that for those with acute respiratory failure, but with less urgency. Similar initial pressures or volumes are used, and since the best candidates have normal lungs with "bellows" problems, oxygen supplementation is often unnecessary. The adaptation period may last weeks to months. Sometimes adaptation is rapid and smooth, and the patient sleeps through the night using NPPV within a few days or weeks. More often, however, problems are encountered. Initially, patients may tolerate the mask only for a few hours at a time, removing it for the remainder of the night. Many complain of discomfort related to mask or air pressure and have difficulty becoming accustomed to the sensation of a foreign object on their face. During this period, the focus must be on optimizing patient comfort and acceptance rather than on improving gas exchange or sleep quality. As long as the patient has fairly stable respiratory insufficiency, there is time to try different straps or masks and adjust pressure. Inspiratory pressure can be increased gradually as adaptation progresses, but abrupt increases in air pressure or duration of use may increase patient discomfort and should be avoided.

16. How should patients using NPPV for chronic respiratory failure be monitored?

Initially, patients should be seen approximately every month to assess symptoms such as morning headache and hypersomnolence, vital signs, signs of cor pulmonale, and daytime arterial blood gas levels. Optimal daytime blood gas values have not been established, but we find that normalization of Pa_{CO_2} may not be achievable and that values ranging from 47–55 mmHg are associated with sustained clinical improvement. Noninvasive monitoring of pulse oximetry and end tidal P_{CO_2} may be useful for following trends, but no method of noninvasive P_{CO_2} measurement is sufficient to replace occasional assessment of arterial blood gases.

In addition to the daytime studies, patients should be monitored nocturnally during ventilator use. This may consist of pulse oximetry at the very least, or home multichannel monitoring. In addition to oximetry, these portable monitors have electrocardiographic, airflow, and chest wall motion channels, which may be useful in identifying obstructive apneas or excessive air leaking. Nocturnal polysomnography in a sleep laboratory is necessary to assess sleep quality, but we recommend screening studies in the home first to determine whether more sophisticated and expensive studies are necessary.

Once patients are fully stabilized, follow-up may be needed only two or three times yearly. In patients who have gradually progressive respiratory dysfunction, upward adjustments in inspiratory pressures, tidal volumes, breathing rates, and hours of daily use may be necessary to maintain stability.

17. What are the potential complications of NPPV?

If candidates for NPPV are carefully selected using available guidelines, the modality is safe and most complications are minor. The most frequently encountered complications are mask-related. Nasal dryness and congestion are common, sometimes occurring in the same patient. Remedies for nasal dryness include use of nasal saline or humidification; for congestion, topical decongestants or steroids and oral antihistamine-decongestant combinations can be used.

Other frequently encountered complications with standard nasal masks include eye irritation caused by air leaking around the mask, and nasal bridge redness or ulceration caused by excessive mask pressure, often during attempts to reduce air leaking. Remedies include minimizing strap tension, switching to masks with pliable sealing, using artificial skin over the bridge of the nose, and switching to an alternative nasal interface such as nasal pillows or seals. Acneiform rashes that develop at areas of mask and skin contact may respond to topical steroids or antibiotics. Gastric insufflation and flatulence are also common but rarely severe enough to warrant discontinuation, probably because insufflation pressures are usually low. Aspiration is a rare complication, as long as NPPV is reserved for patients who can adequately protect their airway.

Some patients (15–30% in most studies) cannot tolerate NPPV, usually because of discomfort from mask or air pressure and less often because of claustrophobia. The practitioner should be willing to make frequent readjustments, try different interfaces, and not give up too easily. Coaching, encouragement, and judicious use of sedation (in acute cases) may be helpful in achieving patient acceptance. In patients with chronic respiratory failure who are unable to tolerate the mask or fail to improve after an adequate trial of NPPV, alternative noninvasive ventilators (e.g., body ventilators) may be successful. In patients with acute respiratory failure, intubation is usually necessary if NPPV fails.

18. When should humidification be used with NPPV?

There are no published data on this issue. Patients using mouthpiece ventilation usually need humidification, but those receiving nasal ventilation usually do not because the nose is an efficient air conditioner. In the acute setting, where use may last for hours to a few days, humidification is rarely necessary. However, when duration of use is anticipated to be longer, humidification may be necessary in some patients who complain of nasal or mouth dryness that fails to respond to local measures such as use of nasal saline. Complaints of dryness are more common during the winter months or in arid climates and are associated with air leaking, particularly through the mouth. If the patient is receiving ventilatory assistance from a portable volume ventilator, a heated cascade type of humidifier can be used.

19. How common is air leaking during NPPV? How much does it compromise efficacy and what should be done about it?

NPPV circuits are leaky by design. Some leaks are intentional, as with exhalation valves on portable pressure-limited ventilators. However, unintentional leaks are also common, depending on the type of mask or interface used. With nasal ventilation, some leaking occurs around the mask, but most occurs through the mouth and may be enough to negate ventilator efficacy. Most of the time, however, patients do well with NPPV despite air leaking through the mouth and may have nearly normal sleep quality. The consequences of air leaking may depend partly on the ventilator mode used. Some pressure-limited ventilators sustain inspiratory air flow to compensate for leaks and maintain mask pressure. Volume-limited ventilators are unable to alter inspiratory air flow in response to leaks, but air leaks may still be compensated by increase in tidal volume. Chin straps may reduce leaking but do not eliminate the problem. Oronasal face masks may be used if excessive air leaks through the mouth with nasal masks, but oronasal masks seal poorly on the chin, replacing leaking through the mouth with leaking around the mask. If so, mouthpiece or total face mask ventilation can be considered.

CONTROVERSIES

20. When should invasive ventilation be used in preference to NPPV?

Most investigators agree that patients who are poor candidates for or fail adequate trials of NPPV and alternative noninvasive ventilators require invasive ventilation. However, there is some disagreement about whether patients requiring continuous ventilatory assistance can be safely managed with noninvasive ventilation. Branthwaite has suggested that patients requiring assisted ventilation most of the time (more than 16 hours per day) should receive invasive ventilation. Bach, on the other hand, recommends mouthpiece NPPV, even for patients with essentially no capacity to breathe spontaneously, as long as upper airway function is intact. Using this approach, many patients have undergone successful decannulation and long-term noninvasive support. It is important to emphasize that success of this approach requires experience and excellent family and caregiver support.

21. Does NIV work in COPD?

During the early 1980s, it was hypothesized that intermittent ventilatory assistance would rest chronically fatigued respiratory muscles in patients with severe COPD, leading to improved muscle function and gas exchange. Several uncontrolled and short-term controlled studies using wrap negative pressure ventilators intermittently during the daytime showed significantly improved maximal inspiratory and expiratory pressures and blood gas levels in patients with severe COPD, consistent with the hypothesis. However, long-term controlled studies have failed to confirm the earlier findings. Shapiro and colleagues, in the largest study, randomized 184 patients to receive either negative-pressure or sham ventilation for 12 weeks and found no improvements in inspiratory muscle strength, daytime gas exchange, exercise tolerance, or symptoms. In addition, negative-pressure ventilation was poorly tolerated by COPD patients in the latter studies.

More recently, NPPV has been used to provide ventilatory assistance to patients with severe COPD, based on favorable findings in uncontrolled studies. However, two recent controlled studies of almost identical design reported virtually opposite results. Strumpf and coworkers observed no benefit of nocturnal NPPV other than in some measures of neuropsychological function; in contrast, Meecham Jones and colleagues found significant improvements in daytime and nocturnal gas exchange, total sleep time, and symptoms of well-being during NPPV therapy. These seemingly conflicting results may be explained by close examination of baseline characteristics of patients entering the respective studies. Patients entering the Strumpf study had an average FEV_1 of 0.54 liters, $PaCO_2$ of 46 mmHg, and no significant sleep desaturation. Those entering the Meecham Jones study had FEV_1 of 0.81 liters, $PaCO_2$ of 56 mmHg, and many nocturnal oxygen desaturations. This suggests that patients with severe COPD but little or no carbon dioxide retention are unlikely to benefit from noninvasive ventilation, whereas the subgroup with marked daytime carbon dioxide retention and nocturnal desaturation may respond favorably. More studies are needed to confirm this possibility.

BIBLIOGRAPHY

1. AARC Clinical Practice Guideline: Intermittent positive pressure breathing. Respir Care 38:1189–1193, 1993.
2. Bach JR: Alternative methods of ventilatory support for the patient with ventilatory failure due to spinal cord injury. J Am Paraplegia Soc 14:158–174, 1991.
3. Bach JR: A comparison of long-term ventilatory support alternatives from the perspective of the patient and the caregiver. Chest 104:1702–1706, 1993.
4. Branthwaite MA: Non-invasive and domiciliary ventilation: Positive pressure techniques. Thorax 46:208–212, 1991.
5. Brochard L, Mancebo J, Wysocki M, et al: Noninvasive ventilation for acute exacerbations of chronic obstructive pulmonary disease. N Engl J Med 333:817–822, 1995.
6. Ellis ER, Bye PT, Bruderer JW, et al: Treatment of respiratory failure during sleep in patients with neuromuscular disease. Positive-pressure ventilation through a nose mask. Am Rev Respir Dis 1135:148–152, 1987.
7. Goldberg R, Sexauer W: Noninvasive ventilation in respiratory failure. Clin Pulm Med 1:313–321, 1994.
8. Hill NS: Noninvasive ventilation. Does it work, for whom, and how? Am Rev Respir Dis 147:1050–1055, 1993.
9. Meduri GU, Abou-Shala N, Fox RC, et al: Noninvasive face mask mechanical ventilation in patients with acute hypercapnic respiratory failure. Chest 100:445–454, 1991.
10. Meecham Jones DJ, Paul EA, Jones PW, et al: Nasal pressure support ventilation plus oxygen compared with oxygen therapy alone in hypercapnic COPD. Am J Respir Crit Care Med 152:538–544, 1995.
11. Meyer TJ, Hill NS: Noninvasive positive pressure ventilation to treat respiratory failure. Ann Intern Med 120:760–770, 1994.
12. Pingleton SK: Complications of acute respiratory failure. Am Rev Respir Dis 137:1463–1493, 1988.
13. Shapiro SH, Ernst P, Gray-Donald K, et al: Effect of negative pressure ventilation in severe chronic obstructive pulmonary disease. Lancet 310:1425–1429, 1992.
14. Strumpf DA, Carlisle CC, Millman RP, et al: An evaluation of the Respironics BiPAP bi-level CPAP device for assisted ventilation. Respir Care 35:415–422, 1990.
15. The Intermittent Positive Pressure Breathing Trial Group: Intermittent positive pressure breathing therapy of chronic obstructive pulmonary disease. Ann Intern Med 99:612–620, 1983.

69. TRADITIONAL INVASIVE VENTILATION

Gregory Diette, M.D., and Roy Brower, M.D.

1. How do hypercapnic and hypoxic respiratory failure differ? When is mechanical ventilation needed in each?

Mechanical ventilation is generally indicated in acute respiratory failure, which may be either hypercapnic, hypoxic, or both. **Hypercapnic respiratory failure**, which reflects inadequate ventilation (movement of air in and out of the lungs), may be caused by various disorders of the CNS, peripheral nerves, muscles, airways, parenchyma, and chest wall. When hypercapnic respiratory failure is acute, the rise in $PaCO_2$ occurs over a relatively short time (minutes to hours), and there is an accompanying drop in arterial pH. Clinical signs may include agitation, tachypnea, accessory muscle use, cyanosis, and decline of consciousness. In such cases, mechanical ventilation may be necessary to prevent death.

In **hypoxic respiratory failure**, there is inadequate arterial oxygenation. This deficit frequently occurs despite the presence of adequate spontaneous ventilation (normal or even low $PaCO_2$). Mechanical ventilation is sometimes helpful in managing hypoxemia, even though ventilation may be adequate. For example, in the acute respiratory distress syndrome (ARDS), use of positive end-expiratory pressure (PEEP) may be necessary to maintain adequate arterial oxygenation. In addition, by assuming some or all of the work of breathing, the ventilator may reduce the oxygen cost of breathing, allowing utilization of blood oxygen by other critical organs, such as the brain and heart.

2. Name some causes of hypercapnic respiratory failure.

Disorders of the CNS with diminished respiratory drive
  General anesthesia
  Narcotic or barbiturate overdose
  Brainstem stroke or trauma
Disorders of spinal cord
  High cervical spinal cord trauma
  Cervical myelitis
  Amyotrophic lateral sclerosis
Disorders of peripheral nerves and muscles
  Myasthenia gravis
  Guillain-Barré syndrome
  Neuromuscular blockade
  Acute intermittent porphyria
  Poliomyelitis
  Muscular dystrophy
  Polymyositis

Disorders of thoracic cage with increased chest wall stiffness
  Kyphoscoliosis
  Morbid obesity
  Flail chest
Disorders of lung parenchyma (increase lung stiffness and physiologic deadspace)
  Pulmonary fibrosis
  Sarcoidosis
Disorders of airways
  Asthma
  Chronic obstructive pulmonary disease (COPD)
  Cystic fibrosis
  Bronchiolitis obliterans

3. In addition to the recognition of respiratory failure, what other three important considerations are needed in the decision to initiate mechanical ventilation?

First, how rapid is the decline in respiratory status? Chronic hypercapnic respiratory failure is generally not an indication for mechanical ventilation. For example, a COPD patient with a $PaCO_2$ of 80 mmHg, arterial pH of 7.37, and PaO_2 of 65 mmHg on FIO_2 of 0.30 has adequate metabolic compensation for the hypercapnia and probably does not require mechanical ventilation. In contrast, a patient with acute asthma whose $PaCO_2$ has risen from 35 to 53 mmHg while in the emergency department might need mechanical ventilation to prevent further deterioration, which could lead to death.

Second, can more conservative measures reverse respiratory failure without resorting to intubation and mechanical ventilation? For example, in the case of opiate overdose, naloxone may rapidly reverse the cause of hypoventilation.

Third, is mechanical ventilation consistent with the patient's overall care goals? For example, some patients with terminal illness may request that mechanical ventilation not be used.

4. What are the usual modes of mechanical ventilation?
  Assist-control (A-C)
  Synchronized intermittent mandatory ventilation (SIMV)
  Pressure support (PS)

5. What is assist-control (A-C) ventilation?

In this mode of ventilation, the physician or therapist selects a minimum respiratory rate, tidal volume, and inspiratory flow rate. If the patient makes no or very weak inspiratory efforts, then the ventilator provides "controlled" breaths by blowing air into the patient's lungs at the prescribed flow rate until the prescribed tidal volume is achieved.

The time interval between controlled breaths is determined by the respiratory rate selected by the clinician. If the patient makes an adequate inspiratory effort during this interval, the machine responds by blowing air at the prescribed inspiratory flow rate until the prescribed tidal volume is achieved. This is an "assisted" breath. In a patient whose intrinsic respiratory rate exceeds the minimum rate for controlled breaths, all breathing will be assisted. With assisted breaths, the work of breathing is shared between the patient and ventilator. With either assisted or controlled breaths, the tidal volume is the same regardless of patient effort.

A-C ventilation is often the mode chosen immediately after initiation of mechanical ventilation. It is useful when the intent is to have the ventilator assume most or all of the work of breathing, as in neuromuscular blockade, respiratory muscle fatigue, or profound neuromuscular weakness.

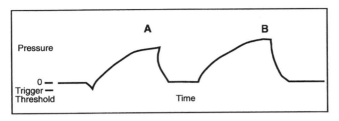

Assist-control ventilation. In Breath *A*, an assisted breath, the initial airway pressure deflection represents the patient's inspiratory effort, before the ventilation begins its positive pressure assist. Breath *B* is delivered by the machine when no inspiratory effort is detected.

6. How does the ventilator "know" that a patient is trying to initiate a breath?

The ventilator monitors pressure at or near the endotracheal tube. A patient's efforts to inspire cause the pressures in the airways to fall below the level that exists at end-expiration, before the beginning of the inspiratory effort. If the airway pressure falls below a trigger threshold, the ventilator responds by raising airway pressure to assist the inspiratory effort. Typically, the trigger threshold is set to 1–2 cm H_2O below the airway pressure at end-expiration.

7. What is synchronized intermittent mandatory ventilation (SIMV)?

As in the A-C mode, with SIMV the physician selects a minimum respiratory rate, tidal volume, and inspiratory flow rate. If there are no inspiratory efforts or very weak efforts, the ventilator provides "controlled breaths" in the same manner as in the A-C mode. Unlike A-C, however, SIMV does not "assist" any patient inspiratory efforts beyond the minimum; the patient must breathe on his or her own. For example, if the physician-selected minimum respiratory rate is 6 breaths/minute (bpm) and the patient makes inspiratory efforts 20 times/min, only 6 bpm will be assisted by the ventilator; the remaining 14 breaths are unassisted. The size of the unassisted breaths will be whatever the patient can achieve on his or her own.

The term *synchronized* means that the machine-assisted breaths occur simultaneously with patient efforts, if any. As with A-C mode, the SIMV ventilator monitors at or near the endotracheal tube to detect the onset of the patient's inspiratory efforts. Synchronization prevents ventilator-delivered breaths from occurring in the middle of a patient-initiated breath.

SIMV was initially developed for weaning, to allow the frequency of assisted breaths to be gradually reduced while the patient resumes an increasing proportion of the work of breathing. SIMV may also be useful in patients requiring substantial ventilatory assistance but whose respiratory rates are too high.

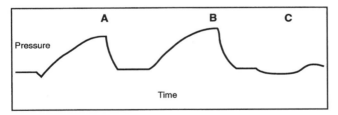

Intermittent mandatory ventilation. Breath *A* is an assisted breath, triggered by the patient's inspiratory effort. Breath *B* is delivered by machine when no inspiratory effort is detected. Breath *C* is a spontaneous, unassisted breath.

8. What is pressure support ventilation?

In the pressure support (PS) mode, the ventilator responds to a patient's inspiratory effort by raising pressure at or near the endotracheal tube to a physician-selected level, such as 15 cm H_2O. The ventilator maintains this pressure until the end of the patient's inspiratory effort, at which point airway pressure returns to the appropriate level for expiration (either zero or the PEEP level, if any). Respiratory rate is determined entirely by the patient.

PS ventilation is often used as an alternative to A-C or SIMV. In the PS mode, the patient has more control over inspiratory flow rate, tidal volume, and duration of inspiration. If the patient feels more dyspneic, he or she may take larger tidal volumes at more rapid inspiratory flow rates. If dyspnea or requirements for ventilation decrease, he or she may take smaller breaths at lower flow rates. This is in contrast to the stereotyped breaths provided in A-C or SIMV. Hence a patient may breathe more comfortably on PS.

Many clinicians also use PS for "weaning." When used for this purpose, the level of PS is gradually reduced in steps (usually over several hours), allowing the patient to gradually resume the work of breathing with each breath.

Pressure support ventilation. Each breath is supported by the ventilator after an inspiratory effort by the patient triggers the ventilator. The pressure during inspiration reaches the clinician-selected level with each breath and is maintained at this pressure until the end of inspiratory effort. The intervals between breaths and the lengths of the inspiratory efforts are variable.

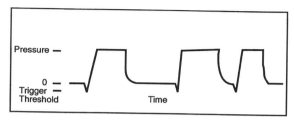

9. Are there contraindications to PS ventilation?

Because the ventilator delivers positive pressure only in response to patient inspiratory efforts, important contraindications to PS ventilation are inadequate respiratory drive and very weak inspiratory effort. These may occur in patients with disorders of the brainstem or profound disorders of the nerve and muscles.

10. What is the right amount of pressure support?

There is no formula to predict or calculate the right amount. Moreover, in some patients, PS is used to assume most of the work of breathing, whereas in other patients, PS is used for smaller amounts of ventilation assistance (as in weaning). When the intent is to assume most of the work of breathing, the right level of PS is one at which the patient is comfortable and receiving adequate ventilation. Comfort can be assessed from the respiratory rate (< 25–30 bpm is usually acceptable), and the level of effort the patient makes with each breath. Use of accessory muscles, diaphoresis, and intercostal retractions are signs of excessive (uncomfortable) effort.

Higher levels of PS are usually necessary when the compliance of the respiratory system is low (as in ARDS), the airway resistance is high (as in asthma or COPD), or the patient is able to make only weak inspiratory efforts (as in neuromuscular diseases). A useful starting level of pressure support is approximately 10–15 cm H_2O. Adjustments in this level should be made quickly (within minutes) after assessing patient comfort and adequacy of ventilation.

11. In a paralyzed patient, what minute ventilation can be expected with each of the following ventilator settings:

A. A-C, tidal volume = 750 ml, minimum respiratory rate = 10 bpm
B. SIMV, tidal volume = 750 ml, minimum respiratory rate = 10 bpm
C. PS, 20 cm H_2O

A. 7.5 liters/min. The patient will receive 10 bpm, each of 750 ml. All of the breaths will be "controlled."

B. 7.5 liters/min. As with A-C, the SIMV mode will deliver the pre-set tidal volume of 750 ml 10 times/min. There will be no additional, unsupported breaths. In paralyzed patients, A-C and SIMV are identical.

C. Zero! PS only supports breaths initiated by the patient. A patient who is unable to make inspiratory effort will not be ventilated in the PS mode. (Most, but not all, ventilators have volume-cycled backup modes that automatically turn on when apnea is recognized.)

12. In a patient making 20 inspiratory efforts per minute, what ventilation can be expected with each of the following settings:

A. A-C, tidal volume = 750 ml, minimum respiratory rate = 10 bpm
B. SIMV, tidal volume = 750 ml, minimum respiratory rate = 10 bpm
C. PS, 10 cm H_2O

A. 15 liters/min. Each inspiratory effort will be assisted, and each tidal volume will equal 750 ml. The minute ventilation will be 20 bpm × 0.75 liters/breath = 15 liters/min

B. > 7.5 liters/min. It is not possible to know the exact amount. Ten breaths of 750 ml will be assisted by the ventilator. The volume of the other 10 spontaneous breaths will be determined by patient effort and mechanics of the lungs and chest wall. Each spontaneous breath may be a different tidal volume and can be less than, equal to, or greater than 750 ml.

C. Impossible to calculate. We know the respiratory rate will be 20 bpm, but we do not know the size of the tidal volumes. The three factors that determine tidal volume in patients on PS are (1) level of pressure support, which we know; (2) amount of patient effort (muscle force); and (3) lung mechanics (resistance of the airways and compliance of the lungs and chest wall). Minute ventilation can be assessed in patients on PS by observing the size of the tidal volumes and multiplying by the rate. Most ventilators report the size of each tidal volume at the end of each breath. Many ventilators also report a value for minute ventilation.

13. What are the static compliance and plateau pressure?

Static compliance of any structure represents its distensibility: i.e., how easy or difficult it is to increase its volume. In mathematical terms, compliance equals the change in volume divided by the change in transmural pressure. Static compliance of the respiratory system represents the combined distensibility of the lungs and chest wall.

It is easy to measure this compliance in a patient on a ventilator by dividing the tidal volume by the change in alveolar pressure that occurs from end-expiration to end-inspiration. The alveolar pressure at end-expiration is usually the same as the pressure at the endotracheal tube (0 or the level of PEEP). The pressure in the alveoli at end-inspiration is measured by occluding the expiratory conduit from the ventilator at the end of the tidal volume inspiration and waiting approx 0.5–1.0 sec. The pressure that the ventilator reports after this brief interval is called the **plateau pressure** and represents the average pressure in the alveoli at end-inspiration.

Static compliance of the respiratory system is then calculated as follows:

$$\text{Static compliance} = \text{tidal volume} \div (\text{plateau pressure} - \text{PEEP, if any})$$

For example, if the tidal volume = 800 ml, PEEP = 5 cm H_2O, and plateau pressure = 25 cm H_2O, then the respiratory system compliance is 800 ml/(25 cm H_2O – 5 cm H_2O) = 40 ml/cm H_2O. Normal respiratory system compliance for an average-sized adult is approx 80–100 ml/cm H_2O. Conditions associated with low respiratory system compliance are pulmonary edema (cardiogenic and noncardiogenic), severe pneumonia, pulmonary fibrosis, kyphoscoliosis, and marked obesity.

14. Define PEEP.

Positive end-expiratory pressure. When no PEEP is applied, the ventilator allows airway pressure to fall to atmospheric pressure during expiration. When PEEP is used, the ventilator maintains airway pressure at the physician-selected level of PEEP during expiration.

15. Who needs PEEP?

PEEP is helpful in maintaining oxygenation in many patients in whom intrapulmonary shunt is responsible for hypoxemia. PEEP improves oxygenation in these patients by recruiting and stabilizing alveoli which tend to collapse. PEEP may allow adequate oxygenation without resorting to potentially toxic concentrations of inspired oxygen (FiO$_2$). In some patients, PEEP may be necessary to maintain adequate oxygenation even with high levels of FiO$_2$.

16. How much PEEP should be used in patients with hypoxemic respiratory failure?

PEEP can have deleterious effects. For example, the risks of pneumothorax and other forms of barotrauma increase when PEEP is applied, because the airway pressures and distending forces in the lungs increase. Cardiac output also decreases when PEEP is applied because pressures in the chest rise, diminishing venous return; when cardiac output decreases, the delivery of oxygen to peripheral tissues decreases.

Because of these and other deleterious effects of PEEP, most clinicians use only enough PEEP to achieve adequate oxygenation (oxyhemoglobin saturation of approx 90%) at levels of FiO_2 that are believed to be safe (approx $\leq$ 50–70%). Recently, some investigators have recommended using additional amounts of PEEP in patients with ARDS to prevent the shear forces associated with opening and reclosing of the unstable alveoli.

17. What is CPAP?

Continuous positive airway pressure. With CPAP, a constant level of positive pressure is applied throughout inspiration and expiration. It is most useful, as is PEEP, in situations in which shunt contributes to hypoxemia. PEEP and CPAP work by recruiting and stabilizing alveoli which tend to collapse.

Some clinicians use CPAP during weaning when hypoxemia is still a problem, yet ventilatory assistance is not required. Also, setting the ventilator to CPAP = 0 cm H_2O will allow a patient to "breathe on his own" but still be connected to the ventilator circuit and its alarms.

18. What is auto-PEEP?

Auto-PEEP (synonymous with intrinsic PEEP) exists when the pressure in the alveolar spaces exceeds pressure in the airway opening (mouth or endotracheal tube). Normally, the pressure in the alveoli at the end of expiration equals the pressure in the airway opening. The lungs stop emptying when their inward recoil equals the outward recoil of the chest wall. Thus, a normal functional residual capacity (FRC) is determined by the relaxation volume of the respiratory system (lung and chest wall combined). Since this relaxation volume is reached normally before the beginning of the next inspiration, there is a period of time, approx 1 sec, when there is no air flow and airway opening and alveolar pressures are identical.

However, in some patients there is insufficient time for the respiratory system to empty down to the relaxation volume. For example, high airway resistance in asthma slows expiratory airflow, leaving insufficient time for the respiratory system to empty down to the normal FRC. The pressure in the alveoli at end-expiration remains greater than airway opening pressure. Rapid respiratory rates and large tidal volume also contribute to the development of auto-PEEP.

Alveolar pressure during the respiratory cycle in a normal patient (*solid line*) and a patient with 5 cm H_2O auto-PEEP (*dashed line*). The patient with auto-PEEP must lower his alveolar pressure by 6 cm H_2O (from 5 to –1 cm H_2O) to reach the trigger threshold, while the normal patient must generate only 1 cm H_2O negative pressure (from 0 to –1 cm H_2O).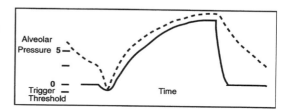

19. Who gets auto-PEEP?

Auto-PEEP is especially likely to occur in patients with airways diseases such as asthma if the ventilator is set to deliver generous tidal volumes. Moreover, patients with acute respiratory failure frequently have rapid intrinsic respiratory rates.

20. What are the effects of auto-PEEP?

When auto-PEEP occurs, there are deleterious effects on the respiratory and circulatory systems. Venous return and cardiac output decrease because, as with external PEEP, the pressures in the chest surrounding the heart rise. Auto-PEEP also increases pulmonary vascular resistance because the high alveolar pressures tend to compress alveolar capillaries. This increases the work of the right ventricle to pump blood through the pulmonary circulation.

The work required to trigger the ventilator increases when there is auto-PEEP because the inspiratory muscles must first contract with enough force to lower alveolar pressure to 0 (or the external level of PEEP) before the patient can trigger the ventilator. Consider a patient with auto-PEEP of 7 cm H_2O (alveolar pressure at end-expiration 7 cm H_2O greater than the pressure in the endotracheal tube) and a ventilator trigger threshold of 1 cm H_2O below atmospheric pressure. This patient must generate 8 cm H_2O negative pressure with his or her inspiratory muscles before the pressure in the endotracheal tube decreases to the trigger threshold. In contrast, if this patient had no auto-PEEP, the ventilator could be triggered with only 1 cm H_2O negative pressure.

21. How do you detect auto-PEEP in a ventilated patient?

Auto-PEEP is not typically measured or reported by the ventilator. To measure auto-PEEP in a patient on a ventilator, it is necessary to occlude the exhalation port of the ventilator a moment before the next inspiration would occur. When the exhalation port is occluded, any expiratory airflow ceases and the pressure the ventilator measures and displays on its manometer equals the pressure everywhere throughout the ventilator tubes, bronchi, and alveoli. Hence, this pressure equals auto-PEEP. This is, unfortunately, difficult to perform, especially in patients with rapid respiratory rates.

22. How can auto-PEEP be minimized or eliminated?

There are three general approaches to managing auto-PEEP:

1. Treat any reversible airways constriction and inflammation. By so doing, airway resistance may decrease, leading to increased expiratory flow rates.

2. Decrease tidal volume. This maneuver may cause hypercapnia, which may have deleterious effects that must be considered in relation to those of auto-PEEP.

3. Increase the time available for exhalation. This can be accomplished in two ways: (a) shorten the duration of inspiration by increasing the inspiratory flow rate; or (b) decrease the respiratory rate. To lower the respiratory rate, it may be necessary to sedate or paralyze the patient. As with decreased tidal volume, the decreased respiratory rate may lead to hypercapnia.

23. What do all those ventilator alarms do?

The alarms on the ventilator are designed to alert people caring for the patient that there may be a harmful situation. The types of alarms are group according to three functions:

	Implication of Alarm
Inadequate ventilation	
Low exhaled volume	Air leak
Low minute ventilation	Air leak, low respiratory rate
Low airway pressure	Air leak
Apnea	Loss of patient respiratory drive; disconnection from ventilator
Harmful physiology	
High airway pressure	Increased risk of barotrauma; mucous plug
High respiratory rate	Patient agitated; risk of overventilation; risk of auto-PEEP
High I:E ration (> 1:1)	Consider adjusting the inspiratory flow rate, respiratory rate
Failure of the ventilator	
Power disconnect	Check the power supply
Low back-up battery	Check the back-up battery
Low pressure at the oxygen inlet	Check the oxygen supply

24. Why are the ventilator alarms always going off?

Each ventilator alarm has a threshold value that is set by the therapist or clinician, depending on specific characteristics of individual patients. Because serious consequences may result if problems are not quickly recognized and corrected, the alarms' thresholds are usually set at levels that make them very sensitive to potential problems. A perfect alarm would be 100% sensitive (sound whenever there is a real problem) and also 100% specific (never sound when there is no problem). Unfortunately, in practical terms, high sensitivity usually comes at the expense of diminished specificity (false alarms). Thus, the tradeoff for detecting all or nearly all dangerous situations is having to respond to many false alarms.

25. What is peak inspiratory pressure?

Peak inspiratory pressure is the highest pressure that occurs during the inspiratory portion of the cycle, usually seen at or near the end of inspiration. High peak inspiratory airway pressures usually reflect either narrowed airways (high airways resistance) or decreased respiratory compliance (stiff lungs or chest wall). Common causes of airway narrowing are bronchospasm (as in asthma and bronchitis), bronchial obstruction from secretions, or kinking of the endotracheal tube. Causes of decreased respiratory system compliance include ARDS, pulmonary edema, kyphoscoliosis, marked obesity, and tension pneumothorax. Peak inspiratory pressures also tend to rise, sometimes to alarming levels, when high inspiratory flow rates are used.

26. Why do we have a high peak inspiratory pressure alarm?

When a high peak pressure alarm is first heard, each of the potential causes should be considered quickly. Sometimes, a problem such as excessive secretions, kinked endotracheal tube, or pneumothorax can be identified and rectified quickly. At other times, it is impossible to intervene to quickly decrease the peak inspiratory pressure without causing other, perhaps worse, problems. For example, in severe asthma, the high airway pressures are likely attributable to the high airway resistance and high inspiratory flow rates (selected to allow sufficient time for exhalation). If the peak flow rate is reduced, auto-PEEP will be worse. Under such circumstances, the best solution may be to increase the alarm threshold to decrease the number of subsequent false alarms.

27. What causes a low exhaled volume alarm?

The exhaled volume alarm is designed to sound when the volume of air that comes out during exhalation is less than a lower limit threshold. Two serious conditions should come to mind quickly when this alarm sounds: First, if the patient is receiving a volume-cycled breath, this alarm should suggest that there is a leak in the system that allows some part of the intended tidal volume to escape without entering the patient's lung. Leaks such as this may be caused by malposition of the endotracheal tube, a ruptured or inadequately inflated endotracheal cuff, endotracheal tube disconnection from the ventilator tubing, or a leak at one of the ventilator circuit connections. Second, if the patient is receiving PS, this alarm may sound if the tidal volume the patient receives is less than some acceptable volume chosen by the respiratory therapist or physician. This may signify that the patient is too weak to ventilate sufficiently at the current PS setting.

28. How should we monitor for the adequacy of gas exchange?

An arterial blood gas sample can be used to assess PO_2. Oxygenation can also be assessed by continuous or intermittent pulse oximetry, which has advantages of being noninvasive and relatively inexpensive. When an adequate signal cannot be obtained on the pulse oximeter (as when extremities are cold and hypoperfused), an arterial blood gas must still be used periodically. An arterial blood gas measurement of PCO_2 provides an assessment of the adequacy of ventilation.

29. What patient position is ideal in mechanical ventilation?

While a patient can be ventilated in virtually any position, the traditional position has been **supine**. There is an emerging trend to considering the **prone** position in patients with diffuse lung injury (e.g., ARDS). Some clinicians have noticed improved oxygenation in the prone position, probably reflecting decreased shunt in dorsal (posterior) lung regions and possibly more advantageous removal of airway secretions.

BIBLIOGRAPHY

1. Grum CM, Chauncey JB: Conventional mechanical ventilation. Clin Chest Med 9:37–46, 1988.
2. Kreit JW, Eschenbacher WL: The physiology of spontaneous and mechanical ventilation. Clin Chest Med 9:11–21, 1988.
3. Pierson DJ, Kacmarek RM (eds): Foundations of Respiratory Care. New York, Churchill Livingstone, 1992.
4. Slutsky AS, et al: ACCP Consensus Conference: Mechanical ventilation. Chest 104:1833–1859, 1993.
5. Tobin M (ed): Principles and Practice of Mechanical Ventilation. New York, McGraw-Hill, 1994.
6. Tobin MJ: Mechanical ventilation. N Engl J Med 1056–1061, 1994.

70. NEW INVASIVE VENTILATORY STRATEGIES

Inchel Yeam, M.D., and Catherine S. H. Sassoon, M.D.

1. Name some of the new invasive ventilatory strategies. Why were they developed?

The goals of mechanical ventilation are to improve gas exchange and to unload the excessive work of the respiratory muscles while avoiding ventilator-induced complications. In general, conventional mechanical ventilation is adequate to achieve these goals. Under special circumstances, however, such as in severe asthma or diffuse lung injury, ventilatory support with conventional volume targeted positive-pressure ventilation (CPPV) may lead to high peak airway pressures. This results in further lung injury. New ventilatory strategies have been introduced with the intention of improving oxygenation while minimizing the risk of lung injury. *Alternative ventilatory strategies* is a better term than *new* because many of these strategies have been employed for several years in pediatric patients. Alternative invasive ventilatory strategies include pressure control ventilation (PCV), inverse ratio ventilation (IRV), permissive hypercapnia, and tracheal gas insufflation (TGI). A fundamentally different mode of mechanical ventilation is high-frequency ventilation (HFV).

2. Explain the terms *pressure control ventilation* and *inverse ratio ventilation*.

Pressure control ventilation (PCV) is a positive-pressure ventilation mode in which the ventilator delivers a breath until a set target pressure and a set inspiratory time is reached, at which time the ventilator cycles off. Tidal volume varies with each breath, depending on lung compliance and airway resistance. A low lung compliance or a high airway resistance (or both) result in small tidal volumes. In addition, when the patient actively triggers the ventilator with a rapid respiratory rate, expiratory time may be curtailed because inspiratory time is preset. This situation results in air trapping or dynamic hyperinflation.

During normal respiration, inspiratory time (I) is about one-half to one-third of expiratory time (E); that is, the I:E ratio usually equals 1:2 to 1:3. Inverse ratio ventilation (IRV) is a reversal of this pattern in which inspiratory time is greater than expiratory time. IRV can be used with either pressure control or volume control ventilation. With pressure control ventilation, a prolonged inspiratory time is set. With volume control ventilation, a low peak flow rate with or without inspiratory pause is set. Most clinicians use pressure control when employing IRV (PC-IRV).

3. What is the indication for PCV?

With CPPV, patients with severe lung injury or ARDS may manifest poor oxygenation despite high levels of inspired oxygen concentration (FIO_2), positive end-expiratory pressure (PEEP), and peak airway pressure. The high peak airway pressures result from the severely decreased lung compliance that occurs in ARDS. In experimental animals, high peak airway pressures of 30 cm H_2O or more have been associated with parenchymal lung injury. Patients with ARDS may benefit from PCV because this mode of ventilation sets a target pressure and thereby decreases elevated peak airway pressures. Lower peak airway pressure protects the lungs from further injury.

4. How does PC-IRV improve oxygenation in patients with ARDS?

Oxygenation is one of the major physiologic derangements in patients with ARDS. Oxygenation is determined by FIO_2 and the mean pressure distending the alveoli (mean alveolar pressure). If FIO_2 requirements remain high (more than 50%) in ARDS despite high levels of PEEP (15 cm H_2O or more), oxygenation may be improved by an increase in mean alveolar pressure. The major determinant of mean alveolar pressure is mean airway pressure. Mean airway pressure can be increased by increasing PEEP, tidal volume, or the duration of inspiratory phase (i.e., by the use of IRV). Progressive increases in tidal volume or PEEP are limited by the excessive rise in airway pressure that occurs with their use.

IRV can increase mean airway pressure above values observed with CPPV even when peak airway pressures are the same. This occurs because a greater proportion of the respiratory cycle is spent in the inspiratory phase with IRV. With higher mean airway pressures, and therefore higher mean alveolar pressures with the use of IRV, oxygenation may improve and toxic levels of FIO_2 can be avoided. IRV is initiated when oxygenation remains inadequate despite high levels of FIO_2 and PEEP or when peak airway pressures are excessive.

5. What are some of the concerns with the use of PC-IRV?

Patients are generally uncomfortable and difficult to synchronize with the ventilator during the use of PC-IRV because this mode of ventilation causes an unnatural pattern of breathing. Patients often require sedation with paralytic agents for this mode to be effective. Unfortunately, prolonged paralysis with residual skeletal muscle weakness has been observed with the use of paralytic agents. With PC-IRV, intrathoracic pressure can increase significantly because of both the prolonged positive intrathoracic pressure and dynamic hyperinflation resulting from the relatively short expiratory time. This compromises venous return to the heart, leading to a decrease in cardiac output. The insertion of a pulmonary artery catheter allows close hemodynamic monitoring. Finally, barotrauma is a concern because of the risk of dynamic hyperinflation.

6. What is dynamic hyperinflation?

Dynamic hyperinflation is a condition in which lung volume increases above the static equilibrium volume of the respiratory system (i.e., functional residual capacity, or FRC) and is associated with increased alveolar pressure at the end of exhalation. The increase in alveolar pressure at end exhalation is referred to as *auto-PEEP* or *intrinsic PEEP*. This phenomenon occurs when expiratory time is short or airway resistance, especially expiratory resistance, is high. A prolonged expiratory time is required for full exhalation. With patient-triggered mechanical ventilation, expiratory time is set by the respiratory rate and the fraction of inspiratory time. When expiratory time is inadequate for full exhalation, the FRC progressively readjusts to a larger lung volume. In other words, at end exhalation, the chest wall continuously recoils, producing positive pressure in the alveoli relative to mouth pressure, while the next breath is delivered by the ventilator. Consequently, the ventilator delivers the next tidal volume at a higher FRC than the previous breath. After a period of "stacking breaths," a new equilibrium is eventually reached at which the inspiratory and expiratory tidal volume are the same. This equilibrium develops when the hyperinflated lungs enlarge airway caliber, thereby decreasing resistance to expiratory flow, and the expanded chest wall increases elastic recoil pressures and promotes expiratory flow. Dynamic hyperinflation occurs most commonly in patients with severe asthma or emphysema.

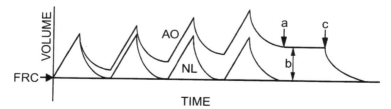

Theoretical time-volume tracing in a controlled mechanical ventilation in normal lung (NL) and lung with airway obstruction (AO). In AO, incomplete exhalation leads to progressive rise in functional residual capacity (FRC). When respiratory muscles are completely relaxed (or paralyzed), airway occlusion pressure can be obtained at end expiration (**a**). With respiratory muscles completely relaxed, opening of the airway (**c**) will gradually bring the volume down to the original FRC. a = airway occlusion at end of expiration and beginning of apnea; b = increase in FRC due to auto-PEEP; c = release of airway occlusion, lungs empty to FRC. (Modified from Tuxen DV: Permissive hypercapnic ventilation. Am J Respir Crit Care Med 150:870–874, 1994.)

7. Why is dynamic hyperinflation or auto-PEEP dangerous?

Patients who experience dynamic hyperinflation are forced to breathe at higher lung volumes, resulting in overdistension of alveolar units and high peak airway pressures. These overdistended alveolar spaces are subject to barotrauma. The increased intrathoracic pressure associated with dynamic hyperinflation can also decrease venous return to the heart, causing hemodynamic compromise.

8. How is the ventilator checked for the presence of auto-PEEP?

Auto-PEEP can be detected by occlusion of the ventilator expiratory port at the end of exhalation by closing the airway occlusion valve and noting the ventilator's display of the end-expiratory occlusion pressure. Normally, end-expiratory pressure is similar to the level of applied PEEP. In the presence of auto-PEEP, end-expiratory airway pressure rises above applied PEEP.

If the ventilator does not have an airway occlusion valve, auto-PEEP can be detected in the absence of applied PEEP by momentarily disconnecting the patient from the ventilator. A continuous expiration of air, which can be quantified using a spirometer, and relaxation of the thoracic cavity beyond the expected time of expiration suggest presence of dynamic hyperinflation. Accurate measurement of auto-PEEP requires the patient to be completely relaxed or paralyzed.

9. How can dynamic hyperinflation be prevented?

Dynamic hyperinflation is usually suspected in the following setting: when airway pressure rises progressively while tidal volumes remain constant or blood pressure progressively decreases in a patient with airway obstruction. With controlled mechanical ventilation in completely passive or paralyzed patients, dynamic hyperinflation can be prevented or minimized by decreasing the tidal volume or decreasing the respiratory rate, allowing for extended expiratory time. This approach, however, may decrease ventilation and lead to hypercapnia (see question 11).

10. What is the emerging strategy in the ventilatory management of patients with ARDS?

It has been suggested that repetitive opening and closing of recruitable alveoli in the setting of ARDS produces shear stress that leads to further lung injury. By increasing end-expiratory lung volume and preventing recruitable alveoli from collapsing, applied PEEP may reduce lung injury caused by shear stress.

The application of PEEP is aided by considering pressure-volume relationships of patients with ARDS. The ideal static pressure-volume curve in early acute lung injury changes its slope in two points, which are referred to as the lower (LIP) and upper inflection points (UIP):

1. LIP is the point at which lung compliance improves as a result of recruitment of collapsed alveolar spaces.
2. UIP is the point at which compliance begins to decrease (flattening of the curve) because of relative hyperinflation of alveolar spaces. UIP usually occurs near airway pressures of 35 cm H_2O.

Ideally, PEEP should be increased until the pressure reaches a level on the static pressure-volume curve just above the LIP; tidal volume should be adjusted downward to maintain the pressure below the UIP.

These maneuvers decrease shear stress and prevent alveolar overdistension, serving as a form of "lung rest." Decreasing tidal volume, however, may lead to hypoventilation and hypercapnia. Because the hypercapnia occurs as a result of purposeful ventilator adjustments, it is termed *permissive hypercapnia*. In some clinical situations, such as severe acute asthma and ARDS, in which the risk of ventilator-induced morbidity is high, the $PaCO_2$ may be allowed to rise gradually to levels above 60 mmHg and even 90 mmHg to avoid potentially devastating lung damage. Ventilation with low tidal volumes may cause breathing discomfort, necessitating sedation with or without paralytic agents in some patients.

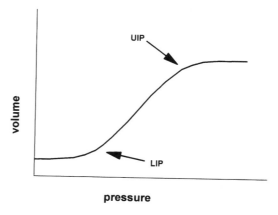

Ideal static pressure-volume curve in early acute lung injury. Lower inflection point (LIP) reflects improvement of lung compliance as a result of recruitment of collapsed alveoli. Upper inflection point (UIP) and flattening of upper portion of the curve represents reduction of compliance from hyperinflation of alveolar spaces.

11. How safe is permissive hypercapnia?

Maintenance of normal levels of $Paco_2$ in ventilated patients is desirable in most clinical situations. However, when peak airway pressures rise and the risk of barotrauma appears to be high, permissive hypercapnia has become an acceptable clinical approach. Increasing experience with this mode of ventilation indicates that high levels of $Paco_2$ are not as dangerous as previously thought, as long as the arterial pH stays at or above 7.20. Carbon dioxide freely diffuses from the blood into the intracellular compartment, but a very efficient buffering system keeps pH relatively constant within the cell. The kidneys eventually readjust the acid-base status by retaining more bicarbonate, further correcting the acidemia. Bicarbonate infusion has been recommended when the pH drops below 7.20 during permissive hypercapnia.

12. What systemic responses occur during permissive hypercapnia from increased $Paco_2$?

High $Paco_2$ causes several systemic responses. Hypercapnia induces cerebral vasodilation, headache, and increased intracranial pressure. Consequently, permissive hypercapnia is contraindicated in patients with cerebral edema or high intracranial pressure. High levels of $Paco_2$ also increase serum catecholamine levels, resulting in tachycardia, sweating, and anxiety. Excessive catecholamine levels may increase the risk of arrhythmia. Hypercapnia also decreases peripheral resistance, reduces myocardial contractility, and increases pulmonary vascular resistance. Poor cardiac output states and pulmonary hypertension, therefore, represent relative contraindications to permissive hypercapnia.

13. What is the role of tracheal gas insufflation in permissive hypercapnia?

Tracheal gas insufflation (TGI) is a technique for reducing dead space ventilation. During the expiratory phase of breathing, gas within the airways is high in carbon dioxide. Upon inspiration, the gas in the upper airways is rebreathed as part of the next tidal volume. A cannula placed in the lower trachea that provides a constant or intermittent fresh gas flow can flush out gas containing carbon dioxide, effectively decreasing the dead space. With higher $Paco_2$ values, greater reduction in $Paco_2$ is observed, thereby making TGI more effective during permissive hypercapnia. Because of reduction in dead space, TGI has been shown to decrease the need for minute ventilation and tidal volume. There are technical difficulties with this procedure, however, such as placement of the cannula, drying of mucosa, or potential for tracheal irritation. Investigations are underway to improve the technique so that TGI may become an important adjunct to mechanical ventilation during extreme hypercapnia.

14. Is there any role for extracorporeal oxygenation and carbon dioxide removal?

The concept of lung rest and avoidance of high peak airway pressures are important evolutionary changes in mechanical ventilation. Despite these advances, poor oxygenation and severe hypercapnia remain serious clinical challenges. Extracorporeal membrane oxygenation (ECMO) and extracorporeal carbon dioxide removal ($ECCO_2R$) are two techniques for patients with serious gas exchange abnormalities. As the names imply, both ECMO and $ECCO_2R$ employ extracorporeal circulation; however, ECMO aims at oxygenation, whereas $ECCO_2R$ aims at carbon dioxide removal. Both offer opportunities to minimize FIO_2 and allow the impaired lungs to heal.

Uncontrolled studies have suggested that outcome is improved in patients with ARDS who are treated with these modalities. However, in a randomized prospective study by Morris and coworkers of 40 patients with severe ARDS, 19 patients were supported with CPPV and the remainder with PC-IRV followed by a combined low frequency positive-pressure ventilation with extracorporeal carbon dioxide removal (LFPPV-$ECCO_2R$).[11] The survival rate for both LFPV-$ECCO_2R$ and CPPV groups were not significantly different. These techniques are invasive, technically complex, and very labor intensive. At present, they do not appear to offer any added advantage, and their routine use in the clinical management of acute lung injury is not recommended.

15. Is survival in ARDS improved when patients receive PCV with limited peak airway pressures?

In a recent study by Amato and coworkers of 28 patients with early ARDS, the survival of 15 patients randomized into pressure targeted ventilation with permissive hypercapnia (VT less than 6 ml per kg) was similar to that of the control group receiving CPPV with a VT of 12 mg per kg. However, the success rate of patients discontinued from mechanical ventilation was 87% in the group receiving pressure targeted ventilation compared with 46% in the group receiving CPPV. Although this study does not show any improvement in survival, it does suggest that a combination of new strategies (i.e., PCV and permissive hypercapnia) does enhance lung recovery and the possibility of early discontinuation from mechanical ventilation. Similar studies with a larger number of patients are needed to confirm these findings.

16. What is high-frequency ventilation?

High-frequency ventilation (HFV) encompasses three different modes of ventilation: high frequency positive-pressure ventilation (HFPPV), high frequency jet ventilation (HFJV), and high frequency oscillation (HFO). In the United States, HFJV and HFO are available for clinical use. Generally, HFV refers to a mode of ventilation using a frequency range between 300 and 3,000 cycles per minute at small tidal volumes (50–100% of dead space). HFJV uses volumes of gas under pressure connected to an injector placed within the endotracheal tube. A high-frequency control valve provides jet pulses at a set frequency and inspiratory time. Tidal volume is generated by the injected gas plus the entrained gas, and exhalation is passive. HFO, used in the pediatric population, operates with a to-and-fro application of pressure in the airway opening that is generated by a piston, membrane, or microprocessor controller. Because of rapid to-and-fro gas movement, the column of air in the proximal airways is compressed and decompressed and no net transfer of gas takes place distally. It is important to understand that in HFV, ventilation does not depend on bulk gas transport and the concepts of tidal volume and respiratory rate become less meaningful.

17. Describe some clinical uses of HFV.

HFV has the theoretical advantage of generating a lower peak airway pressure and thereby reducing the risk of barotrauma. HFO often improves gas exchange in critically ill neonates in whom conventional mechanical ventilation has failed; HFO also can successfully support neonates at high risk for barotrauma. Case reports and clinical series suggest that HFO can improve clinical outcome in neonates with respiratory distress syndrome. Unfortunately, large randomized trials of HFO in premature infants have shown an increased incidence of adverse effects without any improvement in survival. Although experience with HFV in adults has been limited, no reports to date indicate that outcome is improved with this mode of ventilation. HFJV, however, appears to have several limited potential applications. Because the mechanism of gas exchange is via non-bulk flow, HFJV may be useful in patients with large bronchopleural fistulas. HFJV is also associated with reduced thoracoabdominal motion, which allows it to be used, combined with general anesthesia, for extracorporeal lithotripsy and intrabronchial laser therapy. HFJV has also been used in upper airway surgeries because jet ventilation does not require an exhalation valve or tight-fitting endotracheal tube for adequate ventilatory support. It can also serve as an emergency mode of ventilation through a transtracheal catheter when airway access cannot be obtained in an emergency.

18. List some general strategies for difficult ventilatory problems.

Problem	Strategy
Poor oxygenation	Increase FIO_2 Increase PEEP Use inverse ratio ventilation
Hypercapnia	Observe and let body equilibrate (permissive hypercapnia) IV bicarbonate, if pH less than 7.20 Tracheal gas insufflation Extracorporeal carbon dioxide removal
High peak airway pressure	Lower tidal volume (volume cycled ventilation) Pressure targeted ventilation
Large dead space ventilation	Increase tidal volume (only when peak airway pressure permits) Allow carbon dioxide to rise (permissive hypercapnia) Tracheal gas insufflation
Dynamic hyperinflation	Decrease tidal volume Decrease respiratory rate Increase expiratory time Use bronchodilators/steroids (if indicated) Neuromuscular blockade
Bronchopleural fistula	High frequency jet ventilation (if available) Pressure targeted ventilation

BIBLIOGRAPHY

1. Amato MBP, Barbas CSV, Medeiros DM, et al: Beneficial effects of the "open lung approach" with low distending pressures in acute respiratory distress syndrome. Am J Respir Crit Care Med 152:1835–1846, 1995.
2. Bergofsky EH, Hurewitz AN: Airway insufflation: Physiologic effects on acute and chronic gas exchange in humans. Am Rev Respir Dis 140:885–890, 1989.
3. Chang HK: Mechanism of gas transport during ventilation by high frequency oscillation. J Appl Physiol 56:553–563, 1984.
4. Clark RH, Yoder BA, Sell AS: Prospective, randomized comparison of high-frequency oscillation and conventional ventilation in candidates for extracorporeal membrane oxygenation. J Pediatr 124:447–454, 1994.
5. Gattinoni L, Pesenti A, Sascheroni D, et al: Low-frequency positive-pressure ventilation with extracorporeal CO_2 removal in severe acute respiratory failure. JAMA 256:881–886, 1986.
6. Hickling KG, Walsh J, Henderson S, et al: Low mortality rate in adult respiratory distress syndrome using low-volume, pressure-limited ventilation with permissive hypercapnia: A prospective study. Crit Care Med 22:1568–1578, 1994.
7. The HIFI Study Group: High-frequency oscillatory ventilation compared with conventional mechanical ventilation in the treatment of respiratory failure in preterm infants. N Engl J Med 320:88–93, 1989.
8. The HIFO Study Group: Randomized study of high-frequency oscillatory ventilation in infants with severe respiratory distress syndrome. J Pediatr 122:609–619, 1993.
9. Jonson B, Similowski T, Levy P, et al: Expiratory flushing of airways: A method to reduce dead space ventilation. Eur Respir J 3:1202–1205, 1990.
10. Marcy TW, Marini JJ: Inverse ratio ventilation in ARDS: Rationale and implementation. Chest 100:494–504, 1991.

11. Morris AH, Wallace CJ, Menlove RL, et al: Randomized clinical trial of pressure-controlled inverse ratio ventilation and extracorporeal CO_2 removal for adult respiratory distress syndrome. Am J Respir Crit Care Med 149:295–305, 1994.
12. Sassoon CSH: Positive pressure ventilation, alternative modes. Chest 100:1421–1429, 1991.
13. Shanholtz C, Brower R: Should inverse ratio ventilation be used in adult respiratory distress syndrome? Am J Respir Crit Care Med 149:1354–1358, 1994.
14. Tuxen DV: Permissive hypercapnia. In Martin TJ (ed): The Principles and Practice of Mechanical Ventilation. New York, McGraw Hill, 1994, pp 371–392.
15. Tuxen DV: Permissive hypercapnic ventilation. Am J Respir Crit Care Med 150:870–874, 1994.

71. WEANING

Anthony M. Cosentino, M.D.

1. Define *weaning* according to Webster.

To accustom a child or young animal to food other than its mother's milk; to free from a habit or attitude.

2. Define *weaning* as the term applies to critically ill patients undergoing mechanical ventilation.

Process of preparing for and eventually carrying out the removal of external ventilatory support.

3. Do the majority of ventilator patients require a gradual progressive decrease in ventilatory support before mechanical ventilation can be terminated?

No. At least 75% of all ventilated patients are ready to be extubated after a brief trial of spontaneous ventilation without a prolonged period of gradually diminishing ventilatory support.

4. What is the rationale proposed for a gradual decrease in ventilatory support and how well documented is this belief?

Proponents of weaning believe that a period of respiratory muscle reconditioning is required. There is no good clinical or experimental data to justify this belief.

5. Is intermittent mandatory ventilation with diminishing pressure support superior to assist-control ventilation with intermittent trials of unassisted spontaneous breathing for weaning patients from mechanical ventilation?

A recent investigation performed by the Spanish Lung Failure Collaborative Group concluded that assist-control ventilation with brief (up to 2 hours), once daily periods of unassisted breathing (T tube trials) was superior to intermittent mandatory ventilation (IMV) and IMV with pressure support as a means for discontinuing ventilator support. A study by Brochard and coworkers is the only report to conclude that IMV with pressure support is a superior weaning mode. This study, however, has been criticized because the prolonged T tube trials that were used may have resulted in patient fatigue.

6. List indices that have been used to predict the outcome of weaning trials.

Vital capacity	Dynamic compliance
Tidal volume	Static compliance
Minute ventilation	Respiratory frequency and Pao_2:Fio_2 ratio,
Dead space ratios	frequency to tidal volume ratio,
Maximum inspiratory pressure ($P_i$max)	gastric intramural pH

7. Which weaning index is generally regarded as having the best negative *and* positive predictive value?

Yang and Tobin demonstrated that simple is best. The f:VT ratio was the best predictor of successful weaning and $P_i$max and f:VT ratios were the best predictors of failure. Furthermore, a value of 100 is easy to remember, which is fortunate because that is the magic ratio for f:VT that predicts weaning success or failure. A value above 100 predicts failure, and a value below 100 predicts success.

8. How early in a weaning trial is rapid, shallow breathing detected in subjects who are not ready to be weaned?

Almost immediately. Consequently, T tube trials or equivalent methods of unassisted spontaneous breathing may be extremely brief (e.g., 30 minutes) and almost certainly should not exceed 2 hours.

9. In evaluation of weaning circuitry (e.g., IMV, T tube, and continuous positive air pressure), what is the major difference between work of breathing and time-pressure product?

Work of breathing is the product of pressure times volume, which is the correlate of force times distance. Work is not accomplished until the ventilator valve is opened and air flows. The patient's effort to trigger the ventilator system is not included in the work formula. The time-pressure product, on the contrary, includes muscular effort to initiate air flow.

10. How does the time-pressure product compare in the following modes: IMV with pressure support, T tube breathing, and continuous positive airway pressure with 5 cm H_2O of pressure with continuous flow?

A recent study demonstrated that continuous positive airway pressure (CPAP) with continuous flow required slightly less effort (lower time-pressure product) than T tube breathing, and both of these modes required significantly less effort than pressure support. In the CPAP mode, the ventilator valve is always open and requires no triggering effort. All of the subjects in this study, regardless of the mode of weaning, were successfully extubated.

11. Why is the time-pressure product less in the CPAP 5 cm H_2O with continuous flow mode compare with the T tube mode of breathing?

CPAP for all practical purposes does not provide an inspiratory assist because inspiratory pressure does not rise above end-expiratory pressure. CPAP reduces the effort required to initiate air flow only if the subject has a certain amount of intrinsic or auto-PEEP. In this setting, alveolar pressure remains above atmospheric pressure at end expiration and inspiratory air will not flow until alveolar pressure is less than mouth pressure. The application of CPAP increases mouth pressure, thereby compensating for auto-PEEP and promoting inspiratory air flow.

12. Subjects in left ventricular failure often are difficult to wean. Why might the weaning process per se aggravate heart failure? (Hint: What is the effect of spontaneous breathing on left ventricular performance?)

Spontaneous breathing is associated with a decrease in intrapleural pressure (P_{PL}) and thus creates an increase in left ventricular (LV) afterload. Left ventricular afterload equals LV transmural pressure ([Aortic root pressure − intrapleural pressure] × radius ÷ 2 h, where h = wall thickness). Associated with this increase in afterload, pulmonary capillary occlusion pressure rises and favors the formation of pulmonary edema. The effects of P_{PL} on preload in spontaneously breathing patients are negligible because patients in heart failure are maximally preloaded. Positive-pressure breathing has the opposite effect in increasing P_{PL} and decreasing LV afterload. The withdrawal of positive-pressure ventilation during weaning in patients with LV dysfunction, therefore, may increase LV afterload, raise the pulmonary capillary occlusion pressure, and promote pulmonary edema.

13. Define *fledging***.**

To raise a young bird until it is able to fly. I submit that most patients are "fledged" and not weaned from mechanical ventilation.

BIBLIOGRAPHY

1. Brochard L, Rauss A, Benito S, et al: Comparison of three methods of gradual withdrawal from ventilatory support during weaning from mechanical ventilation. Am J Respir Crit Care Med 150:896–903, 1994.
2. Esteban A, Frutos F, Tobin MJ: A comparison of four methods of weaning patients from mechanical ventilation. N Engl J Med 332:345–350, 1995.
3. Lemaire F, Teboul JL, Cinotti L, et al: Acute left ventricular dysfunction during unsuccessful weaning from mechanical ventilation. Anesthesiology 69:171–179, 1988.
4. Marini JJ: Weaning from mechanical ventilation. 138:1043–1046, 1988.
5. Mohsenifar Z, Hay A, Hay J, et al: Gastric intramural pH as a predictor of success or failure in weaning patients from mechanical ventilation. Ann Intern Med 119:794–798, 1993.
6. Permutt S: Circulatory effects of weaning from mechanical ventilation: The importance of transdiaphragmatic pressure. Anesthesiology 69:157–160, 1988 (Editorial).
7. Sassoon CS, Light RW, Lodia R, et al: Pressure-time product during CPAP, PSV and T piece during weaning from mechanical ventilation. Am Rev Respir Dis 143:469–475, 1991.
8. Smith TC, Marini JJ: Impact of PEEP on lung mechanics and work of breathing in severe airflow obstruction. J Appl Phys 65:1488–1499, 1988.
9. Tobin MJ, Perez W, Guenther SM, et al: The pattern of breathing during successful and unsuccessful trials of weaning from mechanical ventilation. Am Rev Respir Dis 134:1111–1118, 1986.
10. Weinberger SE, Weiss JW: Weaning from ventilatory support. N Engl J Med 332:388–389, 1995 (Editorial).
11. Yang KL, Tobin MJ: A prospective study of indexes predicting the outcome of trials of weaning from mechanical ventilation. N Engl J Med 324:1445–1450, 1991.

72. CHRONIC VENTILATORY SUPPORT

Enrique Fernandez, M.D., and Mary Gilmartin, B.S.N., R.R.T.

1. Define chronic ventilatory support.

Chronic ventilatory support is long-term mechanical ventilation in a patient who has recovered from acute respiratory failure and does not require care in an ICU. Requirements for diagnostic, therapeutic, or close monitoring are minimal and noninvasive.

The introduction of portable and compact ventilators along with advances in general respiratory care, rehabilitation, and homecare services have made chronic ventilatory support available in the patient's home with a subsequent decrease in costs and improvement in the patient's quality of life.

2. What are the goals of chronic ventilatory support?

According to the guidelines for long-term mechanical ventilation published by a task force of the American College of Chest Physicians, the goals of chronic ventilatory support, either in the home or elsewhere, must include the following:

Extend life	Reduce morbidity
Enhance the quality of life	Improve physical and physiologic
Provide an environment that will	function
enhance individual potential	Be cost effective

3. How many patients in the United States require chronic ventilatory support?

The actual number of ventilator-assisted individuals in the United States is unknown. However, insight into the dimensions of the problem are provided by a survey study performed in

Minnesota in the years 1986 and 1992. In 1986 there were 103 patients undergoing long-term ventilatory support in Minnesota. By 1992, the number of ventilated patients had increased to 216, of whom 65% were ventilated at home and 35% in long-term care facilities. Extrapolating these findings to the United States as a whole estimates that there were 5,777 patients undergoing long-term ventilatory support in 1986 and 12,279 in 1992. These estimations are probably imprecise, however, because utilization of resources and technology differ in different regions of the country. As of 1992, no registry existed to track this information.

4. Are there economic benefits to placing chronically ventilated patients in a homecare setting?

A 1992 economic analysis done for Bach and coworkers demonstrated a significant cost advantage of homecare for patients without a tracheostomy who did not need tracheal suctioning by a licensed nurse compared with care provided in long-term care units in the community. The reimbursement for a patient in a community long-term unit was $719 per day, whereas the estimated cost of daily care for chronically ventilated patients in a homecare setting was $213. The cost of care for patients who require tracheal suctioning may be as much as $64,000 a month in 1986 dollars if admission to an ICU is required. The economic advantages of placement of chronically ventilated patients in a homecare setting have been supported in many other published articles through the years.

5. When is long-term mechanical ventilation used for life support?

When the lungs of a patient are incapable of sustaining normal gas exchange, long-term mechanical ventilation constitutes a life support system. Most patients on long-term life support ventilation have survived an episode of acute respiratory failure but have failed repeated attempts at weaning. The acute respiratory failure is usually caused by a severe illness such as a pneumonia or a postoperative complication that compromises the respiratory system. Other patients may have experienced an acute illness superimposed on a chronic respiratory disorder. Another group of patients requiring continuous life support are those who do not have adequate spontaneous breathing effort because of central alveolar hypoventilation, spinal cord injuries, intracranial hemorrhage, or stroke. A last group of patients have disorders causing progressive chronic respiratory failure that requires repeated admissions to an ICU or that severely limits their functional status. Examples of such patients include those with kyphoscoliosis, sequelae of old tuberculosis, COPD, or progressive neuromuscular disorders.

6. Which patients are the best candidates for long-term mechanical ventilation used as life support?

Some diagnostic conditions are more suitable than others for the application of long-term mechanical ventilation. Patients with these diagnoses can achieve an improved quality of life, greater medical stability, and longer survival.

In general, a good candidate for long-term mechanical ventilation is young and otherwise healthy except for an isolated disorder of the respiratory system that limits ventilation. Patients with slowly progressive or stable disorders and patients with sequelae of poliomyelitis or traumatic high cervical spinal cord injury are also good candidates for long-term ventilatory support. Because not all neuromuscular disorders progress slowly, the decision to ventilate must be individualized and discussed at length with each patient in a timely manner.

Controversy exists regarding the use of long-term ventilation for patients with primary pulmonary diseases. Management of patients with COPD, for example, is complicated by advanced age, cor pulmonale, severe and often unrelenting dyspnea, and rapid fluctuations in airflow obstruction with resultant hypercapnia and hypoxemia. Chronic ventilatory support for these patients should be carefully evaluated, and patients should be fully aware of the potential benefits and disadvantages of long-term mechanical ventilation. Patients with cystic fibrosis are also considered poor candidates for chronic ventilatory support, because they have copious secretions and frequent infections. Noninvasive positive-pressure ventilation, however, has been used in patients with cystic fibrosis who are awaiting lung transplantation. Patients with pulmonary fibrosis undergoing mechanical ventilation may still experience dyspnea and increased work of breathing even when arterial blood gases are maintained at an acceptable level with the administration of high concentrations of inspired oxygen and high inflating pressures.

The presence of comorbid medical conditions such as cardiac disease, complex medical conditions, psychiatric disorders, cancer, or terminal diseases make long-term mechanical ventilation less feasible. Some patients with active coexisting conditions may require the creation of a hospital ICU environment in the home to achieve chronic ventilatory support, which is not compatible with the goals of home ventilator care.

Suitability of Patients for Long-Term Mechanical Ventilation Related to Underlying Diagnosis

SITE OR TYPE OF DEFECT	FAVORABLE DIAGNOSIS	UNFAVORABLE DIAGNOSIS
Ventilatory drive	Central hypoventilation syndrome Ondine's curse Arnold-Chiari malformation	Cardiovascular accident (stroke) Malignancy
Neural transmissions to the ventilatory muscle	High cervical spinal cord injury Poliomyelitis Guillain-Barré syndrome Bilateral phrenic paralysis	Amyotrophic lateral sclerosis Multiple sclerosis
Ventilatory muscles	Muscular dystrophy Congenital myopathies	
Bony thorax	Kyphoscoliosis After thoracoplasty	
Lung and airways	Bronchopulmonary dysphasia	COPD Bronchiectasis Cystic fibrosis Interstitial lung disease Adult respiratory distress syndrome

From Pierson DJ: Kalmarek RM: Home ventilator care. In Casaburi R, Petty TL: Principles and Practice of Pulmonary Rehabilitation. Philadelphia, W.B. Saunders, 1993; with permission.

7. List the important criteria for success of chronic ventilator support at home.

For optimal long-term ventilation at home, the patient should be clinically and physiologically stable for several weeks before hospital discharge and emotionally stable. The following conditions should be met:

Major organ systems stable
Dyspnea controlled or absent
No acute infections
Acid-base and metabolic stability
Stable ventilatory settings (e.g., ventilatory mode, tidal volume, ventilatory rate)
FIO_2 of 0.40 or less
Arterial blood gas levels acceptable
Minimal fluctuations in airway resistance and compliance
Peak pressure varies ± 5 cm H_2O or less
Positive end-expiratory pressure of 10 cm H_2O or less
Adequate nutrition
Ability to clear secretions and protect the airways
A tracheostomy is placed if an artificial airway is necessary
Management at home expected to be stable, without the need for readmission within at least 1 month
Patient is not managed with intermittent mandatory ventilation

8. What is the expected outcome of patients undergoing chronic ventilatory support?

Reported series indicates that patients with neuromuscular diseases and skeletal conditions experience a better outcome from long-term mechanical ventilation than patients with chronic primary pulmonary diseases. Robert and coworkers reported their experience in 222 patients who were mechanically ventilated at home 11 to 17 hours per day for a variety of conditions associated with chronic ventilatory failure, using tracheostomy and positive-pressure ventilation. Some patients were followed for up to 20 years. The results were excellent both for length of survival as well as day-to-day morbidity (need for recurrent hospitalization, ability to leave home on regular basis, other aspects of quality of life) for all of the patients with chest wall problems (neurologic, muscular, or restrictive syndrome due to chest deformity). Patients with sequelae of poliomyelitis had the best 5- and 10-year survival rates. The results were not as favorable for patients with intrinsic pulmonary conditions, such as chronic airflow limitation.

In a recent multicenter study, Muir and coworkers reviewed prognostic factors and long-term survival associated with chronic mechanical ventilation, via tracheostomy with positive-pressure ventilation, at home in 259 patients with advanced COPD. The survival rate for the overall study population was 70% at 2 years, 44% at 5 years, and 20% at 10 years. These results are better than those observed in other published series and compare favorably with the prognosis of nonventilated COPD patients managed with long-term oxygen therapy. Age less than 65 years, use of an uncuffed cannula, and a PaO_2 of more than 55 mmHg on room air during the 3 months after tracheostomy were the variables that most closely correlated with survival for more than 5 years.

Reported Survival of 222 Patients with Various Respiratory Diseases Undergoing Long-Term Ventilation

	NUMBER	SURVIVAL	
		5 YEARS	10 YEARS
Post-polio	41	95%	87%
Kyphoscoliosis	53	77%	55%
Tuberculosis	55	70%	36%
Myopathy	15	62%	
COPD	50	18%	
Bronchiectasis	10	0%	

From Robert D, Gerard M, Leger P, et al: Domiciliary mechanical ventilation by tracheostomy for chronic respiratory failure. Rev Mal Respir 11:923–936, 1983; with permission.

9. How does ventilatory muscle fatigue contribute to chronic respiratory failure?

Muscle fatigue is a condition in which there is a loss in the capacity for developing force, the velocity of muscle contraction, or both, resulting from muscle activity under load, which is reversible by rest. Progressive muscle fatigue is an important contributor to the development of respiratory failure. The load imposed on respiratory muscles by any chronic respiratory disease frequently worsens with time and increases the work of breathing. Consequently, a higher proportion of the maximal force that the respiratory muscles can develop is required for each breath. When the ventilatory load can no longer be supported, chronic respiratory muscle fatigue develops followed by hypercapnic respiratory failure.

10. How are patients with ventilatory muscle fatigue best managed?

Regardless of the mechanism of fatigue, rest is the best treatment. It allows the ventilatory muscles to recover from the fatigue, which subsequently improves their contractile force and endurance. Rest interrupts the vicious circle of progressive and continuous blood gas deterioration, which further worsens respiratory muscle performance.

Clinical signs of ventilatory muscle fatigue can be reduced or eliminated after a period of controlled ventilation, which rests ventilatory muscles. Rochester, Braun, and Laine were the first to show that negative-pressure respiratory support reduces or abolishes the electrical activity of the respiratory muscles, which affords rest and relieves dyspnea. Prolonged daily intermittent use of negative- or positive-pressure ventilation reverses fatigue, contributes to stabilization of the clinical course, restores sleep, prevents recurrent episodes of hypercapnic respiratory failure, and increases daily function and even employability of patients with hypercapnic respiratory failure of various causes. Thus, there is considerable interest in selectively resting the ventilatory muscles for several hours each day in an effort to improve ventilatory function between periods of rest. This mode of ventilation is termed *elective intermittent ventilation.*

11. List the criteria for elective (noninvasive) intermittent negative- or positive-pressure ventilation in chronic respiratory failure.

Clinical criteria
- Slowly progressive, irreversible respiratory failure caused by neuromuscular diseases,* thoracic wall deformities, COPD†
- Frequent readmission to hospital for respiratory failure
- Deterioration after successful weaning
- Obstructive sleep apnea
- Obesity hypoventilation, idiopathic hypoventilation
- Dyspnea, increasing tachypnea, paradoxical or dysynchronous breathing
- Cor pulmonale despite conventional treatment
- Motivated and cooperative patient with intact upper airway function and minimal secretions

* In amyotrophic lateral sclerosis, bulbar function should be intact.
† If continuous positive airway pressure (CPAP) alone fails. Efficacy still controversial.

Pulmonary function criteria
- VC   < 25% predicted
- FEV_1 < 25% predicted   < 900 ml in males
                                       < 600 ml in females
- MVV   < 25% predicted   < 40 L/minute, males
                                       < 25 L/minute, females
- PI_{Max} < –50 cm H_2O
              < –25 cm H_2O neuromuscular diseases
- PE_{Max} < 40 cm H_2O
- $Paco_2$ < 45 mmHg or increases with oxygen use

Modified from Braun NMT: Intermittent mechanical ventilation. Clin Chest Med 9:153–162, 1988.

12. What are the goals for intermittent elective mechanical ventilation?
- To preserve or increase the functional capacity for daily living activities
- To prevent deterioration of function
- To decrease the rate of clinical deterioration
- To avoid acute respiratory failure

13. How is elective long-term mechanical ventilation delivered?
Initially, elective long-term mechanical ventilation is delivered noninvasively. Many patients with progressive disorders eventually require a tracheostomy, which is usually performed when respiratory failure has progressed to the point at which ventilatory assistance is needed for more than 16 hours daily.

14. Which patients should be offered elective intermittent long-term mechanical ventilation?
The best candidates for elective, intermittent mechanical ventilation are patients with slowly progressive respiratory failure who are otherwise not seriously ill. The ideal patient is

able to initiate and terminate the periods of ventilator assistance himself or herself, relieving family members of the responsibility for continuous ongoing care. In most cases, the period of assistance is timed to coincide with or include the patient's hours of sleep. As in the case of chronic mechanical ventilation provided for life support, patients with primary lung disease (e.g., COPD, cystic fibrosis) are less suitable candidates, although recent studies indicate better results than previously observed, especially in patients with chronic airflow limitation.

15. Which patients benefit most from elective long-term mechanical ventilation?

In 1989, Leger and coworkers demonstrated that intermittent positive-pressure ventilation via a nasal mask improved resting blood gas results during spontaneous breathing 1 year later in a group of patients with neuromuscular disorders, kyphoscoliosis, and old tuberculosis. Indices of quality of sleep and quality of life were similarly improved. In 1994 the same group reported the experience with intermittent positive-pressure ventilation in patients with kyphoscoliosis, posttuberculosis sequelae, Duchenne muscular dystrophy, COPD, and bronchiectasis followed for 2 to 3 years. Patients with kyphoscoliosis and posttuberculosis sequelae had the most favorable outcome, as determined by improved values for PaO_2 and $PaCO_2$ and reduction in days of hospitalization for respiratory illnesses. Patients with Duchenne muscular dystrophy also had fewer days of hospitalization during use of nasal intermittent positive-pressure ventilation, but only 56% of patients continued using ventilatory support for the duration of follow-up. Benefit was more short term for patients with COPD and bronchiectasis.

16. Does intermittent elective noninvasive ventilation play a role in the management of patients with COPD?

The efficacy of intermittent elective noninvasive ventilation in severe stable COPD is controversial. Braun and Marino reported benefits in 16 patients with COPD who were ventilated 5 hours daily over a 5-month period using negative-pressure ventilation with a poncho wrap device. Other investigators have shown that elective ventilation does not need to be given daily to achieve persistent improvement in blood gas levels, quality of life parameters, hospitalization rate, inspiratory muscle strength, and endurance. Still other studies have not showed improvement in any parameter being measured. In a study sponsored by the NIH, 184 patients with stable severe COPD were randomized to use of a poncho wrap or a sham ventilator in a 12-week trial. Only 29% of ventilated patients achieved the study objective of 50% suppression of the diaphragmatic electromyographic signal during ventilator use; no improvement in exercise tolerance, arterial blood gas values, respiratory muscle strength, dyspnea index, or quality of life was shown.

Subgroups of patients with COPD, however, may benefit from elective intermittent mechanical ventilation. Existing data suggest that patients with severe hypercapnia and those with severe nocturnal gas exchange abnormalities be considered for a therapeutic trial.

17. What are the complications of intermittent mechanical ventilation with nasal mask?

Complication	% of Treated Patients
Mouth dryness	58
Nasal dryness	50
Gastric distension	50
Belching-increased flatulence	24
Nasal congestion	24
Eye irritation	24
Gum pain	20
Soreness in the bridge of the nose	19
Epistaxis	9

18. What is the mechanism of action of long-term intermittent mechanical ventilation?

The mechanism by which patients receiving elective intermittent mechanical support for as little as 4–6 hours a day experience sustained improvement in daytime gas exchange, respiratory symptoms, and variables of respiratory muscle function remains unknown and controversial.

Three potential mechanisms have been suggested:

- Improvement of respiratory center sensitivity to carbon dioxide. Patients with chronic progressive ventilatory failure have a gradual progression of nocturnal hypoventilation that blunts the respiratory center response to increasing levels of carbon dioxide. Improved ventilation at night may reset the respiratory center sensitivity to carbon dioxide, resulting in daytime improvement in gas exchange.
- Intermittent mechanical ventilation may increase lung compliance by increasing vital capacity and thereby improving gas exchange without enhancing respiratory muscle strength. In some patients, however, daytime gas exchange improves even though vital capacity remains unchanged.
- If chronic respiratory failure is associated with chronic respiratory muscle fatigue, resting the respiratory muscle via intermittent ventilatory assistance may restore their function and improve daytime gas exchange.

19. Does intermittent ventilation unload respiratory muscles and eliminate respiratory muscle fatigue?

Intermittent mechanical ventilation unloads respiratory muscles as demonstrated by a reduction of integrated diaphragmatic electrical activity and an improved pressure-time index. Not all studies, however, have demonstrated that respiratory muscles are rested or respiratory muscle strength and endurance are improved.

Belman and coworkers recently compared intermittent positive-pressure ventilation (PPV) with intermittent negative-pressure ventilation (NPV) in providing respiratory muscle rest. Integrated electromyograms, transdiaphragmatic pressure, pressure-time integral, and average coeffficient of variation in the tidal volume were consistently lower during PPV compared with NPV. Positive-pressure ventilation, therefore, is more effective than negative-pressure ventilation in reducing diaphragmatic electrical activity. It appears that to unload respiratory muscles is to rest respiratory muscles.

20. What has been the traditional technique for long-term positive-pressure ventilation?

Positive-pressure ventilation via a tracheostomy has been the standard approach in this country to chronic ventilatory support. A tracheostomy provides a secure airway and ready access to the lower airway for removal of secretions. Recently, however, noninvasive long-term ventilation has supplanted tracheostomy in many clinical settings.

21. Describe the major methods for negative-pressure noninvasive ventilation.

Several methods are available for providing patients with noninvasive ventilation. Negative intermittent pressure ventilation encloses the whole body or thoracic cage in a rigid container that generates cyclic negative pressure and promotes inspiratory airflow. Available devices include the iron lung, which is more efficient than a cuirass, which is a plastic shell that encloses only the thorax and upper portions of the abdomen. A jacketed suit or poncho is a nylon garment worn over a rigid shell that is closed by straps around the neck, wrists, and legs and generates intermittent negative pressure. Negative-pressure ventilators are control rather than assist devices, making coordination between patient and ventilator difficult.

Musculoskeletal back and shoulder pain are the main side effects of negative-pressure ventilation. Air leaks are common, especially around the neck. The generation of obstructive apneas and oxygen desaturation during sleep is a major limitation of these devices. This complication occurs commonly in patients with COPD. Patients with neurologic or neuromuscular disorders are most amenable to this form of ventilation.

22. What is a pneumobelt?

A pneumobelt is a cloth corset with an inflatable rubber bladder. The bladder is fitted over the patient's abdomen and inflated intermittently, exerting a positive pressure that forces abdominal contents inward, displacing the diaphragm upward and assisting exhalation. Tidal volume is proportional to the pressure applied to the abdomen, usually 30–50 cm H_2O; any positive-pressure generator capable of producing more than 50 cm H_2O and delivering a 2.0-L volume may be used to power the pneumobelt.

Because the downward motion of the diaphragm relies mainly on gravity, the pneumobelt functions effectively only when the patient is sitting or standing at an angle of approximately 30° or more. Optimal function occurs at 75°, which limits the use of this device during sleep. With a proper fit, the patient's functional residual capacity is reduced, tidal volume increased, and work of breathing decreased. Tidal volumes of 300–500 ml are attainable.

23. What is a rocking bed?

A rocking bed functions by moving the patient in a vertical axis over an arc of 40–45°, using the force of gravity upon the abdomen to effect diaphragmatic motion. When the head of the bed rocks downward approximately 15°, gravity pulls the patient's abdomen and diaphragm toward the head, assisting exhalation. Rocking upright approximately 30° moves the diaphragm caudally, assisting inhalation. A tidal volume of 250–400 ml can be generated with this motion. The rate of tilt may be adjusted to 8–34 per minute. This device is best for patients who have diaphragmatic paralysis or weakness and also some accessory muscle use but who do not have primary pulmonary disease. Its bulkiness, lack of portability, and relative inefficiency limit its application. Both the rocking bed and the pneumobelt function as controllers and may not be tolerated by anxious patients who frequently desire to change their ventilatory rate. They also function poorly in excessively obese patients and those with severe kyphoscoliosis.

24. Can positive-pressure ventilation be delivered through a mouthpiece?

Positive-pressure ventilation has been successfully delivered through a mouthpiece (non-sealed during the day, sealed at night), particularly in postpoliomyelitis patients.

25. Can a nasal mask provide adequate positive-pressure ventilation?

Intermittent positive-pressure ventilation administered via a nasal mask can markedly improve nocturnal oxygen saturation in some patients. Nasal positive-pressure ventilation, used mainly for elective ventilatory assistance, is successful in the majority of patients. All commercially available positive-pressure ventilators may be used through a nasal mask. To be successful, patients must tolerate a nasal mask strapped to the face for 6–8 hours daily. Optimal settings call for assist-control back-up rates set high enough to eliminate the patient's need to trigger the ventilator, allowing complete respiratory muscle rest. This set-up results in mild hyperventilation and a decrease in ventilatory drive. It also requires the mask to be close-fitting and strapped to the face, because air leaks are the principal problem. Other problems are discomfort and pressure sores over the bridge of the nose. Nightly application requires no more than a few minutes of time on the part of the patient or one attendant.

26. What is continuous positive airway pressure ?

Continuous positive airway pressure (CPAP) applied through a nasal mask has been the main treatment of obstructive sleep apnea. Positive pressure in the upper airways prevents pharyngeal collapse and increases functional residual capacity (FRC). The aim is to prevent or abolish apnea or snoring at every sleep stage and in every body position. The treatment has proved effective in relieving symptoms, reducing mortality, and reducing cardiovascular complications associated with the disease. The main side effects are rhinitis and mucosal dryness, which are usually reversed by the addition of a humidifier. Skin irritation or abrasions from the facial mask, conjunctivitis due to mask leakage, and aerophagia are other frequent side effects.

27. What is bilevel positive airway pressure?

Bilevel positive airway pressure (BiPAP) ventilators cycle between two levels of positive airway pressure. The higher level assists ventilation during inspiration (IPAP) and the lower level maintains airway patency during expiration (EPAP); the latter is effectively a positive end-expiratory pressure (PEEP). The cycle is initiated through a flow trigger to a preset pressure able to increase the spontaneous tidal volume (VT) of patients commensurate with their effort.

Termination of inspiration is triggered by low inspiratory flow (approximately 30% of the maximum flow) or by time sequence. Because they maintain high air flow to sustain mask pressure, these pressure-limited ventilators may compensate for mask leaks better than volume ventilators. The ventilator can be set in control mode, in assist mode, or in an intermittent mandatory position, and applied both via tracheostomy and nasal mask.

The two main problems with BiPAP are the absence of alarms, which make them dangerous in patients who depend completely on mechanical ventilatory support, and mucosal dryness, especially when the patient keeps the mouth open while receiving substantial air through the nose. The efficacy of BiPAP is doubtful in patients with poor compliance of the thoracic cage.

28. What patient characteristics predict success in home ventilator care?

Patient Characteristics that may Predict Success in Home Ventilator Care

CHARACTERISTIC	IDEAL	ACCEPTABLE	UNACCEPTABLE
Individual coping style	Optimistic Motivated Resourceful Flexible Adaptable Sense of humor Directive	Optimistic Motivated Sense of humor	None
Support systems	Close family and social supports	Social supports	Lack of family and social supports
Education	College degree Ability to learn	Ability to learn Mechanically astute	Altered mental status Unable to learn
Financial resources	Adequate personal assets Optimal health insurance	Adequate health insurance	Lack of personal assets Lack of health insurance
Medical condition	Stable neuromuscular disease Adequate free time off ventilator No other illnesses	Stable neuromuscular or obstructive disease Limited or no time off ventilator	Unable to care for self or direct others
Self-care ability	Able to provide self-care and/or direct others	Able to provide self-care	Unable to care for self or direct others

From Gilmartin M: Long-term mechanical ventilation. Patient selection and discharge planning. Other mediators of success. Respir Care 36:205–216, 1991; with permission;

29. What other factors are predictors of success with home ventilation?

There are several other predictors of successful outcome of home ventilation care in addition to the patient's characteristics. These predictors should be carefully evaluated before home mechanical ventilation is initiated.

Predictors of Success for the Ventilator-Dependent Patient at Home

Primary diagnosis	Nutritional status
Clinical and physiologic stability	Aspiration potential
Comorbidity	Team: physicians, primary caregivers,
Mode of ventilation—ventilator settings	home care providers
Age	Equipment maintenance and supply

30. What is the importance of discharge planning?

Well-coordinated discharge planning is the key for successful placement of a ventilator-dependent patient in the home; this requires a team of individuals that should include the patient and family in addition to the physician, nurse, respiratory therapist, social worker, physical therapist, occupational therapist, speech therapist, nutritionist, and psychiatric services. Make and Gilmartin describe a 6-step approach to the discharge process:

• Stabilization of the patient's medical condition
• Evaluation and development of realistic goals
• Rehabilitation planning to set the stage for training
• Rehabilitation training to increase strength and endurance
• Discharge planning to ensure success
• Home care and follow-up to decrease medical complications

The home care company and equipment should be selected and completed before discharge. Regardless of who is on the team, communication among team members is essential; they should meet on a regular basis and discuss short-term goals, progress of the patient, and family concerns. With the patient and family present, the physician should discuss specific issues regarding treatment and discharge, using language that ensures understanding.

31. What skills are needed by patient and caregivers before discharge?

Self-care techniques	Equipment maintenance
Airway management	Ventilator
Tracheotomy and stoma care	Humidifier
Cuff care	Suction machines
Tracheal suctioning	Battery and charger
Changing the tracheostomy tube	Oxygen administration
Changing the tracheostomy ties	Manual resuscitator
Chest physical therapy techniques	Troubleshooting for problems
Percussion	Cleaning and disinfection
Vibration	Emergency measures
Coughing	Ventilator failure
Medication administration	Power failure
Oral	Dislodged tracheostomy tube
Inhaled	Obstructed airway
Bed-to-chair transfers	Cuff leaks
Feeding tube care	Shortness of breath
Indwelling-catheter care	Ventilator circuit problems
Implantable IV line care	Infection
Bowel care	Falls
Switching from ventilator	Bleeding
to weaning device	Cardiac arrest

From Gilmartin M: Long-term mechanical ventilation. Patient selection and discharge planning. Other mediators of success. Respir Care 36:205–216, 1991; with permission.

32. How should patients undergoing home ventilation be monitored?

The monitoring needs of both the patient and the equipment should be defined clearly before the patient is discharged from the hospital. Physicians managing home care patients should receive frequent updates regarding the patient's status and understand the home care plan. Being the team leader the physician should regularly set realistic expectations, coordinate the patient's self-care, remind patient and family about respiratory care, and expect good communication among other members of the team. If more acute care is not needed, a patient on chronic ventilatory support should have an evaluation every 3–6 months.

Monitoring Needs of Patients Undergoing Home Ventilation

Patient monitoring
 SpO_2 intermittently
 Arterial blood gases intermittently
 Clinical status
  Vital signs
  Lung sounds
  Sputum production
 Compliance
 Airway resistance, before and after bronchodilator
 Presence of intrinsic PEEP
 $PetCO_2$ intermittently by therapist
 Spontaneous ventilatory parameters (selected patients)
  Tidal volume
  Vital capacity
  Maximum inspiratory pressure
 Tracheostomy site
 Tracheostomy cuff
  Pressure
  Volume

Equipment monitoring
 Ventilator function at routine therapist visit
 Alarm setting daily
 Alarm function daily
 Peak inspiratory pressure daily and at routine therapist visit
 Ventilator settings daily
  V_T machine delivered
  Rate
  Sensitivity
  FIO_2 monthly, at routine therapist visit
  Flow rate and inspiratory time
 Leaks in the systems
 Integrity of the circuit
 Hours of use at routine therapist visit
 Inlet filters per manufacturer's recommendations
 Bacteria filters monthly
 Accessory equipment function

From Gilmartin M: Monitoring in the home and the outpatient setting. In Monitoring in Respiratory Care. St. Louis, Mosby, 1993, pp 767–787.

BIBLIOGRAPHY

1. Adams AB, Whitman J, Marcy T: Surveys of long-term ventilatory support in Minnesota: 1986 and 1992. Chest 103:1463–1469, 1993.
2. Belman MJ, SooHoo GW, Kuli JH, et al: Efficacy of positive vs negative pressure ventilation in unloading the respiratory muscles. Chest 98:850–856, 1990.
3. Braun NMT: Intermittent mechanical ventilation. Clin Chest Med 9:153–162, 1988.
4. Donner CF, Howard P, Robert D: Patient selection and techniques for home mechanical ventilation. Monaldi Arch Chest Dis 48:40–47, 1993.

5. Ellis ER, Bye PTP, Bruderer JW, et al: Treatment of respiratory failure during sleep in patients with neuromuscular disease. Am Rev Respir Dis 135:148–152, 1987.
6. Gilmartin M: Transitions from the intensive care clinic to home: Patient selection and discharge planning. Respir Care 39:456–480, 1994.
7. Goldstein RS, DeRosie JA, Avendana MA, et al: Influence of non-invasive positive pressure ventilation in respiratory muscles. Chest 99:408–415, 1991.
8. Leger P, Bedicam JM, Cornette A, et al: Nasal intermittent positive pressure ventilation. Long-term follow-up in patients with severe chronic respiratory insufficiency. Chest 105:100–105, 1994.
9. Meyer TJ, Hill NS: Non-invasive positive pressure ventilation to treat respiratory failure. Ann Intern Med 120:760–770, 1994.
10. Muir JF, Girault C, Cardinaud JP, et al: Survival and long-term follow-up of tracheostomized patients with COPD treated by home mechanical ventilation. A multicenter French study in 259 patents. Chest 106:201–209, 1994.
11. Pierson DF, Kalmarek RM: Home ventilator care. In Casabari R, Petty TL: Principles and Practice of Pulmonary Rehabilitation. Philadelphia, W.B. Saunders, 1993.
12. Piper AJ, Parker S, Torzillo PJ, et al: Nocturnal nasal IPPV stabilizes patients with cystic fibrosis and hypercapnic respiratory failure. Chest 102:346–350, 1992.
13. Robert D, Gerard M, Leger P, et al: Domiciliary mechanical ventilation by tracheostomy for chronic respiratory failure. Rev Mal Respir 11:923–936, 1983.
14. Rochester DR, Braun NMT, Laine S: Diaphragmatic energy expenditure in chronic respiratory failure: The effect of assisted ventilation with body respirators. Am J Med 63:223–232, 1977.
15. Renston JP, DiMarco AF, Supinski GS: Respiratory muscle rest using nasal BiPAP ventilation in patients with stable severe COPD. Chest 105:1053–1060, 1994.
16. Unterborn JN, Hill NS: Options for mechanical ventilation in neuromuscular diseases. Clin Chest Med 15:765–781, 1994.

XV. Pleural Disorders

73. PLEURAL EFFUSIONS

Steven A. Sahn, M.D.

1. What are the mechanisms responsible for the clinical accumulation of pleural fluid?

Pleural effusions accumulate when production of fluid exceeds absorption of fluid from the pleural space. Mechanisms responsible are:

An increase in hydrostatic pressure in the microvascular circulation (congestive heart failure)

A decrease in oncotic pressure in the microvascular circulation (hypoalbuminemia)

A decrease in pressure in the pleural space (atelectasis)

Increased permeability of the microvascular circulation (pneumonia)

Impaired lymphatic drainage from the pleural space (malignancy)

Movement of fluid from the abdomen into the pleural space (cirrhosis)

2. What is the indication for diagnostic thoracentesis?

Diagnostic thoracentesis is performed when a pleural effusion of unknown cause is present. Unless the diagnosis is clinically secure, such as in a patient with classic congestive heart failure with no atypical features, a thoracentesis should be done to definitively or presumptively establish the cause of the effusion.

3. Are there are absolute contraindications to thoracentesis?

No. If clinical judgment dictates that the information gained from pleural fluid analysis may help in diagnosis and therapy, thoracentesis should be done.

4. What are the relative contraindications to thoracentesis?

A bleeding diathesis, anticoagulation therapy, a small amount of pleural fluid, and mechanical ventilation are relative contraindications.

5. Is the patient on mechanical ventilation at increased risk for pneumothorax with thoracentesis?

The patient is probably not at increased risk of a pneumothorax but is at greater risk for developing a tension pneumothorax if the lung is punctured.

6. What are the complications of diagnostic thoracentesis?

Pneumothorax is the most common clinically important complication. Other complications include pain at the needle insertion site, bleeding (local, intrapleural, or intra-abdominal), empyema, and spleen or liver puncture.

7. What are the complications of therapeutic thoracentesis?

Complications of therapeutic thoracentesis are the same as those of diagnostic thoracentesis; however, three other complications are unique to therapeutic thoracentesis: hypoxemia, unilateral pulmonary edema, and hypovolemia. Hypoxemia, which may occur despite relief of dyspnea, results from worsening of ventilation-perfusion relationships in the ipsilateral lung or from clinically occult unilateral pulmonary edema. Patients with an endobronchial obstruction or trapped lung may develop a precipitous drop in intrapleural pressure when fluid is removed, thus increasing the likelihood of unilateral pulmonary edema.

8. Which patients are most likely to develop unilateral pulmonary edema after thoracentesis?

Patients with a mainstem endobronchial lesion causing atelectasis and patients with a trapped lung from malignancy or previous pleural space infection are at risk. When fluid is removed from the pleural space, pleural pressure drops precipitiously, increasing the pressure gradient across alveolar capillary vessels and promoting pulmonary edema. The chest radiograph in these patients shows a large pleural effusion without contralateral mediastinal shift and suggests an increased risk of developing pulmonary edema.

9. What criteria are used to classify transudates and exudates?

If any one of the following three criteria is present, the fluid is almost always an exudate:
• Pleural fluid total protein:serum total protein ratio more than 0.5
• Pleural fluid lactate dehydrogenase (LDH):serum LDH ratio more than 0.6
• Absolute serum LDH value more than two-thirds of the upper limit of normal
If none of the three criteria are present, the fluid is almost always a transudate.

10. Why is it important to distinguish transudates from exudates?

Establishing the presence of a transudate limits the diagnostic possibilities, which are usually discernible from the clinical presentation. Transudates are caused by imbalances in hydrostatic and oncotic pressures, including congestive heart failure, hepatic hydrothorax, nephrotic syndrome, peritoneal dialysis, and hypoalbuminemia. The differential diagnosis of exudates is more extensive and at times problematic for the clinician.

11. Describe the typical chest radiograph of a patient with pleural effusions from congestive heart failure.

The chest radiograph shows cardiomegaly, bilateral pleural effusions (more copious on the right than on the left), evidence of interstitial or alveolar edema, and sometimes the presence of Kerley B lines.

12. Do all patients with hepatic hydrothorax have clinical ascites?

The majority of patients with hepatic hydrothorax have clinical ascites, but a number of patients have been reported with large hepatic hydrothoraces in the absence of clinical ascites. In this situation, all the ascitic fluid that is produced is immediately mobilized into the chest through a large diaphragmatic defect.

13. What is the best therapeutic option for the patient with a symptomatic hepatic hydrothorax refractory to maximal medical therapy?

Thoracoscopic repair of the diaphragmatic defect followed by pleural abrasion and talc pleurodesis.

14. What diagnosis is suggested by the presence of a unilateral hemorrhagic exudative pleural effusion with blood in a patient with nephrotic syndrome?

Pulmonary embolism. Patients with nephrotic syndrome are hypercoagulable and have a 30% incidence of pulmonary embolism resulting from loss of clotting inhibitors in the urine and abnormal platelet aggregation.

15. How is the diagnosis of urinothorax established?

Urinothorax, a pleural effusion ipsilateral to an obstructed kidney, is diagnosed by the finding of a pleural fluid:serum creatinine ratio greater than 1.0.

16. What is a trapped lung? How is it diagnosed?

A trapped lung results from pleural inflammation or malignancy when a pleural peel does not allow a portion of the lung to expand to the chest wall. Pleural pressure decreases and promotes the accumulation of pleural fluid. The diagnosis can be confirmed by the finding of a pleural liquid pressure of –7 cm H_2O or less at the initial entry of the needle into the pleural fluid. Pleural liquid pressure decreases rapidly when a relatively small volume of fluid is removed.

17. What pleural fluid criteria suggest that a parapneumonic effusion can be treated successfully with observation and appropriate antibiotic therapy directed at the pneumonia?

A pleural fluid pH of more than 7.30, a glucose level of more than 60 mg per dl, and an LDH value of less than 700 IU per liter suggest a good outcome without manipulation of the pleural space.

18. Can patients with empyema be treated with antibiotics alone?

No. Empyema (pus in the pleural space) needs to be treated in the same way that pus anywhere in the body is treated, i.e., with appropriate drainage. A contrast-enhanced CT scan should be done to assess the extent of empyema and the number of loculations before a decision is made about specific therapy. A patient who has a single loculus with minimal pleural enhancement may be drained with a CT-guided chest tube or catheter. Multiloculated empyema requires either empyemectomy and decortication or a radiologic-guided catheter or chest tube with a thrombolytic agent.

19. Are there clinical variables that can differentiate patients with complicated from those with uncomplicated parapneumonic effusions?

No. Peak temperature, presence of pleuritic pain, number of lobes involved with pneumonia, or peripheral leukocyte count cannot make this differentiation. Only pleural fluid analysis can help make the distinction.

20. Does a negative tuberculin skin test exclude the diagnosis of tuberculous pleurisy?

No. Up to 30% of patients in the acute phase of tuberculous pleurisy have a negative tuberculin skin test with purified protein derivative (PPD). In most the skin test becomes positive in 6–8 weeks. The negative skin test is the result of circulating mononuclear cells that suppress the sensitized T-lymphocyte in the peripheral blood and skin but not in the pleural space.

21. What is the usual pleural fluid lymphocyte percentage in patients with tuberculous pleurisy?

Patients with tuberculous pleurisy usually have 90–95% lymphocytes. Other diagnoses with high percentages of pleural fluid lymphocytes include chylothorax, lymphoma, yellow nail syndrome, chronic rheumatoid pleurisy, and sarcoidosis.

22. What diseases are associated with a low pleural fluid pH (less than 7.30)?

The finding of a pleural pH of less than 7.30 narrows the differential diagnosis of the exudative pleural effusion. Empyema, rheumatoid pleurisy, malignancy, tuberculous pleurisy, lupus pleuritis, and esophageal rupture have all been reported with pleural fluid acidosis.

23. What is the significance of pleural fluid eosinophilia?

Pleural fluid eosinophilia (ratio of pleural fluid eosinophils to total nucleated cells more than 10%) suggests a benign disease commonly associated with air or blood in the pleural space. The differential diagnosis includes pneumothorax, hemothorax, pulmonary infarction, benign asbestos pleural effusion, parasitic disease, fungal infection, and drug reaction.

24. Is measurement of pleural fluid glucose a helpful diagnostic test?

Yes. Pleural fluid glucose levels less than 60 mg per dl or a pleural fluid:serum ratio less than 0.5 narrows the differential diagnosis of the exudative effusions to the same diagnoses associated with a low pleural fluid pH, namely, empyema, esophageal rupture, rheumatoid pleurisy, malignancy, tuberculous pleurisy, and lupus pleuritis. Empyema, esophageal rupture, and rheumatoid pleurisy commonly have a pleural fluid glucose concentration less than 30 mg per dl.

25. In the absence of esophageal rupture, what is the most likely diagnosis for a patient with an amylase-rich fluid that is predominantly salivary isoamylase?

Malignancy, most likely adenocarcinoma of the lung or ovary. These tumors secrete a salivary isoamylase responsible for this finding.

26. What is the clinical significance of mesothelial cells in pleural fluid?

Mesothelial cells are found in small numbers in normal pleural fluid, are prominent in transudative effusions, and vary in exudative effusions. Pleural fluid that contains more than 5% mesothelial cells is unlikely to be caused by tuberculous pleurisy.

27. Does finding a non-milky pleural fluid at thoracentesis exclude the diagnosis of chylothorax?

No. Chylothoraces may be milky, bloody, turbid, or serous. Trauma that produces a hemorrhagic effusion can mask the milky appearance. Malnourished patients or patients who have not eaten a meal may present with a turbid or serous effusion. Measurement of triglycerides establishes the diagnosis if the concentration is more than 100 mg per dl.

28. What are the characteristic pleural fluid findings in spontaneous esophageal rupture?

When the esophagus ruptures and the mediastinal pleura is violated, the characteristic findings are a high salivary amylase concentration and a low pleural fluid pH (frequently 6.00). The latter is caused by an anaerobic empyema.

BIBLIOGRAPHY

1. Adelman M, Albelda SM, Gottlieb J, et al: Diagnostic utility of pleural fluid eosinophilia. Am J Med 77:915–920, 1984.
2. Good JT Jr, Taryle DA, Maulitz RM, et al: The diagnostic value of pleural fluid pH. Chest 78:55–59, 1980.
3. Kramer MR, Cepero RJ, Pitchenik AE: High amylase in neoplasm-related pleural effusion. Ann Intern Med 110:567–569, 1989.
4. Light RW, MacGregor MI, Luchsinger PC, et al: Pleural effusion: The diagnostic separation of transudates and exudates. Ann Intern Med 77:507–513, 1972.
5. Sahn SA: The pleura. Am Rev Respir Dis 138:184–234, 1988.
6. Sahn SA: Thoracentesis and pleural biopsy. In Shelhamer J, Pizzo PA, Parrillo JE, et al (eds): Respiratory Disease in the Immunosuppressed Host. Philadelphia, J.B. Lippincott, 1991, pp 118–129.
7. Sahn SA: The diagnostic value of pleural fluid analysis. Semin Respir Crit Care Med 16:269–278, 1995.
8. Staats BA, Ellefson RD, Badahn L, et al: The lipoprotein profile of chylous and non-chylous pleural effusions. Mayo Clin Proc 55:700–704, 1980.

74. PNEUMOTHORAX

Michael E. Hanley, M.D.

1. How are pneumothoraces classified?

Pneumothoraces are classified as either spontaneous or traumatic. Traumatic pneumothoraces result from direct or indirect injury to the chest and are further classified as iatrogenic or noniatrogenic. Spontaneous pneumothoraces occur without obvious cause. They are termed *primary* if they occur in previously healthy individuals. *Secondary* spontaneous pneumothoraces occur as complications of underlying lung disease.

2. What is the differential diagnosis of spontaneous pneumothorax?

Patients with pneumothoraces present with acute onset of respiratory symptoms, including focal pleuritic chest pain, dyspnea, and dry cough. The differential diagnosis includes musculo-skeletal chest pain (chest trauma, costochondritis, rib fracture), myocardial ischemia or infarction, pulmonary embolism or infarction, infectious pneumonia, and viral pleuritis.

3. List the risk factors for primary spontaneous pneumothorax.

History of smoking
Positive family history of primary spontaneous pneumothorax
A tall, thin body habitus

4. Name some uncommon causes of spontaneous pneumothoraces.

- **Catamenial pneumothoraces** occur in association with menstruation. The two mechanisms that have been proposed for their development are movement of air from the peritoneal cavity to the pleural cavity through diaphragmatic defects and development of air in the pleural cavity from pleural endometriosis.
- **Neonatal pneumothoraces** occur spontaneously in 1–2% of newborns and may be asymptomatic in 50% of cases.
- Spontaneous pneumothoraces are a frequent complication in patients with **lymphangioleiomyomatosis** (LAM) and **eosinophilic granulomatosis**.

5. List the most common causes of iatrogenic pneumothoraces.

Common causes of iatrogenic pneumothoraces include:

Percutaneous pulmonary transthoracic needle aspiration and biopsy	Supraclavicular fine-needle aspiration
	Subclavian central venous catheter placement
Thoracentesis	Cardiovascular resuscitation
Transbronchial biopsy	Rarely, pneumothoraces complicate
Pleural biopsy	placement of an internal jugular central
Positive-pressure ventilation	venous catheter

6. What are the typical clinical manifestations of pneumothorax?

Chest pain or dyspnea (or both) occur in virtually all patients with pneumothorax. Although symptoms occur acutely in most patients, up to 20% of patients delay seeking medical consultation for more than 7 days. Physical signs include tachycardia and hyperexpansion of the ipsilateral chest with decreased tactile fremitus, hyperresonance, and decrease in or absence of breath sounds.

The clinical diagnosis of a secondary spontaneous pneumothorax can be especially difficult. Although the combined physiologic effects of pneumothorax and underlying lung disease make symptoms more severe, the physical signs of the pneumothorax are frequently masked by those of the underlying lung disease. This is especially true with pneumothoraces complicating COPD.

7. How do you estimate the size of a pneumothorax?

The size of a pneumothorax is the percentage of the hemithorax occupied by the pneumothorax. The absolute volume (V) of a pneumothorax is the difference between the total volume of the hemithorax and the volume of air remaining in the collapsed lung. The volume of air in the lung and hemithorax is proportional to the cube of their diameters (D). Therefore, assuming the lung retains a constant shape when it collapses, a rough estimate of the size of the pneumothorax can be calculated by the following formula:

$$\% \text{ Pneumothorax} = \frac{(V_{\text{Hemithorax}} - V_{\text{Lung}})}{V_{\text{Hemithorax}}} \times 100\%$$

or

$$\% \text{ Pneumothorax} = \frac{(D^3_{\text{Hemithorax}} - D^3_{\text{Lung}})}{D^3_{\text{Hemithorax}}} \times 100\%$$

8. What is the role of supplemental oxygen in the management of pneumothorax?

Reabsorption of pleural air is determined in part by the pressure gradient between the pleural space and pleural capillaries for each gas. If the patient is breathing room air, the sum of the pressure gradients for each gas (assuming the pneumothorax is not under tension) is only 54 mmHg, which results in reabsorption of about 1.25% of the volume of the hemithorax per day. Administration of 100% oxygen decreases the capillary partial pressure of nitrogen and increases the partial pressure of oxygen. However, the decrease in P_{N_2} is much greater than the increase in P_{O_2}, resulting in a large increase in the net pressure gradient for all gases. Pneumothoraces are reabsorbed four times faster if patients are treated with high concentrations of supplemental oxygen.

9. Do all pneumothoraces require tube thoracostomy?

No. Asymptomatic patients with small (less than 15%) primary spontaneous pneumothoraces or iatrogenic pneumothoraces in patients not being mechanically ventilated may be managed conservatively with either oxygen and radiologic observation alone or simple aspiration with a small-bore catheter followed by observation. Spontaneous secondary pneumothoraces, traumatic pneumothoraces, and pneumothoraces in the setting of mechanical ventilation all require tube thoracostomy.

10. What is a tension pneumothorax?

A tension pneumothorax occurs when significant positive pressure exists in the pleural space, resulting in severe compression of the ipsilateral lung, contralateral shift of the mediastinum, and caudal depression of the ipsilateral hemidiaphragm. It generally results from a ball or one-way valve bronchopleural fistula, especially during positive-pressure ventilation. Many patients who have tension pneumothoraces are clinically unstable with refractory hypoxemia and hypotension.

Tension pneumothoraces are medical emergencies that require immediate treatment. If a tube thoracostomy tray is not readily available and the patient is hemodynamically unstable, an 18- or 20-gauge angiocatheter should be inserted into the ipsilateral second intercostal space in the midclavicular line to relieve tension and stabilize the patient pending more definitive therapy.

11. Should a confirmatory chest roentgenogram be obtained before definitive therapy?

Generally, a confirmatory chest roentgenogram should be obtained before placement of a tube thoracostomy. However, a chest tube should be placed immediately (without delay for a roentgenogram) if a tension pneumothorax is suspected and the patient is clinically unstable.

12. Which patients should be considered for sclerotherapy?

The recurrence rate for both primary and secondary pneumothoraces is 40–50%. Sclerotherapy prevents recurrence by obliterating the pleural space. Studies evaluating the long-term safety of this therapy do not exist. Therefore, it should not be used for primary spontaneous pneumothorax unless it recurs. Because the physiologic consequences of secondary pneumothoraces are greater, early sclerosis (i.e., after the first occurrence) should be considered in this setting.

13. How is a persistent bronchopleural fistula evaluated?

A persistent bronchopleural fistula manifests as a nonresolving "air leak" that is evident after tube thoracostomy has been performed. Patients with large volume air leaks who have experienced chest trauma should be emergently evaluated for tracheobronchial lacerations. This is done via direct visualization of the tracheobronchial tree with fiberoptic bronchoscopy. Disruption of the endobronchial mucosa is confirmed by either observation of localized effervescence after application of hydrogen peroxide to suspicious lesions or appearance of methylene blue that has been instilled in the pleural space in the tracheobronchial tree.

The presence of an external air leak should be excluded in all patients with a persistent bronchopleural fistula. The insertion site of the tube thoracostomy as well as all external catheter connections should be inspected visually for leaks. In addition, extrathoracic tube placement (including extrathoracic location of any of the tube's ports) should be excluded by evaluating the tube's position with posteroanterior and lateral chest roentgenograms.

14. How is a persistent bronchopleural fistula managed?

Conservative treatment of a persistent bronchopleural fistula is generally indicated because most eventually close spontaneously. In the immediate period three options are available: (1) continue current management, (2) increase the suction applied to the pleural space to -35 cm H_2O, or (3) reposition the chest tube. Successful closure of bronchopleural fistulas after instillation of 50–60 ml of the patient's fresh blood into the pleural space has also been reported. However, the efficacy and safety of this technique (termed a *blood patch*) has not been studied in a rigorous fashion.

More definitive therapy should be considered if a bronchopleural fistula persists beyond 5–7 days. If the patient is a good surgical candidate and is at risk for recurrent pneumothoraces, thoracotomy with suturing or resection of the fistula and scarification of the pleura should be performed. Prolonged chest tube drainage with conversion to an outpatient one-way Heimlich valve or intrabronchial bronchoscopic instillation of materials designed to occlude the fistula (such as solubilized absorbable gelatin sponge or fibrin and cyanoacrylate-based glues) should be considered in patients deemed poor surgical risks or not desiring surgery.

15. How do you determine if the tube thoracostomy can be removed?

Removal of the tube thoracostomy should not be considered if a persistent air leak exists. Absence of a visible air leak during inspection of the tube thoracostomy does not guarantee that the leak has resolved because air may bubble out intermittently. Therefore, when there is no longer a visible leak the tube should be placed under water seal for 4–24 hours. The chest tube can generally be safely removed if a subsequent chest roentgenogram demonstrates complete reexpansion of the involved lung. In rare instances a persistent air leak may not be apparent under water seal because positive-pressure maneuvers such as coughing or talking may vent accumulated air out of the tube thoracostomy. If the physiologic consequences of a recurrent pneumothorax are severe (such as in the setting of significant underlying lung disease) it may be prudent not to remove the chest tube until complete reexpansion of the lung has been radiographically demonstrated 4–24 hours after the tube has been clamped.

BIBLIOGRAPHY

 1. Archer GJ, Hamilton AAD, et al: Results of simple aspiration of pneumothorax. Br J Dis Chest 79: 177–182, 1985.
 2. Bense L: Spontaneous pneumothorax. Chest 101:891–892, 1992.
 3. Chadha TS, Cohn MA: Non-invasive treatment of pneumothorax with oxygen inhalation. Respiration 44:147–152, 1983.
 4. Dumire R, Crabbe MM, Mappin FG, et al: Autologous "blood patch" pleurodesis for persistent pulmonary air leak. Chest 101:64–66, 1992.
 5. Engdahl O, Toft T, Boe J: Chest radiograph—a poor method for determining the size of a pneumothorax. Chest 103:26–29, 1993.
 6. Gammon BR, Shin MS, Buchalter SE: Pulmonary barotrauma in mechanical ventilation. Patterns and risk factors. Chest 102:568–572, 1992.
 7. Light RW, O'Hara VS, Mortiz TE: Iatrogenic pneumothorax: Etiology and morbidity. Results of a Department of Veterans Affairs cooperative study. Respiration 59:215–220, 1992.
 8. Liu H, Lin PJ, Hsieh M, et al: Thoracoscopic surgery as a routine procedure for spontaneous pneumothorax. Results from 82 patients. Chest 107:559–562, 1995.
 9. Milanez JRC, Vargas FS, Filomeno LTB, et al: Intrapleural talc for the prevention of recurrent pneumothorax. Chest 4:1162–1165, 1994.
10. Miller KS, Sahn SA: Chest tubes: Indications, technique, management and complications. Chest 91:258–263, 1987.
11. Schoenenberger RA, Haefeli WE, Weiss P, et al: Evaluation of conventional chest tube therapy for iatrogenic pneumothorax. Chest 104:1770–1772, 1993.
12. Wait MA, Dal Nogare AR: Treatment of AIDS-related spontaneous pneumothorax: A decade of experience. Chest 106:693–696, 1994.

75. MESOTHELIOMA

Thomas J. Donnelly, M.D., and York E. Miller, M.D.

1. What is the incidence of malignant mesothelioma?

Fortunately, mesothelioma is relatively rare; 1,500 to 3,000 cases occur yearly in the United States. Specific groups and geographical areas have higher case rates, however.

2. What are the risk factors for mesothelioma?

Exposure to asbestos is the major risk factor for mesothelioma. More than 80% of patients have a clear history of exposure to asbestos. Additional patients may have had unknown asbestos exposure. Chest wall radiation has also been implicated as a risk factor, as has exposure to erionite, a fibrous mineral found in certain regions of Turkey. The latency period between asbestos exposure and disease development is typically more than 20 years. Occupations associated with asbestos exposure include shipbuilding, seafaring, brake repair, and the construction and insulation industries. Family members of asbestos workers have sometimes developed mesothelioma, presumably because of asbestos fibers brought home on work clothes. Individuals who lived in proximity to factories or mines in which asbestos was prominent have also been reported with the disease. A male predominance is seen, probably because of greater exposure rather than gender differences in susceptibility.

3. Do patients have to have asbestosis (i.e., asbestos-induced lung disease) for mesothelioma to occur?

No. Asbestos-induced pulmonary fibrosis or pleural plaques are not necessary for development of mesothelioma.

4. Is mesothelioma always a malignant disorder?

No. A very small group of patients may present with benign, localized disease. Benign mesothelioma has also been termed *localized mesothelioma*, *localized fibrous tumor of the pleura*, and *solitary fibrous tumor of the pleura*. The latter two names recognize the fact that this benign tumor actually arises from cells in submesothelial tissue rather than mesothelial cells themselves. No association exists with asbestos exposure. Benign mesothelioma is often a pedunculated tumor arising from the parietal pleura found incidentally on chest radiograph. Benign mesothelioma may be associated with an exudative effusion and may recur after surgical resection. Between 5 and 20% of patients will have several recurrences, some of which may be unresectable because of local invasion of critical intrathoracic structures. In these cases, the behavior of the tumor could be considered malignant. Benign mesothelioma is frequently associated with hypertrophic pulmonary osteoarthropathy and rarely with hypoglycemia.

5. How do patients with malignant mesothelioma commonly present?

Presentation patterns vary depending on the stage of disease. Asymptomatic patients may present with chest radiographic abnormalities only, usually a pleural effusion. The earliest symptom is often dyspnea caused by pleural effusion. As the tumor progresses and invades local structures, chest pain is frequent. Extensive invasion of local structures can result in Horner's syndrome; vocal cord paralysis; dysphagia; and severe, unremitting dyspnea. Cardiac involvement is common, with myocardial dysfunction and tamponade or restriction. Subdiaphragmatic invasion can result in abdominal pain or intestinal obstruction. Rarely, mesothelioma can arise from the peritoneum.

6. What is the typical clinical course of malignant mesothelioma?

The disease is progressive and relentless. The tumor grows and encases the lung, producing volume loss and functional restriction. The patient usually dies from local disease and its effect on pulmonary function. Distant metastases usually occur late in the course of disease. Death typically occurs within 18 months of diagnosis; rare patients survive 3–4 years.

7. Describe the radiographic features of malignant mesothelioma.

Pleural effusion is often the earliest radiographic feature of malignant mesothelioma. Occasionally an area of progressive pleural thickening is seen on serial films. Pleural changes tend to be irregular and located on the lateral chest wall. They may be large, nodular projections originating from the chest wall and extending medially, compressing thoracic structures. As the disease progresses, the affected side contracts and opacifies. Evidence of asbestos exposure, such as pleural plaques, calcifications and parenchymal fibrosis, should be noted.

8. What pleural fluid characteristics are typical in mesothelioma?

Pleural fluid is exudative, mononuclear cell predominant, and often bloody. Pleural fluid cytologic studies can suggest malignancy, but a firm diagnosis of mesothelioma almost never can be made on pleural fluid cytologic findings alone. Mesothelioma can be excluded if the pleural fluid cytology is diagnostic for another malignancy, such as squamous cell carcinoma, adenocarcinoma, or small cell carcinoma.

9. What other disorders must be considered in the differential diagnosis?

Metastatic adenocarcinoma is probably the diagnosis most commonly confused with mesothelioma. Other diagnoses that should be considered include benign asbestos pleural effusion, pleural tuberculosis, collagen vascular disease, and pulmonary embolism. The diagnosis of mesothelioma may be difficult to establish, particularly if small specimens are obtained, and both false-negative and false-positive diagnoses are possible.

10. Should open or closed pleural biopsy be used for diagnosis?

Closed pleural biopsy (Cope or Abrams needle) is often nondiagnostic or may yield a diagnosis of malignancy, exact cell type uncertain. Video-assisted thoracoscopic biopsy is diagnostic in more than 80% of cases and open thoracotomy is diagnostic in approximately 90%.

11. What special tests are useful in the diagnosis of mesothelioma?

If a definite diagnosis of malignancy is made, but uncertainty exists as to whether it is mesothelioma or metastatic adenocarcinoma, the following special studies may be diagnostic: acid–Schiff stain (with and without diastase treatment), mucicarmine stain, immunohistochemistry with carcinoembryonic antigen or cytokeratin, and electron microscopy. Before either a closed or an open biopsy is performed the clinician should discuss the appropriate stains, fixation, and handling of the tissue with the pathologist.

12. Are medicolegal issues involved in diagnosis of mesothelioma?

In many patients, it may not be clinically important to make the diagnosis of mesothelioma versus metastatic adenocarcinoma for treatment decisions. However, a significant number of patients (and their survivors) may wish to pursue workers' compensation or liability lawsuits for which the diagnosis of mesothelioma is critical. Therefore, a firm tissue diagnosis may be desired for medicolegal reasons.

13. Name the pathologic subsets of mesothelioma. What impact do they have on outcome?

Three pathologic subsets have been defined: epithelial, sarcomatous, and mixed epithelial-sarcomatous. Long-term outcome is universally dismal, but the short-term survival may be better for epithelial mesothelioma. The sarcomatous variant is more likely to metastasize.

14. Is staging useful in mesothelioma? What is the most efficient approach?

Several staging systems have been proposed, but none is universally accepted. Distant metastases are rare and should be pursued with imaging studies only if symptoms or physical examination is suggestive. The extent of local involvement is most critical for planning possible surgical therapy and is best delineated by CT scans of the chest and abdomen.

15. Are single-modality therapies available for mesothelioma? How effective are they?

All therapies for malignant mesothelioma are primarily palliative; cure is rare. Surgery, radio-therapy, and chemotherapy are the single-modality therapies that have received attention in meso-thelioma. Because local disease is bulky and attainment of clear surgical margins is not feasible, none of the single-modality therapies have shown benefit.

16. What are the different surgical options in mesothelioma?

- **Extrapleural pneumonectomy** is a major operation in which the lung and pleura are re-moved en bloc and the hemidiaphragm and pericardium are also removed. Initial reports of operative mortality were 30%, but more recent series at centers that specialize in this pro-cedure are approximately 5%.
- **Pleurectomy and decortication** also can remove all gross tumor in selected cases (the mesothelioma cannot have invaded the lung for this to be feasible) and carries a low mor-tality (2%). Neither this procedure nor extrapleural pneumonectomy is expected to yield microscopically clear margins because vital structures such as the aorta, esophagus, and heart are frequently involved and cannot be widely resected.
- **Limited pleurectomy** is useful in controlling pleural effusion.
- **Thoracoscopy with talc poudrage** is effective for controlling effusion and is palliative for symptoms of pleural effusion.

Extrapleural pneumonectomy and pleurectomy and decortication may yield modest benefit in properly selected patients in terms of prolonging survival, but neither is curative.

17. What is the role of pleurodesis in the palliation of mesothelioma?

Chemical pleurodesis is frequently ineffective in mesothelioma and may complicate addi-tional surgical therapy. Only after a decision has been made to forego surgical or multimodality therapy should chemical pleurodesis be attempted.

18. What multimodality therapies are available for mesothelioma?

Extrapleural pneumonectomy or pleurectomy and decortication followed by radiation and chemotherapy are under investigation at selected centers with an interest in mesothelioma. Gene therapy protocols are also under investigation. Combined modality therapy at the present time does not not lead to cure but may prolong survival in selected patients.

19. Which patients should be considered for aggressive multimodality therapy and where should they be treated?

Only patients with good performance status and in whom gross tumors can be removed should be considered. Because initial mortalities for extrapleural pneumonectomy were 30% and dropped to 5% in centers specializing in this procedure, it is likely that patients will benefit by re-ferral to centers with significant experience with this procedure.

BIBLIOGRAPHY

1. Aisner J: Current approach to malignant mesothelioma of the pleura. Chest 107(Suppl):332S–345S, 1995.
2. Briselli M, Mark EJ, Dickerson GR: Solitary fibrous tumors of the pleura: Eight new cases and review of 360 cases in the literature. Cancer 47:2678–2689, 1981.
3. Light RW: Tumors of the pleura. In Murray JF, Nadel JA (eds): Textbook of Respiratory Medicine. Philadelphia, W.B. Saunders, 1988, pp 1170–1774.
4. Okike N, Bernatz PE, Woolner LB: Localized mesothelioma of the pleura: Benign and malignant variants. J Thorac Cardiovasc Surg 75:363–372, 1978.
5. Rusch V: Clinical features and current treatment of diffuse malignant pleural mesothelioma. Lung Cancer 12(Suppl):S127–S146, 1995.
6. Sugarbaker DJ, Jaklitsch MT, Liptay MJ: Mesothelioma and radical multimodality therapy: Who bene-fits? Chest 107(Suppl):345S–350S, 1995.

XVI. Diseases of the Mediastinum, Chest Wall, and Diaphragm

76. DISORDERS OF THE MEDIASTINUM

Polly E. Parsons, M.D.

1. What structures are in the anterior mediastinum?
Thymus gland
Anterior mediastinal lymph nodes
Aortic arch

2. What structures are in the middle mediastinum?
Heart
Pericardium
Trachea and main bronchi
Paratracheal and tracheobronchial lymph nodes
Phrenic and recurrent laryngeal nerves

3. What are the structures in the posterior mediastinum?
Sympathetic chain
Vagus nerve
Esophagus
Thoracic duct
Posterior mediastinal lymph nodes
Descending aorta

4. Name the common causes of an anterior mediastinal mass.
Remember the four Ts:
   Thymoma
   Teratoma
   Thyroid (intrathoracic goiter)
   "Terrible" lymphoma (or "T-cell" tumors)
Hodgkin's disease, as a form of lymphoma, invariably involves the anterior mediastinum prior to or simultaneously with involvement of hilar or other mediastinal lymph nodes. Patients with mediastinal masses due to lymphoma usually have evidence of disease elsewhere, and the mediastinal adenopathy is detected during staging procedures.

5. How often do patients with lymphoma have radiographic evidence of mediastinal masses?
Up to 50% of patients with Hodgkin's disease have radiographic evidence of intrathoracic lymph nodes on plain chest radiographs at the time of clinical presentation. This proportion increases to 85% if CT scanning is used to examine the mediastinum. Only 24–43% of patients with non-Hodgkin's lymphoma have evidence of mediastinal involvement when evaluated with plain chest radiographs and CT.

In most patients with Hodgkin's lymphoma, mediastinal lymph nodes become involved progressively from contiguous, neighboring nodes. The lymph nodes protrude asymmetrically into both the right and left hemithoraces. Unilateral nodal disease is uncommon. The lymphadenopathy of non-Hodgkin's lymphoma tends to be less bulky and frequently spreads in an unpredictable and noncontiguous fashion.

6. What diagnosis should you think of if you see teeth in the anterior mediastinum on a chest x-ray?

Teratoma

7. What anterior mediastinal mass is associated with myasthenia gravis?

Tumors of the thymus. In some series, up to 15% of patients with myasthenia gravis have thymic tumors, and 35% of patients with thymic tumors have myasthenia gravis. Myasthenia gravis can develop years before or after the appearance of the tumor of the thymus.

Remember that thymic enlargement can also occur in patients with mediastinal Hodgkin's disease. The thymus becomes enlarged because of lymphomatous involvement of the gland. These patients, however, invariably have radiographic evidence of associated lymphadenopathy elsewhere in the mediastinum.

8. What is the most common cause of a posterior mediastinal mass?

Neurogenic tumors. These actually account for 21% of all mediastinal masses and are therefore the most common cause of a mediastinal mass.

9. How does Boerhaave's syndrome present?

As the spontaneous perforation of the esophagus. The patient may complain of the acute onset of chest pain and shortness of breath following vomiting. This condition is a potentially life-threatening one, so recognition and diagnosis are critical. Physical examination may be nonspecific. Chest x-ray findings may include mediastinal and/or pleural air and a pleural effusion. Pleural fluid characteristically has a low pH and a high salivary amylase concentration. The presence of food particles in the pleural fluid is essentially diagnostic for esophageal perforation. The diagnosis is usually made with a radiographic contrast study of the esophagus.

10. What are the common etiologies of acute mediastinitis?

Esophageal rupture
Perforation of the trachea or large bronchi
Direct extension of infection for adjacent structures such as the pleura, retropharynx, lung, pericardium
Infection of a median sternotomy

11. What is Hamman's sign?

Also known as **mediastinal crunch**, Hamman's sign is a crunching sound made from air in the mediastinum (pneumomediastinum). It is heard over the anterior thorax and is synchronous with the heart beat.

12. Name the major causes of pneumomediastinum.

There are three major mechanisms by which air or gas enters the mediastinal space:
1. Spontaneous rupture of alveoli
2. Trauma
3. Rupture of the esophagus or trachea

13. Describe some of the clinical settings in which pneumomediastinum may occur spontaneously.

Pneumomediastinum can occur following any maneuver that increases lung volume or results in rapid changes in alveolar pressure. Pneumomediastinum has been reported as occurring in some individuals following "benign" activities, such as performing pulmonary function tests, yelling, singing, or playing a musical instrument. Individuals who intentionally valsalva or breath-hold while smoking marijuana or inhaling crack cocaine are also at risk. Patients with lung diseases such as asthma and COPD may develop pneumomediastinum if significant alveolar air trapping occurs. In addition, the external application of increased lung volume and/or pressure with mechanical ventilation or continuous positive airway pressure as well as externally applied forces during trauma can also cause pneumomediastinum.

14. How is pneumomediastinum treated?

Pneumomediastinum itself is usually self-limiting and does not cause any clinically important physiologic changes. However, air can extend into the pleural space and produce a pneumothorax that often requires drainage. In addition, air can enter the pericardial space and cause a pneumopericardium with associated clinical manifestations of tamponade.

15. What are the common benign causes of superior vena cava obstruction?

Granulomatous mediastinitis and fibrosing mediastinitis. The occurrence of benign etiologies underscores the importance of establishing a firm diagnosis of the underlying disease before initiating therapy in patients presenting with superior vena cava syndrome.

BIBLIOGRAPHY

1. Abolnik I, Lossos IS, Bruer R: Spontaneous pneumomediastinum: A report of 25 cases. Chest 100:93–95, 1991.
2. Berkman N, Breuer R, Kramer MR, Polliack A: Pulmonary involvement in lymphoma. Leukemia Lymphoma 20:229–237, 1996.
3. Cummings RG, Wesley RLR, Adams DH, et al: Pneumopericardium resulting in cardiac tamponade. Ann Thorac Surg 37:511–518, 1984.
4. Diseases of the mediastinum. In Fraser RG, Pare JAP, Pare PD, et al (eds): Diagnosis of Diseases of the Chest. Philadelphia, W.B. Saunders, 1991, pp 2794–2920.
5. Jantz MA, Pierson DJ: Pneumothorax and barotrauma. Clin Chest Med 15:75–91, 1994.
6. Maunder RJ, Pierson DJ, Hudson LD: Subcutaneous and mediastinal emphysema: Pathophysiology, diagnosis, and management. Arch Intern Med 144:1447–1453, 1984.
7. Mole TM, Glover J, Sheppard MN: Sclerosing mediastinitis: A report on 18 cases. Thorax 50:280–283, 1995.
8. Morgenthaler TI, Brown LR, Colby TV, et al: Thymoma. Mayo Clin Proc 68:1110–1123, 1993.
9. Pierson DJ: Pneumomediastinum. In Murray JF, Nadel JA (eds): Textbook of Respiratory Medicine. Philadelphia, W.B. Saunders, 1994.
10. Seaman ME: Barotrauma related to inhalational drug abuse. J Emerg Med 8:141–149, 1990.
11. Silverman NA, Sabiston DC: Mediastinal masses. Surg Clin North Am 60:757–777, 1980.

77. CHEST WALL DISORDERS

Polly E. Parsons, M.D., and John E. Heffner, M.D.

1. What is a flail chest?

Patients with a flail chest have paradoxical chest wall movement with inspiration and expiration. A flail chest can occur following the fracture of multiple ribs, fracture of the sternum, or disruption of the costochondral junction of several ribs.

2. Do patients with flail chest require mechanical ventilation?

Flail chest alone is not an indication for mechanical ventilation. That therapy should be reserved for patients with respiratory failure as evidenced by hypercapnia or hypoxia.

3. What are the pulmonary complications of ankylosing spondylitis?

The most common complication is chest wall restriction from the fusion of the costovertebral joints. This causes a decrease in both total lung capacity and vital capacity. Functional residual capacity, residual volume, and airflows are generally preserved. In addition to chest wall restriction, parenchymal involvement, manifested as bilateral apical infiltrates and cavities on chest x-ray, is seen in a small number of patients. These x-ray findings are often indistinguishable from those of pulmonary tuberculosis.

4. What causes hemoptysis in patients with ankylosing spondylitis?

The apical cavities can become secondarily superinfected with organisms such as *Aspergillus*, which cause focal inflammation and bleeding.

5. Which tests can be used to evaluate respiratory muscle strength?

1. **Maximum inspiratory pressure** (MIP) and **maximum expiratory pressure** (MEP): These tests can be performed at the bedside and are often abnormal before other measurements of lung function, including arterial blood gases.

2. **Vital capacity**: This can also be performed at the bedside. However, vital capacity does not correlate as well with arterial blood gas measurements as MIP and MEP do.

Other tests, including measurements of transdiaphragmatic pressure and electromyograms of the diaphragms, can also quantitate respiratory muscle weakness, but they are not available in all clinical settings.

6. What degree of impairment of maximal inspiratory pressure is usually associated with an elevated PCO$_2$ on an arterial blood gas?

Less than -30 cm H$_2$O

7. Which disorders of the neuromuscular junction can cause respiratory muscle weakness?

Myasthenia gravis, botulism, and organophosphate poisoning. In addition, some antibiotics, such as the aminoglycosides, can affect the neuromuscular junction and contribute to respiratory muscle weakness, and neuromuscular blocking agents can have prolonged effects. Thus, it is important to carefully evaluate the medication list of all patients.

8. Why do some patients with kyphoscoliosis develop respiratory failure?

Severe kyphoscoliosis causes decreases in lung volumes, the pulmonary vascular bed, and chest wall compliance. This combination leads to hypoventilation and ventilation-perfusion mismatch such that some patients ultimately develop pulmonary hypertension and respiratory failure.

9. Do patients with pectus excavatum develop pulmonary disease?

Pectus excavatum is a skeletal deformity in which the sternum is depressed. Although the deformity may appear to be severe, pulmonary function is preserved in all but a minority of patients.

10. What happens to respiratory muscle function in patients who have a traumatic cervical spinal cord injury at level C3 or above?

These patients have no innervation of the diaphragm or intercostal muscles. They may be able to generate very small tidal volumes using accessory muscles, but they will require ventilatory support.

11. Can patients who have a spinal cord injury between C5 and C8 breathe?

Yes, because the diaphragmatic muscle function and some accessory muscle functions are still intact. Immediately after injury, vital capacity may be reduced to one-third of normal, but within the first few months after injury, some improvement in function usually occurs such that the vital capacity approaches 50% of the pre-injury value. Therefore, these patients usually do not require ventilatory support during the day. Because pulmonary function is affected by the supine position, some patients may require nocturnal mechanical ventilation.

12. What is Tietze's syndrome?

Also known as costochondral osteochondritis, Tietze's syndrome is pain and swelling of the costochondral joints. Patients may complain of pain over the anterior chest which is exacerbated by movement, cough, and breathing. On physical examination, there is usually focal tenderness over one or more costochondral joints. Occasionally, erythema and swelling may be evident. The symptoms last for weeks to months, though they are often alleviated with nonsteroidal anti-inflammatory medications.

13. What are the respiratory effects of obesity?

Although obesity is defined as body weights in excess of 110–120% ideal body weight, most of the studies that examine the impact of weight on respiratory function have studied patients who are 150–200% ideal body weight. The weight of body mass pressing against the thorax and abdomen increases chest wall stiffness and decreases its compliance. Lung compliance may also be decreased, possibly through the effects of increased pulmonary vascular blood volume and increased closure of dependent airways. All of these effects combine to increase mechanical work and oxygen cost of breathing.

Obese patients also have a larger CO_2 production, which requires them to work hard to eliminate CO_2 due to the relative low compliance of their respiratory system. Obesity also overstretches ventilatory muscles, placing them at a mechanical disadvantage. For this and perhaps other reasons, severely obese patients have decreased ventilatory muscle strength and may be at increased risk for ventilatory muscle fatigue. And, of course, obese patients may develop nocturnal (with or without daytime) hypoventilation in the condition called **obesity hypoventilation syndrome.**

14. Does obesity affect pulmonary testing results?

Obesity can produce a restrictive ventilatory deficit in the setting of severe obesity when the weight (kg) to height (cm) ratio is > 1. The compressive effects of chest wall fat decrease functional residual capacity, expiratory reserve volume, and total lung capacity. Impaired respiratory muscle function and decreased compliance of the respiratory system both contribute to decreased vital capacity and maximal voluntary ventilation. Extreme obesity also produces ventilation-perfusion mismatching that can produce hypoxemia with an increased $(A–a)PO_2$.

BIBLIOGRAPHY

1. Appebrouth D, Gottlieb NL: Pulmonary manifestations of ankylosing spondylitis. J Rheumatol 2:446–451, 1975.
2. Bergofsky EH: Respiratory failure in disorder of the thoracic cage. Am Rev Respir Dis 119:643, 1979.
3. Fraser RG, Pare JAP, Pare PD, et al: Diagnosis of Diseases of the Chest. Philadelphia, W.B. Saunders, 1991, pp 2921–2973.
4. Hollingsworth HM, Irwin RS: Extrapulmonary causes of respiratory failure. In Rippe JM, Irwin RS, Fink MP, Cerra FB (eds): Intensive Care Medicine. Boston, Little, Brown, and Co., 1996, pp 628–641.
5. Luce J: Medical management of spinal cord injury. Crit Care Med 13:126, 1985.
6. O'Donohue WJ, Baker JP, Bell GM, et al: Respiratory failure in neuromuscular disease: Management in a respiratory intensive care unit. JAMA 235:733–742, 1976.
7. Ray C, Sue D, Bray G, et al: Effects of obesity on respiratory function. 128:501–506, 1983.
8. Romaker AM: Disorders of the thoracic spine. In Bordow RA, Moser KM (eds): Manual of Clinical Problems in Pulmonary Medicine. Boston, Little, Brown, and Co., 1985, pp 301–304.
9. Watling SM, Dasta JF: Prolonged paralysis in intensive care unit patients after the use of neuromuscular blocking agents: A review of the literature. Crit Care Med 22:893, 1994.

78. DIAPHRAGMATIC FUNCTION AND ASSOCIATED DISORDERS

Antonio Anzueto, M.D., and Shawn Wright, M.D.

1. What is the major function of the respiratory muscles?

The respiratory muscles include the diaphragm, intercostal muscles, and accessory muscles (sternocleidomastoid, scalene, abdominal). The respiratory muscles are unique because breathing depends upon their contractions. They are the only skeletal muscles essential to life. The major function of these muscles is expansion of the thoracic cavity to develop negative intrathoracic pressure and thus facilitate air flow.

2. What is the role of the respiratory accessory muscles in the overall function of respiration?

The accessory muscles include the intercostal, sternocleidomastoid, scalene, and abdominal muscles. The intercostal muscles consist of external and internal muscle groups; the latter are divided into the paraexternal (intercartilaginous) and interosseous muscles. Traditionally, external intercostals were thought to have an inspiratory action and internal intercostals, an expiratory action. Recently, some investigators have shown that both groups have an expiratory action at high volumes and an inspiratory action at low volumes. The sternocleidomastoid and scalene muscles have conventionally been considered accessory muscles. Vigorous respiratory efforts such as when minute ventilation is increased to more than 75% of vital capacity recruit the sternocleidomastoid muscle. Abdominal muscles are the primary muscles of expiration. They may facilitate expiration by three mechanisms. First, during expiration, muscle contraction causes lung volume to drop below atmospheric pressure at end-expiratory level. This pushes the diaphragm into the rib cage and lengthens its fibers, allowing them to function over a more favorable portion of the length-tension curve. Second, upward motion of the diaphragm causes it to become more curved, and the resulting decrease in the radius of its curvature may improve mechanical efficacy. Third, during respiration, elastic energy is stored in abdominal muscles. Release of energy during inspiration can enhance inspiratory efforts.

3. Do the respiratory muscles have other functions?

Other functions of the respiratory muscles include explosive efforts, such as coughing, vomiting, and expectoration. They also stabilize the rib cage and abdomen for posture.

4. Define respiratory muscle fatigue.

Respiratory muscle fatigue has been defined as a loss in the capacity for developing force resulting from muscle activity under load. It is reversible by rest. Generally, fatigue is considered relatively acute loss of contractile force from which the muscle usually recovers spontaneously.

5. What are the mechanisms leading to respiratory fatigue?

The major physiologic mechanisms leading to respiratory fatigue include:
Inhibition of neural drive
Impaired transmission across the neuromuscular junction
Excessive force and duration of contraction
Impaired muscular blood supply
Impaired excitation-contraction coupling
Depletion of muscle energy stores and failure of the contracting machinery, resulting from destructive changes such as muscle dystrophies or disuse atrophy, also may contribute to fatigue.

6. List the conditions that predispose patients to respiratory muscle fatigue.

From a clinical standpoint, conditions that predispose to respiratory muscle fatigue can be divided into two types: conditions that increase the respiratory load and conditions that cause muscle weakness.

Conditions that Predispose Patients to Respiratory Muscle Fatigue

INCREASED LOAD	NEUROMUSCULAR WEAKNESS
Airway obstruction	Neuromuscular disease
	Antibiotic toxicity
	Botulism
	Myasthenia gravis
	Organophosphate poisoning
Parenchymal disease	Hypoperfusion
Chest bellows disease	Hypoxemia
	Hypercapnia
	Malnutrition
	Electrolyte imbalance
	Hyperinflation
	Muscle atrophy, myopathies
	Postoperative phrenic nerve or diaphragm dysfunction
	Anterior horn cell diseases
	Amyotrophic lateral sclerosis
	Poliomyelitis
	Trauma
	Advanced age

7. How does hyperinflation affect respiratory muscle function?

Hyperinflation, a characteristic finding in patients with COPD, has a number of adverse effects on respiratory muscle function. These effects are mainly associated with a decrease in the radius of diaphragm curvature. Such a decrease reduces the muscle's pressure generation efficiency. During contraction of the diaphragm, the medial orientation of the muscle fibers results in rib cage deflation and no expansion. In the hyperinflated chest, thoracic elastic recoil is directed inward, which poses an additional elastic load. The zone of apposition between the diaphragm and the rib cage is decreased in hyperinflation, and this reduced apposition lessens the efficiency of chest wall expansion. Finally, greater variations in transdiaphragmatic pressure may impair diaphragmatic blood supply and limit its efficiency when increased loads are applied.

8. Describe the clinical findings of respiratory muscle fatigue.

The clinical features that suggest respiratory muscle dysfunction include dyspnea, altered breathing pattern, disturbed sleep, cor pulmonale, impaired cough, aspiration, and generalized evidence of neuromuscular disease. It has been considered possible to diagnose inspiratory muscle fatigue with reasonable certainty when the following specific sequence of clinical signs is observed: tachypnea, paradoxical inward motion of the abdomen during inspiration (respiratory paradox), and finally, an increase in carbon dioxide tension and a drop in both the respiratory rate and minute ventilation.

9. How is respiratory muscle weakness assessed in critical care patients?

Respiratory muscle weakness is a relatively common problem in ICU patients, particularly in those requiring ventilatory support for prolonged periods. Some patients have neuromuscular disorders before ICU admission, but in most cases, weakness is a consequence of the underlying illness. The two most frequently used measurements of respiratory muscle strength in the ICU are vital capacity (VC) and maximal respiratory pressures.

A reduction in VC to less than 30% of predicted normal is usually necessary before patients develop an increase in arterial carbon dioxide tension. VC is an index of respiratory muscle strength that is easy to assess but is nonspecific. Although a normal supine VC excludes moderate to severe muscle weakness, reduced VC can be the result of muscle weakness, respiratory disease, or both. In patients with substantial diaphragmatic weakness, VC is further reduced in the supine posture. The maneuver to determine VC has to be done in a patient who is alert and cooperative.

Overall muscle strength is more precisely measured by the maximal inspiratory and expiratory pressures that the respiratory muscles can generate. Maximal inspiratory pressure (MIP or Pimax) is assessed by a pressure manometer with the patient inspiring against a closed airway, initiating the maneuver at residual volume. Normal values for MIP are approximately -100 cm H_2O. Maximal expiratory pressure is easily measured by having the patient exhale forcefully against a closed valve. Normal values are approximately 200 cm H_2O. MIP is normally used as an indicator for weaning during mechanical ventilation. Unfortunately, the thresholds for determining success of weaning (generation of more negative pressure than -30 cm H_2O) or failure of weaning (cannot generate pressure of -20 cm H_2O) are neither sensitive nor specific. The use of MIP in the ICU is further limited by the inability of critically ill patients to make maximal inspiratory efforts.

In some cases, more detailed evaluation of diaphragmatic strength may be needed. This entails measurement of the transdiaphragmatic pressure and the diaphragm's response to phrenic nerve stimulation. Chest and abdominal plethysomographic measurements of rib cage and abdominal movement provide aid in identifying impaired diaphragmatic function. Other techniques, including diaphragmatic electromyography (EMG) signals and maximal relaxation rate of the respiratory muscle, have been examined in ICU patients and can be used to detect muscle failure. Most of these techniques have not been validated, and their use is limited to research purposes.

10. How is respiratory muscle fatigue treated?

Several measures can be used to manage respiratory muscle dysfunction. First, the underlying cause should be removed if possible. In addition, any electrolyte disturbance should be corrected and underlying medical problems that increase metabolic demands on the patient should be treated. It is also important to reduce the respiratory load by reducing any abnormality in pulmonary mechanics, such as bronchospasm. Resting the respiratory muscles (with mechanical ventilation) is the only satisfactory method for managing respiratory muscle fatigue. Although optimal duration of rest is unknown, it is thought to be at least 24 hours. Ironically, however, prolonged rest may result in respiratory muscle atrophy.

11. Is there any drug therapy available for diaphragmatic fatigue?

Aminophylline has been shown to increase diaphragmatic contractility in animal experiments. The usual therapeutic level, however, provides only minimal improvement in ventilatory endurance. Because of this marginal effect and the drug's potential toxicity, the role of aminophylline in managing respiratory muscle dysfunction remains controversial. Correction of electrolytes, especially serum phosphate, has been shown to be beneficial. Other therapies that have been utilized with limited success include calcium channel blockers, digitalis, and vasopressors.

12. What are the common causes of unilateral diaphragmatic paralysis?

An exact cause for unilateral diaphragmatic paralysis can be determined in approximately 50% of cases. The other 50% are idiopathic. The various known causes are outlined below.

Bronchogenic carcinoma	Unusual medical conditions
Surgical trauma	Cervical spine disease
Cervical operations	Thoracic or aortic aneurysm
Thoracic operations	Poliomyelitis
Nonsurgical trauma	Herpes zoster virus
Penetrating trauma	Mediastinitis
Blunt trauma	Others
Traction injury	

13. Is function of the phrenic nerve and diaphragm impaired after coronary artery bypass grafting?

Although improvement in cardiopulmonary bypass technique and reduction in total bypass time have reduced the occurrence of severe postoperative respiratory complications, pulmonary dysfunction still contributes significantly to the morbidity associated with coronary artery bypass grafting (CABG). Patients undergoing this operation often develop a severe reduction in lung volume and left lower lobe atelectasis in the early postoperative period. The cause of this condition is not clear, but it may be the result of trauma to the lung caused by retraction during the surgery, postoperative gastric distention, or intraoperative phrenic nerve injury. Unilateral phrenic nerve palsy as confirmed by electrophysiologic studies occurs in up to 10% of patients after CABG surgery. Unilateral diaphragmatic paralysis is often asymptomatic, although it can lead to left lower lobe atelectasis. Bilateral diaphragmatic paralysis resulting from bilateral phrenic nerve damage is rare and normally requires prolonged ventilatory support. Two major causes of phrenic nerve injury have been postulated. One is stretch injury resulting from surgical manipulation and the other is cold-induced injury related to topical ice or slush placed in the pericardial sac during cold cardioplegia. The incidence of phrenic nerve injury from either cause is further increased when the internal thoracic artery is harvested; phrenic nerve injury also appears to be more common in patients with diabetes, perhaps because of microvascular disease.

14. What are the common causes of diaphragmatic rupture?

Rupture of the diaphragm most often results from blunt or penetrating trauma to the abdomen or lower thorax. Motor vehicle accidents and gunshot or stab wounds are the major causes of injury in most patients. Rupture of the diaphragm has been reported to occur during pregnancy, both iatrogenically and spontaneously. Although mortality from diaphragmatic rupture is reported to be between 10 and 30%, it is rarely an isolated injury. In the acute setting, patients often die of associated trauma rather than the rupture. Although congenital diaphragmatic hernias (Bochdalek and Morgagni types) are not uncommon entities in pediatric populations, such nontraumatic diaphragmatic hernias are exceedingly rare in the adult population. Only about 100 cases have been reported in the world literature.

Cadaver studies and case reviews have established a left-sided predominance to herniation. The diaphragm may be injured at any point; however, most ruptures occur on the left and in a radial, posterolateral direction corresponding to a point of embryologic weakness. The relative infrequency of right-sided herniation is believed to be the result of the protective presence of the liver. Bilateral diaphragmatic rupture is becoming rare. The pathophysiologic effects of diaphragmatic rupture result from the herniation of abdominal contents into the thoracic cavity. The colon is the most common organ that herniates, followed by the omentum and spleen. The herniated organs may be damaged by the explosive force of the injury or later may become strangulated and undergo infarction. Herniation may not occur at the time of rupture. A delayed diagnosis of diaphragmatic rupture in this situation is, unfortunately, common.

15. How is diaphragmatic rupture diagnosed?

It is often difficult to diagnose diaphragmatic rupture. Diagnosis and management of associated trauma often overshadow initial detection of diaphragmatic injury. The first step in diagnosis is recognizing the mechanisms of injury that predispose to injury of the diaphragm. Clinical clues to the diagnosis of diaphragmatic rupture include dyspnea and chest and abdominal pain. Physical examination findings may reveal diminished breath sounds and, rarely, peristalsis over the involved hemithorax. Traumatic ileus often obscures the latter finding. The chest radiograph is abnormal in 75–95% of patients with diaphragmatic rupture but highly suggestive (demonstrating a hollow viscus in the pleural space) in only about 25%. CT scanning is extremely accurate in the detection of herniated viscera but often fails to demonstrate a simple rupture. Contrast studies may be helpful; however, they have a significant false-negative rate. Thoracoscopy, laparoscopy, and liver-spleen scans have occasionally been used to demonstrate injury.

Chest Radiograph Abnormalities Suggesting Diaphragmatic Hernia

Irregularity of diaphragmatic outline or position
Abnormal gas shadows above and around diaphragm
Mediastinal shift with no obvious pulmonary or intrapleural cause
A supradiaphragmatic opacity or lucency
Presence of intestinal outline into the chest
Presence of a pneumothorax or pneumoperitoneum or both, after thoracic surgery

Adapted from Adamthwaite DN: Traumatic diaphragmatic hernia. Surg Annu 15:73–97, 1983; with permission.

16. How is diaphragmatic rupture managed?

Acute (less than 2 weeks old) diaphragmatic rupture is managed by early operative repair even in the absence of symptoms. A transabdominal approach is usually taken because of the high incidence of associated intraabdominal injuries. Delayed (2–3 weeks) and chronic (more than 3 weeks old) ruptures are most often repaired using a thoracotomy approach because of the dense intrathoracic adhesions that form over time. In cases of chronic diaphragmatic rupture, repair is attempted only if the patient is symptomatic.

17. How is the sniff test performed and interpreted?

The sniff test evaluates diaphragmatic movement during a forceful inspiratory effort. It is recommended that this test be performed with the patient awake, breathing spontaneously, and in the sitting position. In diaphragmatic paralysis, the plain chest radiograph may demonstrate that one or both of the hemidiaphragms appear elevated. Fluoroscopy showing at least 2 cm of paradoxical upward movement of the affected hemidiaphragm during the sniffing maneuver confirms the diagnosis of unilateral diaphragmatic paralysis. In bilateral diaphragmatic paralysis, fluoroscopy can be misleading because patients may be able to push their abdominal wall outward and thereby decrease intraabdominal pressure and move both diaphragms downward during a sniffing effort. Ultrasonographic evaluation of diaphragmatic motion has been used as a noninvasive tool to assess suspected diaphragm paralysis. With this method, the thickness as well as the motion of the diaphragm can be evaluated.

18. Can the respiratory muscles be trained?

Various studies have demonstrated that respiratory muscles can be trained to improve strength and endurance, especially in patients with COPD. Strength training can be achieved with the use of high-intensity, low-frequency stimuli. Inspiratory muscles are trained by inspiring against a closed glottis or a shutter. Endurance training is achieved by low-intensity, high-frequency training. The training programs are of three types: flow resistance loading, threshold loading, and voluntary isocapnic hyperpnea.

19. How does pursed-lip breathing affect diaphragmatic function?

Pursed-lip breathing results in slower and deeper respirations, with a significant increase in oxygenation and shift in voluntary muscle recruitment from the diaphragm to the accessory muscles. During exercise, the shift to pursed-lip breathing results in decreased dyspnea. Unfortunately, this pattern of breathing is used only temporarily by most patients. No data exist as to the long-term effectiveness of pursed-lip breathing or other retraining modalities.

20. What are the indications for a diaphragmatic pacer?

The main indication for the diaphragmatic pacer is a ventilator-dependent patient who has sustained high cervical cord injury, usually caused by a traffic, sporting, or diving accident or a gunshot wound. The second important group of patients are those with central alveolar hypoventilation (CAH) associated with central apneas. CAH may be either idiopathic (Ondine's curse) or secondary to organic lesions in the brain stem, e.g., stroke or encephalitis.

21. What requirements must be fulfilled before a diaphragmatic pacer is placed?

Successful diaphragm pacing requires good phrenic nerve and diaphragmatic muscle function. The best technique for assessing this is documentation of the contractile response of each hemidiaphragm to electrical stimulation of each phrenic nerve by surface electrodes in the neck. The movement of each hemidiaphragm can be assessed by radiographic screening or by ultrasound. Descent of 5 cm or more usually indicates that pacing will be successful.

BIBLIOGRAPHY

1. Adamthwaite DN: Traumatic diaphragmatic hernia. Surg Annu 15:73–97, 1983.
2. Bellemare F, Grassino A: Evaluation of human diaphragm fatigue. J Appl Physiol 53:1196–1206, 1982.
3. Benditt JO: Evaluation of respiratory muscles in the intensive care unit. Clin Pulm Med 2:286–294, 1995.
4. Celli BR: The clinical use of upper extremity exercise. Clin Chest Med 15:339–349, 1994.
5. Celli BR: Pulmonary rehabilitation in patients with COPD. Am J Respir Care Med 152:861–864, 1995.
6. De Troyer A, Kelly S, Macklem PT, et al: Mechanics of intercostal space and action of external and internal intercostal muscles. J Clin Invest 75:850–857, 1985.
7. Estenne M, Yernault JC, De Smet SM, et al: Phrenic and diaphragm function after coronary artery bypass grafting. Thorax 40:293–299, 1985.
8. Grassino A, Clanton T: Respiratory muscle fatigue. Semin Respir Med 12:305–321, 1991.
9. Gibson GJ: Diaphragmatic paresis: Pathophysiology, clinical features, and investigation. Thorax 44:966–970, 1989.
10. Leith DE, Bradley M: Ventilatory muscle strain and endurance training. J Appl Physiol 4:508–516, 1976.
11. Martin JG, Levy RD: Respiratory muscle rest. In Tobin MJ (ed): The Respiratory Muscles. Philadelphia, J.B. Lippincott, 1990, pp 534–541.
12. Mead J: Functional significance of the area of apposition of diaphragm to rib cage. Am Rev Respir Dis 119:31–32, 1979.
13. Moxham J, Gogmstone J: Assessments of respiratory muscle strength in the intensive care unit. Eur Respir J 7:2057–2061, 1994.
14. Moxham J, Shneerson JM: Diaphragmatic pacing. Am Rev Respir Dis 148:533–536, 1993.
15. NHLBI Workshop Summary: Respiratory muscle fatigue. Am Rev Respir Dis 142:474–480, 1990.
16. Roussos C, Macklem PT: The respiratory muscles. N Engl J Med 307:786–797, 1982.
17. Tobin MJ: Respiratory muscles in disease. Clin Chest Med 9:263–286, 1988.
18. Tobin MJ: Respiratory muscle involvement in chronic obstructive pulmonary disease and asthma. In Tobin MJ (ed): The Respiratory Muscles. Philadelphia, J.B. Lippincott, 1990, p 377.
19. Wise L, Connors J, Hwang Y: Traumatic injuries of the diaphragm. J Trauma 13:946–950, 1973.

XVII. Special Considerations

79. PULMONARY DISEASE IN PREGNANCY

Elizabeth L. Aronsen, M.D.

1. Does normal pregnancy affect pulmonary function?

Yes. Both pulmonary mechanics and physiology are affected during normal pregnancy in the following ways:

Mechanics. The diaphragm is progressively displaced upward during pregnancy, to a maximum of about 4 cm. The anteroposterior and transverse diameters of the chest also increase about 2 cm. These anatomic changes decrease total pulmonary compliance and increase work of breathing late in pregnancy because of the decreased chest wall compliance.

Physiology. Residual volume (RV) and expiratory reserve volume (ERV) decrease as the diaphragm elevates during pregnancy, resulting in a decrease in functional reserve capacity (FRC) since FRC equals RV plus ERV. Inspiratory capacity (IC) actually increases, however, thus preserving both vital capacity (VC), which is the sum of IC and ERV, and total lung capacity (TLC), which is the sum of VC and RV. Respiratory muscle function and airflow, as measured by FEV_1 and forced vital capacity (FVC), also remain unchanged in normal pregnancy.

2. Why do so many patients complain of shortness of breath during pregnancy?

"Dyspnea of pregnancy" is a common complaint and is often accompanied by hyperventilation. An increase in tidal volume (Vt) rather than respiratory rate (RR) increases minute ventilation (Ve; Ve = RR × Vt) by as much as 50%. The mechanism is probably respiratory center stimulation by progesterone. An elevated diaphragm can produce lower lung atelectasis resulting in crackles on examination. Decreased colloid oncotic pressure results in peripheral edema. Both of these findings may be present in a patient with benign dyspnea of pregnancy or in one with significant pulmonary disease. One clue to the latter is the presence of significant tachypnea. Differential diagnoses that should be ruled out include pulmonary infections, reactive obstructive airway disease (asthma, pulmonary vascular disease, especially thromboembolism), cardiogenic or noncardiogenic pulmonary edema, and acute lung injury.

3. What pulmonary infections are of particular importance in pregnancy?

The agents that cause bacterial pneumonia in pregnant women include *Pneumococcus, Hemophilus influenzae,* and atypical bacterial organisms. No causative agent is found in as many as one third of presumed bacterial pneumonias. Aspiration of oral flora may result in anaerobic pneumonia that may have a cavitary appearance on chest roentgenograms. Influenza A and varicella are important causes of viral pneumonia in the pregnant patient. Less commonly, fungal or mycobacterial organisms may cause pulmonary disease in pregnant patients at risk. **Mendelson's syndrome** is not a pulmonary infection but the aspiration of liquid or particulate gastric contents by the pregnant patient, resulting in pneumonitis or airway obstruction, respectively.

4. Why are pregnant patients considered at increased risk of pneumonia?

Both immunologic and physiologic changes as well as comorbid illnesses increase the risk of pneumonia during pregnancy, as follows:

Immunologic factors	**Comorbid illness**

Immunologic factors
- Decreased number of T4 cells
- Decreased cell-mediated cytotoxicity
- Decreased lymphokine response to alloantigens
- Decreased lymphocyte proliferative response

Physiologic changes
- Atelectasis from diaphragmatic elevation
- Increased baseline oxygen consumption
- Increased lung water
- Increased risk of aspiration (especially during labor and delivery)

Comorbid illness
- Tobacco use
- Illicit drug use
- HIV infection
- Preexisting heart or lung disease
- Anemia
- Immunosuppressive therapy

5. Why is varicella pneumonia a major concern during pregnancy?

Mortality from varicella pneumonia is markedly increased during pregnancy, approaching 4% in some studies compared with 1–2% in the nonpregnant population. Major fetal complications also occur in these patients, including in utero death, prematurity, or neonatal varicella.

6. How do the pulmonary complications of HIV disease contribute to morbidity in pregnancy?

HIV infection confers additional risks to the pregnant patient of unusual infectious and noninfectious pulmonary complications, including *Pneumocystis carinii* pneumonia (PCP), tuberculosis (TB), toxoplasmosis, and lymphoma. Both the therapy for these diseases and the disease itself can be detrimental to the fetus. For example, PCP is ordinarily treated with trimethoprim-sulfamethoxazole combinations; trimethoprim is a potential teratogen and sulfonamides have been linked to hyperbilirubinemia and kernicterus. Toxoplasmosis, also treated with sulfas, is linked to blindness when acquired in utero. Zidovudine therapy is usually not stopped during pregnancy and, in fact, can reduce vertical transmission of the HIV virus from 25% to about 8%. Hypoxemia, the result of the pulmonary complications, causes decreased uterine blood flow and fetal hypoxia. These, in turn, lead to intrauterine growth retardation (IUGR) and low birth weight or small for gestational age (SGA) infants.

7. How is tuberculosis diagnosed and managed in pregnancy?

TB represents a significant risk to both mother and fetus as well as a public health risk. Diagnosis is often delayed because the patient is asymptomatic or there is a reluctance to expose the fetus to the radiation from a radiologic examination. The result is an increase in the incidence of advanced lesions. Inadequate, incomplete, or irregular therapy leads to increased resistance, increased spread of infection to contacts, and increased fetal morbidity including two-fold increases in prematurity, SGA and low birth weight infants, and a six-fold increase in the risk of perinatal death. Active TB should be treated without delay. Treatment does not need to be modified in lactating mothers. In the case of a normal chest radiograph and recent conversion, isoniazid prophylaxis is started after the third trimester. In the case of a normal radiograph and remote conversion or in the case of an abnormal radiograph in an asymptomatic patient who is not likely to have active TB, INH therapy is started after delivery.

8. How does pregnancy affect asthma?

About 1% of all pregnancies are complicated by asthma; of the patients affected, about 1% have exacerbations serious enough to require hospitalization. Of patients with asthma who become pregnant, about one third experience no change in their disease, slightly more than half find that their asthma is worse during pregnancy, and the rest improve. The majority (nearly 75%) of asthmatic patients return to their nonpregnant baseline within 3 months after delivery. In two-thirds, the course of asthma in subsequent pregnancies is similar to that in the first pregnancy. The reasons for differences in the course of reactive airway disease in different pregnant patients probably involves a delicate balance between bronchodilatory (e.g., cortisol, cyclic adenosine monophosphate, prostaglandins E_1 and E_2) and bronchoconstricting (e.g., estrogen, cyclic guanosine monophosphate, prostaglandin $F_{2\alpha}$) substances elaborated during this time.

9. What are the goals of asthma therapy during pregnancy?

The goals of therapy in the pregnant asthmatic are the same as those in the nonpregnant patient with asthma: monitor symptoms, avoid triggers, medicate appropriately, and educate the patient. The difference is that now fetal health is important as well.

- **Monitor symptoms,** generally via spirometry and peak flow measurement of maternal airflow as well as fetal "kick counts" to track fetal well being.
- **Avoid triggers.** Most patients have a clear idea of what triggers their asthma attacks such as infection, odors, vigorous exercise, dust, pollen, or animal danders. A careful history can elicit these triggers and the patient can be given ideas as to how to avoid them.
- **Medicate appropriately.** The primary goal of medical therapy is to maintain maternal health and thereby fetal oxygenation. Although most medications are FDA-approved without being tested in pregnant populations and some are contraindicated because of adverse fetal effects, poorly controlled asthma is clearly associated with maternal morbidity (hyperemesis gravidarum, toxemia, labor complications) and fetal morbidity (low birth weight, prematurity) whereas well-controlled asthma has no significant morbidity over that of the general population. The medications used in asthma exacerbations during pregnancy are essentially the same as those used in the nonpregnant asthmatic patient, and include the following:

  Antiinflammatory agents (steroids, cromolyn)
  Bronchodilators (β-agonists, theophylline)
  Antihistamines (chlorpheniramine, tripelennamine)
  Decongestants (pseudoephedrine, oxymetazoline)
  Antitussives (guaifenesin, dextromethorphan)
  Antibiotics (amoxicillin)

The medications indicated in parentheses are recommendations given in the report of the NIH Working Group on Asthma and Pregnancy.

- **Educate the patient.** For treatment to be effective, the patient must be educated to avoid precipitants of her asthma, to monitor her peak flows, and to seek early medical intervention when peak flow drops below 80% of her usual best. Medical compliance is greatly enhanced by good physician-patient communication.

10. How should status asthmaticus be managed during pregnancy?

Status asthmaticus is one of the most feared complications of asthma during pregnancy. The treating physician must be aware of the risk factors and therapeutic interventions.

- **Risk factors**

  History of previous intubation for asthma
  Frequent emergency department visits (three per month) for asthma
  Frequent hospitalizations (two per year) for asthma
  Recent corticosteroid withdrawal
  History of syncope or seizure with an asthma attack
  Coexisting psychiatric or psychosocial disease

- **Therapy**

  Oxygen
  Rapid-onset β-agonists
  Magnesium sulfate
  Terbutaline
  Methylprednisolone
  Aminophylline

Some of the therapeutic agents act as tocolytics (β-agonists, terbutaline) and can both inhibit labor and produce pulmonary edema. Close fetal and maternal monitoring is required during an asthma exacerbation, and intubation may be necessary. If mechanical ventilation is required in the management of status asthmaticus, difficult choices must be made regarding paralysis and permissive hypercapnia because of potential adverse effects on uterine muscle tone and uterine blood flow, respectively.

11. How should thromboembolic disease be diagnosed and treated during pregnancy?

Although outcomes in the nonpregnant patient with deep venous thrombosis (DVT) and pulmonary thromboembolic (PE) disease have improved, morbidity and mortality in the pregnant patient have been unchanged in recent studies.

Diagnosis requires high clinical suspicion in the right setting. At risk patients are often multiparous, in the second or third trimester of pregnancy, and may have a family or personal prior history of DVT or PE. The abdominal position of the inferior vena cava results in more frequent left versus right lower extremity DVT. Patients typically present with acute onset of shortness of breath, perhaps with pleuritic chest pain and a pleural rub. Signs are typical and include tachypnea, tachycardia, hypoxemia, and electrocardiographic changes of right axis deviation. Duplex ultrasonography, impedance plethysmography, or a lung ventilation-perfusion ($\dot{V}/\dot{Q}$) scan can be used to support the diagnosis. A $\dot{V}/\dot{Q}$ scan provides less than 0.05 rads to the fetus. A limited venogram with the abdomen shielded or pulmonary angiography using a brachial arterial approach has a fetal radiation risk similar to that of the $\dot{V}/\dot{Q}$ scan, if further diagnostic examination is necessary.

The **therapy** of choice for thromboembolic disease during pregnancy is heparin. Warfarin is associated with fetal abnormalities such as brachydactyly, bone stippling, and nasal cartilage hypoplasia (warfarin embropathy). Vena cava filters or disruption have also been used. Thrombolytic therapy is rarely indicated except when life-threatening hemodynamic instability is present.

12. What is amniotic fluid embolism?

Amniotic fluid embolism is an unpredictable catastrophic peripartum event with an 80–90% mortality that generally occurs during any of the three stages of labor or immediately post partum. Patients develop acute onset of respiratory distress, cyanosis, circulatory collapse, and shock. Risk factors include tumultuous labor, uterine stimulant use, advanced maternal age, multiparity, intrauterine death, meconium amniotic fluid staining, and premature placental separation. A complex mechanism involves pulmonary microcirculatory obstruction with capillary leak secondary to vasoactive and inflammatory cytokine release, and secondary ventilation-perfusion mismatching. Maternal morbidity results from pulmonary edema or hemorrhage, disseminated intravascular coagulation, cardiac failure, and convulsions. The diagnosis, often made at autopsy, can be supported in the antemortem period by finding squamous cells in blood obtained from a pulmonary arterial catheter. Therapy is mainly supportive.

13. What is the differential diagnosis of pulmonary edema in pregnancy?

Pulmonary edema in pregnancy has cardiogenic and noncardiogenic causes, including all the causes in the nonpregnant patient. Tocolytic-induced pulmonary edema is unique to the pregnant patient and occurs during or up to 12 hours after cessation of therapy. Risk factors for pulmonary edema in pregnancy include late gestation infection or concomitant cardiac disease with either left ventricular systolic or diastolic dysfunction. Pulmonary edema is more than twice as common in the postpartum period as it is in preeclampsia. Therapy is the same as for the nonpregnant patient and incudes stopping tocolytics in patients receiving these agents or starting antibiotics in patients with sepsis, and use of oxygen, diuretics, digoxin, and afterload reduction. There is no reason to withhold digitalis therapy in the pregnant patient with heart failure.

BIBLIOGRAPHY

1. Chatelain SM, Quirk JG Jr: Amniotic and thromboembolism. Clin Obstet Gynecol 33:473-481, 1990.
2. Crapo RO: Normal cardiopulmonary physiology in pregnancy. Clin Obstet Gynecol 39:17–35, 1996.

3. Elkus R, Popovich J Jr: Respiratory physiology in pregnancy. Clin Chest Med 13:555-565, 1992.
4. Fidler JL, Patz EF Jr, Ravin CE: Cardiopulmonary complications of pregnancy: Radiographic findings. AJR Am J Roentgenol 161:937-942, 1993.
5. Hollingsworth HM, Irwin RS: Acute respiratory failure in pregnancy. Clin Chest Med 13:723-740, 1992.
6. Hornby PJ, Abrahams TP: Pulmonary pharmacology. Clin Obstet Gynecol 39:17-35, 1996.
7. Jana N, Vasishta K, Jindal SK, et al: Perinatal outcome in pregnancies complicated by pulmonary tuberculosis. Int J Gynaecol Obstet 44:119-124, 1994.
8. Lapinsy SE, Kruczynski K, Slutsky AS: Critical care of the pregnant patient. Am J Respir Crit Care Med 152:427-455, 1995.
9. Management of Asthma during Pregnancy. Report of the Working Group on Asthma and Pregnancy. NIH Publication No. 93-3279, September 1993.
10. McColgin SW, Glee L, Brian BA: Pulmonary disorders complicating pregnancy. Obstet Gynecol Clin North Am 19:697-717, 1992.
11. Moore-Gillon J: Asthma in pregnancy. Br J Obstet Gynaecol 101:658-660, 1994.
12. Perlow JH, Montgomery D, Morgan MA, et al: Severity of asthma and perinatal outcome. Part I. Am J Obstet Gynecol 167:963-967, 1992.
13. Phelan JP: Pulmonary edema in obstetrics. Obstet Gynecol Clin North Am 18:319-331, 1991.
14. Zeldis SM: Dyspnea during pregnancy. Distinguishing cardiac from pulmonary causes. Clin Chest Med 13:567-585, 1992.

80. PULMONARY MANIFESTATIONS OF SYSTEMIC DISEASE

Robert H. Poe, M.D., and Douglas W. Booth, R.R.T.

1. Name some pulmonary manifestations of systemic disease.

Pulmonary Manifestations of Systemic Disease

SYSTEM	DISORDER	MANIFESTATION
Cardiovascular	Congestive heart failure	Decreased expiratory flow
		Reflex bronchoconstriction
		Reduced lung volumes
		Decreased diffusion
		Hypoxemia
		Pleural effusions
	Mitral valve disease	Reduced lung compliance
		Increased work of breathing
		Pulmonary hypertension
	Postcardiac injury syndrome	Pericarditis
		Pleuritis
		Pneumonitis
Endocrine	Thyrotoxicosis	Dyspnea
		Increased oxygen consumption
		Increased carbon dioxide production
		Decreased diffusion
		Decreased lung compliance
		Weakness of respiratory muscles
		Pulmonary hypertension
		Tracheal compression

Table continued on following page.

Pulmonary Manifestations of Systemic Disease (Continued)

SYSTEM	DISORDER	MANIFESTATION
Endocrine	Hypothyroidism	Decreased control of ventilatory response to hypoxia and hypercapnia
		Obstructive sleep apnea
		Pleural effusions
		Weakness of respiratory muscles
	Diabetes mellitus	Staphylococcal and gram-negative pneumonias
		Reactivation tuberculosis
Gastrointestinal	Pancreatitis	Hypoxemia
		Pulmonary infiltrates
		Pleural effusions
		ARDS
	Crohn's disease	Granulomatous lung involvement
	Ulcerative colitis	Purulent bronchitis
		Bronchiectasis
	Cirrhosis	Hypoxemia caused by:
		Intrapulmonary shunts
		Portopulmonary anastomoses
		Pleural "spiders"
		Pulmonary hypertension
		Pulmonary vasoconstriction
		$\dot{V}/\dot{Q}$ mismatching
	Gastroesophageal reflux disease	Cough caused by:
		Sensory cough reflex stimulation
		Aspiration
Hematologic	Sickle cell disease	Acute chest syndrome
		Rib infarctions
		Pneumococcal infections
		Fat embolism
	Bone marrow transplantation	Pulmonary edema
		Cyclosporine lung toxicity
		Transfusion reactions
		ARDS
		Opportunistic infections
		Pulmonary embolism
		Veno-occlusive disease
Renal	End-stage renal disease/ hemodialysis	Hypoxemia

2. How does congestive heart failure affect the results of pulmonary function tests?

Chronic left-sided congestive heart failure results in several changes in lung ventilatory function. The edema in the peribronchial interstitium leads to early airway closure during expiration with air trapping and an increase in residual volume. Reflex bronchoconstriction leads to a decrease in expiratory flow rates, FEV_1, vital capacity and total lung capacity. Increased perfusion of underventilated lung leads to a functional right-to-left shunt. Uneven ventilation of other better perfused areas increases dead space. The resulting ventilation-perfusion mismatch causes an increase in the alveolar-arterial oxygen gradient and a decrease in the carbon monoxide diffusing capacity. Since minute ventilation is typically increased, the ability to exchange carbon dioxide is preserved and the arterial P_{CO_2} is usually reduced.

3. What radiographic features suggest that a pleural effusion is caused by congestive heart failure?

The chest radiograph usually shows additional signs of congestive heart failure (e.g., enlarged cardiac silhouette, vascular redistribution, Kerley B lines and bronchial cuffing) if pleural effusions are related. Unilateral effusions resulting from congestive heart failure are most frequently right-sided. For effusions that are bilateral with a normal-sized heart, loculated on decubitus radiographic films, unilateral and large, or have characteristics of an exudate, other causes should be considered, including malignancy, infection, or pulmonary emboli.

4. How does mitral valve disease affect the lung?

Mitral valve disease causes chronic elevation of left atrial pressure. This, in turn, results in structural and functional alterations in the pulmonary vasculature that eventually lead to a reduction in lung compliance and an increase in the work of breathing. Dyspnea at rest is a common complaint. Pulmonary hypertension is caused over time by hyperplasia and hypertrophy of the pulmonary vessels in concert with passive transmission of pulmonary venous pressure to the pulmonary artery and an active pulmonary vasoconstriction. The changes can be reversed with corrective surgery or catheter balloon valvotomy.

5. What is postcardiac injury, or Dressler's, syndrome?

Postcardiac injury syndrome is the development of pericarditis, pleuritis, and pneumonitis 1–12 weeks after any one of several forms of cardiac injury. It occurs most frequently after cardiac surgery but can be seen after myocardial infarction, chest trauma, pacemaker implantation, and diagnostic left ventricular puncture as well. Fever, leukocytosis, auscultatory evidence of pleural and pericardial friction rubs, and a pronounced elevation of the erythrocyte sedimentation rate are manifestations. The chest radiograph shows a pleural effusion, usually left sided, often with accompanying infiltrate. The cause remains obscure, but antimyocardial antibodies, probably a nonspecific response to cardiac injury, have been identified in patients with the syndrome. The diagnosis remains clinical and one of exclusion.

6. What is the most common respiratory symptom of thyrotoxicosis?

Dyspnea is the most common complaint in thyrotoxicosis. Its severity varies from patient to patient and the cause is unclear, although the following have been implicated as possible causes:

    Increased oxygen consumption and carbon dioxide production
    Increased minute ventilation with tachypnea
    Decreased vital capacity and carbon monoxide diffusing capacity
    Decreased lung compliance
    Respiratory muscle weakness
    Increased ventilatory responses to hypoxia and hypercapnia
    High-output left ventricular failure
    Pulmonary artery dilatation with pulmonary hypertension
    Tracheal compression by the enlarged gland

7. How does hypothyroidism affect the respiratory system?

Hypothyroidism decreases central ventilatory responses to hypoxia and hypercapnia, which can lead to respiratory failure and eventual coma. Upper airway obstruction occurs with an increased incidence of sleep apnea, most often obstructive, because of an enlarged tongue or constricted oropharynx (from soft tissue mucopolysaccharide and protein deposition) or myopathic changes in the muscles of the upper airway. Pleural effusions (both unilateral and bilateral, transudate and exudate), the cause of which remains controversial, have been observed. Lastly, muscle weakness combined with obesity can decrease lung volumes with ventilation-perfusion mismatch leading to hypoxemia and carbon dioxide retention.

8. Why is the diabetic patient susceptible to pulmonary infection?

The mechanisms for the increased susceptibility of the diabetic to infection are incompletely understood. Impaired chemotactic, phagocytic, and bactericidal activity of the neutrophil is believed responsible in some part for infections with staphylococci and gram-negative bacteria. Similar reasons probably account for the observation that diabetes is the single most common underlying condition in patients presenting with community-acquired pneumonia. Hyperglycemia decreases intracellular bactericidal activity of lymphocytes and may explain the increase in infection during hyperglycemia and ketoacidosis. Impaired phagocytic activity of monocytes may increase the risk of fungal infections such as mucormycosis. Reactivation tuberculosis was two to three times more common in diabetics in early surveys, presumably because of poor nutrition and decreased cellular immunity, but currently is not an issue.

9. List the pulmonary effects of acute pancreatitis. What is their significance?

The pulmonary manifestations of acute pancreatitis range from asymptomatic reductions in arterial oxygenation, more significant hypoxemia with a normal chest radiograph, nonspecific parenchymal infiltrates and effusions, to a diffuse pulmonary involvement characteristic of ARDS, which occurs in about 15% of patients with acute pancreatitis. The onset of pulmonary symptoms in the patient with acute pancreatitis portends a poor prognosis. Sixty percent of deaths from acute pancreatitis that occur within the first week are associated with respiratory failure, and only 25% of those requiring mechanical ventilation survive. After the second week, pulmonary complications are usually the result of pancreatic infection or pseudocyst formation.

10. Is there an association between granulomatous bowel disease and sarcoidosis?

Possibly. In bronchoalveolar lavage fluid from patients with Crohn's disease lymphocytes predominate and the T4 subset increases during periods of active intestinal disease, similar to the increase in T4 cells found in patients with sarcoidosis. The granulomatous lung involvement occasionally seen in patients with Crohn's disease improves, as does sarcoidosis, with corticosteroid therapy. A similar immunologic abnormality may be common to both disorders.

11. Is there a relationship between ulcerative colitis and airway disease?

In several series of patients with ulcerative colitis, concomitant bronchial disease, including both bronchiectasis and purulent bronchitis, has been described. These pulmonary manifestations appear to be unrelated to the activity of or therapy for the bowel disease. In these patients, the chest radiograph may be normal and pulmonary function testing has shown no consistent abnormality. Biopsies of lung tissue may show thickening of the epithelium and basement membrane with inflammatory cell infiltration of the underlying connective tissue. A common abnormality in immune regulation affecting both bowel and bronchi has been postulated. High-dose corticosteroid therapy often leads to clinical improvement.

12. Why does the patient with hepatic cirrhosis become hypoxic?

Several factors are responsible. The predominant cause is intrapulmonary shunting associated with vascular dilatations in the lungs. These dilatations occur both at the precapillary level and as direct arteriovenous communications; they are associated commonly with orthodeoxia, platypnea, and spider nevi of the skin and when associated with the other clinical features of cirrhosis constitute the "hepatopulmonary syndrome." Other causes of hypoxia include portopulmonary vein anastomoses, pleural "spiders," pulmonary hypertension, impaired pulmonary vasoconstriction and ventilation-perfusion mismatching.

13. How does gastroesophageal reflux cause cough?

Cough may be the sole presenting symptom of gastroesophageal reflux. Cough is believed to be caused by one of three mechanisms. Reflux of stomach contents may irritate the esophageal mucosa and initiate the cough reflex through vagal sensory pathways. Stomach contents may be aspirated and irritate sensory receptors of the tracheobronchial tree. Lastly, stomach contents may reach the hypopharynx and larynx, irritating the afferent limb of the cough reflex without aspiration. Diagnosis is certain only when the cough goes away in response to antireflux therapy.

14. What is the "acute chest syndrome" of sickle cell anemia?

The combination of pleuritic chest pain, fever, cough, and parenchymal infiltrates on chest radiograph constitutes the acute chest syndrome. Infectious pneumonia and sickling of the abnormal red blood cells, either singly or in combination, are usually responsible. Rib infarctions, which are commonly observed radiologically, may also play a role in the pathogenesis. In situ thrombosis leading to pulmonary infarction may also occur. Manifestations of the involvement of other organs—including hemiplegia and an altered mental status, renal failure, and petechiae—suggest fat embolism, which can occur in these patients. Recurrent episodes of acute chest syndrome may result in the development of chronic lung disease.

15. What pulmonary complications can occur after bone marrow transplantation?

Patients undergoing bone marrow transplantation after aggressive salvage chemoradiation therapy are at high risk for pulmonary disease. Early in the course (within the first 100 days after transplantation), pulmonary edema from fluid overload or myocardial injury, hemorrhagic edema from cyclosporine toxicity, and transfusion reactions are seen. ARDS from sepsis and pneumonia (bacterial, fungal caused by candidiasis or aspergillosis, and viral caused by cytomegalovirus), should also be considered. Interstitial pneumonitis from infections with *Pneumocystis carinii* or cytomegalovirus or due to chemotherapy, pulmonary embolism, and veno-occlusive disease are also possible during this period.

Late complications include bronchopneumonia from the aforementioned infections, fat embolism, veno-occlusive disease, interstitial pneumonitis of a nonspecific nature, bronchiolitis obliterans, lymphocytic interstitial pneumonitis, and graft-versus-host disease.

16. Why would a respiratory therapist be asked to administer nebulized albuterol to a patient with end-stage renal disease?

β-2 Agonists in nebulized form substantially lower plasma potassium levels in normal subjects. Doses four to eightfold higher than those used to treat asthma are effective in treating acute hyperkalemia. A 10-mg dose decreases plasma potassium by 0.6 mmol per liter and 20 mg by 1.0 mmol per liter within 30 minutes; the effect lasts for 2 hours. Potassium is shifted from the extracellular to the intracellular compartment. An additive potassium lowering effect is seen when nebulized albuterol is administered with intravenous insulin plus glucose. In general, this therapeutic modality is well tolerated with little effect on heart rate, blood pressure, or arterial saturation.

CONTROVERSIES

17. Why does hypoxemia occur during hemodialysis?

Transient hypoxemia is sometimes seen within 15 minutes of initiation of hemodialysis and is sometimes severe enough to be symptomatic or exacerbate myocardial ischemia. The mechanism postulated to explain the fall in P_{AO_2} is acetate in the bath causing hypoventilation and increased oxygen consumption. Dialysance of carbon dioxide and bicarbonate causes hypocapnia with a lag in bicarbonate regeneration from acetate metabolism. High bicarbonate baths cause metabolic alkalosis. The compensating hypoventilation causes hypercapnia, which can be prevented by decreasing the bicarbonate concentration in the bath. Hypoxia can also result from complement activation by a bioincompatible dialyzer membrane, which can cause leukostasis and plugging of the pulmonary capillaries with resulting hypoxemia. This effect can be reduced by use of synthetic membranes and citrate anticoagulation. In some cases hypoxemia may persist after dialysis has ended.

18. How much oxygen should be administered to a patient with sickle cell anemia who has acute chest syndrome?

Hypoxemia is frequently a sequela of acute chest syndrome. Maintenance of an adequate level of oxygenation is necessary to reduce the adverse effects of hypoxia. Although oxygen may reduce the further sickling that occurs in these patients when the oxygen tension is reduced, it apparently does not alter the duration of the event, presumably because of the damage caused by vaso-occlusion before its administration. Administration of inspired oxygen at a high concentration, in excess of that necessary to maintain a safe level of saturation, traditionally has not been recommended on the basis that it suppresses erythropoiesis. However, the suppression of erythropoiesis in this situation is poorly defined. The hemoglobin level and reticulocyte count have been shown to fall in patients on oxygen therapy and monitoring is advised, although the current belief is that oxygen concentrations of 50% or less are unlikely to do harm, aside from the discomfort associated with the administration.

BIBLIOGRAPHY

1. Allon M: Treatment and prevention of hyperkalemia in endstage renal disease. Kidney Internat 43:1197-1209, 1993.
2. Beutler E: The sickle cell diseases and related disorders. In Beutler E, Lichtman MA, Coller BS, et al (eds): Williams Hematology, 5th ed. New York, McGraw-Hill, 1995.
3. Castro O, Brambilla DJ, Thorington B, et al: The acute chest syndrome in sickle cell disease: Incidence and risk factors. Blood 84:643-649, 1994.
4. Dawson A: The respiratory system. In Haubrich WS, Schaffner F, Berk JE (eds): Bockus Gastroenterology, 5th ed. Philadelphia, WB Saunders, 1995.
5. Gaasch WH, O'Rourke RH, Cohn LH, et al: Mitral valve disease. In Schlant RC, Alexander RW (eds): The Heart, Arteries and Veins, 8th ed. New York, McGraw-Hill, 1994.
6. Ingbar DH: The respiratory system in thyrotoxicosis. In Braverman LE, Utiger RD (eds): Werner and Ingbar's The Thyroid. A Fundamental and Clinical Text, 6th ed. Philadelphia, JB Lippincott, 1991.
7. Jameson MD, Wiegmann TB: Principles, uses and complications of hemodialysis. Med Clin North Am 74:945-960, 1990.
8. Lange PA, Stoller JK: The hepatopulmonary syndrome. Ann Intern Med 122:521-529, 1995.
9. Musher DM: Streptococcus pneumonia. In Mandell GL, Bennett JE, Dolin R, (eds): Principles and Practice of Infectious Disease, 4th ed. New York, Churchill Livingstone, 1995.
10. Sentochnik DE, Eliopoulous GM: Infections and Diabetes. In Kahn CR, Weir GC, (eds): Joslin's Diabetes Mellitus, 13th ed. Philadelphia, Lea & Febiger, 1994.
11. Smlejan JM, Cosnes J, Chollet-Martin S, et al: Sarcoid-like lymphocytes of the lower respiratory tract in patients with active Crohn's disease. Ann Intern Med 104:17-21, 1986.
12. Zipursky A, Robieux IC, Brown RT, et al: Oxygen therapy in sickle cell disease. Am J Pediatr Hematol Oncol 14:222-228, 1992.

XVIII. Surgical Considerations

81. PREOPERATIVE ASSESSMENT OF THE PULMONARY PATIENT

David J. Tardio, M.D., and Gerald N. Olsen, M.D.

1. Define *postoperative pulmonary complication*.

A *complication* is a factor that changes the management of the patient. In contrast, a *finding* is the result of an investigation and may occur in an asymptomatic patient (for example, a reduction in PaO_2). Examples of postoperative pulmonary complications (PPCs) include atelectasis requiring additional respiratory therapy or bronchoscopy, purulent bronchitis, pneumonia, pulmonary edema, pulmonary embolism, and respiratory failure. Complications that cause death are called *postoperative mortality* and those that increase the length and cost of care are called *postoperative morbidity*.

2. Who is at increased risk for postoperative pulmonary complications?

Obviously, not everyone undergoing surgery is at equal risk for developing PPCs. Patients with a history of cardiovascular disease or obstructive airway disease have a higher risk of perioperative complications. Other reported risk factors include advanced age, male gender, smoking history (particularly if the patient has a history of more than 20 pack-years), chronic cough, prolonged anesthesia, and the location of the incision (a general rule of thumb is that the further from the diaphragm, the lower the risk). Severe obesity has been reported to be a risk factor for PPCs; however, stomach reduction procedures (e.g., stapling), called *bariatric surgery*, may be performed by skilled surgeons with very low mortality rates. Emergency procedures also carry greater risk, because the patient's cardiac or pulmonary disease may not be optimally managed before surgery.

3. How does pulmonary function change postoperatively?

After coronary bypass surgery or upper abdominal surgery vital capacity (VC) is temporarily reduced to 50–60% of the preoperative value. In addition, tidal volume is decreased and respiratory rate is increased, resulting in no net change in minute ventilation. Functional residual capacity (FRC) is also reduced after surgery; FRC normally returns to 90% of its baseline value by the fifth postoperative day. Lower abdominal surgery is also associated with a reduction in VC; however, these changes are less significant and usually resolve after 24 hours.

4. How does diaphragmatic function change after surgery?

After an incision in the thorax and upper abdomen, a reduction in diaphragmatic function occurs and may persist for up to 7 days postoperatively. The same type of dysfunction appears to occur after both open and laparoscopic cholecystectomy, but it is less severe and of shorter duration with the laparoscopic procedure. Research has demonstrated that the inherent contractility of the diaphragmatic muscle is not impaired, and the phrenic nerves function normally when stimulated. Complete relief of incisional pain also does not prevent the decrease in function. It is believed that an inhibitory reflex arising from either the sympathetic or the parasympathetic nervous system causes a reduction in phrenic nerve output, leading to a reduction in the contribution of the diaphragm to respiration. This decrease in diaphragmatic function is now accepted as the probable cause in most instances of postoperative atelectasis.

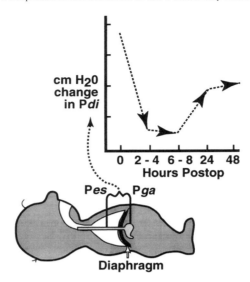

Postoperative diaphragmatic dysfunction is demonstrated as a decrease in transdiaphragmatic pressure (P*di*), which is measured as the difference between the pressure in the esophagus (P*es*) and the pressure in the stomach (P*ga*).

5. Does smoking cessation decrease the risk of PPCs?

A retrospective study of more than 1000 patients and a prospective study of 200 patients who had elective coronary artery bypass grafting (CABG) demonstrated statistically significant reductions in PPCs if the patients had quit smoking for longer than 8 weeks. The incidence of PPCs in patients who refrained from smoking for more than 6 months was similar to that of lifetime nonsmokers. The decreased number of complications has been attributed to decreased sputum production and improved tracheobronchial clearance. It has been suggested that heavy smokers may benefit from smoking cessation even a few hours before surgery, because the reduction in carboyxhemoglobin levels may improve oxygen delivery to the peripheral tissues. Obviously, there is never a bad time to encourage a patient to quit smoking.

6. How should bronchodilators be used before and during surgery?

Several studies have suggested that patients with obstructive airway disease may benefit from at least 48 hours of "tuning up" prior to surgery. Patients should receive bronchodilator therapy throughout the perioperative period to reduce the risk of bronchospasm. β-Agonists such as albuterol can be given every 4 hours before surgery and as needed via the endotracheal tube during the procedure. If acute bronchospasm develops during surgery, terbutaline, 0.25 mg, or 0.3 cc of 1:1000 epinephrine may be used subcutaneously. Epinephrine may precipitate cardiac ischemia in patients with coronary artery disease and is contraindicated in pregnancy.

7. Are perioperative corticosteroids useful?

Yes. Corticosteroid therapy may be useful for patients with severe COPD; it is particularly useful for asthmatic patients, because airway inflammation is a major pathologic feature of their disease. Corticosteroids should be started at least 6–12 hours before surgery to allow enough time to take effect. The optimal dose of corticosteroids has not been established, but 60–125 mg of methylprednisolone is usually given every 6 hours before and during surgery, with a rapid taper postoperatively. Concerns over decreased postoperative wound healing have led some physicians to recommend cessation of corticosteroid therapy for up to 3 days postoperatively.

The decision on wound healing versus respiratory function must be a clinical one based on assessment of the patient's greatest risk.

8. Is use of theophylline perioperatively beneficial?

Theophylline may benefit certain patients with COPD, particularly because of its inotropic effect on respiratory muscles. If the patient was previously on theophylline, its level should be checked preoperatively; if it is therapeutic (8–12 μg per dl), a maintenance intravenous infusion may be used during surgery. If the patient is not on theophylline or if the blood level is subtherapeutic, a loading dose may be given first. Because of the increased risk of cardiac arrhythmias, some would prefer giving only maintenance doses or withholding the drug entirely. Certain medications such as cimetidine and erythromycin may decrease metabolism, thus elevating theophylline levels, and recent tobacco use and other drugs such as phenobarbital may stimulate metabolism, thus lowering the levels.

9. Why is postoperative lung expansion important?

Several prospective studies have demonstrated that the incidence of PPCs can be reduced if techniques designed to increase lung volume are used postoperatively. As noted previously, a reflex inhibition of the diaphragm is thought to occur after thoracic and upper abdominal surgery, leading to a reduction in FRC. The reduced FRC results in alveolar collapse, leading to atelectasis and hypoxia. Lung expansion maneuvers can generate high transpulmonary (alveolar-pleural space) inflation pressures, which can help open the collapsed alveoli.

10. What techniques can be used to promote lung expansion?

Several devices and maneuvers increase lung volume postoperatively. Having the patient inspire to total lung capacity (TLC) is a simple, inexpensive technique that is effective if the patient is cooperative. The disadvantage of deep breathing exercises is that there is no way to assess how well the patient is doing. A commonly used device is the incentive spirometer (IS), which "rewards" the patient by documenting the volume inhaled, thus providing encouragement to improve with each attempt. This inexpensive device has the added advantage of allowing the respiratory therapist to see just how well the patient is doing. Patients should be taught how to perform these techniques before surgery, because patient comprehension may be reduced in the early postoperative period. To be effective, some studies have suggested that the IS must be used at least hourly. There is no evidence that using IS is of any benefit in thoracic procedures or surgery performed on the head, neck, or extremities. If patient cooperation is limited, the lungs may be passively inflated using intermittent positive-pressure breathing (IPPB). A major disadvantage of IPPB is that it is associated with a high incidence of abdominal distension and discomfort. IPPB is also more expensive because it requires specialized equipment and must be administered by a respiratory therapist. Finally, continuous positive airway pressure (CPAP) may be used in an uncooperative patient. The disadvantages of CPAP include the uncomfortable, tight-fitting mask; cost; and need for supervision.

11. Which inflation maneuver is the best?

A randomized study of 172 patients undergoing upper abdominal surgery demonstrated no difference in the incidence of PPCs among patients using IS, IPPB, or deep breathing exercises. Several studies have shown that CPAP is effective in promoting lung expansion postoperatively; however, when compared with IS or deep breathing there was no statistically significant difference in the incidence of PPCs. Thus, no inflation technique is superior to any other in reducing the number of PPCs. The method chosen for a given patient depends largely on patient cooperation and available resources. A cooperative patient may do very well with only deep breathing exercises. IS may be used in an alert patient who would benefit from the feedback provided by the device. Less cooperative patients may require CPAP or IPPB; however, when the latter techniques are used one should watch for the development of abdominal distension, which could lead to aspiration.

12. How should pulmonary function studies be used in the evaluation of patients undergoing lung resection?

Over the past 40 years numerous reports have cited the value of preoperative spirometry, lung volumes, and diffusing capacity in determining who is at increased risk for complications after lung resection, usually performed for lung cancer. The physician who evaluates a lung resection candidate preoperatively should assume that the surgeon may have to perform a pneumonectomy if more extensive disease is found intraoperatively. If a patient has an FEV_1 of more than 2 liters in an adult man, or 60% of the predicted normal value; a maximum voluntary ventilation (MVV) of more than 50% predicted; and a diffusing capacity of the lung for carbon monoxide (DCLO) more than 60% predicted, he or she should be offered surgery without further testing. Although patients who do not meet these criteria are at increased risk of postoperative complications including respiratory insufficiency, they should not be automatically excluded from consideration for potentially life-saving surgery. These higher risk patients should instead undergo further testing to assess whether they can tolerate lung resection.

13. What is quantitative lung scanning?

Quantitative lung scanning, or "split function study," utilizes radioisotopes (Tc 99m–labeled macroaggregates for perfusion and Xe 133 for ventilation) to quantify the fractional contribution each lung or lobe makes to total ventilation and perfusion. The predicted postoperative FEV_1 (FEV_1-ppo) can be calculated using the following formula: FEV_1-ppo = preoperative FEV_1 × (1-fractional contribution of the affected lung). This simple technique has also been used to predict the postoperative diffusing capacity of the remaining lung. These values are often expressed in absolute numbers (e.g., 800 ml or 0.8 liters) or as a percentage of the patient's normal FEV_1. The latter method is more desirable because it takes into account the patient's age, height, and gender; thus, for example, elderly women with small lungs will not be erroneously excluded from surgical therapy. Several studies have shown good correlation between the actual and predicted postoperative values for FEV_1 and DLCO 3–6 months postoperatively.

14. What is the role of exercise testing before lung resection?

Exercise testing assesses the entire oxygen delivery system in the body, which includes the heart, lungs, and pulmonary and systemic vasculature. Many of the changes noted in the lungs during exercise, such as increased ventilation, $\dot{V}O_2$, blood flow, and carbon dioxide excretion ($\dot{V}CO_2$) are also noted after surgery. Therefore, someone who can tolerate a greater level of exercise is probably more likely to tolerate lung resection. Recent studies have estimated the "fitness" of a patient by measuring the maximal oxygen uptake ($\dot{V}O_2$max) during exercise and comparing preoperative $\dot{V}O_2$max to postoperative outcome. Interestingly, patients whose preoperative $\dot{V}O_2$max is reduced have increased postoperative mortality as well as increased morbidity. It is not clear how preoperative exercise testing can predict postoperative complications such as pneumonia and atelectasis, however. In a recent study, exercise testing was combined with quantitative lung scanning, yielding a predicted postoperative $\dot{V}O_2$max ($\dot{V}O_2$max-ppo) that can be used to predict postoperative morbidity and mortality. The study demonstrated good correlation between actual and predicted $\dot{V}O_2$max 3 months postoperatively, although at 6 months the correlation was less impressive. The exercise test may be performed as an inexpensive screening procedure such as climbing stairs. Patients who can climb 3 or more flights of stairs easily may have reduced postoperative complications.

15. How are quantitative lung scanning and exercise tests used in evaluation of a patient for lung resection?

Patients whose preoperative FEV_1 or DCLO is less than 60% of predicted should undergo quantitative lung scanning. If the FEV_1-ppo and DLCO-ppo are more than 40% of predicted, surgery should be offered. Patients with values less than 40% should be considered for exercise testing so that $\dot{V}O_2$max can be measured. During exercise testing electrocardiogram, blood pressure, and oxygen saturation should be monitored in addition to $\dot{V}O_2$max. Patients with a $\dot{V}O_2$max

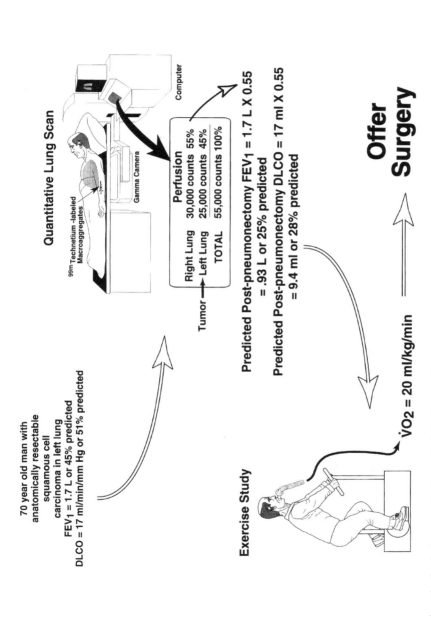

Quantitative Lung Scan

99mTechnetium -labeled
Macroaggregates

Gamma Camera

Computer

**70 year old man with
anatomically resectable
squamous cell
carcinoma in left lung**
FEV₁ = 1.7 L or 45% predicted
DLCO = 17 ml/min/mm Hg or 51% predicted

Tumor ▶

Perfusion

Right Lung 30,000 counts 55%
Left Lung 25,000 counts 45%
TOTAL 55,000 counts 100%

Predicted Post-pneumonectomy FEV₁ = 1.7 L X 0.55
= .93 L or 25% predicted

Predicted Post-pneumonectomy DLCO = 17 ml X 0.55
= 9.4 ml or 28% predicted

Exercise Study

V̇O₂ = 20 ml/kg/min

**Offer
Surgery**

The physiologic evaluation for lung resection in a typical elderly man. The baseline results of pulmonary function tests, FEV₁ and diffusing capacity for carbon monoxide (DLCO) are abnormal. The predicted postoperative values (FEV₁-ppo and DLCO-ppo) are calculated from the percent perfusion emanating from the noncancerous right lung (55%, or 0.55). Because the FEV₁-ppo and DLCO-ppo are both below 40% of predicted, an exercise test is performed. It yields an acceptable value of 20 ml per minute. Surgery is offered.

of more than 15 ml per kg per minute should be offered surgery. Alternatively, exercise testing can be combined with lung scanning to determine $\dot{V}O_2$max-ppo; a value of less than 10 ml per kg per minute has been associated with 100% mortality.

16. True or false: hypercapnia is a contraindication to lung resection?
False. It was once believed that COPD patients with chronic carbon dioxide retention ($PaCO_2$ more than 45 mmHg) could not tolerate lung resection. However, two recent studies have demonstrated that hypercapnic patients can tolerate lung resection without becoming ventilator dependent. Three of the hypercapnic patients who underwent lung resection were able to exercise to a $\dot{V}O_2$max of more than 15 ml per kg per minute.

17. Are other options available to the high-risk lung resection candidate?
Yes. Surgery is the most effective modality by which patients with non–small cell carcinoma of the lung can be cured, so examining all possible surgical techniques is essential. High-risk patients may have fewer complications if they undergo video-assisted thoracoscopic lung resection rather than thoracotomy. Some patients may even opt for tracheotomy and portable, long-term ventilator support in exchange for a cancer cure. Surgical options also exist for improving function in high-risk patients with COPD. Single lung transplantation is being used more and more frequently in patients with severe COPD. Lung reduction surgery may also be useful in rehabilitation of COPD. It is tempting to speculate that given this large number of options, almost no one with lung cancer is truly physiologically inoperable.

BIBLIOGRAPHY

1. Bolliger CT, Wyser C, Roser H, et al: Lung scanning and exercise testing for the prediction of postoperative performance in lung resection candidates at increased risk for complications. Chest 108:341–348, 1995.
2. Celli BR: Perioperative respiratory care of the patient undergoing upper abdominal surgery. Clin Chest Med 14:253–261, 1993.
3. Celli BR, Rodriguez KS, Snider GL: A controlled trial of intermittent positive pressure breathing, incentive spirometry and deep breathing exercises in preventing pulmonary complications after abdominal surgery. Am Rev Respir Dis 130:12–15, 1984.
4. Ford GT, Rosenal TW, Clergue F, et al: Respiratory physiology in upper abdominal surgery. Clin Chest Med 14:237–252, 1993.
5. Gracey DR, Divertie MB, Didier EP: Preoperative pulmonary preparation of patients with chronic obstructive pulmonary disease. Chest 76:123–129, 1979.
6. Hall JC, Tarala R, Harris J, et al: Incentive spirometry versus routine chest physiotherapy for prevention of pulmonary complications after abdominal surgery. Lancet 337:953–956, 1991.
7. Jackson CV: Preoperative pulmonary evaluation. Arch Intern Med 148:2120–2127, 1988.
8. Kearney DJ, Lee TH, Reilly JJ, et al: Assessment of operative risk in patients undergoing lung resection: Importance of predicted pulmonary function. Chest 105:753–759, 1994.
9. Markos J, Mullan BP, Hillman DR, et al: Preoperative assessment as a predictor of mortality and morbidity after lung resection. Am Rev Respir Dis 139:902–910, 1989.
10. Marshall MC, Olsen GN: The physiologic evaluation of the lung resection candidate. Clin Chest Med 14:305–320, 1993.
11. Morice RC, Peters EJ, Ryan MB, et al: Exercise testing in the evaluation of patients at high risk of complications from lung resection. Chest 101:356–361, 1992.
12. Olsen GN: The evolving role of exercise testing prior to lung resection. Chest 95:218–225, 1989.
13. Olsen GN: Lung cancer resection: Who's inoperable? Chest 108:298–299, 1995.
14. Warner MA, Divertie MB, Tinker JH: Preoperative cessation of smoking and pulmonary complications in coronary bypass patients. Anesthesiology 60:380–383, 1984.
15. Warner MA, Offord KP, Warner ME, et al: Role of preoperative cessation of smoking and other factors in postoperative pulmonary complications: A blinded prospective study of coronary bypass patients. Mayo Clin Proc 64:609–616, 1989.
16. Zibrak JD, O'Donnell CR: Indications for preoperative pulmonary function testing. Clin Chest Med 14:227–236, 1993.

82. POSTOPERATIVE PULMONARY CARE

Thomas E. Shaughnessy, M.D., and Jeanine P. Wiener-Kronish, M.D.

1. How does general anesthesia affect pulmonary function?

Exposure to general anesthetic agents may impair pulmonary gas exchange and result in intraoperative and postoperative hypoxemia. The supine position has been shown to cause a 20% decrease in functional residual capacity (FRC). Obesity further worsens FRC, as the increased intraabdominal pressure results in additional cephalad displacement of the diaphragm. With the induction of general anesthesia and muscle relaxation, FRC is further reduced. Patients with elevated closing capacities are more predisposed to the development of atelectasis. Residual effects of both intravenous and inhalation anesthetics blunt the ventilatory responses to hypercapnia and hypoxia. Anesthetic agents also attenuate the protective hypoxic pulmonary vasoconstriction reflex. These effects persist for several hours and may contribute to the intrapulmonary shunting and hypoxia seen in the recovery room. Prolonged pulmonary dysfunction (longer than 24 hours) is usually not caused by anesthesia.

2. How does surgery affect pulmonary function?

The location of the surgery determines whether postoperative pulmonary dysfunction occurs. Immediately after upper abdominal surgery, vital capacity (VC) is reduced to 40% of preoperative values. FRC is reduced to 70% of preoperative values. These pulmonary abnormalities are slow to resolve; the vital capacity and FRC gradually return to normal over 7–14 days. Lower abdominal surgery also decreases ventilation variables to 60–80% of preoperative values over a similar time frame. A thoracotomy decreases vital capacity by almost 4 liters. Superficial and extremity surgery results in little, if any, change in postoperative FRC. Mechanisms thought to be important in causing the decreases in FRC and VC include an increase in negative signaling along the phrenic nerve resulting from stimulation of the abdominal splanchnic nerves. Laparoscopic surgical approaches are associated with significantly less impairment of respiratory function than comparable open procedures, perhaps because of the decrease in splanchnic nerve stimulation.

3. What are the general principles of immediate postoperative pulmonary care?

Postoperative pulmonary dysfunction can be caused by mechanical, hemodynamic, and pharmacodynamic influences related to the surgery and to the anesthesia. The post-anesthesia care unit (PACU) is the area designed for monitoring and care of patients recovering from the immediate effects of these derangements. The drugs and equipment available to provide routine care include supplemental oxygen, suction, vital sign monitors, pulse oximetry, and electrocardiograph. Advanced support equipment (ventilators, intravascular pressure monitors, and defibrillator) must also be available. Airway patency and protection are continuously monitored. Supplemental oxygen therapy is always provided to help ensure that systemic oxygenation is adequate, and oximetry has become the standard of care to document the presence of adequate oxygenation. Maneuvers to facilitate ventilation are frequently employed to prevent potential pulmonary complications such as atelectasis. Examples of such prophylactic measures include early ambulation, coughing, and incentive spirometry.

4. Describe some maneuvers for treatment of postoperative airway obstruction.

Airway obstruction is most commonly caused by the tongue and pharyngeal soft tissues falling backward and occluding the airway. Usually, airway obstruction occurs in a patient who is very sleepy or narcotized. Signs of airway obstruction include a lack of air movement, retractions of the accessory muscles, and a lack of chest wall movement. The following maneuvers are used to reestablish airway patency:

- Neck extension (if not contraindicated) accompanied by a jaw thrust
- Moving the patient into a lateral position may also relieve airway obstruction
- Insertion of an oral or nasal airway, with caution because it may cause vomiting or gagging
- Examination of the oropharynx for obstructing material.

If these conservative measures fail to improve respiration, assistance by mask ventilation or endotracheal intubation may be required. If the patient cannot be intubated, cricothyroidotomy may be necessary. If the patient has undergone a procedure on the neck and intubation has failed, consideration should be given to opening the wound, relieving airway compression, and re-attempting intubation. Laryngospasm is an infrequent cause of air flow obstruction that usually responds to the positive pressure generated by mask ventilation.

5. **What criteria are used to determine when a patient may be extubated after an anesthetic?**
   Think of the mnemonic "When you think the patient will SOAR."

   S   Lower respiratory tract **secretions** are not more excessive than the patient's ability to clear them.

   O   **Oxygenation** is adequate. Usually a PaO_2 of 80 mmHg with an FIO_2 of 0.4 provides for some margin of safety because the maximum FIO_2 that can be dependably delivered to nonintubated patients is approximately 0.5.

   A   The patient is able to protect his or her **airway**. This is easily determined by testing a gag reflex.

   R   **Respiratory effort** is adequate, as assessed by clinical examination or quantified with variables such as a maximum inspiratory pressure more negative than -30 cm H_2O or a vital capacity greater than 10 cc per kg.

6. **What is the differential diagnosis of hypoxemia in the recovery room?**
   Hypoxemia may be caused by splinting, atelectasis, or hypoventilation secondary to residual anesthetic or pain medication. Increased oxygen consumption (because of shivering or hyperthermia) or decreased cardiac output may decrease mixed venous oxygen tension and thus decrease the PaO_2. Hypoxia commonly results from improper delivery of oxygen (Is the patient really receiving oxygen?), ventilation-perfusion abnormalities, or shunting caused by the surgery or the anesthetic. Hypoxia also can be seen when the patient stops adequately ventilating (increasing alveolar carbon dioxide decreases alveolar oxygen and decreases the PaO_2).

   The patient's preoperative pulmonary function should be considered; patients who are hypoxemic preoperatively require oxygen postoperatively, and usually larger quantities of supplemental oxygen will be necessary. Intubation can increase airway reactivity and lead to increased wheezing in asthmatic patients. Untoward events during the procedure that can lead to postoperative hypoxemia include: pneumothoraces; pulmonary edema resulting from volume administration or cardiac malfunction; pulmonary emboli caused by thrombi, air, tumor, or fat; aspiration of gastric contents (usually occurs peri-intubation); sepsis; or hemorrhage. Drugs that significantly increase cardiac output can cause hypoxemia by overcoming the protective hypoxic pulmonary vasoconstriction in diseased or atelectatic areas of the lung. Drugs commonly causing this phenomenon include nitroprusside, nitrates, and dopamine.

7. **What causes inaccurate pulse oximetry readings?**
   Pulse oximeters use the oxyhemoglobin absorption of infrared light transmitted across a pulsatile peripheral vascular bed (i.e., finger, earlobe) to determine the degree of arterial oxygen saturation. Decreases in oxygen saturation are detected only when the arterial oxygen tension falls below the level of full hemoglobin oxygen saturation. Certain situations are associated with inaccurate pulse oximetry readings. Pulse oximetry readings often cannot be obtained from patients who are hypothermic or vasoconstricted because of vasopressor therapy or hypotension. Spurious pulse oximetry readings may be caused by fluorescent or infrared lights (such as those used to warm small infants) or by movement of the extremity where the probe is located. Other causes of inaccurate readings include severe anemia, intravascular dyes (e.g., methylene blue),

fingernail polish, and the presence of other hemoglobin species, such as methemoglobin or carboxyhemoglobin.

Arterial blood gas levels are used to measure arterial oxygen and carbon dioxide tension as well as systemic pH. Venous blood gas levels are useless for determining adequacy of oxygenation; however, the venous blood's carbon dioxide level is only 5 torr above that of arterial blood and the venous blood's pH is decreased only by approximately 0.04 units compared with arterial blood. Thus, venous blood may provide information on adequacy of ventilation and systemic perfusion.

8. What is the differential diagnosis of hypercapnia in the recovery room?

Hypercapnia results from either decreased clearance or increased production of carbon dioxide. Decreased central respiratory drive may result from a neurologic defect or, more commonly, from residual anesthetic effects. Narcotic-induced depression may be reversed by naloxone, whereas benzodiazepines may be counteracted by flumazenil. Impairment of the chest bellows mechanism may occur if residual neuromuscular blockade, chest pain, or abdominal distention is present. Patients with intrinsic lung disease may have greater sensitivity to postoperative stresses, which may cause an exacerbation of hypercapnia. The increased carbon dioxide production associated with shivering or hyperthermia is usually not problematic unless ventilation cannot be appropriately increased.

9. Describe the differential diagnosis of postoperative wheezing.

Wheezing may occur secondary to bronchospastic asthma, exacerbation of COPD or bronchitis, pneumothorax, or congestive heart failure. In the intubated patient, obstruction of the endotracheal tube by mucus, cuff overinflation, a kinked endotracheal tube, an endobronchial intubation, or nasogastric tube misplacement should also be considered.

10. Can you predict which patient with chronic obstructive lung disease will require prolonged mechanical ventilation?

The postoperative complications associated with chronic obstructive lung disease (COLD) include atelectasis, pneumonia, and exacerbation of bronchitis. Identification of patients who will require prolonged postoperative mechanical ventilation has been difficult. In a study of 51 smokers with COLD who were to have elective abdominal vascular procedures, 25% required mechanical ventilation for more than 1 day. These ventilated patients also had longer hospital stays and a higher mortality than the patients who did not require mechanical ventilation. Preoperative data that were predictive of the requirement for prolonged ventilation included an extensive history of smoking (72 pack years versus 44 pack years in the nonventilated group) and a low preoperative arterial oxygen tension (68 mmHg versus 77 mmHg in the nonventilated group). Preoperative spirometry was not helpful in predicting postoperative respiratory failure.

11. Describe the postoperative problems of patients with restrictive lung disease.

There are few recent studies on postoperative problems of patients who have restrictive lung disease from lung fibrosis, interstitial lung disease, or spinal deformities. In contrast, many studies have suggested that irreversible pulmonary failure occurs in patients with scoliosis who have upper thoracic curves exceeding 70 degrees. Pulmonary function is improved in adolescents and children whose scoliosis is surgically corrected. It is unclear whether pulmonary function improves in adults with severe scoliosis after surgical repair of their spinal deformities. Patients with restrictive lung disease have high minute ventilations and may not meet the standard criteria for extubation because of their high respiratory frequencies. Patients with restrictive lung disease have noncompliant lungs that may require positive-pressure ventilation via either mechanical ventilation or intermittent positive-pressure ventilation (IPPB).

12. What complications occur after thoracotomy?

Thoracotomy is associated with the most serious postoperative pulmonary dysfunction because the lungs are affected as well as the rib cage. Furthermore, thoracotomies are often performed on patients who already have severe underlying lung disease. Preoperative evaluation of patients with bronchogenic carcinoma who are candidates for pulmonary resection or pneumonectomy has therefore been extensively investigated. Surgery is the only possible cure for lung cancer but the rate of complications is high (10–15% in patients who have had pneumectomies); the complications seen after thoracotomy include respiratory failure, myocardial infarction, pneumonia, atelectasis, and death. Preoperative evaluation of candidates for lung resection should include exercise studies because several investigators have shown that oxygen consumption levels during exercise are helpful in predicting whether a patient can undergo lung resection and have an uneventful postoperative course. In a recent study, if a patient had a $\dot{V}o_2$max of more than 75% of predicted, the patient had a 90% chance of not having complications, even after a pneumonectomy. The ability to achieve a high $\dot{V}o_2$max during exercise suggests that the patient has good pulmonary and cardiac function and is capable of moderate exercise (i.e., not debilitated). Static pulmonary function studies are not as helpful in predicting postoperative complications in this patient population.

Definition of Postthoracotomy Complications (Within 30 Days of Surgery)

Acute carbon dioxide retention (partial pressure of arterial carbon dioxide > 45 mmHg)	Pneumonia (temperature > 38° C, purulent sputum, infiltrate seen on chest radiograph)
Prolonged mechanical ventilation (> 48 hours)	Pulmonary embolism
Symptomatic cardiac arrhythmias requiring treatment	Lobar atelectasis (necessitating bronchoscopy)
Myocardial infarction	Death

Adapted from Bolliger CT, et al: Exercise capacity as a predictor of postoperative complications in lung resection candidates. Am J Respir Crit Care Med 151:1472–1480, 1995.

13. What causes atelectasis?

Atelectasis usually occurs in the basal lobes of the lung (100% incidence after thoracotomies) and is secondary to trauma to the lung, reduced respiratory effort caused by an increase in negative nervous signals along the phrenic nerve, splinting, obesity, intrathoracic fluid, pulmonary edema, and decreased compliance. These factors and a rapid, shallow respiratory pattern predispose the patient to small airway closure and alveolar collapse. Mucous plugging, inspissated secretions, and a poor cough contribute to persistent atelectasis. The diagnosis is made by clinical examination chest radiograph, and arterial blood gas analysis.

14. How should atelectasis be treated?

The most effective therapy for atelectasis is the use of a respiratory maneuver that increases inspiration and has the patient hold his or her inspiratory breath, allowing the inspired gas to enter collapsed alveoli via the pores of Kohn. No study has shown a benefit of one maneuver over another; IPPB, blow gloves, and incentive spirometers are all equivalent in their ability to treat atelectasis, decrease hospital stays, and decrease respiratory failure. Other therapeutic interventions used for atelectasis include extended mechanical ventilation, chest percussion, coughing, bronchodilators, enhanced analgesia, and nasotracheal suctioning. Patient positioning is also important. The sitting position places the diaphragm at a better mechanical advantage and increases FRC. The lateral decubitus position, with the expanded lung in the dependent position improves ventilation-perfusion matching and facilitates mucus clearance from the atelectatic, nondependent lung. Application of positive end-expiratory pressure (PEEP) has generally been shown to be an effective adjunct. Bronchoscopy has proved to be a controversial therapy (see question 24).

15. What methods may be used to mobilize and remove secretions in postoperative patients?

Inspiratory gases may be humidified. This decreases mucus viscosity and supports ciliary function. Adequate intravascular hydration helps to maintain the humidification capacity of the nasopharynx and tracheal mucosa. Mucolytic agents such as *N*-acetylcysteine have been suggested as a way of decreasing the viscosity of secretions, but their potential for causing bronchospasm limits their utility. Blind nasal suctioning with a soft catheter is an effective way of generating a cough, especially in the uncooperative patient. During suctioning procedure, electrocardiographic monitoring is used to detect reflex arrhythmias and bradycardias. Bronchoscopy is reserved for the most refractory cases of thickened, retained secretions.

16. Describe the various measures for delivery of oxygen therapy in nonintubated patients.

The major considerations in selection of a supplemental oxygen device are patient comfort and compliance, as well as the level of FIO_2 required. Nasal cannulas are well tolerated, but the delivered FIO_2 decreases with increased minute ventilation. Because of poor humidification, flow rates greater than 6 liters per minute may dry nasal mucosa. A venturi mask entrains a controlled amount of room air into a high flow of oxygen, which provides a more constant FIO_2 independent of minute ventilation and inspiratory flow rate. This device is less comfortable and has limited humidification ability. An open face mask, when tightly fitted, can deliver up to 50% FIO_2 and higher levels of humidity because of larger bore tubing. Face tents are more comfortable but vary in the amount of oxygen delivered. Masks with reservoir bags (nonrebreathing masks) have enhanced oxygen delivery capacity (60–80% FIO_2). Combinations of nasal cannulas and face masks are sometimes used. They are able to deliver enriched oxygen concentrations, but the high flows necessary are seldom tolerated for prolonged periods.

17. How can stridor or bronchospasm be reversed?

Stridor (suggested by a wheezing during inspiration) is indicative of partial upper airway obstruction, which is often caused by swelling or paralysis of the laryngeal or supraglottic soft tissues. Therapy should be aimed at reduction of swelling. Nebulized racemic epinephrine is useful if the side effects of tachycardia and hypertension can be tolerated. Dexamethasone is an effective antiinflammatory but requires several hours for effect. If epiglottitis is likely, the patient's airway (especially that of a small child) should be evaluated in the operating room, because the airway may become totally obstructed after being manipulated. In all patients with stridor, equipment should be readily available for intubation or tracheostomy in case clinical deterioration makes one or both of these measures necessary.

Bronchospasm initially should be treated, if possible, by removal of any precipitating agents (e.g., β-blockers). The cornerstones of inhalation therapy are β_2 agonists. Albuterol has the least β_1 effects and may be administered via metered dose inhaler or continuously as an aerosol. The aerosol form of the anticholinergic ipatroprium may also facilitate bronchodilatation. Steroid therapy has become the primary treatment for bronchospasm caused by asthma. In severe asthma, steroids need to be given early and in large amounts, because deaths in asthmatics tend to occur in patients who received too little steroid treatment or were given steroids too late in the attack. In asthmatic patients who have a history of intubation for their disease, preoperative administration of steroids should be considered. Asthmatic patients on steroids, either long term or acutely, are at high risk for prolonged paralysis if they receive more than one dose of nondepolarizing paralytic agents.

18. Describe the commonly used modalities of mechanical ventilation.

Volume ventilation. In assist control (AC) ventilation, when the patient initiates an inspiration, the ventilator delivers a preset tidal volume. If the patient's respiratory rate falls below a preset level, the machine delivers breaths automatically at a back-up rate. With intermittent mandatory ventilation (IMV), the ventilator delivers a preset tidal volume at a preset rate, but the patient may breathe spontaneously between cycles, then assume a greater portion of their ventilatory needs. Synchronization is possible between the expiratory phase of the patient's breath and a mandatory ventilation cycle (SIMV). With volume regulated ventilation, variables such as mode of ventilation, tidal volume, respiratory rate, inspiratory and flow rate must be set.

Pressure ventilation. With pressure-regulated ventilation, inspiratory pressure, inspiratory time, and respiratory rate need to be set. In pressure-regulated ventilation, the tidal volume varies if the patient has an unexpected increase or decrease in lung compliance. For example, a patient with severe bronchospasm whose initial inspiratory pressure was set at 50 cm H_2O to deliver a 500-ml tidal volume would receive a much larger tidal volume when the bronchospasm resolved and compliance increased. All modes of ventilation also require the clinician to dictate the F_{IO_2} and level of desired PEEP.

Continuous positive airway pressure (CPAP) can be used in both intubated and in nonintubated patients; the patient breathes spontaneously through a high-flow system that does not allow the patient's inspiratory pressure to go to zero at any time during the respiratory cycle. If the patient is intubated, preset levels of pressure support may be added during the patient's inspiratory effort. This is intended to overcome the excess work of breathing through demand valves and ventilator tubing as well as that caused by the patient's underlying pathology.

19. What are the variables commonly used in postoperative ventilation?

Common Ventilator Settings in the Postoperative Period

	VOLUME CONTROL	PRESSURE CONTROL
Tidal volume or inspiratory pressure	10 cc/kg	Titrate to maintain 10 cc/kg (10–30 cm H_2O)
Respiratory rate	10–12	10–12
Inspiration:expiration ratio	—	1:2–3
F_{IO_2}	100% with titration to 50% based on Pa_{O_2} or Sa_{O_2}	100% with titration to 50% based on Pa_{O_2} or Sa_{O_2}
PEEP	5 cm H_2O	5 cm H_2O

20. Are there potential hazards to oxygen therapy?

Pulmonary oxygen toxicity is manifest as thickening and edema of the lung interstitium. It is a function of oxygen dose and duration of therapy. Even with 100% oxygen supplementation, days may be required before microscopic damage may be detected. Toxicity is unlikely to develop at levels up to 60% oxygen, even for prolonged periods of exposure. Thus the benefits of oxygen therapy greatly outweigh the risks in the postoperative period.

Because oxygen diffuses into pulmonary capillary blood much faster than nitrogen, periods of 100% oxygen supplementation in smaller alveoli may actually promote their collapse. The resulting atelectasis may cause increased intrapulmonary shunting and hypoxia, despite the enhanced oxygen support. Retrolental fibroplasia is a hazard of oxygen therapy that occurs in neonates of low birth weight or less than 44 weeks of gestational age.

21. What is the difference between a humidifier and a nebulizer?

Nebulizers are devices that generate aerosolized suspensions of particles in a carrier gas. They are categorized as jet (pneumatic) and ultrasonic. The jet nebulizer utilizes the Bernoulli effect of a directed high velocity gas stream drawing surface liquids into the stream as aerosolized particles. They are frequently used to humidify gases and deliver bronchodilator drugs.

Humidifiers are used to provide dry medical gases with a water content similar to that normally present in room air. Passover humidifiers depend on evaporation to add water vapor to gases that pass over a water surface. In bubble-through humidifiers, gas passes as bubbles through a reservoir of heated water. This increases the capacity of the gas to hold water vapor. Humidifiers of this type are frequently used when the humidification function of the upper airway is bypassed, such as during mechanical ventilation.

CONTROVERSIES

22. Does epidural analgesia improve pulmonary function?

Although many studies have demonstrated improved radiologic markers in patients receiving epidural analgesia compared with those receiving general anesthesia and systemic opioids, the effects of epidural therapy on serious pulmonary complications (pneumonia and respiratory failure) remain unclear. The studies that observed a benefit from epidural analgesia examined high-risk patients, used intraoperative epidural anesthesia, and continued epidural analgesia (local or opioid) into the postoperative period. On the other hand, those studies that did not observe a difference used healthy patients, did not study high-risk procedures, or did not control postoperative analgesia. There are data, however, showing that complete pain relief achieved by epidural narcotics will not improve VC or FRC. In contrast, local anesthetics appear to improve pulmonary function after upper abdominal surgery. Thus, epidural analgesia that includes local anesthesia may offer additional benefit to patients at high risk for pulmonary complications.

23. Which is more effective for bronchodilator therapy, jet nebulization or metered-dose inhalers?

Many studies have shown little difference between these two modalities in both intubated and nonintubated patients. However, several studies show (by filter collection and radiolabeled techniques) that in intubated patients, administration of bronchodilators with a metered-dose inhaler attached to a spacing device or delivered by catheter to the distal end of the endotracheal tube results in improvement of deposition by 5 to 20–30%. Metered-dose inhalers with spacing devices have also been shown to improve delivery in the nonintubated patient. It is not clear, however, whether this technique is more effective than nebulized therapy because it is difficult to show dosage equivalency and there are problems with patient cooperation in the acute setting. Metered-dose therapy used appropriately can substantially decease the cost of respiratory care services.

24. Is bronchoscopy effective for the treatment of atelectasis?

Fiberoptic bronchoscopy has been used as a therapeutic modality for selected cases of atelectasis. Atelectasis usually can be managed with vigorous respiratory therapy alone. Many anecdotal reports of the use of bronchoscopy to resolve lobar atelectasis exist in the literature, but prospective studies demonstrate no advantage of bronchoscopy over vigorous pulmonary toilet for these cases. Although not proven prospectively, consideration for bronchoscopy may be given to patients in whom lobar or more widespread atelectasis has not responded to vigorous respiratory care (i.e., suctioning, postural drainage, chest percussion) or those with life-threatening acute whole lung atelectasis. One study suggests that bronchoscopy is useful only when the lung is not totally consolidated, as suggested radiographically by the presence of air bronchograms.

25. How often should ventilation circuits and humidification reservoirs be changed?

The common practice of changing ventilator circuits every 24–48 hours is based upon 1981 recommendations of the Centers for Disease Control that were established before bacteriostatic innovations such as heat moisture exchangers, nonaerosolizing humidifiers, and heated wire circuits. Several studies have shown an increase in bacterial contamination of ventilator circuits over time, as well as an association with the use of unheated bubble-through or nebulizing humidifiers. The bacteria isolated from the condensate usually correlate with organisms previously isolated from the patient's sputum, suggesting that the patient's oropharyngeal flora is the primary source of circuit colonization. Highly contaminated condensate from the patient in the ventilator circuit may be a significant risk factor in the development of nosocomial pneumonia, but studies have failed to reveal an increased incidence of pneumonia even when the interval between circuit changes is as long as 1 week. Based on the apparent lack of significant adverse sequelae, the American Association for Respiratory Care in a practice guideline statement recommends establishment of circuit change intervals based on local surveillance programs. Circuits employing the aforementioned innovations may, in the absence of soilage, require change only every 5–7 days. These recommendations have significant implications in terms of reducing use of ICU resources.

BIBLIOGRAPHY

1. American Association for Respiratory Care. Clinical practice guideline. Ventilator circuit changes. Respir Care 39:797–802, 1994.
2. Bolliger CT, et al: Exercise capacity as a predictor of postoperative complications in lung resection candidates. Am J Respir Crit Care Med 151:1472–1480, 1995.

3. Dodson BA, et al: Changes in acetylcholine receptor number in muscle from critically ill patients receiving muscles relaxants: An investigation of the molecular mechanism of prolonged paralysis. Crit Care Med 23:815–821, 1995.
4. Firestone LL, Lebowitz PW, Cook CE: Clinical Anesthesia Procedures of the Massachusetts General Hospital, 3rd ed. Boston, Little, Brown, 1988.
5. George RB, Light RW, Matthay MA, et al: Chest Medicine, Essentials of Pulmonary and Critical Care Medicine, 3rd ed. Baltimore, Williams & Wilkins, 1995.
6. Jayr C, et al: Preoperative and intraoperative factors associated with respiratory failure following major abdominal vascular surgery. Chest 103:1231–1236, 1993.
7. Liu S, Carpenter RL, Neal JM: Epidural analgesia and anesthesia. Anesthesiology 82:1474–1506, 1995.
8. Maguire GP, Newman T, DeLorenzo LJ, et al: Comparison of a hand-held nebulizer with a metered dose inhaler-spacer combination in acute obstructive pulmonary disease. Chest 100:1300–1305, 1991.
9. Miller RD: Anesthesia, 3rd ed. New York, Churchill Livingstone, 1990.
10. Rau JL, Harwood RJ, Groff JL: Evaluation of a reservoir device for metered-dose bronchodilator delivery to intubated adults. An in vitro study. Chest 102:924–930, 1992.
11. Stoelting RK, Dierdorf SF: Anesthesia and Co-Existing Disease, 3rd ed. New York, Churchill Livingstone, 1993.
12. Stoelting RK, Miller RD: Basics of Anesthesia, 2nd ed. New York, Churchill Livingstone, 1989.
13. Wiener-Kronish JP, Matthay MA: Preoperative evaluation in Murray JF, Nadel JA (eds): Textbook of Respiratory Medicine. Philadelphia, W.B. Saunders, 1994.

83. LUNG TRANSPLANTATION

Nelson C. Yu, M.D., and Janet R. Maurer, M.D.

1. How long has lung transplantation been done?

Long-term success of lung transplantation for selected patients with irreversible pulmonary failure has only been achievable since 1983. Defective healing of the bronchial anastomosis, lack of experience with opportunistic infections, and inadequate immunosuppression contributed to the deaths of most patients who underwent lung transplantation before 1982. In 1983, the Toronto group first achieved long-term success with lung transplantation. They reduced the airway ischemia by wrapping an omental pedicle around the bronchial anastomosis. Since then, improvements in surgical technique and more sophisticated postoperative management have led to successful airway healing without the omental support.

SCREENING AND PREPARATION FOR TRANSPLANTATION

2. Which patients are candidates for lung transplantation?

Untreatable end-stage pulmonary disease of almost any cause
No other significant medical diseases
Substantial limitation of daily activity
Limited life expectancy
Ambulatory with rehabilitation potential
Acceptable nutritional status
Satisfactory psychosocial profile and emotional support system

Modified from Official American Thoracic Society Statement—June 1992: Lung transplantation: Report of the ATS Workshop on Lung Transplantation. Am Rev Respir Dis 147:772–776, 1993.

3. How are patients matched to the various lung transplantation procedures?
Single-Lung Transplant
End-stage fibrotic lung disease
COPD, including α-1-antitrypsin deficiency
Primary and secondary pulmonary hypertension (selected cases)
Miscellaneous diseases (e.g., lymphangioleiomyomatosis, eosinophilic granuloma, sarcoidosis)

Double-Lung Transplant
Pulmonary sepsis (e.g., cystic fibrosis)
COPD, including α-1-antitrypsin deficiency
Primary and secondary pulmonary hypertension (selected cases)
Miscellaneous diseases (e.g., lymphangioleiomyomatosis, eosinophilic granuloma, sarcoidosis)
Heart-Lung Transplant
Pulmonary parenchymal disease with separate cardiac dysfunction
Primary and secondary pulmonary hypertension (selected cases)
Complicated congenital heart disease with Eisenmenger's syndrome
Modified from Judson MA: Clinical aspects of lung transplantation. Clin Chest Med 14:335–357, 1993.

4. Which is the transplant procedure of choice for pulmonary hypertension?

There is presently no standard method to decide whether to perform single-lung, double-lung, or heart-lung transplantation in patients with pulmonary hypertension. These patients were initially thought to require double-lung transplantation or heart-lung transplantation if significant right ventricular dysfunction was present. It was later shown that this condition reverses to a large extent just by single-lung transplantation when the pulmonary artery pressure is lowered. Even patients with Eisenmenger's syndrome are often successfully transplanted with single or double lung grafts and the cardiac defect is repaired at the time of surgery. However, complications such as reperfusion injury or rejection may be more difficult to manage because nearly 100% of the cardiac output flows through the transplanted lung.

5. Why is double-lung transplantation needed for pulmonary sepsis?

Single-lung transplantation is not adequate for this situation because the transplanted lung would be endangered by spillage of organisms from the native lung and sepsis would be a constant problem. Cystic fibrosis with chronic pulmonary infection caused by *Pseudomonas* spp. and diffuse bronchiectasis are two examples of chronic suppurative bronchial diseases that would require double-lung transplantation.

6. What are the potential advantages of lung transplantation over heart-lung transplantation for end-stage pulmonary disease?

Isolated lung transplantation allows the patient to retain his or her own heart, which avoids the development of cardiac rejection. It also leaves the donor heart (and the other donor lung in the case of single-lung transplantation) available for transplantation into another individual.

7. How is bilateral sequential lung transplantation done? How does it compare with previous double-lung transplantation procedures?

This technique involves performance of two single-lung transplants sequentially in a recipient during one visit to the operating room. It represents a significant advance over previous double-lung transplantation procedures because it often avoids the need for placing recipients on cardiopulmonary bypass. Healing of the bronchial anastomosis in this technique is also better than that of the tracheal anastomosis in the original double-lung transplant procedures.

8. What are the criteria for donor lungs?

Age < 55 years
Minimal smoking history
$Pao_2 > 300$ mmHg on $Fio_2 = 1.0$, PEEP = 5 cm H_2O
Normal bronchoscopic examination (without purulent secretions)
Absence of infected sputum
No significant chest trauma or pulmonary contusion
Negative serology for human immunodeficiency virus and hepatitis B surface antigen
Normal chest radiograph before lung harvest (occasionally lungs with infiltrates are used if they can be shown to be noninfectious)
Modified from Egan TM, Kaiser LE, Cooper JD: Lung transplantation. Curr Probl Surg 26:681–751, 1989.

9. What requirements need to be met in the process of matching recipient to donor?

Additional requirements for designated recipients of specific donors include ABO compatibility and lungs that are of proper size. In many centers an attempt is made to provide cytomegalovirus (CMV)-negative lungs for CMV-negative recipients, because such patients have a relatively low incidence of CMV infection. Human leukocyte antigen (HLA) matching is not required because the lungs might deteriorate during the time required for matching. Furthermore, retrospective analysis of HLA compatibility of donors and recipients does not appear to correlate with subsequent episodes of rejection or mortality.

10. How are lungs matched for size?

The ideal donor lungs are those in which the recipient's and donor's predicted total lung capacities are within 500 ml of each other. In a patient with an oversized chest (e.g., one with COPD), however, a slightly larger lung often can be used and vice versa.

11. In unilateral procedures, which side should be transplanted?

The choice of which hemithorax to use for single-lung transplantation is determined by several factors. If there has been a prior major thoracotomy, the nonoperated side is transplanted. If one native lung receives significantly more ventilation and blood flow than the other, the side with poorer function is transplanted. If unilateral bronchiectasis is present, that side must be removed. Sometimes only one lung is available and, of course, barring other absolute contraindications, that lung determines which side is transplanted.

12. How are the selected prospective lung transplant recipients prepared preoperatively?

Patients who are accepted for transplantation must be ambulatory preoperatively (with supplemental oxygen if needed) because they are encouraged to participate in an outpatient pulmonary rehabilitation program to maintain physical fitness. While awaiting surgery, they are often able to significantly improve their distance on the 6-minute walk test. Every effort is made to transplant only applicants who are well enough to function in an outpatient setting. Patients on mechanical ventilators are generally not considered, although exceptions are occasionally allowed.

13. What preoperative conditions in the assessment and work-up of eligible lung recipients are important in the final decision-making process?

Prospective recipients require adequate renal reserve. Screening for coronary artery disease is important for patients who are at risk. Transplantation should not be offered to candidates with the following:

- Poorly controlled systemic illnesses such as collagen vascular diseases (except scleroderma) that affect the lung
- Active sites of infection
- Diabetes mellitus
- Hypertension
- Neurologic diseases

Abnormal hepatic function and active peptic ulcer disease are relative contraindications. Candidates with a history of malignancy should demonstrate a disease-free interval of several years. With regard to corticosteroid therapy, most programs will accept patients who can be maintained long term on 15 mg per day of prednisone or less. Substance use including alcohol is a high risk for noncompliance with posttransplant immunosuppressive regimen. Most centers require abstinence from cigarette smoking for 6 months to 2 years before reconsideration.

INFECTIOUS COMPLICATIONS AFTER TRANSPLANTATION

14. Why is the transplanted lung a common site of infection?

The lung is denervated and there is no cough reflex beyond the bronchial anastomosis. Mucociliary clearance is also decreased in lung transplant recipients. Other local immune surveillance mechanisms may also be impaired. Finally, acute and chronic rejection can result in local inflammation or even bronchiectasis in the lung allograft so that it may become easily infected.

15. What is the role of antimicrobial prophylaxis in lung transplantation?

- **Bacterial pneumonias.** With the use of broad-spectrum antibiotic prophylaxis and routine culturing of the donor's trachea, the incidence has been significantly lessened. If the cultures remain negative, antibiotics are discontinued after 3-4 days.
- ***Pneumocystis carinii* pneumonia (PCP).** In centers where trimethoprim-sulfamethoxazole (TMP-SMX) prophylaxis is routinely used, the incidence of PCP is less than 1%.
- **CMV pneumonia.** The easiest way to reduce CMV infections is to match CMV-negative recipients with CMV-negative donors whenever possible. If either is CMV-positive, prophylaxis with ganciclovir or hyperimmune globulin, or both, is often used.
- **Herpes simplex virus (HSV) infection.** Acyclovir may be administered for 6 months after a ganciclovir regimen is completed. If donor and recipient are CMV-negative, then acyclovir at a lower dose is started immediately and given for 6 months.

16. When do bacterial infections occur in the lung transplant patient?

Bacterial pneumonia is a threat from the early transplant period onward, although most episodes occur within the first 3 months postoperatively. Gram-negative rods of the Enterobacteriaceae family and *Pseudomonas* spp. are the most common pathogens. *Staphylococcus aureus* and *Haemophilus influenzae* account for most of the other bacterial pathogens. Bacterial pneumonia is also a major infectious complication in the intermediate and late postoperative periods and has been responsible for late death of lung transplant recipients. One important difference is that late bacterial pneumonia often develops with concomitant chronic rejection and bronchiectasis.

Bacterial infections also may present outside the transplanted lung. Wound infections, line sepsis, and intraabdominal abscess are not uncommon and may be difficult to detect in patients taking large doses of corticosteroids.

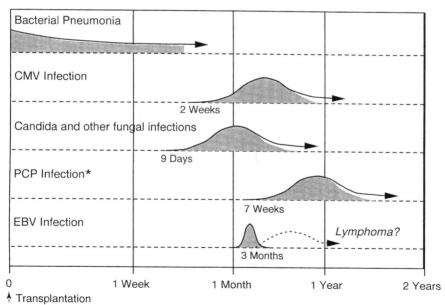

Incidence of infectious complications after lung transplantation. * Incidence of *Pneumocystis carinii* pneumonia (PCP) is now minimal if prophylaxis with trimethoprim-sulfamethoxazole is used. CMV = cytomegalovirus; EBV = Epstein-Barr virus. (Adapted from Judson MA: Clinical aspects of lung transplantation. Clin Chest Med 14:335–357, 1993.)

17. What is the incidence of CMV infection in the transplant recipient?

CMV infection most often occurs between the second and twelfth weeks after transplantation. It is much less common when recipients and donors both have negative blood tests for CMV unless the patient receives blood products that are CMV positive. The most severe CMV infections occur when a CMV-seronegative recipient receives a lung from a CMV-seropositive donor. Approximately 25% of CMV infections are asymptomatic seroconversions detected in cultures of recipient buffy coats or urine in the postoperative period. However, the infection rate approaches 100%. Widespread use of prophylaxis has greatly reduced the number of patients who develop severe disease. Systemic symptoms may include fever, chills, myalgias, malaise, abdominal discomfort, and leukopenia.

18. How often does CMV infection involve the lung?

CMV is the second most common cause of pneumonia in lung transplant patients; bacteria are the most common infectious agents. Patients typically present with fever, cough, hypoxemia, and radiographic infiltrates. Diagnosis of CMV pneumonia usually requires fiberoptic bronchoscopy with bronchoalveolar lavage (BAL). If results of viral culture and cytologic examination are equivocal, a sample of lung tissue from a transbronchial biopsy or open lung biopsy may be required. Although only 4–20% of kidney, liver, or cardiac allograft recipients develop CMV pneumonia, the prevalence rate among lung or heart-lung allograft recipients may be as high as 50%. Preemptive treatment is often employed based solely on positive "shell vial" accelerated centrifugation cultures of BAL fluid in an appropriate clinical setting.

19. What role do other viruses of the Herpesviridae family play in lung transplantation?

Primary infection from Epstein-Barr virus (EBV) can occur between the first and the third month after transplantation. A mononucleosis syndrome can develop from EBV infection with fever, malaise, pharyngitis, and adenopathy. These infections may resolve spontaneously or may result in B cell lymphoproliferative disorders, including lymphoma. Although acyclovir is often given to lung transplant recipients as prophylaxis against herpes simplex virus infections, it may have some prophylactic effect on EBV infection as well.

20. What fungal infections can occur in the posttransplantation period?

The overall incidence of fungal infections with lung or heart-lung transplantation ranges from 10–22%, most of which are caused by *Candida* or *Aspergillus* spp.; more than 80% of these infections occur within the first 2 months. Candidal pneumonia occurs early, probably because it frequently colonizes the donor airway, which may eventually lead to pulmonary infection in the recipient. The presence of numerous candidal organisms is therefore a contraindication to transplantation in some centers because of the high risk of fatal invasive candidiasis with infection. *Aspergillus* spp. may present as an indolent invasive pneumonia or as an acute fulminant infection. Another form of infection with *Aspergillus* spp. that was recently recognized is tracheobronchitis. This locally invasive infection of the upper airways has a propensity for dissemination if not detected early. The overall mortality of fungal infections in heart-lung and lung transplant recipients is reported to be between 40 and 70%. Most fungal infections can be treated successfully with amphotericin B, although *Aspergillus* spp. are especially difficult to eradicate and may cause lethal infection.

IMMUNOSUPPRESSION IN LUNG TRANSPLANTATION

21. What are the principles underlying the postoperative immunosuppressive regimen?

Immunosuppression to avoid rejection is a lifelong requirement of organ transplantation patients. The establishment of a successful regimen is a constant balancing act. Inadequate therapy may result in organ rejection. Excessive doses may result in infection or organ damage from drug toxicity. Chronic rejection and infection are the predominant causes of death.

22. Name the standard immunosuppressive drugs used after lung transplantation.

Cyclosporine, azathioprine, and corticosteroids are used for long-term immunosuppression. In addition, antilymphocyte preparations are sometimes administered as early induction immunosuppressive agents and in cases of resistant rejection. A new more potent drug, tarcolimus (FK 506), may soon become commonly used as an alternative to cyclosporine.

23. List the common toxicities of cyclosporine.

Nephrotoxicity	Seizures	Delirium	Electrolyte disturbances
Hypertension	Stroke syndromes	Hypertrichosis	Photosensitivity
Headaches	Coma	Gingival hyperplasia	Malignancy
Tremor			

Modified from Maurer JR: Therapeutic challenges following lung transplantation. Clin Chest Med 11:279–290, 1990.

NONINFECTIOUS COMPLICATIONS AFTER TRANSPLANTATION

24. What is the pulmonary reimplantation response?

Newly transplanted lungs may develop noncardiogenic pulmonary edema soon after the blood supply has been reestablished. This process has been called the *pulmonary reimplantation response* (PRR). It is believed to be secondary to the effects of free oxygen radicals that are produced after ischemic injury to the donor lung. Additional postulated causes of this response include surgical trauma, denervation, and lymphatic interruption. Because this process nearly always peaks in severity by the fourth postoperative day, any pulmonary process beginning thereafter should be investigated for another cause.

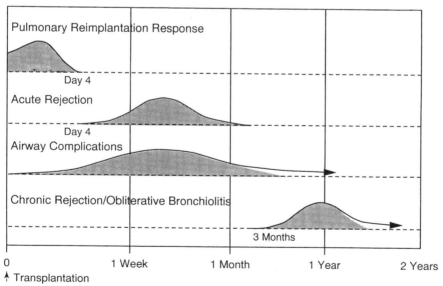

Incidence of noninfectious complications after lung transplantation. (Adapted from Judson MA: Clinical aspects of lung transplantation. Clin Chest Med 14:335–357, 1993.)

25. Why is PRR a diagnosis of exclusion?

The most frequent radiographic finding of the PRR is perihilar and basal consolidation in the transplanted lung. Fluid overload, left ventricular failure, rejection, infection, and atelectasis need to be excluded. Normal pulmonary artery wedge pressures and often bronchoscopy are required to rule out the presence of volume overload, atelectasis, or mucopurulent infected secretions.

26. When does acute rejection occur? How is it diagnosed clinically?

The peak incidence of acute lung allograft rejection is within the first few weeks, but it usually occurs at least several days after transplantation. The clinical diagnosis of acute lung allograft rejection is generally made from the following criteria:

Fever	Exclusion of infection
Dyspnea	Rapid improvement with increased
General malaise	immunosuppression, usually in the
Worsening infiltrates on chest radiograph	form of large intravenous doses
Worsening gas exchange	of corticosteroids

The gold standard for diagnosis of acute rejection is histologic study of a sample usually obtained by transbronchial biopsy.

27. How does acute rejection present radiographically?

The radiographic features of acute rejection are variable. The chest radiograph is usually abnormal during rejection in the first month after transplantation but is abnormal in only 25% of cases after the first month. When infiltrates are present they may be interstitial or alveolar, localized or diffuse. When the infiltrates are localized, they are most common early in the perihilar areas of the transplanted lung. Pleural effusion can be an isolated marker of rejection, especially in children.

28. What is the role of high-dose corticosteroid therapy in acute rejection?

Usually, 1 gm of methylprednisolone is given intravenously each day for 3 days to treat acute rejection. If acute lung allograft rejection has occurred, hypoxemia and pulmonary infiltrates should begin to resolve within 12 hours, and the temperature should return abruptly to normal. A poor clinical response suggests an alternative diagnosis or resistant rejection. Bronchoscopy should be performed before treatment with corticosteroids is begun.

29. What are the expected airway complications after lung transplantation?

Lung transplant recipients may develop airway ischemia and necrosis, which may result in partial airway dehiscence and impaired healing with bronchial stenosis at the anastomotic site. Airways that appear bronchoscopically at risk (persistent dusky or white areas) should be assessed regularly so that appropriate interventions (dilatation or stent placement, or both) can be made if the airway becomes stenotic.

30. What is obliterative bronchiolitis?

Obliterative bronchiolitis (OB) is an inflammatory disorder of the small airways leading to obstruction and destruction of pulmonary bronchioles. This inflammation results in bronchiolar distortion, narrowing, plugging, and scarring that results in severe obstructive airway disease. Often, secondary bronchiectasis or bronchomalacia develops. The clinical course varies but three usual scenarios exist: rapid downhill course; slow, gradual decline in function; abrupt fall in function with subsequent stabilization over time. Patients rarely regain lost function.

31. What causes obliterative bronchiolitis?

By 5 years after transplantation, most large centers now predict at least 50% of patients will have some degree of OB, the causes of which include acute rejection, infection, lung denervation, bronchial ischemia, drug toxicity, altered mucociliary clearance, and impaired lower respiratory tract defense mechanisms. At present it is believed that OB is a manifestation of chronic allograft rejection. Evidence supporting this includes the presence of donor tissue-directed lymphocytes in the airway submucosa early in the development of OB lesions.

32. What then is the bronchiolitis obliterans syndrome?

Although OB is the histopathologic hallmark of chronic rejection, bronchiolitis obliterans syndrome (BOS) clinically connotes graft deterioration secondary to progressive airway disease, which usually begins at least 3 months after lung transplantation. Its development is often insidious. The patient may feel slightly short of breath and have mild malaise. Sometimes only a fall in the forced expiratory volume in 1 second (FEV_1) is detected. Recurrent lower respiratory tract infections often occur later in the course. Pulmonary function first reveals a "scooping" of the midportion of the flow-volume loop with a diminished forced expiratory flow. When this obstructive defect progresses, eventually FEV_1, FEV_1/forced vital capacity (FVC), and FVC are reduced. Airflow obstruction rarely improves spontaneously and enhanced immunosuppression often brings about little change. Hypoxemia may occur. Chest radiographs may be unchanged from baseline or late in the disease may show subpleural fibrosis.

33. How is chronic rejection diagnosed?

Although tissue confirmation has been considered the diagnostic "gold standard," OB often has a patchy distribution that may be missed on transbronchial biopsy. Patients are therefore usually monitored for the development of BOS with frequent pulmonary function tests. Suggestive symptoms mandate immediate investigation. Once worsening airflow obstruction is detected, transbronchial lung biopsies are obtained in an effort to confirm the diagnosis. Patients with a clinical course consistent with chronic rejection will be presumed to have it and be treated as such even if the transbronchial biopsy is negative.

34. How is the severity of BOS in lung transplant recipients graded?

The severity of BOS is based on the degree of fall in FEV_1 from the baseline posttransplantation value defined as the average of the two previous highest consecutive measurements obtained 3–6 weeks apart. Factors other than chronic rejection need to be excluded as a cause of significant change in the FEV_1. The following is the proposed staging system for chronic rejection:

Each numerical stage is further subclassified into a or b, depending on whether pathologic evidence of OB is absent (a) or present (b).

Chronic Rejection Stages

STAGE	VERBAL DESCRIPTION	FEV_1
0	No significant abnormality	80% or more
1	Mild BOS	66–80%
2	Moderate BOS	51–65%
3	Severe BOS	50% or less

35. How is chronic rejection treated?

Many approaches to enhanced immunosuppression have been tried, but none are reliably successful. One approach is "pulse" courses of intravenous corticosteroids for several days after which an oral corticosteroid taper is begun back toward the maintenance dose. Use of antilymphotic agents has also been attempted. Patients who progress in spite of augmented immunosuppression pose a challenging clinical problem. OB accounts for 26% of all lung transplant deaths. Less common causes of late mortality include renal failure, lymphoma and other malignancies, and ARDS.

LIFE AFTER TRANSPLANTATION

36. What are the anticipated changes in pulmonary function after lung transplantation?

Better total lung capacity (TLC), vital capacity (VC), FEV_1, and DLCO occur in all lung transplant recipients. Arterial Po_2 also increases to almost normal values in many patients. Increments in these variables are usually significant at 3 months and may continue to improve over the first year.

37. Do double-lung transplant recipients have better exercise performance than their single-lung transplant counterparts?

Despite the acquisition of superior pulmonary function in double-lung recipients, there is little difference in exercise capacities in patients undergoing single versus double lung transplant.

The distance walked in 6 minutes, $\dot{V}O_2max$, anaerobic threshold, and maximum heart rates are similar. Both groups reach approximately 50% of predicted workload. It is not clear why bilateral lung recipients have this impairment, although it is usually not clinically important. Although a dramatic increase in exercise performance is evident after transplantation, these patients still are significantly incapacitated. The reasons for the incapacity are not known because patients do not seem to be either respiratory or cardiac limited.

38. What is the impact of lung transplantation on the patient's quality of life?
Lung transplant recipients enjoy a much improved quality of life especially if significant complications do not occur. Satisfaction with physical and emotional health was rated good or excellent by more than 80%, and satisfaction with life good or excellent by more than 70% in one survey.

39. What are the relative success rates of lung transplantation in different patient populations?
To date, the best survivals are in COPD patients (more than 75% in 1 year; 55% in 4 years). Pulmonary hypertension and pulmonary fibrosis survivals are around 65% in 1 year and 45–50% in 4 years; however, the number of patients followed out to 4 years is small.

40. What are the inherent problems currently? What future developments are projected in the field of transplantation?
The supply of donor organs remains extremely limited and efficient methods must be developed to maintain the lungs of potential donors to allow for transplantation. Improved techniques of preservation will increase the supply of suitable lungs and considerably simplify the logistics of transplantation. Animals may be genetically engineered to provide tissues that will not be rejected by humans. To improve the long-term outcomes of transplant recipients, new, more selective immunosuppressive agents are being developed and research into the cause and prevention of obliterative bronchiolitis is ongoing.

BIBLIOGRAPHY

1. Egan TM, Kaiser LE, Cooper JD: Lung transplantation. Curr Probl Surg 26:681–751, 1989.
2. Ettinger NA, Bailey TC, Trulock EP, et al: Cytomegalovirus infection and pneumonitis. Am Rev Respir Dis 147:1017–1023, 1993.
3. Griffith BP, Zenati M: The pulmonary donor. Clin Chest Med 11:217–226, 1990.
4. Hosenpud JD, Novick RJ, Breen TJ, et al: The Registry of the International Society for Heart and Lung Transplantation. Eleventh Official Report—1994. J Heart Lung Transplant 13:561–570, 1994.
5. International Society for Heart and Lung Transplantation: A Working Formulation for the Standardization of Nomenclature and for Clinical Staging of Chronic Dysfunction in Lung Allografts. J Heart Lung Transplant 12:713–716, 1993.
6. Judson MA: Clinical aspects of lung transplantation. Clin Chest Med 14:335–357, 1993.
7. Kaiser LR, Cooper JD: The current status of lung transplantation. Ad Surg 25:289–307, 1992.
8. Levine SM, Peters JI, Anzueto A, et al: Aspergillus infection in single lung transplant recipients. Am Rev Respir Dis 147:A599, 1993 (Abstract).
9. Levy RD, Ernst P, Levine SM, et al: Exercise performance after lung transplantation. J Heart Lung Transplant 12:27–33, 1993.
10. Maurer JR: Therapeutic challenges following lung transplantation. Clin Chest Med 11:279–290, 1990.
11. Mohar DE, Bryan CL, Jenkinson SG, et al: HLA matching as a predictor of OB or death in SLT. Chest 104:157S, 1993 (Abstract).
12. Official American Thoracic Society Statement—June 1992: Lung transplantation: Report of the ATS Workshop on Lung Transplantation. Am Rev Respir Dis 147:772–776, 1993.
13. Paya CV: Fungal infections in solid-organ transplantation. Clin Infect Dis 16:677–688, 1993.
14. Peters JI, Levine SM: Lung Transplantation. In George RB, Light RW, Matthay MA, et al (eds): Chest Medicine—Essentials of Pulmonary and Critical Care Medicine, 3rd ed. Baltimore, Williams and Wilkins, 1995, pp 540–559.
15. Peters JI, Levine SM, Anzueto A, et al: Infectious complications in single lung transplant recipients. Am Rev Respir Dis 147:A601, 1993 (Abstract).
16. Trulock EP: Management of lung transplant rejection. Chest 103:1566–1576, 1993.

INDEX

Page numbers in **boldface type** indicate complete chapters.